Introductory
Pathophysiology
for Nursing and Healthcare Professionals

Visit the *Introductory Pathophysiology for Nursing and Healthcare Professionals* Companion Website at **www.pearsoned.co.uk/zelman** to find valuable student learning material including:

- interactive exercises
- self-assessment questions
- an audio glossary
- revision flashcards

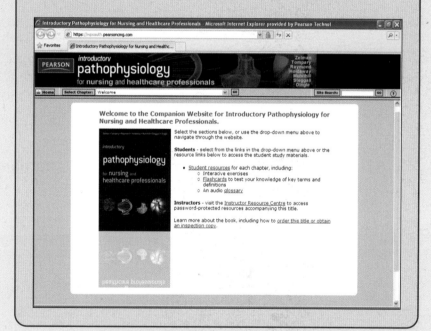

PEARSON

We work with leading authors to develop the strongest educational materials in nursing, bringing cutting-edge thinking and best learning practice to a global market.

Under a range of well-known imprints, including Pearson, we craft high quality print and electronic publications which help readers to understand and apply their content, whether studying or at work.

To find out more about the complete range of our publishing, please visit us on the World Wide Web at: **www.pearsoned.co.uk**

Introductory
Pathophysiology
for Nursing and Healthcare Professionals

Mark Zelman, PhD
Associate Professor, Aurora University,
Aurora, Illinois

Elaine Tompary, PharmD
Outcomes Research, McNeil Consumer and Specialty Pharma,
Fort Washington, Pennsylvania

Jill Raymond, PhD
Professor, Rock Valley College,
Rockford, Illinois

Paul Holdaway, MA
Professor, William Rainey Harper College,
Palatine, Illinois

Mary Lou Mulvihill, PhD
Professor Emeritus, William Rainey Harper College,
Palatine, Illinois

Dr Martin Steggall
Associate Dean, Undergraduate Pre-registration Nursing and Midwifery,
Head of Department, Applied Biological Sciences,
City University, London

Ms Maria Dingle
Senior Lecturer, Department of Applied Biological Sciences,
City University, London

Harlow, England • London • New York • Boston • San Francisco • Toronto
Sydney • Tokyo • Singapore • Hong Kong • Seoul • Taipei • New Delhi
Cape Town • Madrid • Mexico City • Amsterdam • Munich • Paris • Milan

Pearson Education Limited
Edinburgh Gate
Harlow
Essex CM20 2JE
England

and Associated Companies throughout the world

Visit us on the World Wide Web at:
www.pearsoned.co.uk

First published 2011

ISBN: 978-0-273-72386-8

British Library Cataloguing-in-Publication Data
A catalogue record for this book is available from the British Library

Library of Congress Cataloging-in-Publication Data
Introductory pathophysiology for nursing and healthcare professionals / Mark Zelman . . . [et al.].
    p. ; cm.
  Includes index.
  ISBN 978-0-273-72386-8 (pbk.)
  1. Physiology, Pathological.   2. Nursing.   I. Zelman, Mark.
  [DNLM: 1. Disease—Nurses' Instruction.   QZ 140]
  RB113.I58 2011
   616.07—dc22

                                                                    2010041772

10 9 8 7 6 5 4 3 2 1
15 14 13 12 11

Typeset in 10/14pt Giovanni Book by 35
Printed and bound by Graficas Estella, Spain

BRIEF CONTENTS

CONTENTS

Supporting resources

Visit **www.pearsoned.co.uk/zelman** to find valuable online resources

Companion Website for students
- interactive exercises
- self-assessment questions
- an audio glossary
- revision flashcards

For instructors
- PowerPoint slides
- 'Mytest' question testbank for class testing

Also: The Companion Website provides the following features:
- Search tool to help locate specific items of content
- E-mail results and profile tools to send results of quizzes to instructors
- Online help and support to assist with website usage and troubleshooting

For more information please contact your local Pearson Education sales representative or visit **www.pearsoned.co.uk/zelman**

ADAPTERS' PREFACE

We have endeavoured to maintain the style of the original text (*Human Diseases: A Systemic Approach*, 7th edition) but have, where necessary, made changes to more accurately reflect practice in the UK. The text is aimed at 2nd year student nurses studying Adult Nursing who are learning about applied pathophysiology and related pharmacology. We have tried to get across the essential features of the common pathologies that are seen in clinical practice and, as such, have avoided complex detail.

In contemporary nursing, there is a need for a sound knowledge of pathophysiology and related pharmacology, and we hope that this book will help with *introducing* you to this complex subject. Our aim in adapting this book is not to provide all the pathophysiology and pharmacology knowledge that you will ever need throughout your course, or indeed career, but to reduce the anxiety that this subject often instils in people.

Special features

This text contains terminology guides, clinical applications and case studies that we hope you find engaging and supportive as you learn about the myriad of diseases that can affect the human body. The case studies and self-assessment questions are linked to UK-based practice and there is a companion website, which includes interactive material. The key to studying pathophysiology is to adopt a combination approach; a little reading, some practical exercises, some reflection and then further reading, are the essential skills in helping make sense of what is happening in the patient. A knowledge of pathophysiology enables nurses to plan nursing care based on a sound foundation of what is going on in the body.

We hope that you enjoy reading the book!

GUIDED TOUR

Introductory Pathophysiology for Nurses and Healthcare Professionals is a comprehensive visual survey of pathophysiology. Explore and understand common pathologies for each body system, with full colour and learning features which make the potentially complex subject of pathophysiology interesting and accessible.

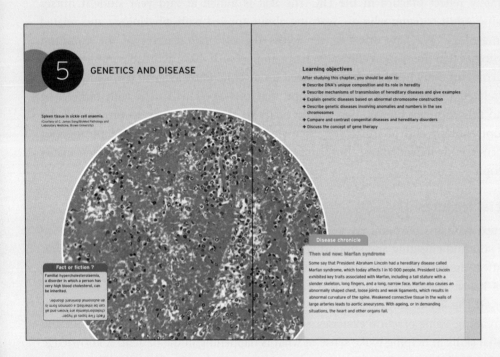

5 GENETICS AND DISEASE

Spleen tissue in sickle cell anaemia.
(Courtesy of C. James Sung/BioMed Pathology and Laboratory Medicine, Brown University)

Learning objectives

After studying this chapter, you should be able to:
✦ Describe DNA's unique composition and its role in heredity
✦ Describe mechanisms of transmission of hereditary diseases and give examples
✦ Explain genetic diseases based on abnormal chromosome construction
✦ Describe genetic diseases involving anomalies and numbers in the sex chromosomes
✦ Compare and contrast congenital diseases and hereditary disorders
✦ Discuss the concept of gene therapy

Fact or fiction ?

Familial hypercholesterolaemia, a disorder in which a person has very high blood cholesterol, can be inherited.

Fact! Five types of hyper-cholesterolaemia are known, and all can be inherited; a common form is an autosomal dominant disorder.

Disease chronicle

Then and now: Marfan syndrome

Some say that President Abraham Lincoln had a hereditary disease called Marfan syndrome, which today affects 1 in 10 000 people. President Lincoln exhibited key traits associated with Marfan, including a tall stature with a slender skeleton, long fingers, and a long, narrow face. Marfan also causes an abnormally shaped chest, loose joints and weak ligaments, which results in abnormal curvature of the spine. Weakened connective tissue in the walls of large arteries leads to aortic aneurysms. With ageing, or in demanding situations, the heart and other organs fail.

The interactive chapter opener includes a brief history of a disease, helping to put it into the context of your studies, while a quick knowledge test is included in **Fact or fiction?** The **Learning objectives** clearly set out what you should be able to do after studying the chapter.

Each chapter includes professionally illustrated **anatomical diagrams** and numerous **medical pictures in full colour**, helping you to understand and recognise diseases as you would see them in real life.

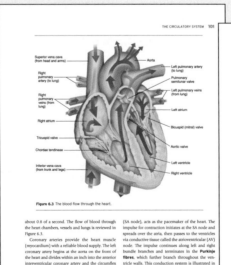

THE CIRCULATORY SYSTEM 101

Superior vena cava (from head and arms)
Aorta
Right pulmonary artery (to lung)
Left pulmonary artery (to lung)
Pulmonary semilunar valve
Right pulmonary veins (from lung)
Left pulmonary veins (from lung)
Left atrium
Right atrium
Bicuspid (mitral) valve
Tricuspid valve
Aortic valve
Chordae tendineae
Left ventricle
Inferior vena cava (from trunk and legs)
Right ventricle

Figure 6.3 The blood flow through the heart.

about 0.8 of a second. The flow of blood through the heart chambers, vessels and lungs is reviewed in Figure 6.3.

Coronary arteries provide the heart muscle (myocardium) with a reliable blood supply. The left coronary artery begins at the aorta on the front of the heart and divides within an inch into the anterior interventricular coronary artery and the circumflex artery, which continues left around the back of the heart. The right coronary artery also branches from the front of the aorta and sends divisions to the right side and back of the heart (Figure 6.4).

Unlike skeletal muscle, cardiac muscle contracts continuously and rhythmically without conscious effort. A small patch of tissue, the **sinoatrial node**

(SA node), acts as the pacemaker of the heart. The impulse for contraction initiates at the SA node and spreads over the atria, then passes to the ventricles via conductive tissue called the atrioventricular (AV) node. The impulse continues along left and right bundle branches and terminates in the **Purkinje fibres**, which further branch throughout the ventricle wall. This conduction system is illustrated in Figure 6.5.

Heart muscle does not depend on nerve stimulation for contraction, but is influenced by the autonomic nervous system and hormones such as adrenaline (epinephrine). Two sets of nerves work antagonistically, one slowing the heart and the other accelerating it. The vagus nerve slows the heart

38 CHAPTER 3 INFECTIOUS DISEASES

Figure 3.3 *Ascaris.*
(Sinclair Stammers/Science Photo Library/Photo Researchers, Inc.)

Figure 3.4 *Necator americanus.* The cutting plates around the mouth are used to tear open blood vessels of the host.
(© David Scharf/Peter Arnold, Inc.)

Figure 3.5 Adult *Enterobius vermicularis.*
(Science Photo Library Ltd/Science Vu/Visuals Unlimited)

America, South East Asia and China. Larvae of the hookworm penetrate the skin of the foot, hand, arm or leg. The larvae travel to the small intestine and mature into adult worms. Females lay several thousand eggs per day. The eggs are shed in faeces and hatch out into larvae in water. There are no specific symptoms or signs of hookworm infection. Stool samples are used for diagnosis, and drugs are available for treatment. Prevention includes not walking barefoot, using toilet facilities, and not using human excrement or raw sewage as fertilizer in agriculture.

Enterobius vermicularis infects an estimated 200 million people worldwide and is probably the most widespread infection in the UK (Figure 3.5). The female pinworm migrates to the anus to deposit her eggs on the skin around the anus. She then secretes a substance that causes a very strong itching sensation, inciting the host to scratch the area and thus transfer some of the eggs to the fingers. Eggs can also be transferred to cloth, toys and the bath, and can survive from 2 to 3 weeks outside the human body. Humans ingest the eggs, which hatch into larvae in the small intestine. The larvae then migrate to the large intestine and mate. Enterobiasis infections are diagnosed by the Graham sticky-tape method. A piece of transparent tape is placed on the skin around the anus so it can pick up eggs that were laid earlier. The tape is microscopically examined for the presence of eggs. Treatment includes drugs and thorough washing of clothing and linens to kill eggs. Prevention includes practising proper personal

an estimated 740 million people in the developing nations of the tropics (Figure 3.4). The largest numbers of cases occur in sub-Saharan Africa, Latin

Each chapter includes specific features to help and inform your study. **Prevention PLUS!** provides information on how disease can be prevented, while links to further resources on the internet are also included. All the diseases covered in each chapter can be easily accessed using the **Diseases at a glance** feature, which provides useful information on disease symptoms through to treatment and prevention.

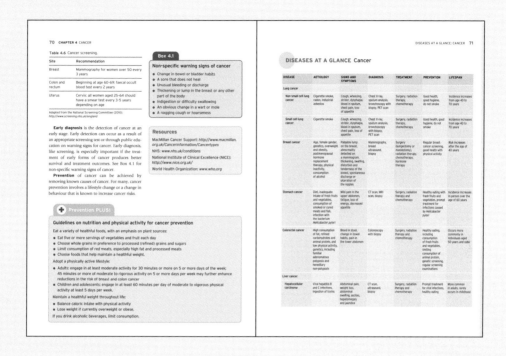

End-of-chapter **Interactive exercises** based on UK practice are designed to test and reinforce your learning. Exercises consist of quick answer questions, including multiple choice questions, longer case studies and also visual exercises, such as labelling questions. Answers to all the exercises are available in an appendix at the end of the book.

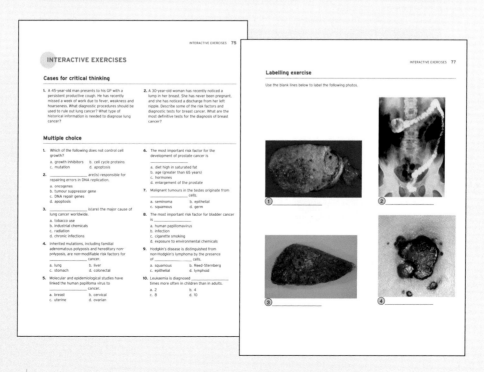

The appendices at the end of the book contain further useful information including a comprehensive **Glossary** containing pronunciation guides (audio version available on the companion website) and an extra appendix on **Laboratory and diagnostic tests**.

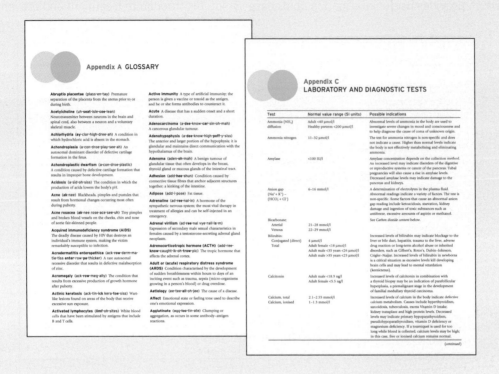

A Premium Companion Website containing further interactive exercises, self-assessment questions, an audio glossary and revision flashcards is also available at **www.pearsoned.co.uk/zelman**.

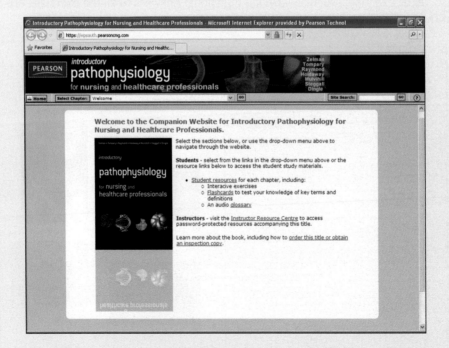

ABOUT THE AUTHORS

Mark Zelman, PhD, is Associate Professor of Biology and Chair of Natural Sciences and Mathematics at Aurora University in Aurora, Illinois. A native of Chicago, Mark received his BS in biology, with minors in psychology and chemistry, at Rockford College. Mark received his PhD from the Department of Microbiology and Immunology at Loyola University Chicago, where he studied bacterial and mammalian antigens in a mouse model for human autoimmune disease. Mark was a postdoctoral fellow at the University of Chicago, where he studied molecular cell physiology. Before coming to Aurora University, Mark was a biology professor, a college administrator and a medical writer. Mark pursues a wide range of interests in biology and he is especially interested in enhancing K–12 science education. He enjoys bird-watching and camping with his sons, Joe and Tom, and wears out quite a few shoes training for marathons and triathlons.

Elaine Tompary, PharmD, received her Doctor of Pharmacy Degree from the University of Illinois at Chicago. Dr Tompary taught courses in pharmacology, pathophysiology, pharmacy law and pharmaceutical calculations at William Rainey Harper College and the College of Lake County in Illinois. She has served as mentor and preceptor for pharmacy students at the University of Illinois and Drake University. She currently works for McNeil Consumer and Specialty Pharmaceuticals as a manager of medical science and outcomes research. She is a dedicated wife to Drew and mother and teacher to her children, Christopher and Andriana.

Jill Raymond, PhD, received her PhD in microbiology from the University of California at Davis. She received and completed a postdoctoral fellowship in infectious diseases at the University of California at San Diego, where she studied the parasite *Giardia lamblia*. She has been teaching for 13 years at Rock Valley College in Rockford, Illinois. In addition to teaching numerous biology courses, both traditional and online, Dr Raymond teaches a human sexuality course and lectures at community education outreach programmes. Dr Raymond enjoys gardening, working with dogs and European travel. Dr Raymond would like to thank her wonderful husband and family for their continuing support through the craziness of writing a textbook.

Paul Holdaway, MA, a native Hoosier, is a graduate of Indiana State University and was an instructor there for 2 years. He is currently the senior member of the Biology Department at Harper College in Palatine, Illinois, where Dr Mary Lou Mulvihill was an admired fellow biologist and friend. Dr Zelman and Dr Tompary are also former departmental colleagues and longstanding friends. Upon Dr Mulvihill's retirement, Professor Holdaway assumed the teaching schedule of Dr Mulvihill, and he has been involved in the anatomy, physiology and human disease curriculum since that time. Paul takes pleasure in a wide range of biological and clinical interests, as well as sports and family activities.

UK adapters

Mr Peter Bentley, Deputy Head of Department and Senior Lecturer, Department of Applied Biological Sciences, City University, London. Adapted Chapters 2 and 5.

Dr William Blows, Lecturer in Mental Health, Department of Applied Biological Sciences, City University, London. Adapted Chapters 13 and 14.

Ms Alison Coutts, Senior Lecturer, Department of Applied Biological Sciences, City University, London. Adapted Chapters 7, 9 and 16.

Ms Maria Dingle, Senior Lecturer, Department of Applied Biological Sciences, City University, London. Adapted Chapters 6 and 12, Appendix B and co-editor.

Ms Lynda Filer, Lecturer, Department of Applied Biological Sciences, City University, London. Adapted Chapter 8.

Dr Sarah Greenwood, Lecturer, Department of Applied Biological Sciences, City University, London. Adapted Appendix C.

Ms Ihinosen Ovbude, Lecturer, Department of Applied Biological Sciences, City University, London. Adapted Chapter 16 and co-adapted Chapter 11.

Dr Martin Steggall, Associate Dean, Undergraduate Pre-registration Nursing and Midwifery, Senior Lecturer and Head of Department, Applied Biological Sciences, City University, London. Adapted Chapters 1, 4 and 10, co-adapted Chapter 11, Appendix A and B; co-editor.

Mr Ugbai Tekley, Education Facilitator, Department of Applied Biological Sciences, City University, London. Adapted Chapter 3.

ACKNOWLEDGEMENTS

To our students who challenge, surprise and enthuse us with their thirst for knowledge. To our families, whose support and tolerance have been invaluable. To David Harrison at Pearson Education for guidance and support. To Ms Johanna Watkinson for expert help and guidance with phonics. Finally, a special thanks to Aiden, William and Harriet for giving us the time to adapt this book.

Publisher's Acknowledgements

We are grateful to the following for permission to reproduce copyright material:

Tables

Table 3.1 from *World Health Report*, World Health Organization (2004); Table 4.3 from *Andreoli and Carpenter's Cecil Essentials of Medicine*, 7th ed., Saunders (Andreoli, T.E., MACP, Carpenter, C.C.J., Griggs, R.C., Benjamin, I. 2007), Copyright Elsevier, 2007; Table 4.5 adapted from material on the Cancer Research UK website, http://www.cancerresearchuk.org/; Table 4.6 adapted from material found on the UK National Screening Committee website, http://www.screening.nhs.uk/england; Table 6.3 adapted from Cardiovascular and Metabolic Risk Factors: How Can We Improve Outcomes in the High-Risk Patient, *The American Journal of Medicine*, 120(9A), pp. S3–S9 (Grundy, S.M. 2007), with permission from Elsevier; Table 12.2 from the American Diabetes Association website, http://www.diabetes.org/diabetes-basics/symptoms/, Copyright 2010 American Diabetes Association. Modified with permission from The American Diabetes Association.

Text

Boxs 14.1, 14.2, 14.4, 14.5 from *Diagnostic and Statistical Manual Text Revision IV*, American Psychiatric Association (2000), Reprinted with permission of the American Psychiatric Association.; Box on page 410 adapted from Taken from the American Cancer Society website, http://www.cancer.org/Cancer/CancerCauses/SunandUVExposure/SkinCancerPreventionandEarlyDetection/skin-cancer-prevention-and-early-detection-skin-exams, Reprinted by the permission of the American Cancer Society, Inc. from www.cancer.org. All rights reserved.

In some instances we have been unable to trace the owners of copyright material, and we would appreciate any information that would enable us to do so.

Photographs

The publisher would like to thank the following for their kind permission to reproduce their photographs:

(Key: b-bottom; c--centre; l-left; r-right; t-top)

C James Sung: 78; Centers for Disease Control and Prevention: 150, 270, 403tr, 404, Dr Brodsky 36l, Dr Ed Ewing 18, 30, 225r, Dr Edwin Ewing 372, 403br, Dr Edwin P Ewing Jr 210, Dr Edwin P Ewing, Jr 52, Dr Gilda Jones 176, Dr Herrman 401tl, Dr Libero Ajello 394, Dr Lucille K Georg 403, Dr N J Fiumara 409r, 426cr, Dr Steve Kraus 420l, Dr Thomas F Sellers 400tl, Dr Weisner 255r, Joe Miller 234, Lucille K Georg 402, Sherry Brinkman 98, Stacey Howard 134; Custom Medical Stock Photo Inc: 81, 411tl, 414tl, 426tl, NMSB 411tr, O J Staats 300, SIU 240r; DK Images: 331; Getty Images: Jonathan Seliq 348; Mediscan: 255l; National Eye Institute: 330, 332, 335t, 335b; National Toxicology Program: 8; Photolibrary.com: Bart's Medical Library / Phototake 413, David Scharf / Peter Arnold 38bl, Dr. Isabelle Cartier / ISM / Phototake 240l, ISM / Phototake 22, 66, 77br, 142r, 149r, 408, Javier Domingo / Phototake , Martin Rotker 198, Sovereign / ISM / Phototake 115tl; Phototake, Inc: NIH 325; Ray Kemp/911 Imaging: 160; Science Photo Library Ltd: 59, 77tl, 379l, Antonia Reeve 115cl, Chris Bjornberg 379r, CMSP 414br, 426bl, Dr E Walker 61, 77bl, Dr Gladden Willis / Visuals Unlimited 36r, 144, Dr Ken Greer / Visuals Unlimited 283, Dr P Marazzi 108, 403cl, 411br, 412, 420r, 426tr, Dr PMarazzi 12, Gilbert S Grant 44, Joaquin Carrillo Farga 137, Lowell Georgia 42, Mike Devlin 416, Molly Borman 183, NIBSC 23, Omikron 141, Patrick Dumas / Look At Sciences 157, Science Vu / Visuals Unlimited 38tr, Scott Camazine 142l, 149l, Simon Fraser, RNC Newcastle 109l, Sinclair Stammers 38, SIU 225l, Sovereign, ISM 60, 77tr, St Bartholomew's Hospital 169, St Bartholomews Hospital 407, Steve Gschmeissner 185l, Zephyr 109r, Zuber / CMSP 415; Sharmyn McGraw: 287l, 287r

All other images © Pearson Education

In some instances we have been unable to trace the owners of copyright material, and we would appreciate any information that would enable us to do so.

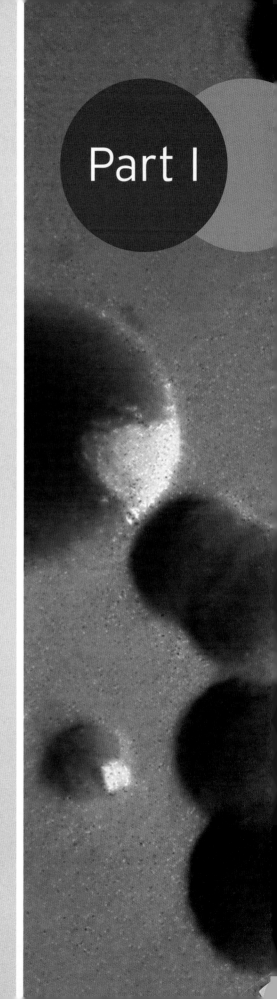

Part I

MECHANISMS OF DISEASE

How do we define and describe disease? What causes disease? In Part I, we discuss the manifestations, terminology, diagnosis and mechanisms of disease.

Chapters

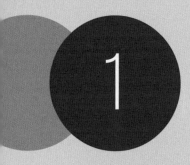

1 INTRODUCTION TO DISEASE

A heart infusion agar culture growing colonies
of *Yersinia pestis* bacteria.
(Courtesy of the CDC/Dr Brodsky, 1966)

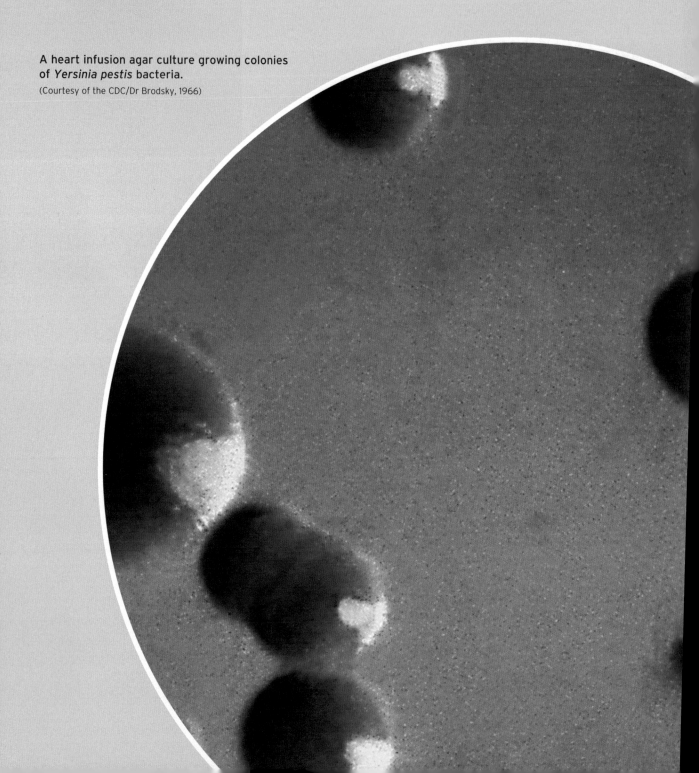

Learning objectives

After studying this chapter, you should be able to:

+ Define disease and disease-related terms
+ Define and discuss the manifestations of disease
+ Define terms used to describe disease
+ Explain diagnosis of disease
+ Define and discuss the chief causes of disease
+ Identify risk factors related to disease

Disease chronicle

The Black Death

...If one were to seek to establish one generalisation...to catch the mood of the Europeans in the second half of the fourteenth century, it would be that they were enduring a crisis of faith. Assumptions which had been taken for granted for centuries were now in question; the very framework of men's reasoning seemed to be breaking up. And though the Black Death was far from being the only cause, the anguish and disruption which it had inflicted made the greatest single contribution to the disintegration of an age.

P. Ziegler, *The Black Death*

The Black Death, also known as the plague, has killed and terrified people through the ages. For much of human history, understanding of disease and knowledge of normal human physiology was extremely limited. Effective control and treatment of most diseases awaited a systematic, scientific approach and a body of medical knowledge and technology.

INTRODUCTION

The human body possesses a remarkable capacity to maintain health. Changes constantly occur within and outside the body, and yet a steady state called **homeostasis** is generally maintained. Although pH, temperature, blood composition, and fluid levels fluctuate, organ systems normally correct these changes before they threaten the body's health. A significant disturbance in the homeostasis of the body triggers a variety of responses that often produce disease. If we consider homeostasis to be a state of equilibrium, **disease** can be defined as a state of functional disequilibrium, a change in function or structure that is considered to be abnormal. Clearly, knowledge of normal structure (**anatomy**) and normal function (**physiology**) are essential to the study of disease. **Pathology** is the study of disease in general, and **pathophysiology** is the study of the physiological processes leading up to disease.

MANIFESTATIONS OF DISEASE

A disease manifests itself through certain signs and symptoms. **Signs** are objective evidence of disease observed on physical examination, such as abnormal pulse or respiratory rate, fever, sweating and pallor; **symptoms** are subjective indications of disease reported by the patient, such as pain, dizziness and itching. Certain sets of signs and symptoms occur concurrently in some diseases, and their combination is called a **syndrome**. These include acquired immunodeficiency syndrome, malabsorption syndrome and Down's syndrome.

DIAGNOSIS

Diagnosis is the use of scientific or clinical methods to determine the nature of a disease. A diagnosis provides the basis for rational and effective treatment of disease and is based on many factors, including the physical examination, signs and symptoms, patient history, laboratory data and

specific diagnostic tests. Signs and symptoms, discussed previously, are familiar manifestations of disease and can be ascertained through physical examination and interviews with a patient or with a patient's family. Frequently the course and history of the signs and symptoms yields important diagnostic information. Likewise, family disease history may give insight into genetic risk for developing certain diseases. Laboratory data are derived from procedures such as urinalysis, blood chemistry, electrocardiography and radiography. Diagnostic imaging techniques such as computed tomography (CT) scan, magnetic resonance imaging (MRI), ultrasound and nuclear medicine allow physicians to visualise structural and functional changes. A biopsy, surgical removal and analysis of tissue samples yields information about changes at the cellular level.

DESCRIBING DISEASE

The physician, having made a diagnosis, may state the **prognosis** of the disease, or the predicted course and outcome of the disease. The prognosis may state the chances for complete recovery, predict the permanent loss of function or give probability of survival. The course of a disease varies; it may have a sudden onset and short duration, in which case it is an **acute** disease. Influenza, measles and the common cold are examples. A disease may have a slower, less severe, onset and a long duration of months or years; such a disease is **chronic**. Such diseases include diabetes, cancers and osteoarthritis. Diseases that will end in death are called **terminal**.

The signs and symptoms of disease at times subside, during a period known as **remission**. They may recur in all their severity in a period of **exacerbation**. Certain diseases (leukaemia and ulcerative colitis, for example) are characterised by periods of remission and exacerbation. A **relapse** occurs when a disease returns weeks or months after its apparent cessation.

A **complication** is a disease or other abnormal state that develops in a person already suffering from a disease. The complication may negatively affect the prognosis or course of the original disease. For example, a person confined to bed with a serious fracture may develop pneumonia as a complication of the inactivity. Infection of the testes may be a complication of mumps, particularly after puberty. Anaemia generally accompanies leukaemia, cancer and chronic kidney disease. The aftermath of a particular disease is called the **sequela**, a sequel (pl. sequelae). The permanent damage to the heart after rheumatic fever is an example of sequela, as is the paralysis of polio. Sterility may be the sequela of pelvic inflammatory disease and sexually transmitted infections.

Public health agencies monitor the impact diseases have on populations by gathering mortality and morbidity data. **Mortality** is a measure of the number of deaths attributed to a disease in a given population over a given period of time. **Morbidity** is a measure of the disability and extent of illness caused by a disease. Each gives public health officials and physicians an idea of how serious a disease is and thus helps direct resources toward prevention and cure. Table 1.1 lists the leading causes of death in the United Kingdom.

Disease occurrence is also described in terms of prevalence and incidence. **Prevalence** describes the number of cases of a disease occurring at a given time in a specified population. Prevalence data allow the determination of the impact and significance of a disease for a given population and these data are used to direct healthcare resources and research. Certain diseases, such as cancer, heart disease and diabetes, are more prevalent in older adults than in adolescents. **Incidence** describes the number of new cases of a disease at a given time in a specified population. Incidence data allow tracking of changes in the occurrence of disease. A disease may increase in incidence seasonally, as influenza does during winter.

Epidemiology is the study of the occurrence, transmission, distribution and control of disease. Epidemiologists use prevalence and incidence data and information about the geographic distribution of disease to develop methods to prevent and control diseases.

CAUSES OF DISEASE

An important aspect of any disease is its **aetiology**, or cause. The source or cause of a disease, together with its development, is its **pathogenesis**. If the cause of a disease is not known, it is said to be **idiopathic**. Most causes of disease fall into one or more categories. At the root of most causes, however, is a **lesion** of some sort. A lesion could be a damaged gene or enzyme, or abnormal cells, tissues or organs. The major causes and mechanisms of disease are discussed in the remaining chapters in Part I of the text. These causes include inflammatory or immune disorders, including allergy; infection; abnormal cell growth (neoplasm); heredity; nutrition; environmental factors; and stress. Table 1.2 lists major causes and examples of associated diseases.

Table 1.1 Leading causes of death in 2007 in the UK.

Disease	Number of deaths
Heart disease	74 184
Cancer	127 719
Stroke	43 539
Chronic lower respiratory disease	64 600
Accidents	10 831

Source: Department of Health: dh.gov.uk/dr_consum/dh_digital assets.

Table 1.2 Major causes of disease.

Cause	Disease
Inflammation/ autoimmunity/allergy	Asthma, systemic lupus erythematosus
Infection	Tuberculosis, influenza
Neoplasm	Lung cancer, malignant melanoma
Heredity	Sickle cell anaemia, cystic fibrosis
Malnutrition	Pernicious anaemia, iron-deficiency anaemia
Stress	Hypertension, heart disease

RISK FACTORS

Risk factors predispose an individual to the development of a disease. Note that a risk factor is not equivalent to a **cause**. While an individual with a risk factor for a certain disease has an increased chance of developing that disease, it may not necessarily cause the disease. Risk factors may be environmental, chemical, physiological, psychological or genetic. A well-known risk factor for lung cancer is cigarette smoking. The development of coronary artery disease has multiple well established risk factors, such as high blood cholesterol and lipids, a history of hypertension, cigarette smoking, physical inactivity, obesity, diabetes and a family history. Knowledge of disease risk factors is important; while eliminating known risk factors for a disease may not prevent disease, it may reduce the chance of developing disease.

TREATMENT OF DISEASE

Treatment includes procedures for the cure or reduction of symptoms of disease. Treatment depends on the nature of the disease, the characteristics of the patient, and goals of the patient and physician.

Treatment may be aimed at curing a disease and/or removing its cause if possible. Not all diseases are curable, and in some cases, the causes are unknown. Thus some treatments are **palliative**, or **symptomatic**, designed to relieve and manage the symptoms of the disease without addressing the cause.

Treatment includes medical (pharmacological) procedures, which use specific drugs to cure or relieve symptoms. Other diseases may require surgery to correct anatomical and physiological abnormalities related to the disease. Some diseases require psychiatric and psychological treatments. In some cases, effective treatment requires the use of several procedures simultaneously.

Readers will apply disease terms and concepts learned in Chapter 1 throughout their study of the text. In Part I, general processes of disease will be discussed, including the roles of heredity, infection, abnormal cell growth (cancer), inflammation and immunity. In Part II of the text, readers will apply concepts and terms from Part I to the study of specific diseases of the body systems.

> **Resources**
>
> Department of Health: *http://www.dh.gov.uk*

INTERACTIVE EXERCISES

Cases for critical thinking

1. Some athletes may develop abnormally high red blood cell counts. Why? In the athlete's case, is this a sign of disease?

2. A patient reports to her nurse practitioner that she feels weak and dizzy. Is this enough information to make a diagnosis? What other sources of information can her nurse practitioner consult?

3. Consult Table 1.1. How can this information be used to direct healthcare research and resources? What is the significance of the information about accidents?

Multiple choice

1. A skin rash is an example of a _____
   a. sign   b. symptom
   c. laboratory result d. syndrome

2. A(n) _____ disease has a sudden onset and short course
   a. acute   b. terminal
   c. chronic   d. idiopathic

3. The cause of a disease is known as its
   _____
   a. pathogenesis   b. complication
   c. sequelae   d. aetiology

4. A steady state maintained within the body is called _____
   a. homeostasis   b. disease
   c. disequilibrium   d. pathology

5. The worsening of signs and symptoms is known as
   _____
   a. remission   b. exacerbation
   c. relapse   d. complication

True or false

_____ 1. Anatomy is the study of normal body function.

_____ 2. Mortality refers to the number of deaths caused by a disease.

_____ 3. Symptoms are objective evidence of a disease.

_____ 4. Signs may be perceived by the physician.

_____ 5. Exacerbation and remission may characterise a chronic disease.

Fill-ins

1. The predicted outcome of a disease is its _____.

2. Damaged tissue, DNA or enzymes are examples of _____ that cause a disease.

3. If the cause of a disease is not known, it is said to be _____.

4. Return of symptoms after their apparent cessation is _____.

5. The signs and symptoms of a chronic disease at times subside during a period known as _____.

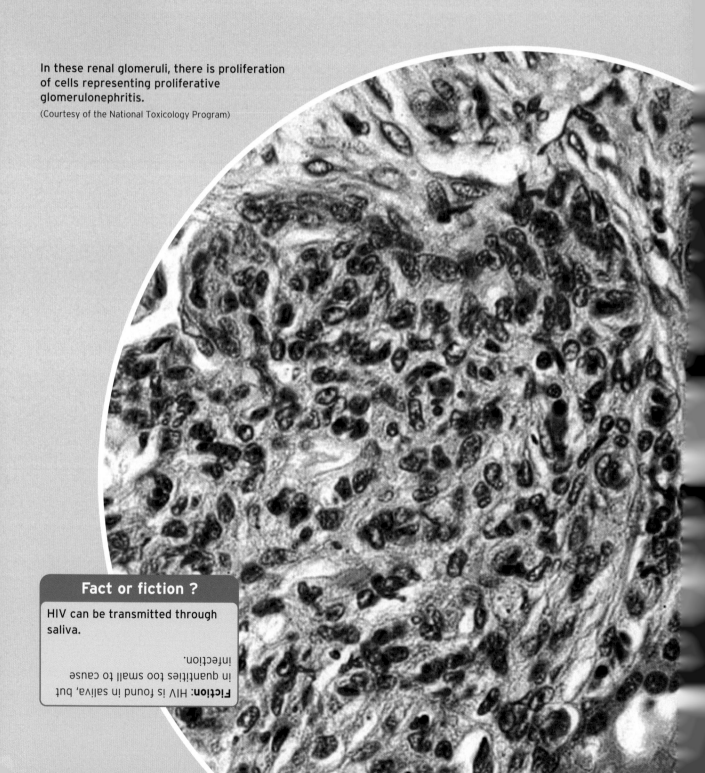

2

IMMUNITY AND THE LYMPHATIC SYSTEM

In these renal glomeruli, there is proliferation of cells representing proliferative glomerulonephritis.
(Courtesy of the National Toxicology Program)

Fact or fiction ?

HIV can be transmitted through saliva.

Fiction: HIV is found in saliva, but in quantities too small to cause infection.

Learning objectives

After studying this chapter, you should be able to:

+ Define immunity
+ Compare and contrast non-specific and specific immunity
+ Describe the normal structure and function of the lymphatic system
+ Identify the four types of hypersensitivities
+ Define autoimmunity and autoantibodies
+ Describe the aetiology, incidence, symptoms, diagnosis and treatment for selected autoimmune diseases
+ Describe the aetiology, incidence, symptoms, diagnosis and treatment for HIV and AIDS
+ Explain AIDS as it relates to immunodeficiency
+ Compare and contrast active and passive immunity

Disease chronicle

Inflammation

Throughout history, humans have undoubtedly observed the inflammatory response even if they understood little of its causes or treatment. Around 1500 BC, Egyptians used dried myrtle leaves to relieve back pain. In 200 BC, the Greek physician Hippocrates prescribed willow bark leaves to relieve fever and pain. One of the early systemic descriptions of inflammation came from the Roman physician Aulus Cornelius Celsus (25 BC–50 AD), who recorded its cardinal signs: heat, redness, swelling and pain. Today, the active ingredient in aspirin, acetylsalicylic acid, is derived from a related anti-inflammatory chemical (salicylic acid) found in myrtle leaves and willow tree bark.

IMMUNITY

Immunity is the ability of the body to defend itself against infectious agents, foreign cells and even abnormal body cells such as cancer cells. Immunity can be acquired naturally by infection, as when chicken pox confers protection against acquiring it again. Immunity can be artificially acquired by immunization, as when the polio vaccine induces immunity against polio. Immunity includes non-specific and specific immunity. Non-specific immunity, also known as innate immunity, is present at birth and provides immediate but general protection against any foreign agent that enters the body. **Specific immunity**, also known as acquired immunity, is effective against particular identified foreign agents and develops in response to contact with that agent. Once established against a foreign agent, specific immunity is able to respond to future exposures to the same agent.

Non-specific immunity

Physical and chemical barriers Intact skin is the body's first line of defence. A physical barrier, skin also produces chemical barriers to infection. Secretions such as tears, saliva, sweat and oil contain chemicals that destroy foreign invaders. Mucous membranes that line body passages open to the exterior produce mucus, which traps foreign material and forms a barrier to invasion. Microscopic cilia hairs that line the respiratory tract sweep out debris and impurities trapped in mucus.

Phagocytosis White blood cells (**leucocytes**) can destroy infectious agents through phagocytosis. In phagocytosis, which means cell-eating, leucocytes engulf and digest bacteria or other material. This process is fairly non-specific, being unable to discriminate among or remember past encounters with various types of infectious agents. While some leucocytes travel in the blood to target foreign material, others remain in tissues.

Natural killer cells Natural killer cells are a type of leucocyte that recognises body cells with abnormal membranes. Cell membranes can become altered from cells being infected with foreign invaders such as viruses. Natural killer cells can destroy abnormal cells on contact by secreting a protein that destroys the cell membrane.

Fever Fever can be a sign that the body is defending itself. When phagocytes find and destroy foreign invaders, they release substances that raise body temperature. Fever aids the immune system by stimulating phagocytes, increasing metabolism and inhibiting the multiplication of some micro-organisms. Hence, fever is a symptom arising from the normal interplay between the immune system and micro-organisms, and can be beneficial. Fever should not always be eliminated; however, fever should be monitored closely.

Interferon **Interferon** is a group of substances that stimulate the immune system. Because interferon boosts the immune system, it has been used to treat infections and cancer. Interferon was first found in cells infected with the flu virus and was named for its ability to interfere with viral multiplication. Virus-infected cells and other agents produce interferon.

Inflammation The cause of inflammation may be a trauma or injury, such as a sprained ankle or a severe blow. A physical irritant in the tissue – a piece of glass, a bee sting, or an ingrown toenail – will trigger the response. Pathogenic organisms such as bacteria, viruses, fungi or parasites will do the same. Figure 2.1 shows various agents that are capable of stimulating an inflammatory response.

The signs and symptoms of inflammation are redness, swelling, heat and pain. Inflammation is a protective tissue response to injury or invasion. Vascular changes occur when tissue is traumatised or irritated. Local blood vessels, arterioles, and capillaries dilate, increasing blood flow to the injured area. This increased amount of blood, **hyperaemia**, causes the heat and redness associated with inflammation. As the blood flow to the site of the injury or infection increases, more and more leucocytes reach the area. Leucocytes called **neutrophils** line up

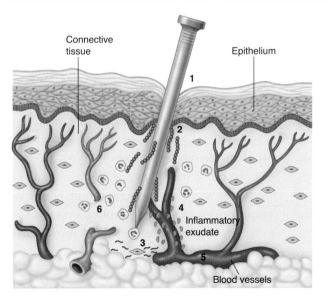

Figure 2.1 Agents capable of stimulating an inflammatory response.

within the capillary walls. Neutrophils are specialised cells that defend the body against invading micro-organisms and speed healing by engulfing cell debris in injured tissues. The damaged tissue releases a substance called **histamine** that causes the capillary walls to become more permeable. This increased permeability enables plasma and neutrophils to move out of the blood vessels into the tissue. The attraction of the white blood cells to the site of inflammation is called **chemotaxis**. The plasma and white blood cells that escape from the capillaries comprise the **inflammatory exudate** (Figure 2.2). This exudate in the tissues causes the swelling associated with inflammation. The excess of fluid in the tissues puts pressure on sensitive nerve endings, causing pain.

Bacterial infection may cause inflammation. The presence of toxin-producing bacteria such as

1. Dirty nail punctures skin
2. Bacteria enter and multiply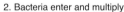
3. Injured cells release histamine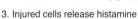
4. Blood vessels dilate and become permeable, releasing inflammatory exudate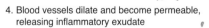
5. Blood flow to the damaged site increases
6. Neutrophils (polymorphs) move toward bacteria (chemotaxis) and destroy them (phagocytosis)

Figure 2.2 Vascular changes that occur with inflammation.

staphylococci and streptococci triggers an inflammatory response. To increase the effectiveness of the inflammatory and immune response, the bone marrow and lymph nodes release very large quantities of leucocytes. The white cell count may rise to 30 000 or more from the normal range of 4000 to 10 000 per cubic microlitre of blood. The excessive production of white cells is called **leucocytosis** and is a sign of infection or inflammation, such as appendicitis.

The neutrophils die soon after ingesting bacteria and toxins, and release substances that liquefy the surrounding tissue, forming pus, a thick yellow fluid consisting of liquefied tissue, dead neutrophils and inflammatory exudate. Other phagocytic white cells, the **monocytes** or **macrophages**, follow the neutrophils in the process of clearing debris. Inflammatory exudate contains a plasma protein, **fibrin**, essential for the blood clotting mechanism. Fibrin forms a clot in the damaged tissue, walling off the infection and preventing its spread.

Bacteria that cause pus formation are called **pyogenic** bacteria. An inflammation associated with pus formation is a **suppurative** inflammation. Abscesses, boils and styes are examples of inflammations with suppuration.

The inflammatory agent may damage tissue. Wound healing occurs in two ways: by regeneration and fibrosis. Whether one or both processes occurs depends on the type of tissue damaged and the severity of the injury. Regeneration is the replacement of destroyed tissue with the same kind of cells. In fibrosis, **fibroblasts**, a type of connective tissue cell, produce collagen fibres. The fibres contract, drawing the cut surfaces together. The healed site consists of a meshwork of collagen fibres known as scar tissue. A scar after surgery or a severe burn is often raised and hard. This development is known as keloid healing and is really a benign tumour (Figure 2.3). Surgery to remove such a scar is usually ineffective, as the subsequent incision will have a tendency to heal in the same way. Sometimes the collagen fibres anchor together adjacent structures, causing **adhesions**, which can interfere with organ functions. The problems associated with adhesions are explained in later chapters.

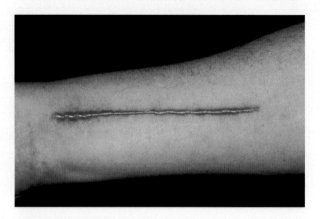

Figure 2.3 Keloid.
(Science Photo Library Ltd/Dr P. Marazzi)

SPECIFIC IMMUNITY AND THE LYMPHATIC SYSTEM

Specific immunity or the immune system is connected to the body via the lymphatic system. The lymphatic system includes a network of **lymphatic vessels**, **lymph nodes** and other **lymphoid organs** (Figure 2.4). Without the lymphatic system the cardiovascular system would cease to function and body defences would be seriously impaired. Because the cardiovascular system is a high-pressure system, fluid leaks out of the capillary beds into tissues. Most of this fluid is reabsorbed, but some, up to 3 litres a day, remains behind in the tissues. The fluid, called **lymph**, must be returned to the bloodstream or it will accumulate in the tissues, producing swelling or oedema, and there will be insufficient blood volume for cardiovascular functioning. Lymphoedema occurs when tissues swell because lymphatic vessels are blocked.

As lymph is transported in the lymphatic vessels toward the heart, it is filtered by lymph nodes. Within lymph nodes, macrophages phagocytose or engulf and digest bacteria, viruses and other foreign material. Swelling of lymph nodes during infection is a result of this filtration function. Lymph nodes produce **lymphocytes**, a type of white blood cell that responds to bacteria, viruses and foreign material in lymph. Lymphocytes play a critical role in specific immunity.

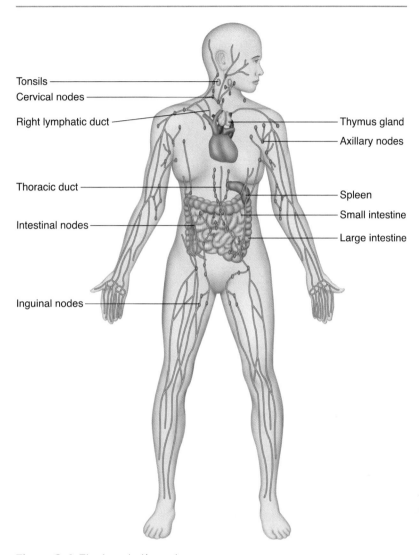

Tonsils

Cervical nodes

Right lymphatic duct

Thymus gland

Axillary nodes

Thoracic duct

Spleen

Small intestine

Intestinal nodes

Large intestine

Inguinal nodes

Figure 2.4 The lymphatic system.

Specific immunity is based on the ability to recognise and respond to foreign elements. The foreign element that triggers the immune response is known as an **antigen**, which often is a protein from micro-organisms or other foreign cells. Antigens differ from each other in structure and are unique. The specificity of acquired immunity is its ability to recognise these different antigens.

Specific immunity against antigens includes humoral and cell-mediated immunity. **Humoral immunity** includes **antibodies**, and **cell-mediated immunity** includes activated lymphocytes. Antibodies and activated lymphocytes comprise acquired immunity (Figure 2.5). Both humoral and cell-

mediated immunity work together to fight a foreign invader. Both are activated by an antigen, such as *Salmonella* bacteria from an undercooked chicken breast. The antigen interacts with lymphocytes in tissues, in lymph or in blood.

Two types of lymphocytes provide immunity: the T and B lymphocytes. The lymphocytes responsible for cell-mediated immunity are processed by the thymus gland; hence they are called **T lymphocytes**. The other type of lymphocyte, **B lymphocytes**, are responsible for humoral immunity. Antibodies and T lymphocytes are each highly specific for one type of antigen. B lymphocytes can play different roles in humoral immunity. Some B lymphocytes interact

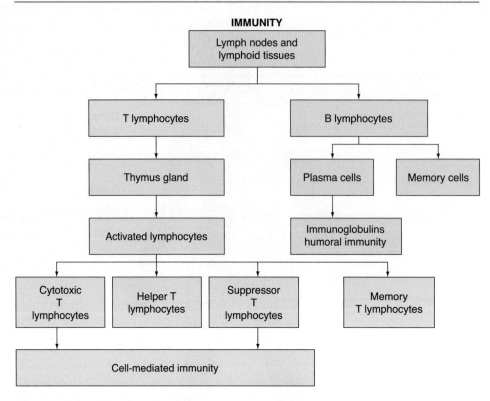

Figure 2.5 Cell-mediated immunity versus humoral immunity.

with antigens and become activated. Some other activated B lymphocytes are transformed into **plasma cells**, which divide rapidly and produce large numbers of antibodies. These agents are secreted into the lymph and travel to the blood to be circulated through the body. The antibodies are plasma proteins, which are gamma globulins called **immunoglobulins** (Ig). Antibodies bind to antigens and tag the antigen for destruction by the immune system. There are several types of immunoglobulins: IgG neutralises toxins and viruses; IgM protects newborns; IgA offers localised protection at mucosal surfaces; IgE is involved in allergy; and IgD activates B lymphocytes. See Table 2.1 for a summary of immunoglobulin functions.

Other B lymphocytes do not become plasma cells but remain dormant until reactivated by the same antigen. These lymphocytes are called **memory cells**

Table 2.1 Types of immunoglobulins.

Type	Function	Location
IgG	Produced in primary and secondary immune responses, neutralises toxins, bacteria and viruses	Blood plasma; crosses the placenta from mother to fetus
IgM	Protects newborns	Bound to B lymphocytes in circulation; usually the first to increase in the immune response
IgA	Localised protection at mucosal surfaces	Mucosal secretions, colostrum (early breast milk)
IgE	Allergy	Trace amounts in serum; secreted by sensitised plasma cells in tissues and locally attached to mast cells
IgD	Activates B lymphocytes	Attached to B lymphocytes

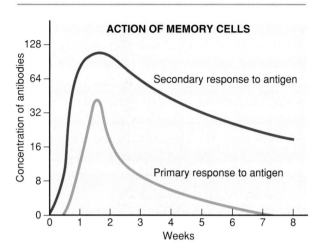

ACTION OF MEMORY CELLS

Secondary response to antigen

Primary response to antigen

Figure 2.6 Secondary response begins more rapidly after exposure to antigen, produces more antibodies and lasts for a longer time than initial exposure.

and are responsible for a more potent and rapid antibody response during subsequent exposures to the same antigen. This secondary response to the antigen produces antibodies faster and in larger quantities and lasts longer than the initial response. This strong secondary response explains why a vaccine protects a person from a subsequent exposure to an infectious agent. The secondary immune response is also the basis for the effectiveness of booster injections, which are given at intervals after initial vaccinations to increase levels of memory cells (Figure 2.6).

There are several different kinds of T lymphocytes, each with different functions: **cytotoxic** or **CD8 T lymphocytes, helper** or **CD4 T lymphocytes,** memory T lymphocytes and **suppressor T lymphocytes**. The cytotoxic T lymphocytes are often called killer lymphocytes because they are capable of killing invading organisms. They have on their surfaces receptor proteins that bind tightly to cells or organisms that contain a specific antigen. Once bound, the cytotoxic T lymphocytes release poisonous substances into the attacked cell. Many organisms can be killed by one killer lymphocyte. The cytotoxic lymphocytes are important in killing cells that have been invaded by viruses. These T lymphocytes can also destroy cancer cells.

The helper T lymphocytes are named for their ability to help the immune system in many ways.

They increase the activity of killer lymphocytes and stimulate B lymphocytes. Activated helper T lymphocytes secrete lymphokines (sometimes called cytokines) that increase the response of other types of lymphoid cells to the antigen. In addition, lymphokines activate macrophages to destroy large numbers of invaders by phagocytosis. After an infection or vaccination, some of the T lymphocytes that participated in the response remain as memory T lymphocytes that can be rapidly mobilised should the same antigen be encountered again. Suppressor T lymphocytes are believed to dampen or suppress the immune response.

HYPERSENSITIVITY - ALLERGIES

Closely related to the concept of immunity is **allergy**, or **hypersensitivity**. Some diseases result from an individual's immune response, which causes tissue damage and disordered function rather than immunity. The immune phenomena are destructive rather than defensive in the individual who is hypersensitive or allergic to an antigen. Hypersensitivity diseases or allergic diseases may manifest themselves locally or systemically.

Abnormal sensitivity to allergens such as pollens, dust, dog hair and certain foods or chemicals is the result of overproduction of IgE and its interaction with the allergens. IgE attaches one end to cells called **basophils** and **mast cells**; its other end points away from the cells, where the IgE can bind to the allergens. Mast cells are found in connective tissue and contain the chemicals **heparin, serotonin, bradykinin**, prostaglandin and histamine.

When allergens enter the body and bind to the IgE antibodies located on the mast cells, the cells break down and release their chemicals. Histamine causes the dilatation of the blood vessels, making them leak plasma into the tissues. This tissue fluid causes oedema, or swelling, which, when localised in the nasal passages, results in the familiar congestion and irritation of hay fever. If the tissue damage and oedema are near the skin, the welts and itching of hives may appear. Antihistamines inhibit the effects

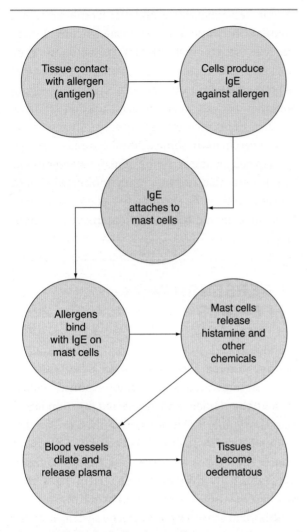

Figure 2.7 Typical allergic reaction.

of histamine and are quite effective in the treatment of hives but less so for hay fever. A typical allergic reaction is illustrated in Figure 2.7.

Skin tests can determine the specific cause of an allergy. This procedure involves injecting a minute amount of antigen intradermally and observing any redness, which indicates a positive skin reaction. Injections of the allergen can desensitise the hypersensitive person. Small amounts of the offending allergen are administered, and concentrations are gradually increased. Desensitisation inoculations work by causing an increase of IgG in the bloodstream. The IgG coats the allergen in the blood, blocking it from binding to IgE in the tissues, subsequently reducing the amount of tissue damage.

Local allergies occur in confined areas such as skin and mucous membranes and are exemplified by the development of a blocked nose after inhaling pollen. In contrast, systemic allergy (anaphylaxis) occurs throughout the body and may be life-threatening.

The underlying cellular mechanisms of the systemic anaphylactic reaction are the same as in the local response. However, during the systemic response, mast cells and basophils throughout the body become involved, triggering a generalised change in capillary permeability that leads to hypotension (low blood pressure) and shock. Smooth muscle contraction in the respiratory tract causes respiratory distress resembling asthma. Fluid in the larynx may obstruct the airways and necessitate a tracheotomy, a surgical opening into the trachea to facilitate passage of air or evacuation of secretions.

Less severe signs may include flushed skin, hives, swelling of lips or tongue, wheezing and abdominal cramps. Life-threatening signs include weakness and collapse owing to low blood pressure, inability to breathe and fits.

Adrenaline (epinephrine), glucocorticoids or cortisone derivatives may be used to reduce the immune response and stabilise the vascular system.

Four types of hypersensitivities are recognised. Type I hypersensitivities are labelled allergic or anaphylactic hypersensitivity. These are triggered by allergen binding to IgE on mast cells, which produces either local severe inflammation or systemic severe inflammation (anaphylactic shock) (Figure 2.8). These are produced by bee venom, foods or pollen.

Type II hypersensitivities are labelled cytotoxic or cytolytic and involve IgM or IgG interacting with foreign cells to cause their destruction. An example of a type II response is an incompatible blood transfusion. A person with type A blood has A antigens on the red cells and antibodies against type B blood in the serum. If such a person receives a type B transfusion, the antigens and antibodies interact. The red blood cells agglutinate, or clump together, and massive haemolysis (rupture) occurs.

Cross-matching for a blood transfusion must match blood type and **Rhesus factor (Rh)**. In addition to antigens that determine blood type, Rh-positive (Rh⁺) individuals have another antigen,

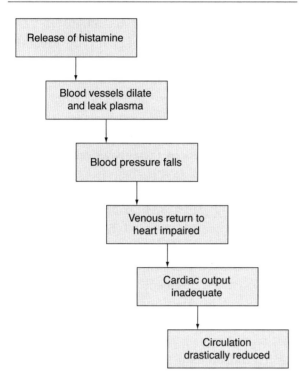

Figure 2.8 Sequence of vascular events in anaphylactic shock.

the Rh factor, on their red blood cells. Rh-negative (Rh⁻) individuals lack the Rh antigen. Another example of the cytolytic allergic response involves the transfusion of Rh⁺ blood to an Rh⁻ recipient. No problems would arise for the Rh⁻ recipient if it were the first such transfusion received, but if the Rh⁻ recipient was previously exposed or sensitised to the Rh factor, the recipient may form antibodies against this foreign protein, causing clumping and rupture of red blood cells.

Rh incompatibility during pregnancy is also a type II hypersensitivity. A Rh⁻ mother can become sensitised to the Rh antigen if the fetus is Rh⁺.

However, maternal antibodies do not form and damage the fetus during the first such pregnancy, because the maternal and fetal blood do not mix. But during birth there may be mixing of blood, exposing the mother to the Rh⁺ antigen. The mother's immune system can recognise this antigen as foreign and produce antibodies against it, which would threaten subsequent pregnancies with an Rh⁺ fetus. To prevent this, Anti-D (Rh₀) immunoglobulin, an injectable medication, is given to Rh⁻ women after the delivery of Rh⁺ babies.

Type III hypersensitivities are labelled immune complex. In this type of hypersensitivity, antigens combine with antibodies, forming immune complexes. These immune complexes deposit in tissues and blood vessels, causing inflammation and tissue destruction. Immune complexes may form in the kidneys (causing glomerulonephritis, triggered after a streptococcal infection) or the lungs (causing farmer's lung, triggered by mould spore inhalation). Types I, II and III are all immediate hypersensitivities; they develop within about 30 minutes of exposure to antigens or allergens.

Type IV hypersensitivities are called cell-mediated or delayed. Initial exposure to an antigen results in activation of a T lymphocyte-mediated immune response, which is slow to develop (delayed). For example, no reaction occurs the first time one contacts the oil of poison ivy. However, T cells may become sensitised to it. On the next exposure, the typical rash and irritation appear, caused by T lymphocyte secretion of cytokines that damage the tissues where the ivy oil has been absorbed. This delayed development is the type of reaction found in contact dermatitis and the significant tuberculin test (Figure 2.9). Table 2.2 summarises the four types of hypersensitivities.

 Prevention PLUS!

Adrenaline treatment for anaphylaxis

The most vital therapy for systemic anaphylaxis is prompt intramuscular injection of adrenaline (epinephrine). Certain allergic individuals must carry adrenaline at all times in an EpiPen®, which can be self-injected in an emergency.

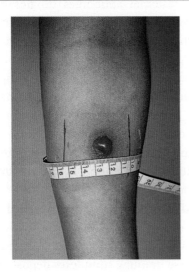

Figure 2.9 Induration measurement in a tuberculin skin test, a type IV hypersensitivity.
(Courtesy of the CDC)

Organ transplantation can be a desirable treatment option for those suffering from serious organ disease. There are currently over 7000 of the population in the UK waiting for an organ transplant and new patients are added to the list every month, with increased demands expected in the future due to factors such as increases in type 2 diabetes impacting on demands for kidney transplants. Every year an estimated 1000 people die while waiting for an organ.

Organs that can be transplanted include heart, kidney, lung, liver, intestine and pancreas. In an **autograft**, tissue grafts are transplanted from one site to another in the same patient; for example, a skin graft. **Isografts** are tissues donated by an identical twin. Autografts and isografts are highly successful because the immune system does not view the graft as foreign. **Xenografts** are tissue grafts

harvested from a different animal species; the use of pig heart valves in humans is an example.

The most common type of graft is an **allograft**, in which tissue is transplanted from one person to another, but the transplant donor and recipient are not identical twins. Before an allograft is attempted, the blood type of both the donor and recipient must be determined and must match. In addition, cell membrane antigens of their tissue cells are typed to determine how closely they match. At least a 75% match in cell membrane antigens is needed to attempt an allograft. Good tissue matches between unrelated people are difficult to find.

Tissue and organ rejections are examples of type IV or delayed hypersensitivity reactions. Organs could be easily transplanted if it were not for the immune system. The immune system recognises the transplanted organ as foreign, and lymphocytes attack it, eventually destroying the transplanted organ. Compounding the problem is that the transplanted organ carries with it donor lymphocytes that react against the recipient's tissues (a graft versus host reaction). For these reasons, donor and recipient antigens are matched as closely as possible to lessen possible rejection. To prevent immune system rejection, the transplant patient receives medications, which may include corticosteroids to suppress inflammation, and immunosuppressants. These drugs have severe side effects, including the suppressed immune system being unable to protect the body against other foreign agents and leaving the patient open to infection and some cancers.

Sepsis and multiple organ failure

The most common cause of inflammation is due to infection from a micro-organism, most commonly

Table 2.2 Types of hypersensitivities.

Type	Mechanism	Effect
I	Excess IgE bound to mast cells and activated by allergens	Inflammation
II	IgM or IgG cause destruction of foreign cells	Cell lysis
III	Immune complexes are deposited in tissue and vessels	Inflammation and tissue destruction
IV	Sensitised T lymphocytes release cytokines	Inflammation and tissue damage

bacteria. Whilst in most cases the inflammation provides an important immune response, by improving the blood supply to the affected area, attracting leucocytes and substances which will aid tissue repair, in a small number of cases the effects of inflammation can be detrimental to the person's health and can sometimes worsen health and in some cases lead to death. What may have begun as a local infection can spread to other regions of the body if the micro-organism responsible has been unresponsive to antimicrobial drugs or the immune system has been overwhelmed. The spread of the micro-organism most commonly occurs via the blood or lymphatic systems. Sepsis refers to an infection that is present in the blood. Signs of sepsis include fever, raised heart and respiratory rates, raised white blood cell count as well as local signs such as abdominal pain if the origin of the infection was from the gut. The term Systemic inflammatory response (SIRS) describes the overwhelming inflammatory events that occur in infections. SIRS can also occur, following injuries due to major trauma, extensive tissue injuries and also due to severe blood loss. The overwhelming inflammatory response is characterised by release of an array of substances that affect the circulation and major organs, lead to damage to the normal circulation which can lead to tissue hypoxia and organ failure. During SIRS there is release of vasoactive substances that cause vasodilatation to occur; this lowers the blood pressure, leading to hypotension and reduced perfusion of organs. Capillary permeability increases and there is increased loss of plasma into the tissues, which further lowers the blood pressure as fluids move from the circulation into the tissues, leading to hypotension.

Compensatory mechanisms from the cardiovascular centre in the brain respond to the reduced venous return to the heart and, in order to compensate, increases heart rate to maintain cardiac output. Increased peripheral resistance and vasoconstriction in blood vessels can increase blood pressure. Blood flow is diverted away from areas such as the gut, kidneys and skin to essential areas such as the heart, lungs and brain. However, maintaining normal blood pressure becomes increasingly difficult owing to vasoactive substances and loss of circulating volume.

Prolonged reduced perfusion to organs can cause organ failure; when more than one organ fails the term multiple organ failure is used. The organs most commonly affected include the lungs, kidneys, heart and liver. Despite advances in treatments, multiple organ failure carries high rates of morbidity and mortality, particularly in vulnerable groups such as the elderly and immunocompromised. There can also be a genetic component to individual responses to sepsis and the subsequent multiple organ failure. At the present time the reasons for this are not fully understood.

These damaging effects of sepsis occur because of a combination of an overwhelming infection and a widespread inflammatory response. Bacteria may contain **endotoxins** and **exotoxins** which may contribute to the inflammatory events. Endotoxins are present in the cell walls of mostly Gram-negative bacteria. They are released when the bacteria die and can trigger damaging immune responses which lead to fever and vascular collapse, with widespread vasodilatation and hypotension. Exotoxins are released by living bacteria. These toxins can paralyse nerves, damage various cells and in some cases are able to digest host tissues. These foreign antigens stimulate the activation of additional leucocytes which further increases the inflammatory response.

During severe inflammation various cytokines are released, which further worsen the situation. Cytokines are chemical messengers released by activated leucocytes and also by the endothelial lining of blood vessels. Well-known families of cytokines include the **interleukins** (IL) and **tumour necrosis factor** (TNF). Some cytokines are mediators of inflammation but there are also cytokines which have the opposite effects and reduce inflammation.

TNF is known to play a role in the hosts response to infection, by activating phagocytes and increasing inflammation. Interleukin 1 (IL1) has some similar actions to TNF, but also contributes to stimulating T helper and cytotoxic T cells. IL6 depresses myocardial function, affecting normal cardiac function, and triggers the release of proteins from the liver, known as acute phase proteins which can be measured in the blood to determine inflammation. The most well known is **C-reactive protein** (CRP), which is elevated in inflammatory responses to infections.

Arachidonic acid is released from cell membranes owing to the enzyme phospholipase A2. Cyclo-oxygenase enzymes convert arachidonic acid to various substances, mostly to thromboxanes and **prostaglandins**. Thromboxanes cause pulmonary vasoconstriction, which can be a contributory factor to respiratory failure.

Prostaglandins have a wide variety of actions, causing both vasoconstriction and vasodilatation, as well as contributing to pulmonary hypertension in some cases. There is recognition that by blocking the cyclo-oxygenase pathway, reduction of inflammation can occur and this can also provide pain relief because of the reduced inflammation. Examples of drugs which work in this pathway are the non-steroidal anti-inflammatory drugs such as ibuprofen and paracetamol. Arachidonic acid can also be converted into leukotrienes by lipo-oxygenases. Leukotrienes are also implicated in inflammatory response as they increase vascular permeability, cause coronary vasoconstriction and lower cardiac output. Knowledge of the actions of leukotrienes in inflammation has led to the development of a family of drugs known as the leukotriene receptor antagonists. This group includes montelukast, which has been used to reduce inflammation in the airways, acting to prevent asthma attacks.

Treatments of sepsis involve administering antimicrobial drugs and intravenous fluids to maintain the circulatory volume and to prevent imbalances of electrolytes. Multiple organ failure requires drugs to maintain the cardiovascular system and specialist treatments such as kidney dialysis when there is kidney failure. After a period with high levels of inflammation and other immune mechanisms, a period of immunosuppression occurs which can make the patient vulnerable to a secondary infection; this may also carry high levels of mortality and morbidity.

AUTOIMMUNITY

The immune response normally recognises the difference between the individual's own tissues and those of invaders; this is known as tolerance. When tolerance fails, an **autoimmune disease** may be the result. **Autoimmunity** occurs when individuals develop antibodies called autoantibodies to their own tissues, or self-antigens. Almost all patients presenting with autoimmunity have some autoantibodies present in their serum. It is not always known whether the autoantibodies play an important role in the disease or are a secondary result of the tissue damage that has been caused by the disease process itself. Autoimmune patients also have autoreactive T cells. Several of these autoimmune diseases are described elsewhere in this book.

Scleroderma

Derived from the Greek words *sclerosis*, meaning 'hardness', and *derma*, meaning 'skin', scleroderma literally means 'hard skin'. Scleroderma or systemic sclerosis is an autoimmune disease of the connective tissue. Scleroderma is characterised by the formation of scar tissue (fibrosis) in the skin and organs of the body. The Scleroderma Society states that 1 in 10 000 of the UK population suffer from scleroderma, with between 6000 and 7000 Britons having scleroderma. Scleroderma is four times more common in women than in men. Scleroderma is categorised into two major classes: localised scleroderma and systemic scleroderma. Both groups include subgroups (Figure 2.10).

Localised types of scleroderma are those limited to the skin and related tissues and in some cases, the muscle below. Internal organs are not affected by localised scleroderma, and localised scleroderma can never progress to the systemic forms of the diseases. There are two generally recognised types of localised scleroderma: **morphea** and **linear scleroderma**. Morphea comes from a Greek word that means 'form' or 'structure'. The word refers to local patches of scleroderma. The first signs of the disease are reddish patches of skin that thicken into firm, oval-shaped areas. The centre of each patch becomes ivory coloured with violet borders. These patches sweat very little and have little hair growth. Patches appear most often on the chest, stomach and back. Morphea can be localised or generalised. Localised

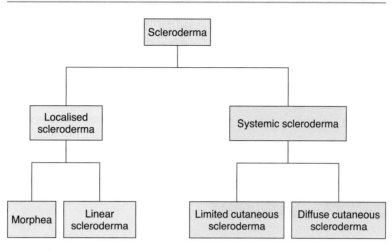

Figure 2.10 Types of scleroderma.

morphea limits itself to one or several patches, ranging in size from half an inch to 12 inches in diameter. The disease is referred to as generalised morphea when the skin patches become very hard and dark and spread over large areas of the body. Regardless of the type, morphea generally fades out in 3–5 years; however, some people are left with darkened skin patches and, in rare cases, muscle weakness. Linear scleroderma is characterised by a single line or band of thickened skin. It usually runs down an arm or leg, but in some patients it runs down the forehead.

Systemic scleroderma involves the skin, tissues under the skin, blood vessels and the major organs. Systemic scleroderma is typically broken down into **limited cutaneous scleroderma** and **diffuse cutaneous scleroderma**. Limited cutaneous scleroderma typically comes on gradually and affects the skin of the fingers, hands, face, lower arms and legs. People with limited disease often have all or some of the signs and symptoms that are referred to as CREST: calcinosis, Raynaud's phenomenon, oesophageal dysfunction, sclerodactyly and telangiectasia. Calcinosis refers to the formation of calcium deposits in the connective tissue. They are typically found on the fingers, hands, face and trunk. When the deposits break through the skin, painful ulcers can result. Raynaud's is a condition in which the small blood vessels of the hands and/or feet constrict in response to cold or anxiety; see Chapter 6 for further information. Oesophageal dysfunction

refers to impaired function of the oesophagus that occurs when smooth muscles in the oesophagus lose normal movement. In the upper and lower oesophagus, the result can be swallowing difficulties; in the lower oesophagus, the result can be chronic heartburn or inflammation. Sclerodactyly refers to thick and tight skin on the fingers, resulting from deposits of excess collagen within skin layers. The condition makes it more difficult to bend and straighten the fingers. The skin may also appear shiny and darkened. Telangiectasia is a condition caused by the swelling of tiny blood vessels, in which red spots appear on the hands and face. While not painful, these red spots can create cosmetic problems.

Diffuse cutaneous scleroderma comes on suddenly; skin thickening begins in the hands and spreads quickly over much of the body in a symmetrical fashion. Skin changes can cause the skin to swell, appear shiny, and feel tight and itchy (Figure 2.11). Internally it can damage key organs such as the intestines, lungs, heart and kidneys; however, less than one-third of patients develop severe organ problems. Patients are often tired, lose appetite and weight, and have joint swelling or pain. The damage of diffuse cutaneous scleroderma occurs over a few years and patients often have periods of exacerbation and remission.

The cause(s) of scleroderma is unknown, but there are immune, genetic, environmental and hormonal factors involved. The immune system is

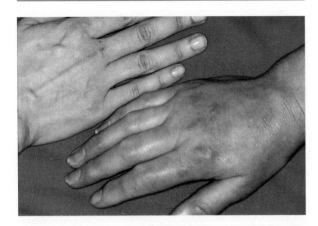

Figure 2.11 Scleroderma of the hand.
(Phototake NYC)

thought to stimulate fibroblasts so they produce too much collagen. The collagen forms thick connective tissue that builds up within the skin and internal organs. Genetics may put certain people at risk for scleroderma. Although no environmental agent has been shown to cause scleroderma, research suggests that exposure to viral infections and certain chemicals may trigger scleroderma in those who are genetically predisposed. By middle to late childbearing years (ages 30–55), women develop scleroderma 7–12 times more often than men; this suggests that the disease may be linked to oestrogen production.

Diagnosis of scleroderma begins with a thorough medical history and physical examination. Finding one or more of the following can aid in the diagnosis: changes in skin appearance and texture; swollen fingers and hands; tight skin around the hands, face, mouth or elsewhere; calcium deposits developing under the skin; changes in the capillaries at the base of the fingernails; thickened skin patches. Autoantibodies against DNA are found in the blood of some scleroderma patients. In some cases a skin biopsy is performed.

Scleroderma has no known cure, and there is no treatment to stop the overproduction of collagen. Scleroderma patients should not smoke and should avoid exposure to cold and stress, protect their skin and moisturise frequently.

Physical therapy and exercise can help to maintain muscle strength but cannot totally prevent joints

from freezing in permanent (usually flexed) positions. Medications, including anti-inflammatory drugs (non-steroidal and corticosteroids) and immunosuppressive drugs, may be necessary. Light therapy may be helpful in treating skin lesions. For some people, scleroderma (particularly the localised forms) is fairly mild and resolves with time. But for others, living with the disease and its effects day to day has a significant impact on their quality of life. A negative prognosis is more likely for those who have early symptoms of heart, lung or kidney damage.

Sjögren's syndrome

Sjögren's syndrome is a chronic autoimmune inflammatory disease of glands and other tissues. In the UK an estimated 500 000 are affected by Sjögren's syndrome and 90% of these are women. About half the time, Sjögren's occurs alone and is known as primary Sjögren's; the other half it occurs with a disease like rheumatoid arthritis, lupus or scleroderma and is called secondary Sjögren's. Sjögren's can be a systemic disease affecting the entire body, including kidneys, gastrointestinal system, blood vessels, lungs, liver, pancreas and nervous system. The most common symptoms of Sjögren's syndrome are dry eyes, dry mouth, dry skin and vaginal dryness.

The cause(s) of Sjögren's syndrome are not known. Genetic factors, hormones and environmental triggers, including viral infections, may play a role. A first-degree relative with autoimmunity increases the risk for Sjögren's syndrome sevenfold. Sjögren's syndrome often affects women during their childbearing years, suggesting a link between the syndrome and female hormones. Sjögren's syndrome is often under diagnosed or misdiagnosed because the signs and symptoms may mimic those of menopause, drug side effects or diseases like lupus, rheumatoid arthritis and multiple sclerosis. The average time from the onset of symptoms to diagnosis is over 6 years. No single test will confirm the diagnosis of Sjögren's syndrome. Tear and salivary gland function are measured. Laboratory tests, including blood chemistry tests, measurement of general levels of inflammation, and autoantibody testing may be performed. Lip or salivary gland biopsy may also be performed.

Currently there is no cure for Sjögren's syndrome. Medications may be used to alleviate different types of dryness. Medications, including anti-inflammatory drugs (non-steroidal and corticosteroids), anti-malarials and immunosuppressive drugs, may be necessary. Sjögren's patients should be aware that the incidence of lymphoma (cancer of the lymph nodes) is significantly higher in Sjögren's patients. The prognosis is generally good. However, if the lungs, kidneys or lymph nodes are damaged by the antibodies, pneumonia, kidney failure or lymphoma may result.

IMMUNE DEFICIENCY

Acquired immunodeficiency syndrome (AIDS)

One of the most deadly diseases to affect today's population is **acquired immunodeficiency syndrome (AIDS)**. AIDS destroys the individual's immune system, making the person remarkably susceptible to infection. AIDS was first noted in the early 1980s among homosexual/bisexual men with multiple sexual contacts with other men and drug users who shared hypodermic needles.

AIDS is now a pandemic. According to the Joint United Nations Programme on HIV/AIDS, at the end of 2007, an estimated 30.8 million adults and 2.5 million children worldwide were living with HIV/AIDS, 2.5 million people worldwide became infected with HIV, and 2.1 million people died an AIDS-related death. Heterosexual transmission accounts for two-thirds of new infections. Mother-to-infant transmission and intravenous drug users each account for approximately 10% of HIV infections. Homosexual transmission and healthcare transmission each account for approximately 5–10% of HIV infections. Of people living with HIV, 95% live in the developing world, with over 60% in sub-Saharan Africa. In the UK in 2007 over 7000 new cases of HIV were diagnosed; most cases were in the heterosexual population, especially in migrants from areas where HIV is common such as

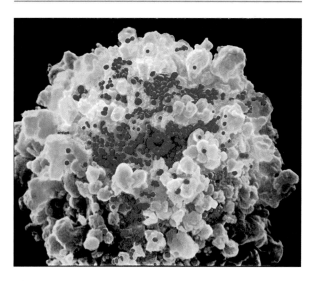

Figure 2.12 Coloured scanning electron micrograph (SEM) of a T lymphocyte (green) infected with HIV (red). The virus has infected the T lymphocyte and instructed the lymphocyte to reproduce many more viruses. Small spherical virus particles (red) are budding away from the T lymphocyte membrane. Viral budding destroys the T lymphocyte. Depletion in the blood of CD4 lymphocytes through HIV infection is the main reason for the destruction of the immune system in AIDS. (National Institute for Biological Standards and Control (U.K.)/Science Photo Library/Photo Researchers, Inc.)

sub-Saharan Africa. Since the 1980s, the UK has seen over 18 000 deaths from AIDS.

The causative agent of AIDS is the **human immuno-deficiency virus (HIV)**, a retrovirus; that is, it carries its genetic information as RNA rather than DNA (Figure 2.12). HIV is transmitted via contaminated body fluids, including blood, semen, vaginal secretions and breast milk. Therefore, HIV is transmitted by unprotected anal, oral or vaginal intercourse, birth, breastfeeding and the sharing of needles. The virus infects primarily helper or CD4 T lymphocytes. The virus replicates within these lymphocytes, killing them and spreading to others. These lymphocytes normally activate B cell lymphocytes; thus, the body's immune response is impaired and the body is susceptible to infections and tumours that a healthy immune system could easily control.

Many people do not develop signs or symptoms immediately after HIV infection. Some people develop signs and symptoms within several days to

Table 2.3 Possible signs and symptoms of initial HIV infection, asymptomatic period and AIDS.

Initial HIV infection	Asymptomatic period	AIDS
HIV+	HIV+	HIV+
Fever	Lack of energy	One of AIDS indicator diseases
Headache	Weight loss	CD4 T lymphocyte count less than 200
Fatigue	Frequent fever and sweats	
Enlarged lymph nodes	Persistent or frequent yeast infection	Cough and shortness of breath
	Persistent skin rashes or flaky skin	Seizures and lack of coordination
	Short-term memory loss	Difficult or painful swallowing
	Mouth, genital or anal herpes sores	Confusion and forgetfulness
		Severe and persistent diarrhoea
		Fever
		Loss of vision
		Nausea
		Abdominal cramps and vomiting
		Weight loss
		Extreme fatigue
		Severe headache with stiff neck
		Coma

weeks after infection, and these usually disappear within a few weeks. The length of an asymptomatic period may last a few months or more than 10 years. The long latent period increases the risk of spreading the infection because individuals may not be aware they have the disease. During this period the virus continues to multiply, infecting and killing CD4 lymphocytes. Once the immune system is weakened by the virus, an HIV-positive person may develop signs and symptoms. Eventually, a threshold is crossed and the HIV-infected person develops AIDS. To move from an HIV-positive diagnosis to an AIDS diagnosis, the patient must have one of the AIDS indicator diseases and have a CD4 T lymphocyte count of less than 200. Table 2.3 shows common signs and symptoms for initial HIV infection, the asymptomatic period and AIDS.

The presence of HIV antibodies in the blood can be detected with the enzyme-linked immunosorbent assay (ELISA), as most people produce antibodies against HIV within 3 months of being infected. If the ELISA test is positive, the test is usually repeated and the result confirmed using a Western blot test. A positive P24 antigen test indicates circulating HIV antigen. Polymerase chain reaction (PCR) can also be used to test for HIV RNA.

Free testing for HIV antibodies is available at local health trusts throughout the UK.

Drug therapy that begins shortly after infection increases the chances that the immune system will not be destroyed by HIV. While there is no cure for AIDS, medications may hinder HIV replication to the extent that the viral load becomes undetectable in some individuals. Anti-HIV medications are used to control replication of the virus and to slow the progression of HIV-related disease. Anti-HIV medications do not cure HIV infection, and individuals taking these medications can still transmit HIV to others. Highly active antiretroviral therapy (HAART) is the recommended treatment for HIV infection. HAART combines three or more anti-HIV medications in a daily regimen. HAART medications target HIV replication and entry. These drugs are very expensive, cause side effects, and the regimen of pill-taking throughout the day is very demanding. If the drugs are not taken as prescribed or if the therapy is stopped, resistance or relapse may occur. AIDS-related deaths have declined as a result of HAART. Most people living with HIV in the developing world have no access to HAART.

There are some exciting experimental HIV drugs on the horizon that target HIV DNA integration transcription and viral assembly. Development of a vaccine to prevent the spread of AIDS has not yet been possible. The genetic make-up of the AIDS virus varies greatly from strain to strain; HIV tends to mutate quickly, which complicates the attempt to develop an AIDS vaccine, and vaccines to date have not been successful in stimulating HIV antibody production. A new area of research involves attempting to stimulate and train killer T cells to recognise and destroy HIV quickly.

The Global HIV Prevention Working Group estimates that by delivering comprehensive HIV prevention to those who need it, annual HIV incidence could be nearly two-thirds lower in 2015. This would mean 4 million fewer infections each year by the middle of the next decade. Sexual transmission can be prevented by abstinence, monogamy and use of condoms. Blood transmission can be prevented by needle exchange programmes and screening of blood. Healthcare workers should use personal protective equipment and safe administration of injections (as discussed in Chapter 3) to protect themselves. Mother-to-child transmission can be prevented by antiretroviral medication. Unfortunately, most people at risk of HIV infection have little or no access to these prevention tools.

VACCINATION

Two types of artificial immunity can be administered: active and passive immunity. In **active immunity**, the person receives a **vaccine** or a **toxoid** as the antigen, and he or she forms antibodies to counteract it. A vaccine is a suspension of whole organisms or pieces of organisms that is used to induce immunity. Attenuated whole-agent vaccines use living but attenuated (weakened) organisms. Organisms can be attenuated by aging or altering their growing conditions. Because the organisms have been specially treated to deactivate them, they cannot cause disease. As proteins foreign to the body, these antigens do trigger antibody production against them. Examples of attenuated vaccines include the Sabin polio vaccine and the MMR (measles, mumps and

rubella) vaccine. Inactivated whole-agent vaccines use organisms that have been killed, usually by formalin or phenol. Examples of inactivated whole-agent vaccines include rabies, influenza and the Salk polio vaccine. A **toxoid** works similarly. It consists of a chemically altered toxin, the poisonous material produced by a pathogenic organism. Having been treated chemically, the toxin will not cause disease. It will, however, stimulate the immune response. Examples of toxoid vaccines include tetanus and diphtheria. Subunit vaccines use only those antigenic fragments of organisms that best stimulate an immune response. Genes for specific disease antigens are inserted into the genetic material of harmless organisms. The antigens produced by these organisms are extracted, purified and used for immunisation. The hepatitis B vaccine is produced in this manner. Active immunity is long-lived. Time is required to build up immunity and, for some vaccines, a booster injection is necessary. Once cells have been sensitised to these viruses, bacteria or toxins, they retain the ability to produce antibodies against them when encountered again.

What if a person is exposed to a serious disease such as hepatitis, tetanus or rabies and has no immunity against it? It takes too much time to build antibodies in response to a vaccination. In this case, the person is given **passive immunity**, doses of preformed antibodies from immune serum of an animal, usually a horse. This type of immunity is short-lived but acts immediately. Table 2.4 contrasts active and passive immunity.

Table 2.4 Differences between active and passive immunity.

Active immunity	Passive immunity
Person forms antibodies	Preformed antibodies received
Vaccine (deactivated bacteria or virus)	Immune horse serum
or	*or*
Toxoid (chemically altered toxin)	Antibodies, cells in breast milk
Long-lived immunity (requires time to act)	Short-lived immunity (acts immediately)

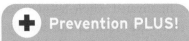
Prevention PLUS!

Disease prevention through vaccination

Without appropriate immunisation, children are susceptible to many serious and life-threatening infections, such as measles, whooping cough, hepatitis and meningitis. Vaccines are effective, particularly when a high proportion of people in a population are immunised. Reactions to the vaccines are usually mild and rarely serious. The risks from these childhood diseases far outweigh the risk of a serious reaction from a vaccine. The following charts include childhood immunisation recommendations from the Department of Health.

Routine childhood immunisation programme in 2009

Each vaccination is given as a single injection into the muscle of the thigh or upper arm.

When to immunise	Diseases protected against	Vaccine given
Two months old	Diphtheria, tetanus, pertussis (whooping cough), polio and *Haemophilus influenzae* type b (Hib) Pneumococcal infection	DTaP/IPV/Hib + Pneumococcal conjugate vaccine, (PCV)
Three months old	Diphtheria, tetanus, pertussis, polio and *Haemophilus influenzae* type b (Hib) Meningitis C	DTaP/IPV/Hib + MenC
Four months old	Diphtheria, tetanus, pertussis, polio and *Haemophilus influenzae* type b (Hib) Meningitis C Pneumococcal infection	DTaP/IPV/Hib + MenC + PCV
Around 12 months	*Haemophilus influenza* type b (Hib) Meningitis C	Hib/MenC
Around 13 months old	Measles, mumps and rubella Pneumococcal infection	MMR + PCV
Three years and four months or soon after	Diphtheria, tetanus, pertussis and polio Measles, mumps and rubella	DTaP/IPV or dTaP/IPV + MMR
Girls aged 12 to 13 years	Cervical cancer caused by human papillomavirus types 16 and 18	HPV
13 to 18 years old	Diphtheria, tetanus, polio	Td/IPV

Non-routine immunisations

When to immunise	Diseases protected against	Vaccine given
At birth (to babies who are more likely to come into contact with TB than the general population)	Tuberculosis	BCG
At birth (to babies whose mothers are hepatitis B positive)	Hepatitis B	Hep B

STRESS AND THE IMMUNE SYSTEM

Stressors such as trauma, infection, surgery, pain and emotional distress all have significant effects on the immune system's ability to function. Stress causes an increased production of the hormone **cortisol**. Cortisol decreases production of antibodies and substances released by leucocytes that stimulate other cells of the immune system.

Cortisol production occurs when noradrenaline and adrenaline are released by the sympathetic nervous system, as happens during the fight-or-flight response. The combined effect of these three hormones increases the total number of neutrophils in the circulation. Lymphocyte maturation in the lymph nodes stops because adrenaline decreases blood flow to the lymph nodes as it increases blood flow to the heart, lungs, brain and muscles. These changes in the immune response brought on by stress leave the body less capable of fighting off the effects of injury, disease and other stress causes.

AGE AND THE IMMUNE SYSTEM

The immune system simply does not function as efficiently in older adults as in younger people. The body becomes less able to distinguish self from non-self and, as a result, autoimmune disorders become more common among the elderly. Common problems related to the immune system in older people include increased infection risk and decreased ability to fight disease. By middle age, the thymus is only about 15% of its maximum size. The total number of T lymphocytes does not decrease with age, but the diversity of T lymphocytes is reduced. This decrease in T lymphocyte population diversity in older adults leads to less effective location and elimination of pathogens. There are fewer lymphocytes capable of responding to new antigens; therefore, when older people encounter a new antigen, the body is less able to recognise and defend against it. It takes longer for macrophages to destroy bacteria, viruses, cancer cells and other antigens. The amount of antibody produced in response to an antigen and the antibody's ability to attach to the antigen are reduced. Because of the reduction in antibody production, vaccines are less likely to produce immunity in older people. While vaccines do not work as well in older adults, vaccinations for diseases such as influenza, pneumonia, hepatitis B, tuberculosis, diphtheria and tetanus have been found to reduce mortality in the elderly and are still worthwhile.

Resources

Department of Health, UK: *www.dh.gov.uk*

Global HIV Prevention Working Group: *www.globalhivprevention.org/index.html*

Health Protection agency, UK: *www.hpa.gov.uk*

Joint United Programme on HIV/AIDS: *www.unaids.org/en*

Scleroderma Society, UK: *www.sclerodermasociety.co.uk*

British Sjögren's Syndrome Association: *www.bssa.uk.net*

Terence Higgins Trust (HIV), UK: *www.tht.org.uk*

INTERACTIVE EXERCISES

Cases for critical thinking

1. Tetanus is caused by bacteria that enter the body through wounds in the skin. The bacteria produce a toxin that causes spastic muscle contraction. Death often results from failure of the respiratory muscles. A patient comes to the Accident and Emergency Department after stepping on a nail. If the patient has been vaccinated against tetanus, he or she is given a tetanus booster injection, which

consists of the toxin altered so that it is harmless. If the patient has never been vaccinated against tetanus, he or she is given an antiserum injection against tetanus. Explain the rationale for this treatment.

2. Explain why identical twins are an ideal case for organ transplantation.

3. A crime scene investigator finds a body of a woman and discovers animal bites on the victim's body. The investigator examines the bites and sees they are not inflamed. Did the animal bites happen before or after the woman died?

4. A baby receives his first dose of oral polio vaccine from his paediatrician. Is this active or passive immunity? What does the polio virus trigger in the body?

5. Some people with decreased IgA exhibit recurrent sinus and respiratory infections. Why?

6. Explain why HIV's attack on helper CD4 T lymphocytes devastates the entire immune system.

Multiple choice

1. Passive immunity is achieved artificially by injection of _____
   a. preformed antibodies
   b. autoantibodies
   c. deactivated viruses and bacteria
   d. toxoids
   e. bacterial toxins

2. Long-lived lymphocytes, which remain dormant until reactivated after an immune response, are the _____
   a. helper lymphocytes
   b. cytotoxic lymphocytes
   c. suppressor lymphocytes
   d. memory lymphocytes
   e. plasma cells

3. Defence against antigens via antibodies is called _____
   a. humoral immunity
   b. cell-mediated immunity
   c. plasma cells
   d. adhesion
   e. suppression

4. Which of the following agents is/are capable of causing an inflammatory response?
   a. allergen   b. trauma
   c. chemical agents   d. all of the above

5. Which is a foreign substance that triggers an immune response?
   a. antigen   b. antibody
   c. antibiotic   d. adhesion

6. Which cells secrete antibodies during the immune response?
   a. T helper   b. B
   c. plasma   d. T killer

7. The response to poison ivy is an example of which type of hypersensitivity?
   a. I   b. II
   c. III   d. IV

8. Which antibody is produced in excess during an allergic response?
   a. IgE   b. IgG
   c. IgM   d. IgA

9. The virus of acquired immune deficiency syndrome invades and damages leucocytes, especially targeting the _____
   a. B lymphocytes
   b. cytotoxic or CD8 T lymphocytes
   c. helper or CD4 lymphocytes
   d. suppressor lymphocytes

10. Which cells are involved in both cellular and humoral reactions during an immune response?
    a. cytotoxic T cells   b. natural killer cells
    c. plasma cells   d. helper cells

True or false

_____ **1.** HIV can be transmitted through saliva.

_____ **2.** Fever is an example of specific immunity.

_____ **3.** Inflammation is an undesirable reaction to injury.

_____ **4.** Antibodies provide humoral immunity.

_____ **5.** Cell-mediated immunity depends on the activities of B lymphocytes.

_____ **6.** T lymphocytes produce antibodies.

_____ **7.** The release of histamine increases the permeability of capillary walls.

_____ **8.** Failure of immune tolerance creates an autoimmune disease.

_____ **9.** Anaphylactic shock is a moderately serious allergic reaction.

_____ **10.** Type I hypersensitivities involve IgM or IgG and cause destruction of foreign cells.

Fill-ins

1. Bacteria that cause pus formation are called _____ bacteria.

2. _____ is a group of substances that stimulate the immune system.

3. A substance that triggers an immune response is an _____.

4. A _____ consists of a low dose of dead or deactivated bacteria or viruses.

5. _____ immunity is effective against any foreign agent.

6. Damaged tissue releases _____.

7. Ig _____ protects newborns.

8. _____ are a type of leucocyte that recognises body cells with abnormal membranes.

9. The causative agent of AIDS is the _____.

10. In _____ immunity, the person is given preformed antibodies.

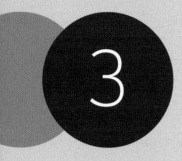

3 INFECTIOUS DISEASES

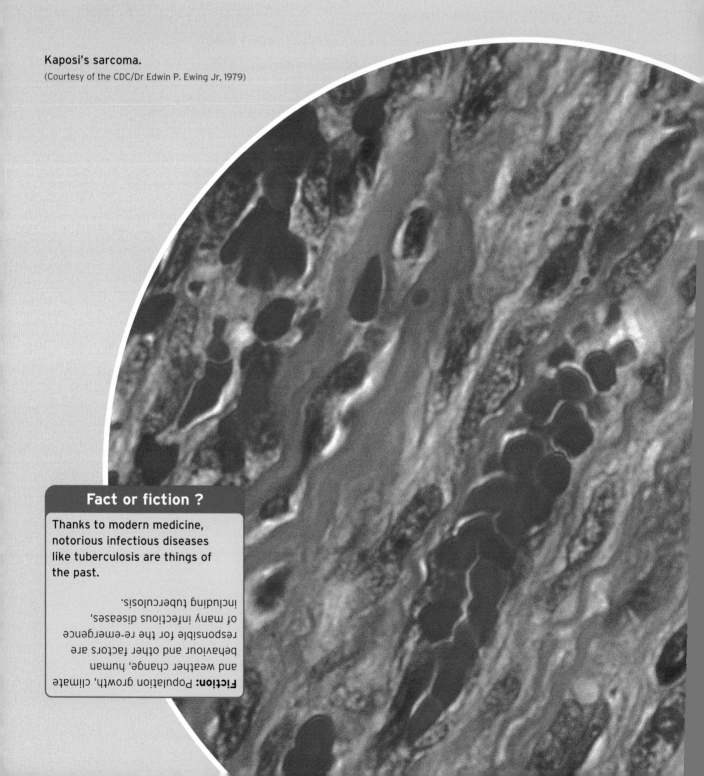

Kaposi's sarcoma.
(Courtesy of the CDC/Dr Edwin P. Ewing Jr, 1979)

Fact or fiction ?

Thanks to modern medicine, notorious infectious diseases like tuberculosis are things of the past.

Fiction: Population growth, climate and weather change, human behaviour and other factors are responsible for the re-emergence of many infectious diseases, including tuberculosis.

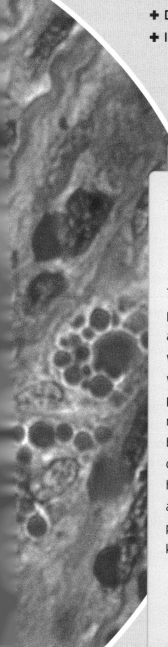

Learning objectives

After studying this chapter, you should be able to:

+ Define infectious disease and its terminology
+ Explain how infectious diseases are transmitted
+ Describe and compare the characteristics of prions, viruses, bacteria, protozoa, fungi and helminths
+ Define nosocomial infections
+ Explain treatment for bacterial, viral, fungal and parasitic infectious diseases
+ Understand the appropriate use of antibiotics and explain the problem of antibiotic resistance
+ Describe examples and causes of emerging and re-emerging infectious diseases
+ Identify common childhood vaccine-preventable infectious diseases

Disease chronicle

Spanish flu pandemic

> If the epidemic continues its mathematical rate of acceleration, civilization could easily disappear from the face of the earth within a few weeks.
> Victor Vaughan, Surgeon General of the Army, October 1918

The influenza pandemic of 1918–1919 has been called the most devastating pandemic in recorded world history. Known as Spanish flu, the pandemic was a global disaster. The pandemic killed an estimated 20–40 million people worldwide and as many as 250 000 in Great Britain and one-fifth of the world was infected. The mortality rate was 2.5% compared to the previous influenza pandemics, which had mortality rates of 0.1%. One of the great unsolved mysteries surrounding the 1918 pandemic is why it tended to kill healthy adults between the ages of 20 and 40. During normal seasonal influenza outbreaks, deaths are most common among the young, elderly and those with chronic health conditions. Scientists believe that even with modern antiviral and antibacterial drugs, vaccines and prevention knowledge, the return of a pandemic virus equivalent in pathogenicity to the virus of 1918 would likely kill more than 100 million people worldwide.

INTRODUCTION

Despite medical advances that have produced drugs and vaccines that are safe and effective against bacteria, viruses, fungi and parasites, **infectious diseases** are still a major cause of death, disability and social and economic upheaval for millions around the world. Illness and death from infectious diseases are particularly tragic because they are largely preventable and treatable. More than 90% of deaths from infectious diseases worldwide are caused by a few diseases (Table 3.1). In developed countries, infectious disease accounts for 1 out of 10 deaths; in developing countries, infectious disease accounts for 6 out of 10 deaths. Poverty, lack of access to healthcare, antibiotic resistance, evolving human migration patterns, new infectious agents, and changing environmental and developmental activities all contribute to the expanding impact of infectious diseases. How many more victims could a lethal strain of influenza similar to the 1918 pandemic claim today with half a billion passengers travelling on planes?

The world's population now exceeds 6 billion people, and most of the growth has occurred in the most densely populated and poorest cities. Crowding, chronic disease, malnutrition and lack of medical resources will become dire. Infectious diseases thrive in these conditions. Scientists must continue research into the cause, transmission, prevention and treatment of infectious diseases for future generations. This chapter describes the nature of infectious diseases, surveys the types of micro-organisms responsible for infections, explains their transmission and discusses treatment.

PRINCIPLES OF INFECTIOUS DISEASE

Some infectious diseases described in this book have been in existence for centuries whereas others have emerged as new pathologies. It is important to have a framework for understanding infectious diseases. Most micro-organisms do not cause disease. A **pathogen** or infectious agent is a disease-causing organism.

Infectious diseases are caused by a pathogen which subsequently grows and multiplies in the body. Diseases transmitted by human contact are said to be **contagious** or **communicable**. Measles and influenza are well-known contagious diseases. Infectious diseases are classified as **non-communicable** if they cannot be transmitted directly from person to person. For example, rabies can be transmitted by the bite of a rabid dog, and cholera is transmitted by drinking faecal-contaminated water.

Epidemiology is the study of the transmission, occurrence, distribution and control of disease. Study of the distribution and frequency of diseases can help predict and prevent disease. The number of new cases of a disease in a population is its **incidence**. Disease incidence may follow a pattern, as when influenza incidence increases in winter and subsides in summer or when Lyme disease increases in summer and subsides in winter. The number of existing cases of a disease is known as its **prevalence**, and this information can tell how significant the disease is in a certain population. When a disease always occurs at low levels in a population, it is said to be **endemic**. Sexually transmitted infections (Chapter 11) are endemic diseases. If a disease occurs in unusually large numbers over a specific area, it is said to be **epidemic**. Influenza occurs as epidemics. When an epidemic has spread to include several large areas worldwide, it is said to be **pandemic**. AIDS is considered to be pandemic. When a disease suddenly occurs in unexpected numbers in a limited

Table 3.1 Leading causes of death owing to infectious diseases.

Disease	Number of deaths
Lower respiratory infections	3.9 million
HIV/AIDS	2.8 million
Diarrhoeal diseases	1.8 million
Tuberculosis	1.6 million
Malaria	1.2 million
Measles	0.6 million

Source: World Health Report, 2004, World Health Organization (WHO).

area and then subsides, this is described as an **outbreak**. Certain diseases are under constant surveillance in the UK and are called **notifiable diseases**. Physicians are required to report the occurrence of these diseases to the Health Protection Agency (HPA). This ensures tracking and identification of disease occurrence and patterns. The notifiable infectious diseases include anthrax, measles, mumps, rubella, polio, tuberculosis, tetanus, rabies, cholera, diphtheria, tetanus, etc.

The 100 trillion micro-organisms in and on our bodies make up our **normal flora**. Normal flora does not harm us and in some cases helps us by preventing overgrowth of harmful micro-organisms and producing vitamins. Normal flora may become harmful if an opportunity to do so arises. In this case, normal flora becomes opportunistic pathogens or opportunists. Opportunists typically do not cause disease in their usual location in a healthy person but may cause disease in a different location or if the host is weakened or immunocompromised (for example, a patient with an HIV infection or AIDS).

TRANSMISSION OF INFECTIOUS DISEASES

The source of an infectious agent is known as a **reservoir**. Reservoirs include humans, animals, insects, soil and water. For example, humans are the reservoir for the measles virus because it does not infect other organisms. Those who harbour an infectious agent but do not have signs or symptoms are known as carriers. Carriers play an important role in the transmission of pathogens like HIV (Chapter 2). Infectious diseases can be transmitted directly from an infected human to a susceptible human. This route is called **horizontal transmission**. Influenza and gonorrhoea are transmitted this way. Other infectious diseases are transmitted from one generation to the next, as when HIV (Chapter 2), syphilis (Chapter 11), or ophthalmia neonatorum (an eye infection; see Chapter 13) are transmitted to newborns from infected mothers. This route is called **vertical transmission**.

To cause disease, micro-organisms must enter the human host. The respiratory tract is the easiest and most frequently used portal of entry for pathogens. Microbes that use the respiratory tract as their portal of entry include the common cold, influenza and tuberculosis. Microbes also use the gastrointestinal and genitourinary tracts as portals of entry. Punctures, injections, bites and surgery can allow micro-organisms to be deposited directly into the tissues below the skin. This is known as the **parenteral** route, and micro-organisms such as HIV and hepatitis B can use this portal of entry.

Infectious agents may be transmitted from the reservoir to the host through either direct or indirect contact. Direct contact occurs when an individual is infected by contact with the reservoir (for example, by touching an infected person, kissing, engaging in sexual contact, or being bitten by an infected animal or insect). Some diseases that are transmitted primarily by direct contact with the reservoir include AIDS (Chapter 2), ringworm (Chapter 16), influenza, rabies and malaria.

Indirect contact occurs when a pathogen can withstand the environment outside its host for a long period of time before infecting another individual. In airborne transmission, droplets containing infectious agents are small enough to remain airborne for prolonged periods and travel more than 3 feet from the reservoir to the host; tuberculosis and measles can be transmitted by airborne droplets. Inanimate objects or **fomites** that are contaminated by direct contact with the reservoir (e.g. a tissue used to wipe the nose of an individual who has a cold, syringes or utensils) may be the indirect contact for a susceptible individual. Intravenous drug users who share needles can transmit infectious agents like hepatitis and HIV via indirect contact transmission.

Ingesting food and beverages contaminated by contact with a disease reservoir is another example of disease transmission by indirect contact. The faecal–oral route of transmission, in which sewage-contaminated water is used for drinking, washing or preparing foods, is a significant form of indirect transmission, especially for gastrointestinal diseases such as cholera, rotavirus infection and giardiasis. Every year there are 1.8 million diarrhoeal deaths related to unsafe water, sanitation and hygiene worldwide. More than 1 billion people lack access to an improved water source. In the UK, serious outbreaks of foodborne illness that caused the death of over 35 people in the 1980s and 1990s from bovine spongiform encephalopathy (BSE; 'mad cow' disease) and *E. coli* were precursors to the establishment of the Food Standards Agency. Control of infectious diseases can be achieved by preventing transmission. **Isolation** of infected persons in hospitals and self-imposed isolation, such as when a person with influenza remains home in bed, can be effective. **Quarantine** is the separation of persons who may or may not be infected from healthy people until the period of infectious risk is passed. **Disinfection** of potentially infectious materials is necessary to prevent transmission. Medical and dental implements need disinfection to remove human pathogens after use.

SURVEY OF INFECTIOUS AGENTS AND PATHOGENIC MICRO-ORGANISMS

Humans can be infected by a variety of pathogens, ranging from tiny, single-celled bacteria to macroscopic, complex worms (Figure 3.1).

Prions

A **prion**, short for proteinaceous infectious particle, is an infectious agent composed only of protein. Prions cause a number of diseases in animals and

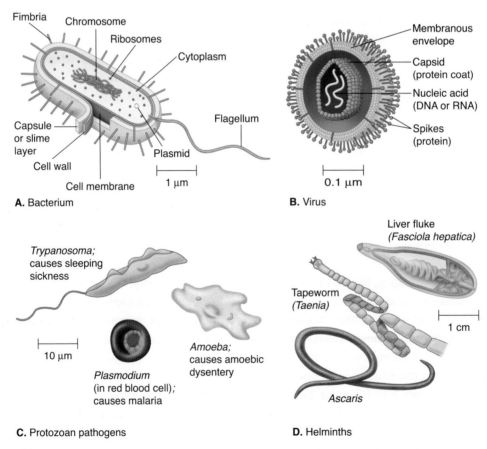

Figure 3.1 Pathogenic micro-organisms include bacteria (A), viruses (B), protozoa (C) and helminths (D).

humans known as spongiform encephalopathies, in which the brain becomes riddled with holes. All known prion diseases affect the structure of the brain or other neural tissue by inducing abnormal folding of normal cellular proteins in the brain, leading to brain damage. Prion diseases usually progress rapidly and are currently untreatable and fatal. Human prion diseases include Creutzfeldt–Jakob disease (CJD), familial Creutzfeldt–Jakob disease (fCJD) and kuru. Although CJD is the most common human prion disease, it is still rare and only occurs in about one in every one million people.

Viruses

Viruses are infectious particles made of a core of genetic material (either RNA or DNA) wrapped in a protein coat (**capsid**). Some viruses also have a lipid membrane surrounding their capsid that plays a role in host cell recognition, and spikes that aid in attachment. Viruses may be classified into several different morphological types, including helical or rod-shaped, polyhedral or many-sided, enveloped or complex. Viruses are not considered living organisms because they do not independently grow, metabolise or reproduce. Viruses must carry out their life processes by entering cells and directing the cells' energy, materials and organelles for these purposes.

Certain viruses infect and grow in only certain types of human cells. Some viruses, like cold viruses, target only cells of the respiratory epithelium. Others, like herpes viruses, reproduce in nervous tissue. Signs and symptoms of infection result from the way these viruses reproduce in cells or from the way the immune system responds to viral infection. Some viruses cause the cells they infect to lyse, or rupture. This is the case when HIV infects and reproduces within T cells. The resultant T cell deficiency leads to the immunodeficiency in AIDS. Other viruses sustain a **latent infection**, whereby the viruses insert themselves in cells and do not reproduce. At this time, no signs and symptoms may be present. Later, a trigger, such as stress, infection with another pathogen or a weakened immune defence, activates the viruses. Signs and symptoms of the disease then manifest themselves as the viruses reproduce. This pattern is seen in the recurrence of herpes infections. Other viruses cause abnormal cell growth because the viral genetic material interferes with the cell's growth control genes. Abnormal growth of tissues is discussed further in Chapter 4. Such growth may be benign, as in a dermal wart (Chapter 16). However, the result may be a malignant growth; that is, a cancer. For example, human papillomavirus infection is linked to cervical cancer (Chapter 11).

Bacteria

Bacteria are microscopic, single-celled organisms. A simple structure (no nucleus or membranous organelles) and small size (1–10 μm) are key characteristics that differentiate bacteria from other single-celled organisms. Although often described as simple, they are far from primitive, for they have adapted to a wide variety of habitats and have evolved complex strategies for infecting and surviving in the human body.

Bacteria have **cell walls**, a rigid layer of organic material surrounding their delicate cell membranes. These walls give bacteria their characteristic shapes. Bacteria may have spherical, round cells called **cocci**, rod-shaped cells called **bacilli**, spiral-shaped cells called **spirilla**, corkscrew-shaped cells called **spirochaetes**, or comma-shaped cells called **vibrios**. The walls protect these cells; should walls be disrupted, cells are susceptible to bursting. This is the action of the antibiotic penicillin. Penicillin interferes with correct cell wall construction of certain types of bacteria. The bacteria cell walls may be thick, thin or absent. The thickness and chemical composition of the cell wall accounts for the way certain cells stain during the **Gram stain** procedure. During the Gram stain, thick-walled cells turn blue–purple and thin-walled cells become red; thus, bacteria can be identified using this technique (Figure 3.2). Identification is critical to obtain an accurate diagnosis and effective treatment of an infection. Other bacteria that do not fit into the above categories of shape and Gram stain properties include the chlamydias and rickettsias, which are intracellular parasites. *Chlamydia trachomatis* causes a sexually transmitted infection (Chapter 11). Rickettsias are transmitted

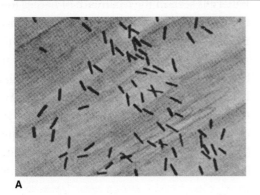 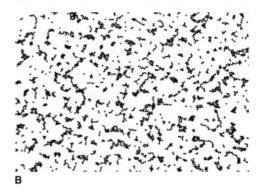

Figure 3.2 Gram-stained bacteria on a microscope slide: (A) Red rod-shaped cells are *Escherichia coli* (Courtesy of the CDC, 1979); and (B) Blue-purple cocci are *Staphylococcus aureus* (Science Photo Library Ltd/Dr Gladden Willis/Visuals Unlimited)

by ticks and cause diseases such as typhus and Rocky Mountain spotted fever.

Many bacteria secrete on their surface a substance called **glycocalyx** or sugar coat. The bacterial glycocalyx is sticky and lies outside the wall. If the glycocalyx is organised and firmly attached to the wall, it is described as a **capsule**. Capsules often protect bacteria from phagocytosis by host cells. If the glycocalyx is unorganised and loosely attached to the wall, it is described as a **slime layer**. Slime layers aid in attachment to surfaces. *Streptococcus mutans*, an important cause of dental decay, attaches itself to the surface of teeth using a slime layer.

Some bacteria, like *E. coli*, have **flagella** that can be used for locomotion. Motility enables bacteria to move toward a favourable environment or away from an adverse environment. Many Gram-negative bacteria contain short, hair-like appendages called **fimbriae** and **pili**. Fimbriae can occur at the ends of bacteria or they can cover the entire surface of the bacteria. Fimbriae enable bacteria to attach to surfaces; *Neisseria gonorrhoea* uses fimbriae to attach to the reproductive tract (Chapter 11). Pili are usually longer than fimbriae, and bacteria have only one or two pili. Pili join bacteria in preparation for the transfer of DNA from one cell to another; because of this they are also called sex pili. Transfer of DNA between bacteria can aid in antibiotic resistance.

Some bacteria produce **endospores**, commonly called spores. The endospore contains the genetic material of the cell packaged in a tough outer coat that is resistant to desiccation, acid, extreme temperature and even radiation. Endospores germinate and form growing cells when conditions are correct. Certain diseases, like tetanus and botulism, can be caused by endospores that contaminate food, water or wounds.

Bacteria cause illness in humans in a variety of ways. A particularly potent toxin called **endotoxin** causes life-threatening shock. This toxin is released into tissues when Gram-negative cells die. Some bacteria produce other types of toxins that interfere with normal physiology. For example, tetanus is caused by the toxin produced by the bacterium *Clostridium tetani*. The tetanus toxin interferes with the ability of muscle cells to relax, resulting in frozen, rigid muscles characteristic of the disease. Other toxins are enzymes that enable the bacteria to spread through tissues and to obtain nutrients.

In addition to the bacterial chromosome, bacteria often contain small circular, double-stranded DNA molecules called **plasmids**. Plasmids contain extra genetic material that replicates independently of the bacterial chromosome. Plasmids may carry genetic information for antibiotic resistance, the production of toxins, tolerance to toxic metals and the synthesis of enzymes.

Bacteria grow rapidly and reproduce by splitting in half, a process known as **binary fission**. Under favourable conditions, this process may take only

30 minutes, which means that a small number of cells may increase to a very large number in a relatively short time. The reproduction of a cell and its genetic material occurs with very few errors or mutations. Still, this rapid growth rate virtually guarantees that mutations will arise, and some of these will favour survival of the bacteria under certain conditions.

Protozoa

Protozoa are single-celled eukaryotic micro-organisms. They are much larger than bacteria and have complex internal structures, including a nucleus and membranous organelles. Protozoa are found in nearly every habitat, and most do not cause disease; however, they may invade and destroy certain tissues, or they may provoke damaging inflammatory responses. Protozoa are classified as **amoeboids**, **flagellates**, **ciliates** and **sporozoans**.

Amoeboids move by means of cell membrane extensions called **pseudopodia**. An amoeba of great health concern is *Entamoeba histolytica*, the cause of amoebic dysentery (Chapter 9), an intestinal infection acquired from faeces-contaminated food or water. The flagellates swim by using one or more whip-like appendages called flagella. Pathogens in this group include *Trichomonas vaginalis*, the cause of trichomoniasis, a sexually transmitted infection (Chapter 11), and *Giardia*, the cause of giardiasis, an intestinal infection. Ciliates move by means of numerous short, hair-like projections called **cilia**. There are few pathogens among the ciliates.

Sporozoans are not mobile. *Plasmodium* is the most notorious among them because it causes malaria. Every year, more than 500 million people worldwide become severely ill with malaria and more than 1 million people die as a result. Malaria kills mostly infants, young children and pregnant women, largely in Africa. *Plasmodium* is transmitted via the bites of infected mosquitoes.

Fungi

Fungi are single-celled or multicelled organisms with cell walls that contain a special polysaccharide called **chitin**. Fungi use specialised filaments called **mycelia** to absorb nutrients from their surroundings. They also have reproductive structures bearing **spores**, which are known allergens.

Fungal infections are known as **mycoses**. Healthy human tissue is relatively resistant to fungal infections but may be susceptible under certain circumstances. Fungi can more easily infect damaged tissue than intact healthy tissue. Also, immunocompromised hosts may be unable to resist fungal infections. Fungi cause disease by producing toxins, interfering with normal organ structure or function, or inducing inflammation or allergy. Some common fungal diseases include candidiasis, an infection of skin or mucous membranes caused by the yeast *Candida* (Chapter 16); *Pneumocystis*, an opportunistic pathogen and one of the diagnostic indicator diseases for AIDS (Chapter 2); and a variety of ringworm infections of the skin, hair and nails (Chapter 16).

Helminths

Helminths are parasitic worms. Like other animals, helminths are complex multicellular motile organisms. They often have well developed reproductive systems capable of producing large numbers of offspring. Many helminths have also evolved complex life cycles and strategies for infecting new hosts. Infections with these organisms are often called **infestations**.

Ascaris infects an estimated 1.4 billion people (Figure 3.3). Ascariasis is found worldwide, but the largest numbers of cases occur in tropical and sub-tropical regions. The eggs of the worm are found in soil contaminated by human faeces or in uncooked food contaminated by soil. A person becomes infected by ingesting the eggs. The eggs hatch into larvae in the small intestine and mature into adult worms. The female adult worm lays eggs that are then passed into faeces. Infections are usually asymptomatic. Stool samples are used for diagnosis, and drugs are available for treatment. Prevention includes the use of toilet facilities, hand washing, safe stool disposal, protection of food from dirt and soil, and thorough washing of produce.

Hookworms like *Necator americanus* are a leading cause of anaemia and protein malnutrition, afflicting

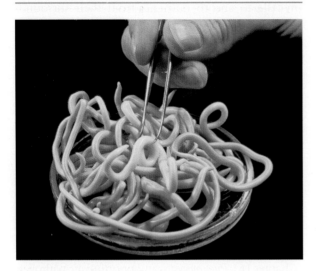

Figure 3.3 *Ascaris.*
(Sinclair Stammers/Science Photo Library/Photo Researchers, Inc.)

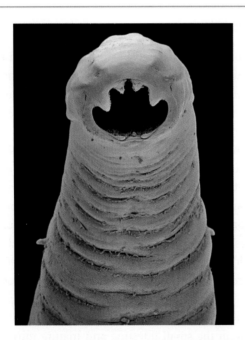

Figure 3.4 *Necator americanus.* The cutting plates around the mouth are used to tear open blood vessels of the host.
(© David Scharf/Peter Arnold, Inc.)

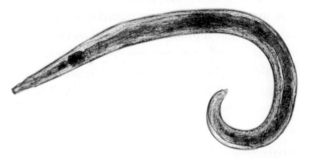

Figure 3.5 Adult *Enterobius vermicularis.*
(Science Photo Library Ltd/Science Vu/Visuals Unlimited)

an estimated 740 million people in the developing nations of the tropics (Figure 3.4). The largest numbers of cases occur in sub-Saharan Africa, Latin America, South East Asia and China. Larvae of the hookworm penetrate the skin of the foot, hand, arm or leg. The larvae travel to the small intestine and mature into adult worms. Females lay several thousand eggs per day. The eggs are shed in faeces and hatch out into larvae in water. There are no specific symptoms or signs of hookworm infection. Stool samples are used for diagnosis, and drugs are available for treatment. Prevention includes not walking barefoot, using toilet facilities, and not using human excrement or raw sewage as fertilizer in agriculture.

Enterobius vermicularis infects an estimated 200 million people worldwide and is probably the most widespread infection in the UK (Figure 3.5). The female pinworm migrates to the anus to deposit her eggs on the skin around the anus. She then secretes a substance that causes a very strong itching sensation, inciting the host to scratch the area and thus transfer some of the eggs to the fingers. Eggs can also be transferred to cloth, toys and the bath, and can survive from 2 to 3 weeks outside the human body. Humans ingest the eggs, which hatch into larvae in the small intestine. The larvae then migrate to the large intestine and mate. Enterobiasis infections are diagnosed by the Graham sticky-tape method. A piece of transparent tape is placed on the skin around the anus so it can pick up eggs that were laid earlier. The tape is microscopically examined for the presence of eggs. Treatment includes drugs and thorough washing of clothing and linens to kill eggs. Prevention includes practising proper personal hygiene, frequent changing and washing of linens and clothing, keeping nails trimmed, and not scratching the bare anal area.

NOSOCOMIAL INFECTIONS

Nosocomial or hospital-acquired infections are infections acquired in a healthcare facility. About 1 in 10 inpatients in the UK acquire a nosocomial infection; the incidence is highest in surgical wards and intensive care units, and lowest in medical units. Lower respiratory tract and urinary tract represent 23% each, surgical wound 11%, skin 10%, bacteraemia 6%, gastrointestinal 5%, intravascular device 4%, other and unknown 13% and 5%, respectively. Rates of nosocomial infections are markedly higher in developing countries owing to lack of supervision, poor infection practices, inappropriate use of limited resources and overcrowding of hospitals. The micro-organisms that cause nosocomial infections can come from the patient's normal flora, contact with healthcare staff, contaminated instruments or needles, and the healthcare environment. Because hospital stays are short, patients are often discharged before the infection becomes apparent. As a consequence, it is often difficult to determine the source of the infection.

Healthcare facilities are a major reservoir for a variety of opportunistic pathogens that can cause nosocomial infections. A weakened patient is an ideal target for an opportunistic pathogen. The weakened patient's resistance to infection can be reduced as a result of disease, compromised non-specific defences and a suppressed immune system. Burns, surgical wounds, injections, invasive diagnostic procedures, ventilators, intravenous therapy and catheters increase the risk of infection. The principal routes of transmission of nosocomial infections are direct contact transmission from healthcare staff to patient and indirect contact transmission through fomites and the hospital's ventilation system.

According to the Health Protection Agency (HPA), hand washing is one of the most important ways of controlling the spread of nosocomial infections. Education of healthcare facility staff and visitors about basic infection control measures, isolation of patients, sterilisation of equipment, use of disposable materials and prescription of antibiotics only when necessary can help to control nosocomial infections.

Occupational exposure to blood

Data collected through the HPA Centre for Infections scheme (Eye of the needle) indicate that workers in the healthcare industry and related occupations are at risk of occupational exposure to bloodborne pathogens, including human immunodeficiency virus (HIV), hepatitis B virus (HBV) and hepatitis C virus (HCV). In its report Eye of the needle: 2008, 914 incidents were reported to the scheme between 2006 and 2007.

The rate of HBV transmission to susceptible healthcare workers ranges from 6% to 30% after a single needlestick exposure to an HBV-infected patient. However, such exposures are a risk only for

 Prevention PLUS!

Advice for travellers

Travelling out of the country? Have you considered how you will protect yourself and your family from infectious diseases? In a different country, you will be faced with different infectious diseases to which you are unlikely to be immune. Will you need vaccinations or prophylactic medications? The Department of health (DH) and HPA can provide advice to travellers.

Prevention PLUS!

Hand washing

According to the HPA, hand washing is the single most important means of preventing the spread of infection. The HPA provides the following instructions for correct hand washing:

- Wet hands first
- Apply soap and cover all surfaces
- Rinse with water
- Dry hands thoroughly with disposable paper towel
- Use the paper towel to turn off the tap.

healthcare workers who are not immune to HBV; healthcare workers who have antibodies to HBV either from pre-exposure vaccination or prior infection are not at risk. In addition, if a susceptible worker is exposed to HBV, post-exposure prophylaxis with hepatitis B immune globulin and initiation of hepatitis B vaccine is more than 90% effective in preventing HBV infection. The average risk for infection after a needlestick or cut exposure to HCV-infected blood is approximately 1.8%. There is no vaccine against HCV, and there is no post-exposure prophylaxis treatment available that reduces transmission. The average risk of HIV infection after needlestick exposure or cut exposure to HIV-infected blood is 0.3%. There is no vaccine against HIV; however, the use of antiretroviral drugs after occupational exposures may reduce the chance of HIV transmission.

TREATMENT OF INFECTIOUS DISEASE

The effective treatment of an infectious disease depends on the type of causative pathogen. Bacterial infections can be treated with a variety of **antibiotics**. Penicillin and related drugs act on the cell wall, and they are especially useful in controlling Gram-positive bacteria. Some antibiotics target the bacterial cell membrane, causing lysis. Other antibiotics target the protein synthesis machinery of the cell; this is effective because the ribosomes and enzymes involved in bacterial protein synthesis are sufficiently different from those in human cells. Other antibiotics interfere with bacterial metabolism or with DNA and RNA synthesis. Antibiotic resistance plays an important role in the increased incidence of bacterial infections.

Correct use of antibiotics can prevent the development of **antibiotic resistance**. Some staphylococcus species, streptococcus species and enterococcus species, among others, have developed resistance to several antibiotics. Resistance arises when bacteria adapt to antibiotics and the adaptation becomes common in the bacterial population, soon rendering the antibiotics ineffective. An antibiotic should be used only for bacterial infections. A number of infections, including influenza and the common cold, are viral and are not treatable with antibiotics. Some viral ailments closely mimic bacterial infections. For example, it turns out that group A streptococci cause only 15% of pharyngitis cases, so only a small proportion of sore throats are really 'strep' throat. Most sore throats are really caused by viral infections, some of which closely mimic strep throat because the signs and symptoms include swelling and exudate. If antibiotics are used for many of these viral infections, bacterial populations will more likely evolve resistance to those antibiotics. In the UK, there are national and regional guidelines that have evolved to help GPs identify and treat patients who are likely to have group A streptococcus, and these are promoted for use by the National Health Service (NHS) and HPA. Physicians need to take a throat swab and perform a rapid strep antigen test to confirm the presence of group A streptococci before prescribing antibiotics. If prescribed, the appropriate antibiotic must be selected. Patients need to follow through on the prescription and use the antibiotics for the entire time prescribed, should not end treatment early, and should not save antibiotics for use in subsequent illnesses.

Viruses do not have the cell walls and cell membranes of bacteria, nor do they have metabolic or protein synthesis machinery. Viruses are not susceptible to antibiotics. Viruses need human cells to reproduce and decode their genetic material. Some antiviral drugs interfere with this process by acting as **nucleic acid analogues**, substances that mimic the correct DNA or RNA bases. These analogues are used to manufacture the viral genetic material but, in fact, do not function as the normal DNA or RNA bases. Viruses are not replicated correctly and are eventually reduced in number or eliminated. Other antiviral drugs interfere with the assembly of new virus particles inside cells or interfere with the attachment of viruses to host cells and thus prevent infection before disease begins.

Antifungal drugs target fungal walls and membranes but can affect human cells as well, leading to serious toxic side effects. Topical agents are effective for skin infections, such as infections of nails or ringworm, and pose fewer adverse effects. A systemic infection, however, requires systemic treatment, which entails the risk of serious side effects. Systemic treatment requires careful dosing and monitoring for side effects.

Protozoa are treated with drugs that interfere with protein synthesis and metabolism. Certain antibiotics may be used to treat protozoal infections. Helminths are susceptible to drugs that paralyse their muscles or interfere with their carbohydrate metabolism.

Although effective treatments have been discovered and used for many important infections, certain problems remain. One complication is that resistant micro-organisms can evolve, rendering existing treatments useless. Another difficulty is that some treatments are accompanied by unacceptable toxic side effects or allergies. For these reasons,

preventive measures are the best choice for long-term control of certain diseases.

EMERGING AND RE-EMERGING INFECTIOUS DISEASES

In 1963, the respected physician and anthropologist T. Aidan Cockburn said, 'We can look forward with confidence to a considerable degree of freedom from infectious diseases at a time not too far in the future. Indeed . . . it seems reasonable to anticipate that within some measurable time . . . all the major infections will have disappeared.' Infectious diseases are not only spreading faster, they appear to be emerging more quickly than ever before. Since the 1970s, newly emerging diseases have been identified at the unprecedented rate of one or more per year.

Emerging infectious diseases include outbreaks of previously unknown diseases or known diseases whose incidence in humans has significantly increased in the past two decades. Table 3.2 lists emerging infectious diseases. **Re-emerging infectious diseases** are known diseases that have reappeared after a significant decline in incidence. Table 3.3 lists re-emerging infectious diseases. Human demographics and behaviour, technology and industry, economic development and land use, international travel and commerce, microbial adaptation and change, breakdown of public health measures, and climate change can play a role in emergence or re-emergence of infectious diseases.

Human behaviour (failing to vaccinate, for example) can play a role in the re-emergence of infectious diseases. Worldwide, more than 20 million people are affected each year by measles. In 2005, it was estimated that there were 345 000 measles deaths globally; the primary reason for continuing high childhood measles morbidity and mortality is the failure to deliver at least one dose of measles vaccine to all infants. In countries that are able to keep vaccination coverage high, around 95%, measles is very rare. Immunisation controls most infectious diseases in the UK. However, whilst the vaccinations aren't compulsory in the UK, a number

Table 3.2 Examples of pathogenic microbes identified since 1973.

Microbe	Type	Disease
Rotavirus	Virus	Infantile diarrhoea
Ebola virus	Virus	Acute haemorrhagic fever
Legionella pneumophila	Bacterium	Legionnaires' disease
Human T-lymphotrophic virus I	Virus	T cell lymphoma/leukaemia
Toxin-producing *Staphylococcus aureus*	Bacterium	Toxic shock syndrome
Escherichia coli O157:H7	Bacterium	Haemorrhagic colitis; haemolytic uraemic syndrome
Borrelia burgdorferi	Bacterium	Lyme disease
Human immunodeficiency virus	Virus	Acquired immunodeficiency syndrome
Helicobacter pylori	Bacterium	Peptic ulcer disease
Hepatitis C	Virus	Hepatitis
Vibrio cholerae O139	Bacterium	Cholera
Hantavirus	Virus	Respiratory distress syndrome
Cryptosporidium	Protozoa	Enteric disease
nvCJD	Prion	New variant Creutzfeldt–Jakob disease
HVN1	Virus	Influenza
Nipah	Virus	Severe encephalitis
SARS coronavirus	Virus	Severe acute respiratory syndrome

of parents avoid vaccinating their children on the grounds of religion and philosophy. Unimmunised children are usually the cause of outbreaks and this seems to be particularly the case for measles.

Climate changes can alter the breeding ranges of arthropod vectors like mosquitoes and flies. Malaria, Dengue fever and yellow fever, all mosquito-borne infections, show sensitivity to climate. Even in areas where malaria is endemic, it occurs with less frequency in higher and cooler elevations.

Lyme disease, which is caused by a bacterium carried by ticks, is not a common infection but recently started to occur more regularly in the UK. As urban centres grow, human and deer populations inevitably come in contact with more frequency, giving the Lyme disease ticks ample opportunity to attach to humans and their pets. In addition, people

Table 3.3 Re-emerging pathogens.

Microbe	Type	Disease
Paramyxovirus	Virus	Mumps
Prion	Prion	Prion disease
Streptococcus, group A	Bacterium	Strep throat, impetigo
Staphylococcus aureus	Bacterium	Pneumonia, meningitis
Clostridium difficile	Bacterium	Colitis
Enterovirus 71	Virus	Hand, foot, mouth disease
Coccidioides immitis	Fungus	Valley fever
Mycobacterium tuberculosis	Bacterium	Tuberculosis
Vibrio cholerae	Bacterium	Cholera
Plasmodium	Protozoa	Malaria
Dengue virus	Virus	Dengue haemorrhagic fever

who walk in the countryside, mainly on wild areas with grasses and vegetation, are more at risk.

Emerging antimicrobial resistance demonstrates the potential of microbial adaptation. XDR-TB is the abbreviation for extensively drug-resistant tuberculosis (TB). One in three people in the world is infected with dormant TB bacteria; only when the bacteria become active do people become ill with TB. Bacteria become active as a result of anything that can reduce the person's immunity, such as HIV, advancing age or some medical conditions. TB can usually be treated with a course of four standard, or first-line, anti-TB drugs. If these drugs are misused or mismanaged, multidrug-resistant TB (MDR-TB) can develop. MDR-TB takes longer to treat with second-line drugs, which are more expensive and have more side effects. XDR-TB can develop when these second-line drugs are also misused or mismanaged and therefore also become ineffective. Because XDR-TB is resistant to first- and second-line drugs, treatment options are seriously limited. It is therefore vital that TB control is managed properly. Multidrug-resistant strains of *Enterococcus, Staphylococcus, Streptococcus*, HIV and *Plasmodium* are growing global threats.

International travel aids in the emergence of infectious disease. Severe acute respiratory syndrome (SARS) is a viral respiratory illness caused by a coronavirus, called SARS-associated coronavirus (SARS-CoV), first reported in Asia in February 2003. Over the next few months, the illness spread to more than two dozen countries in North America, South America, Europe and Asia before the SARS global outbreak of 2003 was contained.

COMMON CHILDHOOD VACCINE-PREVENTABLE INFECTIOUS DISEASES

Vaccine-preventable childhood infectious disease levels are rare in the UK. However, owing to reduced levels of MMR (measles, mumps and rubella) vaccine coverage, there were over 1300 confirmed cases of measles across England and Wales during 2008. The global picture is very different. Every year 1.4 million

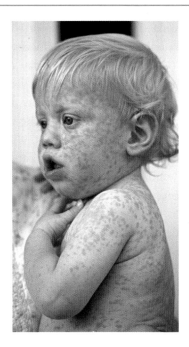

Figure 3.6 Measles rash.
(© Lowell Georgia/Science Source/Photo Researchers, Inc.)

children worldwide die from vaccine-preventable diseases before they reach the age of 5.

Measles is a highly contagious disease caused by the rubeola virus. The rubeola virus is spread by respiratory droplets or airborne transmission. Early signs and symptoms include fever, cough, runny nose and fatigue, followed by a rash that usually begins on the head and spreads to cover the body (Figure 3.6). Greyish spots, called Koplik spots, often develop inside the mouth before the rash appears. Diagnosis is based on history of exposure, Koplik spots and rash. There is no cure for measles, and it usually runs its course in 7–10 days. Treatment is supportive and may include pain relievers and fever reducers.

Mumps is caused by the paramyxovirus and is spread by direct contact with respiratory secretions or saliva or through fomites. Cases of mumps may start with a fever of up to 39°C as well as a headache and loss of appetite. The well-known hallmark of mumps is swelling and pain in the parotid glands, the largest of the salivary glands. Mumps in adolescent and adult males may also result in the development of orchitis, an inflammation of the testicles.

Diagnosis is based on history of exposure and signs and symptoms. Treatment is supportive and may include pain relievers and fever reducers.

Rubella (German measles or 3-day measles) is caused by the rubella virus. The rubella virus is highly contagious and is spread by respiratory droplets, by airborne transmission and can also be transmitted from pregnant women to their fetus. When rubella occurs in a pregnant woman, it may cause congenital rubella syndrome, with potentially devastating consequences for the developing fetus. Many people with rubella have few or no signs or symptoms. Some rubella patients develop a rash that appears as either pink or light red spots, which may merge to form evenly coloured patches. Other signs and symptoms of rubella, which are more common in teens and adults, may include headache, loss of appetite, mild conjunctivitis (inflammation of the lining of the eyelids and eyeballs), a stuffy or runny nose, swollen lymph nodes in other parts of the body, and pain and swelling in the joints (especially in young women). Diagnosis is based on history of exposure, signs and symptoms, and throat culture for the rubella virus. Treatment is supportive and may include pain relievers and fever reducers.

Whooping cough is a highly contagious bacterial infection caused by *Bordetella pertussis*. The bacteria are spread by direct contact with respiratory droplets. The first signs and symptoms of whooping cough include runny nose, sneezing, mild cough and low-grade fever. After 1–2 weeks, the cough develops into coughing spells that end with a whooping sound when the patient breathes in. Diagnosis is based on signs and symptoms and bacterial cultures of the nose and throat. Antibiotics are used for treatment. Pertussis is part of the diphtheria, tetanus, pertussis vaccine.

Diphtheria is a highly contagious bacterial disease caused by *Corynebacterium diphtheriae*, which is primarily spread by respiratory droplets; transmission by fomites is rare. Early signs and symptoms include low-grade fever and a sore throat. The bacteria produce a toxin that can cause a thick coating in the nose, throat or airway that may hinder breathing and swallowing. In the bloodstream the toxin can cause damage to the heart, kidneys and nervous system. Up to 50% of patients who do not get treatment die.

Diagnosis is based on a throat culture. Treatment includes antibiotics and antitoxin. Diphtheria is part of the diphtheria, tetanus, pertussis vaccine.

Tetanus is a bacterial infection caused by *Clostridium tetani*. The bacterium is found in contaminated soil and animal excrement and enters the body via wounds. Once the bacteria are in the body, they produce a toxin that affects the nervous system, causing stiff neck, lockjaw, muscle spasms and difficulty swallowing. Diagnosis is based on history of exposure, signs and symptoms. Treatment includes antibiotics and injection of tetanus immunoglobulin to neutralise the tetanus toxin. Tetanus is part of the diphtheria, tetanus, pertussis vaccine.

Chickenpox is a highly contagious viral infection caused by the varicella zoster virus. There are an estimated 60 million cases worldwide each year. The virus is spread by direct contact, droplet transmission and airborne transmission. Symptoms begin with a runny or stuffy nose, sneezing, fever and a cough. A few days later an itchy rash appears, usually on the chest and face (Figure 3.7). At first,

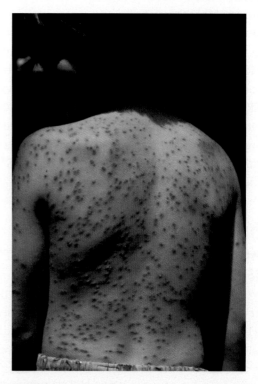

Figure 3.7 Chickenpox rash.
(Science Photo Library Ltd/Gilbert S. Grant)

the rash looks like pinkish dots that quickly develop a small blister on top. After about 24–48 hours, the fluid in the blisters gets cloudy and the blisters begin to crust over. Chickenpox blisters show up in waves, so after some begin to crust over, a new group of spots may appear. A person is contagious from up to 48 hours before the initial rash occurs until all blisters have burst and crusted over. Diagnosis is based on history of exposure and the rash. Treatment is supportive and can include treatments to control scratching (calamine lotion and antihistamines), pain relievers and fever reducers. Dehydration can be avoided by ensuring a good fluid intake. A vaccine is available for varicella zoster.

Haemophilus influenzae type b (Hib) is a bacterium that causes diseases including meningitis and pneumonia. There are an estimated 3 million cases and nearly 400 000 deaths worldwide each year. The bacterium lives in the human respiratory tract and can be recovered from the nasal and throat passages of up to 90% of all healthy individuals. Hib disease is spread by respiratory droplets, and signs and symptoms include cough, fever, chills, lack of appetite, extreme sleepiness, severe headache and stiff neck or back. More serious signs are mental confusion, convulsions, shock and coma. Diagnosis is based on signs and symptoms, lumbar puncture and bacterial culture. Antibiotics are used for treatment, and there is a vaccine available for Hib.

Poliomyelitis is caused by the polio virus. Transmission of the virus occurs either by direct person-to-person contact or by indirect contact with infectious saliva or faeces or with contaminated sewage or water. Polio is asymptomatic in approximately 95% of cases. In the cases in which there are symptoms, the illness appears in two forms: non-paralytic polio and paralytic polio. Patients with non-paralytic polio do not develop paralysis. Signs and symptoms can include sore throat, fever, nausea, vomiting and constipation. Non-paralytic

aseptic meningitis is another type of non-paralytic polio. In addition to the flu-like signs and symptoms just mentioned, it causes stiffness of neck, back or legs. Paralytic polio occurs in 0.1–2.0% of polio cases. Paralytic polio usually begins with fever; other symptoms, including headache, neck and back stiffness and constipation, generally appear a few days later. Acute flaccid paralysis, which causes the limbs to appear loose and floppy, often comes on suddenly and usually affects only one side; if both sides are affected, typically one side is worse than the other. Diagnosis is based on history of exposure, signs and symptoms, isolation of the virus from the throat or faeces, and lumbar puncture if the nervous system is involved. Treatment is supportive and may include pain relief. A vaccine is available for polio.

Streptococcus pneumoniae is a bacterium that causes diseases including meningitis and upper and lower respiratory disease. Worldwide each year *S. pneumoniae* is estimated to kill approximately 1 million children under the age of 5 years. *S. pneumoniae* is present in the upper respiratory tract of about half the population and is transmitted by respiratory droplets. Signs and symptoms may include fever, chills, headache, ear pain, cough, chest pain, disorientation, shortness of breath and occasionally stiff neck. Diagnosis is based on bacterial culture of body fluids. Antibiotics are used for treatment, although antibiotic resistance is a problem. There is a vaccine available for *S. pneumoniae*.

Resources

Occupational Safety and Health Administration (OSHA): *www.osha.org*

World Health Organization: *www.who.org*

Health Protection Agency Homepage (HPA): *http://www.hpa.org.uk/*

Department of Health (DH): *http://www.dh.gov.uk/en/index.htm*

DISEASES AT A GLANCE Pathogens

PATHOGEN	DISEASE	SIGNS AND SYMPTOMS	DIAGNOSIS	TREATMENT	PREVENTION
Ascaris	Ascariasis	Asymptomatic	Stool sample	Medication to paralyse helminth muscles or interfere with their carbohydrate metabolism	Use of toilet facilities, hand washing, safe stool disposal, protection of food from dirt and soil, thorough washing of produce
Necator americanus	Anaemia and protein malnutrition	Asymptomatic	Stool sample	Medication to paralyse helminth muscles or interfere with their carbohydrate metabolism	Not walking barefoot, use of toilet facilities, not using human excrement or raw sewage as fertiliser in agriculture
Enterobius vermicularis	Enterobiasis	Itching	Graham sticky-tape method	Medication to paralyse helminth muscles or interfere with their carbohydrate metabolism	Personal hygiene, frequent changing and washing of linens and clothing, keeping nails trimmed, not scratching the bare anal area
Rubeola virus	Measles	Fever, cough, runny nose, fatigue, Koplik spots, rash	History of exposure, Koplik spots, rash	Supportive pain relievers, fever reducers	Vaccine
Paramyxovirus	Mumps	Fever, headache, loss of appetite, swelling and pain in parotid glands	History of exposure, signs and symptoms	Supportive pain relievers, fever reducers	Vaccine
Rubella virus	Rubella or German measles	May be asymptomatic; rash; other symptoms in teens and adults may include headache, loss of appetite, mild conjunctivitis, a stuffy or runny nose, swollen lymph nodes in other parts of the body, and pain and swelling in the joints	History of exposure, signs and symptoms, throat culture	Supportive pain relievers, fever reducers	Vaccine
Bordetella pertussis	Whooping cough	Runny nose, sneezing, low-grade fever, coughing spells with whooping sound when breathing in	Signs and symptoms, bacterial culture of nose and throat	Antibiotics	Vaccine
Corynebacterium diphtheriae	Diphtheria	Low-grade fever, sore throat, coating in the nose, throat or airway	Throat culture	Antibiotics and antitoxin	Vaccine
Clostridium tetani	Tetanus	Stiff neck, lockjaw, muscle spasms and difficulty swallowing	History of exposure, signs and symptoms	Antibiotics and tetanus immunoglobulin	Vaccine
Varicella zoster virus	Chickenpox	Stuffy nose, sneezing, fever, cough, rash	History of exposure, rash	Supportive to control itching, pain relievers, fever reducers	Vaccine

DISEASES AT A GLANCE Pathogens (continued)

PATHOGEN	DISEASE	SIGNS AND SYMPTOMS	DIAGNOSIS	TREATMENT	PREVENTION
Haemophilus influenzae type b	Meningitis and pneumonia	Cough, fever, chills, lack of appetite, extreme sleepiness, severe headache, and stiff neck or back. More serious signs are mental confusion, convulsions, shock and coma	Signs and symptoms, lumbar puncture, bacterial culture	Antibiotics	Vaccine
Polio virus	Poliomyelitis	Non-paralytic polio: sore throat, fever, nausea, vomiting and constipation. Non-paralytic aseptic meningitis: sore throat, fever, nausea, vomiting and constipation, stiffness of neck, back or legs. Paralytic polio: fever, headache, neck and back stiffness, constipation, acute flaccid paralysis	History of exposure, signs and symptoms, isolation of the virus from the throat or faeces, and lumbar puncture if the nervous system is involved	Supportive pain relief	Vaccine
Streptococcus pneumoniae	Meningitis and lower respiratory diseases	Fever, chills, headache, ear pain, cough, chest pain, disorientation, shortness of breath and, occasionally, stiff neck	Culture of body fluids	Antibiotics	Vaccine

INTERACTIVE EXERCISES

Cases for critical thinking

1. Based upon what you learned about transmission and control of infectious diseases, compare how one would approach the control of influenza with the control of malaria. Explain which methods would be useful for each disease.

2. Explain why antibiotics are ineffective against viral infections. What problems can arise when viral infections are treated with antibiotics?

3. Explain why vaccination is a particularly effective method for controlling infectious disease.

4. About a week or two ago, Joe, a 3-year-old boy, had a runny nose, a mild cough and a low fever. Joe is now having coughing spells and he is having a difficult time inhaling during these coughing spells. What is your diagnosis? How is this transmitted? What treatment is available? Is a vaccine available?

5. Mason, a 5-year-old boy, had a runny nose, fever and cough after attending a birthday party. A few days later a rash appeared on his chest and face. The rash began as pinkish dots but quickly developed a small blister on top. The blisters are appearing in waves. What is your diagnosis? How is this transmitted? What treatment is available? Is a vaccine available?

6. Marion, a 3-year-old girl, has a thick coating in her throat that hinders her breathing and swallowing. What is your diagnosis? How can this diagnosis be confirmed? What treatment is available?

Multiple choice

1. A glycocalyx that is organised and firmly attached to the wall is a _____
   a. flagella   b. pili
   c. capsule   d. slime layer

2. These contain the genetic material of a bacteria packaged in a tough outer coat.
   a. pili   b. toxins
   c. endospores   d. fimbriae

3. Small, circular DNA molecules that some bacteria have in addition to the bacterial chromosome are called _____
   a. pili   b. endospore
   c. plasmid   d. glycocalyx

4. Bacteria reproduce by _____
   a. mitosis
   b. meiosis
   c. binary fission
   d. none of the above

5. Single-celled eukaryotic organisms are called _____
   a. bacteria   b. helminths
   c. viruses   d. protozoa

6. German measles is caused by _____
   a. *Bordetella pertussis*
   b. rubeola virus
   c. rubella virus
   d. varicella zoster virus

7. Whooping cough is caused by _____
   a. *Bordetella pertussis*
   b. rubeola virus
   c. rubella virus
   d. varicella zoster virus

8. The protein coat of a virus is its _____
   a. nucleus   b. capsid
   c. core   d. mycelia

9. The most common worm infection in the UK is _____
   a. *Enterobius vermicularis*
   b. Lymphatic filariasis
   c. Ascariasis
   d. Shistosomiasis

10. Which of the following is not an example of contact transmission?
    a. kissing   b. touching
    c. sexual contact   d. a needlestick

True or false

_____ 1. Infectious diseases are not a major cause of death and disability in the world today.

_____ 2. Rabies is a communicable disease.

_____ 3. Antibiotics are effective against viruses.

_____ 4. The respiratory system is the most frequently used portal of entry.

_____ 5. Ascariasis is the most common type of roundworm infection in humans.

_____ 6. More than 90% of deaths from infectious diseases worldwide are caused by a few diseases.

_____ 7. Prions are composed of protein and nucleic acid.

_____ 8. Hand washing is the single most important means of preventing the spread of nosocomial infections.

_____ 9. Antibiotics are effective treatments for helminth infestations.

_____ 10. Chickenpox is transmitted by the parenteral route.

Fill-ins

1. Micro-organisms in and on our bodies make up our _____.

2. _____ diseases are known diseases that have reappeared after a significant decline in incidence.

3. Measles is caused by the _____ virus.

4. _____ infections are acquired in a hospital.

5. In _____ transmission, infectious diseases can be transmitted directly from an infected human to a susceptible human.

6. The bacterial _____ is sticky and lies outside the cell wall.

7. _____ are short, hair-like appendages that enable bacteria to attach to surfaces.

8. _____ are infectious agents composed only of protein.

9. Mumps is caused by the _____.

10. Chickenpox is caused by the _____ virus.

Labelling exercise

Fill in the blanks below to label the protozoan pathogens and helminths pictured.

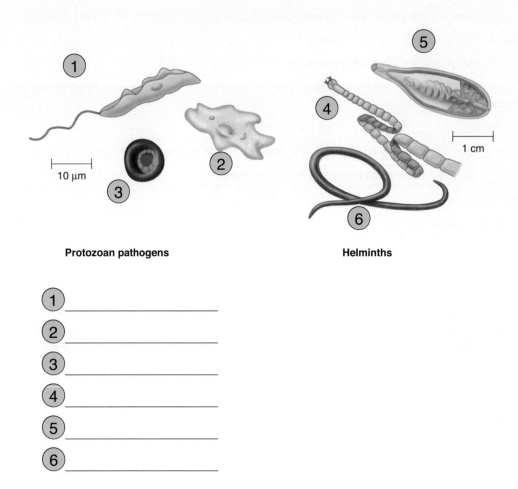

Protozoan pathogens   **Helminths**

1 _____

2 _____

3 _____

4 _____

5 _____

6 _____

4 CANCER

Histopathology of papillary carcinoma, thyroid.
(Courtesy of the CDC/Dr Edwin P. Ewing Jr, 1973)

Fact or fiction ?

From a public health perspective, there is an overwhelming case to justify the development of a human papillomavirus (HPV) vaccine.

Fact: At least 50% of sexually active adults have had a genital HPV infection. Low-risk HPV infections cause benign lesions or genital warts, whereas high-risk HPV infection is the main cause of cervical cancer.

Learning objectives

After studying this chapter, you should be able to:

+ Describe cancer classification
+ Explain the biology of human cancer and the role of oncogenes, tumour suppressor genes and DNA repair genes
+ Identify the aetiologies of cancer
+ Describe the epidemiology, symptoms, aetiology, diagnosis and treatment of the most common cancers
+ Demonstrate understanding of the value of cancer prevention, early detection and screening in reducing cancer
+ Develop an understanding of cancer staging

Disease chronicle

Roy Castle: lung cancer

Roy Castle was a dancer, singer, comedian, actor, television presenter and musician. In January 1992 he was diagnosed with lung cancer, undergoing chemotherapy and radiotherapy before going into remission in autumn 1992. He was a non-smoker and attributed his illness to years of playing the trumpet in smoky jazz clubs. His illness returned a year later and he underwent further treatment. He carried out the high profile 'Tour of Hope' to raise funds for the erection of the building that would become the Roy Castle Lung Cancer Foundation (www.roycastle.org); this is the only British charity entirely dedicated to defeating lung cancer. He died on 2 September 1994, two days after his 62nd birthday. His widow worked with the charity for many years after her husband's death, and was a key figure in campaigning for the British smoking ban which came into effect during 2007 and has seen smoking banned in virtually all enclosed public places.

INTRODUCTION

Cancer or **malignancy** is not a single disease. Over 100 different types and subtypes of human cancer affect the young and old and involve nearly every tissue or organ in the body. Cancer has a profound emotional and physical impact for the patient and is associated with significant **morbidity** or complications and possible **mortality** or death.

Cancer is the leading cause of death worldwide and afflicts two of every three families. Of a total of 58 million deaths worldwide in 2005, cancer claimed the lives of 7.6 million people. The main types of cancer leading to overall cancer mortality include:

- Lung (1.3 million deaths/year)
- Stomach (almost 1 million deaths/year)
- Liver (662 000 deaths/year)
- Colon (665 000 deaths/year)
- Breast (502 000 deaths/year).

Deaths from cancer worldwide are projected to continue to rise, with an estimated 9 million deaths projected in 2015 and 11.4 million deaths in 2030, according to the World Health Organization.

In the UK, cancer is responsible for 126 000 deaths per year and one in four people die from cancer. The most common cancers in the UK are:

- Breast cancer
- Prostate cancer
- Lung cancer
- Cancer of the colon or rectum
- Bladder cancer
- Cancer of the uterus.

CLASSIFICATION OF CANCER

Other terms used to describe cancer are **tumours** and **neoplasms**. A **tumour** fundamentally means swelling, and **neoplasia** refers to new growth. A tumour or neoplasm can be either **benign** or **malignant**. A benign neoplasm is non-cancerous and is usually localised to a tissue or organ. Malignant neoplasms, or cancer, consist of rapidly dividing cells that accumulate uncontrollably, invade normal

Table 4.1 Classification of tumours.

T (Tumour)

Tx	Tumour cannot be adequately assessed
T0	No evidence of primary tumour
Tis	Carcinoma in situ
T1-4	Size and/or extent of primary tumour

N (nodes)

Nx	Regional lymph nodes cannot be assessed
N0	No evidence of regional lymph node involvement
N1-3	Involvement of regional lymph nodes (number and/or extent of spread)

M (metastasis)

Mx	Distant metastasis cannot be evaluated
M0	No distant metastasis
M1	Distant metastasis (cancer has spread to different parts of the body)

tissue, and have the ability to **metastasise** or generate tumours at distant sites (see Table 4.1).

Both benign and malignant tumours are classified according to the tissue in which they develop (Table 4.2). Benign tumours are generally encapsulated with clearly defined edges, which makes their removal from surrounding tissues relatively

Table 4.2 Nomenclature of selected benign and malignant tumours.

Tissue of origin	Benign	Malignant
Epithelial cells	Adenoma	Adenosarcoma
	Papilloma	Papillary adenocarcinoma
	Squamous cell papilloma	Squamous cell carcinoma
	Liver cell adenoma	Hepatocellular carcinoma
	Renal tubular adenoma	Renal cell carcinoma
Connective tissue	Fibroma	Fibrosarcoma
	Lipoma	Liposarcoma
	Chondroma	Chondrosarcoma
	Osteoma	Osteosarcoma
	Haemangioma	Angiosarcoma
	Rhabdomyoma	Rhabdomyosarcoma
	Leiomyoma	Leiomyosarcoma

easy. Benign tumours do not metastasise, nor do they recur after surgical removal. Unlike benign tumours, cancer cells continue to grow and form abnormal cells.

BIOLOGY OF CANCER

Normal cell growth

In normal tissues, cells are reproduced according to the need of the organism. Four factors regulate cell growth: growth factors, growth inhibitors, cell cycle proteins called **cyclins**, and programmed cell death or **apoptosis**. In response to injury, cell growth is accelerated by growth factors. Once damaged tissue has been repaired, inhibitory growth factors decrease cell growth. Cell cycle proteins, or cyclins, regulate specific phases of the cell cycle. If a cell has not completely and accurately replicated its DNA or does not have the full complement of substances required to complete cell division, the cell is either repaired or undergoes cell death.

Carcinogenesis

Carcinogenesis, the development of cancer, is a multi-step process that involves a complex sequence of genetic mutations. A **mutation** is a change in the biochemistry of a gene, resulting in the production of abnormal cells. Genes within DNA and its product RNA hold key information for cell replication. Most invasive cancers develop only when several genes are mutated. Generally, mutations in three classes of genes are responsible for the development of cancer: oncogenes, tumour suppressor genes and DNA repair genes (Table 4.3).

Oncogenes An oncogene is a gene that, when mutated or expressed at abnormally high levels, contributes to converting a normal cell into a cancer cell. Oncogenes are derived from proto-oncogenes or growth-promoting genes and are activated genetic alterations induced by retroviruses. Normally, oncogenes encode for proteins that regulate cell growth, differentiation and apoptosis. Activation or over-

Table 4.3 Cancers associated with selected genetic mutations.

Gene	Major tumour type
Oncogene	
BCR_ABL translocation	Chronic myelogenous leukaemia
BCL-2	Chronic lymphocytic leukaemia
KT, PDGFRA	Gastrointestinal tumours
Tumour suppressor gene	
P53	Breast cancer, sarcoma, brain
APC	Colon, stomach, intestine
VHL	Kidney
DNA repair gene	
BRCA1	Breast, ovary
MSH2, MLH1	Colon, uterus, stomach

Source: *Andreoli and Carpenter's Cecil Essentials of Medicine*, 7th edn, 2007, Elsevier.

production of an oncogene leads to dysregulation of cell growth, increased proliferation and a loss of apoptosis. Over 100 different types of oncogenes have been identified.

Tumour suppressor genes The transformation of a normal cell to a malignant cell takes place not only by activation of oncogenes but also by inactivation or deletion of tumour suppressor genes (TSGs). The protein products of TSGs are involved in a number of cellular functions, such as cell cycle control, checkpoint control, cell signalling, promotion of apoptosis and DNA repair. Inactivation or loss of TSGs by a mutation or deletion leads to a loss of function, reduced restrictions on cell growth and division (ultimately causing genetic instability and loss of apoptosis), and enhanced possibility of malignant behaviour.

DNA repair genes DNA repair genes, also known as caretaker genes, are responsible for the repair of errors in normal DNA replication. Mutations in DNA repair genes result in persistent DNA damage and consequent further mutations and genetic instability. This may lead to a loss of tumour repair genes and conversion of a proto-oncogene to an oncogene, resulting in an increased susceptibility to cancer.

AETIOLOGY OF CANCER

Understanding the causes of human cancer requires both laboratory or **in vitro** research and **epidemiological** or population-based studies. Laboratory research provides information on the development of cancer after exposure to a carcinogen, whereas epidemiological studies provide measures of cancer rates in relation to people and their environment. Population measures of cancer rates in epidemiological studies identify **endogenous** and **environmental** aetiologies of cancer.

Endogenous

The genetic make-up of the individual, including age, sex, race, heredity, hormones and immunity, is among the endogenous non-modifiable aetiologies associated with cancer. Cancer can occur at any age; however, carcinomas are more common around the fifth to seventh decades of life. Sex differences in the aetiology of cancer are often due to differences in hormone levels among males and females. Hereditary differences in cancer occur in both males and females, with either autosomal dominant or autosomal recessive inheritance (Table 4.4).

Environmental

The variations among different types of cancer as well as differential rates of cancer based on geography explain the importance of environmental factors in the development of cancer. Tobacco, industrial chemicals and radiation are among the most significant environmental human carcinogens. Other causes of human cancer include diet, alcohol consumption, chronic infections and certain medicinal drugs.

Tobacco Cigarette smoke is the major cause of lung cancer throughout the world. The risk of cancer is 20-fold greater in long-term heavy smokers than it is in non-smokers. Smoking cessation decreases the risk of cancer to one-third the risk observed in continuing smokers. Smoking and chewing tobacco are the leading causes of head and neck cancer. Tobacco exposure is also a major factor in the development of cancers of the stomach, pancreas, kidney, bladder and cervix. Exposure to second-hand smoke is also associated with an increased risk of lung cancer in non-smoking women married to heavy smokers.

Industrial chemicals Asbestos exposure is the most common cause of occupational cancer. Exposure to asbestos increases the risk for **mesothelioma** (cancer of the membrane that covers and protects most of the internal organs of the body), lung cancer and other cancers, such as those of the larynx and kidney. Rates of asbestos-related cancers are declining with a decrease in workplace-related exposure.

Miners exposed to radon are at a 20-fold increased risk for lung cancer. Other chemical compounds linked to human cancer include benzene (leukaemia); benzidine (bladder cancer); arsenic, soot and coal tars (lung and skin cancer); and wood dust (nasal cancer). Chemical carcinogens have also been identified in water and air pollution.

Radiation Exposure to ionising radiation from natural, industrial and medical sources can cause a variety of neoplasms, including **leukaemia** (cancer of white blood cells), breast cancer and thyroid cancer.

Sunlight is the most significant source of ultraviolet radiation and causes several types of skin cancer. The development of skin cancers depends on the level of skin exposure, the position of the sun

Table 4.4 Autosomal genes and associated cancers.

Inheritance	Associated cancer
Autosomal dominant	
Familial adenomatous polyposis of the colon	Carcinoma of the colon
Familial retinoblastoma	Retinoblastoma and osteogenic sarcoma
Von-Hippel-Lindau syndrome	Renal cell carcinoma
Autosomal recessive	
Xeroderma pigmentosum	Skin cancer
Bloom syndrome	Lymphoid malignancies
Fanconi's anaemia	Leukaemia

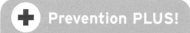

Prevention PLUS!

Cigarettes and cancer

It is estimated that nearly one-third of all cancers can be prevented by lifestyle modification. Cigarette smoking accounts for at least 30% of all cancer deaths. It is a major cause of cancers of the lung, larynx (voice box), oral cavity, pharynx (throat) and oesophagus, and is a contributing cause in the development of cancers of the bladder, pancreas, liver, uterine cervix, kidney, stomach, colon and rectum, and some leukaemias. A lifestyle without smoking is a life with a significantly reduced risk of cancer.

Source: NHS Choices: www.nhs.uk/conditions/cancer

and skin type. Highly exposed populations, those experiencing acute sunburn, and those with fair skin are particularly at risk for skin cancers.

Diet After smoking, diet and obesity is the next largest contributor to cancer deaths. There is evidence that eating more than five portions of fruits or vegetables per day reduces cancer risk, especially colon and stomach cancer. Physical exercise reduces cancer risk, especially colon cancer, and is helpful in reducing obesity.

Alcohol Alcohol abuse, along with tobacco use, has been strongly associated with the development of cancers in the mouth, pharynx, larynx and oesophagus. Alcohol has also been linked to liver, rectal and breast cancers.

Chronic infections Almost 20% of cancers are associated with chronic infections. The most frequently associated organ sites are the liver, cervix, lymphoid tissue and stomach. Chronic hepatitis B and C viral infections have been linked with the development of liver cancer. A universal vaccination programme directed against hepatitis B has been shown to decrease the incidence of childhood hepatic cancer in Taiwan. Human papillomaviruses have been linked with cervical cancers, and a vaccine has recently been developed. The human immunodeficiency virus can lead to Kaposi's sarcoma and certain lymphomas. Chronic infection with the bacterium *Helicobacter pylori* can cause certain gastric lymphomas and gastric adenocarcinoma.

Medicines Various medicines have been associated with an increased risk of specific cancers. For example, synthetic oestrogens such as diethylstilboestrol, which was given to mothers during pregnancy in the 1960s and 1970s, was strongly associated with the development of vaginal cancer in their offspring. Cancer chemotherapy agents not only fight cancer but can also be carcinogenic. Successful treatment of primary malignancies with cancer chemotherapy and radiation has been associated with the development of secondary cancers.

HUMAN CANCERS BY ORGAN SITE

Lung

Lung cancer is the most common malignant disease worldwide and is the major cause of death from cancer. It was a rare disease until the beginning of the twentieth century, becoming more common owing to an increase in the consumption of tobacco. In both men and women, the incidence of lung cancer is low before age 40 and increases up to at least age 70. Lung cancer is the second most common cancer (after skin cancer) in England and Wales, with an estimated 31 000 new cases being diagnosed every year. In 2007, there were 29 660 deaths in England and Wales as a result of lung cancer.

Smoking is the single biggest risk factor for lung cancer, accounting for an estimated 85–90% of cases. People who smoke more than 20 cigarettes a day are 20 times more likely to develop lung cancer than non-smokers. In addition to cigarette smoke, household exposure to radon as well as industrial exposures to asbestos and other airborne chemicals increase lung cancer risk.

Most lung cancers are clinically silent, with symptoms presenting once the disease is advanced. Cough is the most common presenting symptom in lung cancer and is reported along with shortness of breath, blood in sputum, chest pain and loss of appetite. Additional symptoms include wheezing; **stridor**, or a high pitch during respiration; hoarseness; and **dysphasia**, or difficulty speaking.

The two major types of lung cancer include non-small cell lung cancer (NSCLC) and small cell lung cancer (SCLC). NSCLC includes different cellular types, such as squamous cell carcinomas, adenocarcinomas and large cell tumours. Squamous cell carcinomas are usually located in the bronchi and are commonly associated with abnormal increases in blood calcium. Adenocarcinomas are the most common lung cancers and the type most often diagnosed in non-smokers. Large cell tumours are the least common form of lung cancer. SCLC is significantly linked to exposure to cigarette smoke. SCLCs often occur as large central tumours and are associated with endocrine abnormalities such as syndrome of inappropriate antidiuretic hormone production and Cushing's syndrome.

A number of different medical tests are required to diagnose lung cancer accurately. A screening diagnosis of lung cancer begins with a patient history, chest X-ray, sputum analysis and various blood tests. CT scans are essential tools for **staging** or evaluating the extent of disease and for surgical evaluation for removal of the tumour. Positron emission tomography (PET) scans are useful for assessing metastases or distant dissemination of the disease. Bronchoscopy provides a tool for obtaining local tissue, or **biopsy**, for examination under a microscope for assessment of the **histology**, or cell structural abnormalities.

Early stage tumours are treated with surgery. Radiation therapy is also used to treat early stage tumours in patients who are considered poor candidates for surgery. More advanced stages of lung cancer may be treated with a combination of chemotherapy and radiation therapy. Using multiple chemotherapy agents often provides better treatment outcomes than using each respective agent alone. Chemotherapy agents commonly used to treat lung cancer include cisplatin, cyclophosphamide, doxorubicin, paclitaxel, vincristine and vinblastine.

Despite the availability of multiple agents to treat lung cancer, relapse rates occur frequently and survival rates are poor. In light of poor survival rates, prevention of lung cancer remains a global priority. Lung cancer is a largely preventable disease that has declined owing to anti-smoking campaigns and cancer prevention programmes. According to the World Health Organization, decreasing current smoking rates by half could prevent 20–30 million deaths before 2025 and 150 million deaths by 2050.

Breast

Breast cancer is the most frequently diagnosed cancer in women, with more than one million cases occurring worldwide annually. More than 45 500 cases of breast cancer are diagnosed every year in the UK, usually in women over 50 who have reached menopause. However, it is possible for women of any age to get breast cancer and, in rare cases, the condition can affect men.

The earliest sign of breast cancer is often an abnormality detected on a mammogram or breast self-examination. Large tumours are usually felt as a mass on or around the breast. Less common symptoms include changes to the breast such as thickening, swelling, distortion, tenderness and skin irritation, and nipple changes such as spontaneous discharge or ulceration.

Age, female gender and personal family history are the most important risk factors for breast cancer. Reproductive factors such as a long menstrual history, oral contraceptive use, never having children, or having a first child after age 30 have also been linked to breast cancer. Being overweight, obesity after menopause, postmenopausal hormone replacement therapy, physical inactivity and excess consumption of alcohol are risk factors that can be modified to potentially reduce risk. Changes in certain genes increase the risk of breast cancer, including *BRCA1*, *BRCA2* and others. Tests may show the presence of specific gene changes in families with a history of breast cancer.

The diagnosis of breast cancer is currently made by assessment of breast lumps, clinical history and physical examination, mammography and/or breast ultrasound, plus a fine needle aspiration biopsy. Breast cancer screening has been associated with a 30% reduction in breast cancer mortality in populations where mammography has been adopted. Treatment of breast cancer depends on the tumour size and stage, as well as patient preferences. Surgical treatment may involve a lumpectomy (surgical removal of a tumour) or mastectomy (surgical removal of the breast) with removal of some of the axillary (underarm) lymph nodes. In early stages of the disease, lumpectomy followed by radiation therapy will allow for breast conservation. Mastectomies are often necessary for large tumours. Chemotherapy, hormone therapy or targeted biological therapy are also used alone or in combination with surgery and radiation.

Stomach

Stomach cancer was the fourth most common malignancy in the world in 2000 and is steadily becoming less common. The incidence of stomach cancer in Europe, for example, has fallen by more than 60% during the past 50 years. There is good evidence that the advent of refrigeration of food protects against stomach cancer by facilitating year-round consumption of fruits and vegetables. Vitamin C, contained in fruits and vegetables and other foods of plant origin, is protective, and so too are diets high in whole grain cereals.

Dietary risk factors for stomach cancer include inadequate intake of fresh fruits and vegetables, high salt intake and consumption of smoked or cured meats or fish. The infectious bacterium *Helicobacter pylori* triggers excess cell proliferation within the stomach with chronic gastritis, and ulceration is also considered a risk factor for stomach cancer.

Early forms of stomach cancer are usually asymptomatic. The most common symptom is a mild pain

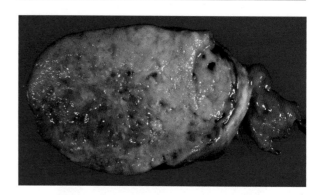

Figure 4.1 Stomach cancer.
(Science Photo Library Ltd)

in the upper abdomen, which is often confused with simple indigestion. Generalised and non-specific symptoms include fatigue, loss of energy and a decrease in appetite.

Like all forms of cancer, the definitive diagnosis of stomach cancer is performed by taking a biopsy. CT or MRI scans provide information on size, location and spread of the cancer.

Surgery is the most important treatment for stomach cancer. The extent of surgical removal of the stomach depends on the location of the tumour and extent of tissue involvement. Often a large part of the stomach or all of the stomach will need to be removed. Radiation therapy is especially important in cases where the tumour cannot be removed. The most commonly used chemotherapy agents for treating stomach cancer include 5-fluorouracil, folinic acid, etoposide, adriamycin, methotrexate, cisplatin or carboplatinum (Figure 4.1).

Colorectal

Cancers of the colon and rectum are most common in western societies where consumption of high-fat food, refined carbohydrates and animal protein combined with low physical activity is common. In England, bowel cancer is the third most common type of cancer, with an estimated 30 800 new cases diagnosed each year. Approximately 14 000 cases of bowel cancer are diagnosed in women, making it the second most common cancer in women after

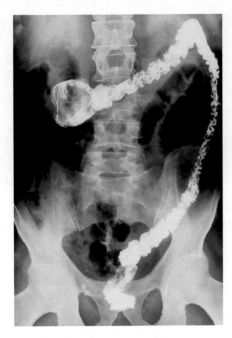

Figure 4.2 Radiograph of colon cancer.
(Science Photo Library Ltd/Sovereign, ISM)

breast cancer. It is the third most common cancer in men after prostate and lung cancer. In England, there are an estimated 13 000 deaths as a result of bowel cancer annually. Two-thirds of bowel cancers develop in the colon, with the remaining third developing in the rectum.

Screening is necessary to detect colorectal cancer in its early states. Advanced forms of colorectal cancer may cause rectal bleeding, blood in the stool, a change in bowel habits, and pain in the lower abdomen (Figure 4.2). Colonoscopy enables visual inspection of the entire large bowel and rectum. The procedure is a safe and effective means of evaluating the large bowel. The technology for colonoscopy has evolved to provide a very clear image of the mucosa through a video camera attached to the end of the scope. The camera connects to a computer, which can store and print colour images selected during the procedure. Colonoscopy is especially useful in detecting small adenomas; however, the main advantage of colonoscopy is that it allows for identification and removal of cancerous lesions or polyps as well as for biopsy of suspect tissue.

The risk of colorectal cancer increases with age; more than 80% of cases are diagnosed in individuals aged 60 years and older. Certain inherited genetic mutations, including familial adenomatous polyposis and hereditary non-polyposis colorectal cancer, are non-modifiable risk factors for colorectal cancer. Modifiable risk factors include obesity, physical inactivity, smoking, heavy alcohol consumption, a diet high in red and processed meat, and inadequate intake of fruits and vegetables.

Surgery is curative for colorectal cancers that have not spread. A permanent **colostomy**, or the creation of an abdominal opening for elimination of body waste, is rarely needed for colon cancer and is frequently required for rectal cancer. Chemotherapy alone or in combination with radiation therapy is used to treat invasive tumours prior to and after surgery. Chemotherapeutic agents used to treat colorectal cancer include oxaliplatin and 5-fluorouracil.

Liver

Hepatocellular carcinoma (HCC), or malignancy of the liver cells, accounts for 80% of all primary cancers in the liver. Liver cancer accounts for almost 4% of all cancers worldwide and affects men three times more frequently than women. HCC is responsible for approximately 1500 deaths in the UK annually. It is more common among men, and those over the age of 60 are more likely to be affected by it. The liver is the second most commonly involved organ in metastatic disease, after the lymph nodes.

In vitro studies have demonstrated the carcinogenic effects of hepatitis B and C viruses on **hepatocytes**, or liver cells. Viral replication in infected cells and the consequent immune response result in persistent inflammation that progresses toward chronic liver disease and malignant changes. In developing countries, dietary ingestion of toxins produced by mould is causally associated with HCC.

Common symptoms of HCC are abdominal pain, weight loss, fatigue, abdominal swelling and **anorexia**, or loss of appetite. Other signs include impaired liver function, **ascites** (accumulation of fluid in the abdominal cavity), **hepatomegaly**

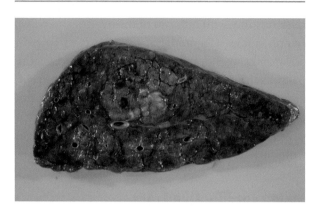

Figure 4.3 Cancer of the liver.
(Dr E. Walker/Science Photo Library/Photo Researchers, Inc.)

(enlarged liver) and **jaundice** (yellowish discolour-ation of the skin, sclera and bile). Liver cancer follows a rapid and progressive course, with only around 5% surviving at 5 years.

Most cases of liver cancer can be diagnosed by computed tomography (CT) and ultrasound. A defini-tive diagnosis depends on identification of cellular abnormalities obtained by a biopsy (Figure 4.3).

The treatment of malignant tumours of the liver depends on the extent of disease and the underlying liver function. Surgical removal of the tumours with defined margins is the primary treatment for malig-nant liver neoplasms. Most hepatocellular cancers are not sensitive to chemotherapy. Radiation ther-apy can be used to control symptoms by shrinking the tumour. Liver transplantation is recommended when chemotherapy and radiation are ineffective.

Female reproductive tract

Cervical Cervical cancer is a relatively rare type of cancer. In the UK, approximately 2800 women are diagnosed with it each year. The incidence and mortality have declined in the last 40 years in western societies with the development of extensive screening programmes.

Molecular and epidemiological studies have shown that certain human papillomavirus types (HPV) are central to the development of cervical cancer. High-risk sexual behaviour, such as multiple sexual partners, and early age at initiation of sexual

activity potentially reflect the probability of infec-tion with HPV and associated cervical cancer.

Precancerous changes in the cervix can be readily detected with the Pap test. Additional tests include a colposcopy (endoscopic examination of the cells of the cervix) and biopsy for a definitive diagnosis.

Moderate to severe precancerous changes to the cervix can be treated by killing the diseased tissue via freezing, or **cryosurgery**, or applying heat via **cautery** or **laser**, which vaporises cells. If a larger area of the cervix needs to be removed, it is removed by a surgical procedure called a **cone biopsy**. Invasive cervical cancers are treated with radiation therapy and chemotherapy.

Uterine Cancer of the uterus or **endometrium** (endometrial cancer) is the most commonly occur-ring cancer of the female reproductive system. It is the fourth most common cancer that affects women, after breast cancer, lung cancer and can-cer of the colon and rectum. In 2006 in England and Wales, 6056 new cases of endometrial cancer were registered and there were 1039 deaths from endometrial cancer. Approximately 75% of cases of endometrial cancer are in women who have had the menopause (postmenopausal), mostly in women aged 60–69.

Endometrial cancer is linked to reproductive life, with a higher rate among women who have never been pregnant and women in late menopause. Oral oestrogen therapy and prior removal of the ovaries also increase the risk for endometrial cancer. This disease is also associated with obesity, diabetes and hypertension.

The most common sign of uterine cancer is uterine bleeding, especially after menopause. Other signs of the disease are those linked to a mass in the abdomen: these are **dysuria** (difficult urinating), constipation or bloating.

Endovaginal echography and hysteroscopy are useful in identifying the tumour. Histological exam-ination provides a more definitive diagnosis.

Precancerous lesions of the endometrium are treated by surgical removal of the uterus or **hys-terectomy**. A total abdominal hysterectomy with removal of the ovaries is the definitive treatment

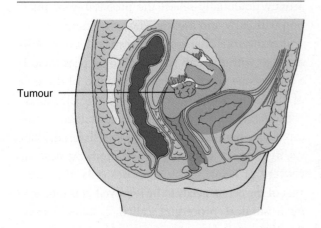

Figure 4.4 Tumour on ovary.

for carcinoma of the uterus. Postsurgical radiation therapy is also recommended in patients at risk for relapse following surgery. In inoperable cases, pelvic radiation therapy may be the sole treatment.

Ovarian Cancer of the ovary may develop in one or both ovaries and may spread to other parts of the abdomen. Because the ovaries are situated deep within the pelvis, the early stages may cause no symptoms, so that ovarian cancer is frequently diagnosed in advanced stages of the disease (Figure 4.4).

A family history is the single most important risk factor for ovarian cancer. Cancer of the ovary is influenced by hormones and reproductive factors, and the risk is greater among women with a prior history of breast cancer and no history of pregnancy. A history of pelvic inflammatory disease, polycystic ovary disease and endometriosis has also been associated with increased risk.

The majority of patients with ovarian cancer usually present after the disease has spread outside the ovary. Symptoms include abdominal discomfort, bloating, abnormal vaginal bleeding and gastrointestinal or urinary tract abnormalities.

Abdominal and vaginal ultrasound are used to detect the presence of an ovarian tumour; however, a definitive diagnosis requires surgical examination and a biopsy.

Surgery is often the first option for diagnosis via biopsy and treatment of ovarian cancer. Surgical

treatment of the disease includes a total abdominal hysterectomy with removal of the ovaries and pelvic lymph nodes. Chemotherapy agents used to treat advanced stages of ovarian cancer include cisplatin, paclitaxel, vincristine, actinomycin, bleomycin, etoposide and cyclophosphamide in various cycles and duration. Despite treatment, the overall 5-year survival rate for all stages of ovarian cancer ranges from 30% to 50%.

Male reproductive tract

Prostate Prostate cancer is the third most common cancer in men worldwide, with approximately 543 000 new cases each year. It is the most common cancer in men, and is responsible for 25% of newly diagnosed cases of cancer in England and Wales. The incidence and the mortality rate increases with age and peaks around the seventh decade of life. Thus, approximately three-quarters of the cases occur in men aged 65 years and older.

Age is the leading risk factor for prostate cancer, although ethnicity is also implicated. For reasons that are not understood, prostate cancer is more common in men who are of Afro-Caribbean or African descent and less common in men of Asian descent. Dietary pattern studies suggest that a diet high in saturated fat is a significant risk factor, whereas ingestion of micronutrients such as vitamins A, D, E, selenium, lycopene and calcium has a protective effect. The role of hormones in the development in prostate cancer has been suggested, though the exact role of hormones in prostate carcinogenesis is still not understood.

There are no symptoms that are absolutely specific to prostate cancer. The symptoms, including urinary hesitancy, frequency, urgency, dribbling, weak stream, blood in the urine and pain in the lower abdomen, resemble symptoms of a urinary tract infection or a benign growth of the prostate, also called **benign prostatic enlargement**.

Digital rectal examination is the simplest way to detect abnormalities of the prostate gland (Figure 4.5). A blood test for **prostate-specific antigen (PSA)** may support the diagnosis of prostate cancer. Ultrasound-guided biopsy studies establish the

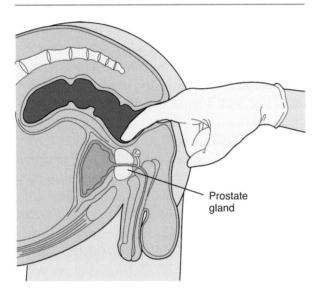

Figure 4.5 Digital rectal examination to detect abnormalities of the prostate gland.

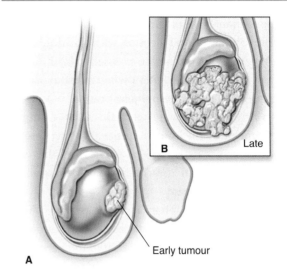

Figure 4.6 Early and late stage testicular tumours.

dimensions of the tumour. Radiological examinations such as CT scans and MRI are performed to help stage a diagnosed prostate cancer.

Surgery to remove the prostate is recommended for those with localised disease and a life expectancy greater than 10 years. Radiation therapy is recommended for men who are not suitable for surgery. Advanced disease is treated with radiation therapy and endocrine therapy. Endocrine therapy is aimed at reducing hormone levels that may continue to foster growth of the tumour.

Cancer of the testes Cancer of the testes accounts for 0.7% of all cancers. It is the most common cancer in men between the age of 20 and 35 although can occur in men of all ages. Approximately 1960 men are diagnosed with the condition each year in the UK.

The most common malignant tumours of the testes originate from germ cells. **Germ cells** are cells that have the potential to grow and develop into many different types of tissues. There are two types of germ cell tumours: **seminomas**, or cancer of sperm-producing cells, and **non-seminomas**, cancers of embryonic cells. Seminomas are slow growing tumours and are sensitive to radiation therapy (Figure 4.6).

Environmental causes of testicular cancer have not been established. There is an increased incidence of the disease in men with a history of undescended testicles and those with a close family history of testicular cancer. In utero exposure to exogenous oestrogen may increase the risk of undescended testes, also known as **cryptorchidism**.

Cancer of the testes is usually detected as a painless lump on the testicle. Rarely, the first noticeable symptoms of a non-seminomatous cancer are a lump in the neck, pain or discomfort in the back, or shortness of breath due to metastases in the lungs.

Current management of germ cell tumours includes surgical resection, radiation therapy and chemotherapy. Approximately 80% of patients with advanced disease respond to all three treatments.

Oesophageal cancer

Cancer of the oesophagus is relatively rare in the UK, although it has become more common in the past 30 years. Currently, it accounts for approximately 3% of all cancer cases. Approximately 7560 people are diagnosed with the condition each year, with males over the age of 55 years most commonly affected.

Consumption of tobacco and alcohol, associated with low intake of fresh fruits and vegetables, is causally associated with cancer of the oesophagus. Greater than 90% of oesophageal cancer is attributable to tobacco and alcohol, with an additive risk among individuals who are exposed to both factors. Longstanding oesophagitis owing to reflux disease increases the risk of oesophageal cancer.

Difficulty swallowing or pain with eating or drinking are the most noticeable symptoms. Unexplained weight loss, hoarseness of the voice and bleeding from the throat may be associated with advanced disease.

Diagnosis of oesophageal cancer requires microscopic examination of the diseased tissue, or biopsy. CT scan and endoscopic ultrasonography are useful in determining the extent of the tumour and whether there is spread to neighbouring tissues. Barium medium X-rays provide information on how well the oesophagus is functioning as well as the location of the tumour.

Primary treatment for local disease is surgical removal of the oesophagus. Replacement with a prosthetic tube or a stent across the tumour **stenosis** (narrowing) may help restore swallowing in patients not suitable for surgery. Radiation therapy, as well as multiple chemotherapy regimens, have been used alone or combined with surgery, though these approaches are rarely curative. Despite the availability of treatment, the overall 5-year survival rate for oesophageal cancer ranges from 10% to 20%.

Bladder cancer

Bladder cancer is the seventh most common cancer in the UK, with an estimated 10 000 new cases diagnosed annually. In the UK it is estimated that 3300 men and 1600 women die annually from bladder cancer.

The most important risk factor for bladder cancer is cigarette smoking, which accounts for approximately 65% of male cases and 30% of female cases. Upon cessation of cigarette smoking, a substantial decrease in risk of bladder cancer is observed. Exposure to certain industrial chemicals, such as rubber, aromatic hydrocarbons, asbestos and solvents used in paint and hairspray, is correlated with

an increased risk. In certain endemic regions, infection with a worm, *Schistosoma haematobium*, is linked with up to a fivefold risk of bladder cancer.

The most common symptom of bladder cancer is **haematuria**, or blood in the urine. Pain is rarely associated with haematuria. Increased urinary frequency is also reported but is often mistaken for a less serious condition.

Surgery alone or in combination with radiation or chemotherapy is used to treat greater than 90% of cases. Localised tumours can be treated with immune therapy or chemotherapy administered directly into the bladder. For all diagnosed cases and stages combined, the 5-year survival rate of bladder cancer is 90%.

Head and neck cancer

Cancer in the upper aerodigestive tract (which extends from the surface of the lips to the neck region), larynx and pharynx comprise head and neck cancer. These cancers are among the eleventh most common worldwide, with 390 000 new cases of oral cancer, 65 000 new cases of pharyngeal cancer, and 160 000 cases of laryngeal cancer reported worldwide per year. The incidence rate is more than twice as high in men as women in the UK.

Smoking and excess alcohol consumption are the major risk factors for head and neck cancer. Smoking accounts for about 14% of laryngeal and oral/pharyngeal cancer cases in men and about 15% of cases in women worldwide. Tobacco smoking has also been found to be an important risk factor for nasopharyngeal cancer.

Symptoms of oral cancer include head or neck pain; bleeding; difficulty in opening the mouth, chewing, swallowing and talking; and pain in the neck. Early disease is often painless and present as elevated, red mucosal patches or hardened ulcers or growths. With advanced disease, large masses with areas of **necrosis**, or death to surrounding tissue, may extend to the bone, muscle and skin.

There are no general screening tests for head and neck cancers. Frequently these cancers are detected by dentists or primary care physicians as abnormal changes in oral tissue. Endoscopic examination to obtain a biopsy is useful for laryngeal and pharyngeal tumours.

Like many other forms of cancer, tumour resection is aimed at removing the tumour while preserving optimal tissue function. Radiation therapy along with surgery is a mainstay treatment for most head and neck cancers. Chemotherapy is applied for advanced stages of disease.

Lymphoma

Lymphoma covers a heterogeneous group of neoplasms of lymphoid tissue. Lymphomas are categorised as either Hodgkin's disease or non-Hodgkin's lymphoma. Within each of these two categories are a range of diverse subtypes. There are around 9000 new cases of non-Hodgkin's lymphoma and 1500 new cases of Hodgkin's lymphoma diagnosed annually in the UK.

Hodgkin's disease Hodgkin's disease comprises approximately 23% of malignant lymphomas worldwide, and approximately 45% of cases can be attributed to Epstein–Barr virus (EBV). Hodgkin's disease is distinguished from non-Hodgkin's lymphoma by a particular type of cell termed the **Reed-Sternberg cell**.

Hodgkin's disease most often occurs in young adults. The risk for Hodgkin's disease has been explained by infections with EBV, HIV and chronic exposure to wood or wood products. The most common presenting symptom is a painless swelling of the lymph nodes in the neck, armpit or groin. Other symptoms include fatigue, unexplained fever, night sweats and indigestion in cases of gastric lymphoma.

Hodgkin's disease is often treated with chemotherapy with combinations of several different agents. Survival of Hodgkin's disease is related to the extent of disease at diagnosis; however, 5-year survival for all stages of the disease combined is estimated at 100% in young people, but in individuals aged 50 years or more, the survival rate is nearer 75–80%.

Non-Hodgkin's lymphoma Patients with HIV/AIDS or those who have received immune suppressive therapy are at a higher risk for developing non-Hodgkin's lymphoma. In addition to HIV, viral infections with HTLV1 and EBV are also associated with non-Hodgkin's lymphoma. Infection in the stomach with the bacterium *Helicobacter pylori* is linked with gastric lymphoma.

The most common presenting symptom of non-Hodgkin's lymphoma is painless swelling of the lymph nodes. Similar to Hodgkin's disease, non-specific feelings of fatigue, night sweats and fever are also reported. Accurate diagnosis requires microscopic evaluation of lymphoid tissue. X-rays, CT scans, MRI, bone marrow sampling and lymphograms are useful in determining the extent of disease.

Indolent or slow growing lymphomas often present as advanced disease. Treatment with radiation and or chemotherapy can be administered as needed over a period of many years. The goal in treating advanced, slow growing lymphomas is to obtain a cure. This is accomplished with several doses and combinations of chemotherapeutic agents alone or in combination with radiation therapy. Recurrent lymphomas have been treated with bone marrow transplantation with some success.

Leukaemia

Leukaemia, which causes massive proliferation of immature forms of white blood cells, occurs in more than 250 000 individuals worldwide each year. These cancers are further classified on the basis of malignancy involving either **lymphoid** (B cells or T cells in lymph tissue) or **myeloid** (bone marrow) cells and whether the disease is acute or chronic.

Leukaemia is diagnosed 10 times more often in adults than in children, although it is often thought of as a childhood cancer. Symptoms include fatigue, paleness, weight loss, repeated infections, fever, bruising easily and nosebleeds or other haemorrhages. These signs often appear suddenly in acute leukaemia, whereas chronic leukaemia can progress slowly with few symptoms.

Because the symptoms often resemble less serious conditions, leukaemia is difficult to diagnose early. Blood tests and bone marrow biopsy provide definitive evidence for this disease.

Chemotherapy is the most effective method for treating leukaemia. Supportive treatment with blood transfusions and antibiotics is needed to treat anaemia and infections. Bone marrow transplantation from a matched donor is one form of therapy for late stages of this disease. Survival in leukaemia depends on type, ranging from a 5-year survival of 20% for those with acute myeloid leukaemia to 74% for people with chronic lymphocytic leukaemia.

Pancreatic cancer

Pancreatic cancer is a difficult disease to detect and treat. Approximately 7000 people are diagnosed with this form of cancer annually in the UK, accounting for 3% of all cancer diagnoses.

About 30% of cases of pancreatic cancer are attributed to smoking. Cigarette smokers develop this disease two to three times more often than non-smokers. Diets low in fibre and high in consumption of red meat and fat are also associated with this disease.

The diagnosis of pancreatic cancer is rarely made during early stages of the disease. It is frequently diagnosed once patients present with clinical symptoms, including weight loss, nausea, diarrhoea, weakness, jaundice and upper abdominal pain.

Ultrasonography is useful for initial diagnoses. CT scanning allows for clearer images of the head and tail of the pancreas as well as the extent of the involvement of surrounding tissues.

Currently, surgery offers patients the only chance for a cure. Palliative treatment is often needed for the treatment of jaundice and gastric obstructions. Simultaneous chemotherapy may provide a survival benefit. Survival from pancreatic cancer is poor, and the majority of patients with this condition die within 1 year of diagnosis.

Melanoma

Melanoma is a malignant proliferation of pigment-producing cells or **melanocytes**. This disease occurs primarily in white-skinned individuals. Malignant melanoma accounts for 10% of all cancer diagnoses, with 1500 people dying annually from the disease.

The risk factors for melanoma vary by skin type; sensitivity to sunlight; extent of sun exposure; exposure to industrial chemicals such as coal tar, arsenic and radium; and past history of skin cancer. Melanomas can occur anywhere on the skin, though the majority of melanomas in men appear on the back, while in women the majority appear on the legs.

Early detection of skin cancer is possible by personal examination of the skin. Melanomas usually start as small, mole-like growths that increase in size and change in colour (Figure 4.7). A simple ABCD rule outlines the warning signs of the most common forms of melanoma: asymmetry, border irregularity, colour and diameter.

The diagnosis of a melanoma is made by a biopsy. If the lesion is found to be a melanoma, surgery is required to remove the lesion. Radiation therapy is used to treat recurrent disease or metastases. In general, melanomas are not very responsive

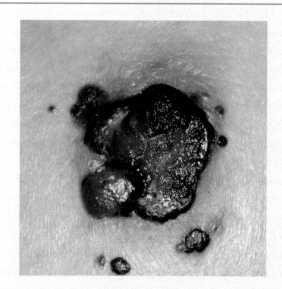

Figure 4.7 Malignant melanoma.
(ISM/Phototake NYC)

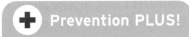

Prevention PLUS!

The ABCDs of skin cancer

Perform skin examination regularly, and check for the ABCDs:

- A is for asymmetry; one-half of the mole does not match the other half
- B is for border irregularity
- C is for colour; the pigmentation of the cancer is not uniform
- D is for diameter greater than 6 millimetres

to chemotherapy drugs. Biological therapy with interferon-alpha and interleukin-2 produces treatment responses in some patients that last many years.

Thyroid cancer

Cancer of the thyroid gland is relatively rare, with an incidence of about 1200 new cases in the UK annually. In general, thyroid cancer can occur at any age, including young adults and teens.

Radiation exposure, iodine deficiency and radioactive iodine exposure are among known risk factors for thyroid cancer. This cancer grows slowly and in many cases is cured by complete surgical removal of the thyroid gland.

Thyroid cancer commonly causes no obvious symptoms in its early stages. The vast majority of cancers become clinically palpable as thyroid nodules, although a minority of all thyroid nodules are malignant. Hoarseness, dyspepsia and dysphagia may reflect local invasion to the larynx, trachea or oesophagus. A definitive diagnosis is achievable by biopsy.

Kidney cancer

The most common type of kidney cancer, renal carcinoma, occurs twice as frequently in men as in women. Renal carcinoma accounts for approximately 3% of cancers in the UK annually, with 5700 cases diagnosed in 2004.

Kidney cancer has consistently been found to be more common in cigarette smokers than in non-smokers. An increased risk has been linked to obesity, especially in women. Leather tanners, shoe workers and dry cleaning employees have an increased risk, as do workers exposed to asbestos.

Kidney cancer commonly causes no obvious symptoms in its early stages. Advanced disease symptoms include haematuria, flank pain and a palpable kidney mass. Systemic symptoms of renal carcinoma result from overproduction of normal kidney proteins and hormones that cause hypertension, fevers, anaemia, **erythrocytosis** (elevated number of red blood cells), abnormal liver function and hypercalcaemia (abnormally high calcium levels).

Urine tests are used as a screening tool to confirm the presence of blood cells in the urine. An intravenous urogram (IVU) is an X-ray in which a special contrast medium is injected into a vein and X-ray pictures are taken as the medium passes through the kidneys. Ultrasound and CT scans are useful for evaluating the size, location and spread of disease.

Surgery is the mainstay treatment for cancer of the kidney. Surgery can be curative for early disease and may help prevent further spread of disease when the disease has advanced. Renal cell carcinoma is responsive to treatments with immune modifiers such as interferon and interleukin-2 in combination with chemotherapy.

Cancers of the nervous system

The majority of adult tumours of the central nervous system (CNS) are derived from **glial** cells, which are support cells in the nervous system. These cancers are rare and account for less than 2% of all malignancies worldwide. Brain tumours have two peaks of incidence. The first is in childhood, with a peak between 3 and 12 years of age. The second group is older adults, with a peak between 60 and 70 years of age.

Some brain tumours are associated with inherited cancer syndromes. The brain is also a frequent site of metastases from primary tumours that occur elsewhere in the body. Childhood brain tumours are thought to result from defects in cell cycle control mechanisms originating from fetal development. Rare cases of brain tumours are caused by therapeutic radiation. Children who have received preventative brain radiation for acute leukaemia seem to have an increased risk of developing malignant gliomas.

The signs and symptoms largely depend on the location of the neoplasm and may include **paresis** or a slight paralysis, speech disturbances and personality changes. Some patients have long histories of epileptic seizures. Large tumours can cause life-threatening pressures to build up in the CNS that may lead to unconsciousness and respiratory arrest. Headaches occur when the tumour infiltrates the **meninges** or membranes covering the brain.

CT scans of the brain will often show the position of a tumour, whether it is causing swelling around the brain, and whether it is blocking the flow of the cerebrospinal fluid. The MRI scan may provide additional information about tumour location, size and spread. An **EEG** (electroencephalogram) or electrical brain activity recording device is useful for identifying seizure activity. If possible, a brain biopsy will provide a definitive diagnosis of the tumour type.

Surgical removal of the tumour usually involves a **craniotomy**, in which a flap of bone is temporarily removed. In some circumstances, the tumour may be surgically removed by use of a laser. Dexamethasone is a steroid medication that is very helpful in reducing swelling around brain tumours. Radiation therapy is often applied to the specific areas of the brain that are affected.

Paediatric cancers

Although uncommon, childhood cancer is the second leading cause of death in children. Approximately 1400 children (aged 0–14 years) were diagnosed with cancer in 2004 in the UK. The majority of childhood cancers are leukaemia.

Like many adult forms of cancer, symptoms of early disease in children are often mistaken for less serious conditions. Common general symptoms include loss of energy, pallor, easy bruising, persistent pain, prolonged fever, frequent headaches, profuse vomiting, sudden changes in vision and weight loss (Table 4.5).

Childhood forms of cancer are treated by a combination of therapies: surgery, radiation and chemotherapy. The number of treatment cycles as well as the agents used depend on the type and stage of cancer. Long-term survival from childhood cancer has improved, though many patients experience cancer treatment effects. Late effects of paediatric cancer treatment include organ damage and malfunction, secondary cancers and cognitive impairments.

Cancer and ageing

Cancer is more common with increasing age. With the expansion of the aging population, the number of cancer survivors over the age of 65 is likely to continue to increase. Coupled with this cancer health risk, older adults are often living with chronic diseases of older adulthood and are likely to have concomitant health problems. These coexisting health conditions often affect prognosis and treatment outcomes in older adults.

The most common cancers of older adulthood are prostate, breast, colon, pancreas, bladder, stomach and lung. Chronic illnesses that often accompany aging, such as heart problems, vision loss, decline in memory, hearing difficulties, decreased kidney function and weight loss, may interfere with the older adult's ability to handle a stressful illness like cancer.

Cancer treatment in older adults is the same as in young and middle-aged adults. The goals of cancer treatment in persons of all ages include curing the primary tumour, allowing the patient to live longer with good quality of life, reducing cancer symptoms and maintaining functions of daily living. In older

Table 4.5 Childhood cancers.

Childhood cancer	Childhood cancer (%)	Disease description	Disease signs and symptoms
Leukaemia	32	Proliferation of abnormal white blood cells	Severe anaemia, haemorrhages, slight enlargement of the lymph nodes or the spleen. Weakness, bone and joint pain, bleeding and fever
Brain, nervous system	30	Mostly medulloblastoma, which are undifferentiated primitive cells that appear on the cerebellum, brainstem and spinal cord	Headache, nausea, vomiting, blurred or double vision, dizziness, and difficulty handling objects
Neuroblastoma	11	Cancer of the sympathetic nervous system; consists of immature embryonic-like cells	Occurs most frequently in the mediastinal and retroperitoneal abdomen. Recognised by a lump or swelling on the abdomen
Lymphomas	5	Affects the lymph nodes but may spread to the bone marrow and other organs	May cause swelling of the lymph nodes of the neck, armpit and groin. Fever and weakness may also be present
Osteosarcoma	4	Occurs on the surface of bone and usually presents in adolescents	Most frequent site of occurrence is in the long bones of the lower limbs. Osteosarcomas are associated with pain, tenderness and inflammation of the affected limb(s). Symptoms become persistent and worse with pain occurring at rest
Wilms' tumour	3	Malignant renal tumour that is composed of small spindle cells and cells that resemble embryonic glomeruli; often inherited as an autosomal dominant trait	May occur in one or both kidneys. Symptoms include swelling or palpable mass in the flank as well as moderate to severe pain
Retinoblastoma	1	Eye cancer that occurs in children under the age of 4. May be familial form that is caused by autosomal dominant mutation of the retinoblastoma gene, which is a tumour suppressor gene	In familial cases the disease is usually bilateral, with multiple lesions within the eye

Adapted from *Cancer Research UK, 2010*.

adulthood, unlike other stages in life, the availability of a carer to assist with the effects of treatment may be lacking. Often assistance is sought from children, extended family and friends. Caregivers, along with the patient, experience emotional distress from the stress of cancer treatment and the inability to maintain a 'normal' routine. Like their younger counterparts, older adults respond to cancer treatment, and with continued support can lead a fulfilling life.

CANCER SCREENING, EARLY DIAGNOSIS AND PREVENTION

Cancer screening refers to early testing in individuals with risk factors for cancer. For example, the Pap test is recommended for all females who have been sexually active. The ideal screening test is one that can detect cancer at an early stage (Table 4.6).

Table 4.6 Cancer screening.

Site	Recommendation
Breast	Mammography for women over 50 every 3 years
Colon and rectum	Beginning at age 60-69: faecal occult blood test every 2 years
Uterus	Cervix: all women aged 25-64 should have a smear test every 3-5 years depending on age

Adapted from the National Screening Committee (2010): http://www.screening.nhs.uk/england

Early diagnosis is the detection of cancer at an early stage. Early detection can occur as a result of an appropriate screening test or through public education on warning signs for cancer. Early diagnosis, like screening, is especially important if the treatment of early forms of cancer produces better survival and treatment outcomes. See Box 4.1 for non-specific warning signs of cancer.

Prevention of cancer can be achieved by removing known causes of cancer. For many, cancer prevention involves a lifestyle change or a change in behaviour that is known to increase cancer risks.

Box 4.1

Non-specific warning signs of cancer

- Change in bowel or bladder habits
- A sore that does not heal
- Unusual bleeding or discharge
- Thickening or lump in the breast or any other part of the body
- Indigestion or difficulty swallowing
- An obvious change in a wart or mole
- A nagging cough or hoarseness

Resources

MacMillan Cancer Support: *http://www.macmillan.org.uk/Cancerinformation/Cancertypes*

NHS: *www.nhs.uk/conditions*

National Institute of Clinical Excellence (NICE): *http://www.nice.org.uk/*

World Health Organization: *www.who.org*

 Prevention PLUS!

Guidelines on nutrition and physical activity for cancer prevention

Eat a variety of healthful foods, with an emphasis on plant sources:

- Eat five or more servings of vegetables and fruit each day
- Choose whole grains in preference to processed (refined) grains and sugars
- Limit consumption of red meats, especially high fat and processed meats
- Choose foods that help maintain a healthful weight.

Adopt a physically active lifestyle:

- Adults: engage in at least moderate activity for 30 minutes or more on 5 or more days of the week; 45 minutes or more of moderate to rigorous activity on 5 or more days per week may further enhance reductions in the risk of breast and colon cancer
- Children and adolescents: engage in at least 60 minutes per day of moderate to vigorous physical activity at least 5 days per week.

Maintain a healthful weight throughout life:

- Balance caloric intake with physical activity
- Lose weight if currently overweight or obese.

If you drink alcoholic beverages, limit consumption.

DISEASES AT A GLANCE Cancer

DISEASE	AETIOLOGY	SIGNS AND SYMPTOMS	DIAGNOSIS	TREATMENT	PREVENTION	LIFESPAN
Lung cancer						
Non-small cell lung cancer	Cigarette smoke, radon, industrial asbestos	Cough, wheezing, stridor, dysphagia, blood in sputum, chest pain, loss of appetite	Chest X-ray, sputum analysis, bronchoscopy with biopsy, PET scan	Surgery, radiation therapy, chemotherapy	Good health, good hygiene, do not smoke	Incidence increases from age 40 to 70 years
Small cell lung cancer	Cigarette smoke	Cough, wheezing, stridor, dysphagia, blood in sputum, chest pain, loss of appetite	Chest X-ray, sputum analysis, bronchoscopy with biopsy, PET scan	Surgery, radiation therapy, chemotherapy	Good health, good hygiene, do not smoke	Incidence increases from age 40 to 70 years
Breast cancer	Age, female gender, genetics, overweight and obesity, postmenopausal hormone replacement therapy, physical inactivity, consumption of alcohol	Palpable lump on the breast, abnormality detected on a mammogram, thickening, swelling, distortion and tenderness of the breast, spontaneous discharge or ulceration of the nipples	Mammography, breast ultrasound, biopsy	Surgery (lumpectomy or mastectomy), radiation therapy, chemotherapy, hormone therapy	Regular breast cancer screening, good health with physical activity	Risk increases after the age of 40 years
Stomach cancer	Diet, inadequate intake of fresh fruits and vegetables, consumption of smoked or cured meats and fish, infection with the bacterium *Helicobacter pylori*	Mild pain in the upper abdomen, fatigue, loss of energy, decreased appetite	CT scan, MRI scan, biopsy	Surgery, radiation therapy and chemotherapy	Healthy eating with fresh fruits and vegetables, prompt treatment for infections caused by *Helicobacter pylori*	Incidence increases in person over the age of 60 years
Colorectal cancer	High consumption of fat, refined carbohydrates and animal protein, and low physical activity, genetics, including familial adenomatous polyposis and hereditary non-polyposis	Blood in stool, change in bowel habits, pain in the lower abdomen	Colonoscopy with biopsy	Surgery, radiation therapy and chemotherapy	Healthy eating, including consumption of fresh fruits and vegetables, limiting consumption of animal protein, genetic screening, regular screening examinations	Occurs more commonly in individuals aged 50 years and older
Liver cancer						
Hepatocellular carcinoma	Viral hepatitis B and C infections, ingestion of toxins	Abdominal pain, weight loss, abdominal swelling, ascites, hepatomegaly and jaundice	CT scan, ultrasound, biopsy	Surgery, radiation therapy and chemotherapy	Prompt treatment for viral infections, healthy eating	More common in adults, rarely occurs in childhood

DISEASES AT A GLANCE Cancer (continued)

DISEASE	AETIOLOGY	SIGNS AND SYMPTOMS	DIAGNOSIS	TREATMENT	PREVENTION	LIFESPAN
Female reproductive tract						
Cervical cancer	Human papilloma virus infections, high-risk sexual behaviour, early age at initiation of sexual activity	Usually asymptomatic	Pap test, colposcopy with biopsy	Precancerous changes are treated with cryosurgery or laser	Practise safe sex, use condoms to prevent infections	Second most common cancer in women; all women are at risk
Uterine cancer	Oral oestrogen therapy, no history of pregnancy, removal of the ovaries, history of obesity, diabetes or hypertension	Vaginal bleeding after menopause, dysuria, constipation and bloating	Endovaginal echography, hysteroscopy and biopsy	Abdominal hysterectomy, radiation therapy	Healthy lifestyle, regular cancer screening examinations	Occurs most commonly in women of middle age or older, with a peak incidence around 50–60 years
Ovarian	Family history, prior history of breast cancer, no history of pregnancy, polycystic ovary disease, pelvic inflammatory disease, endometriosis	Abdominal discomfort, bloating, abnormal vaginal bleeding, gastrointestinal or urinary symptoms	Abdominal or vaginal ultrasound, biopsy	Surgery, including a total abdominal hysterectomy, removal of the ovaries, appendectomy, removal of the pelvic lymph nodes and chemotherapy	Healthy lifestyle, treatment of polycystic ovary disease and pelvic inflammatory disease, especially in individuals with a prior family history of ovarian cancer	All women are at risk
Male reproductive tract						
Prostate	Diet high in saturated fat, age	Urinary symptoms, including hesitancy, frequency, dribbling, poor urine stream, blood in the urine, pain in the lower abdomen	Digital rectal examination, PSA test, ultrasound, biopsy	Surgery, radiation therapy, endocrine therapy	Exercise, diet low in saturated fats	Incidence and mortality increases with age; most cases occur in men aged 65 years or older
Cancer of the testes	History of undescended testes (cryptorchidism), family history of testicular cancer, prenatal exposure to exogenous oestrogen	Painless lump on the testicle	Biopsy, physical examination of the testicles	Surgery, radiation therapy and chemotherapy	Self-examination of testicle, annual cancer screening examination, surgical treatment of cryptorchidism	Can occur at all ages, risk is greatest in men during the third or fourth decades of life
Oesophageal cancer	Tobacco smoke, or chewing tobacco, consumption of alcohol, history of oesophagitis	Difficulty swallowing, pain with eating or drinking, weight loss, hoarseness of the voice	Biopsy, endoscopic ultrasound	Surgery, radiation therapy and chemotherapy	Do not smoke or chew tobacco, avoid excessive consumption of alcohol, treatment of reflux disease to prevent oesophagitis	More common in individuals over the age of 60 years

DISEASES AT A GLANCE Cancer (continued)

DISEASE	AETIOLOGY	SIGNS AND SYMPTOMS	DIAGNOSIS	TREATMENT	PREVENTION	LIFESPAN
Bladder cancer	Cigarette smoke, exposure to industrial chemicals such as rubber, aromatic hydrocarbons, asbestos and solvents, infections with *Schistosoma haematobium*	Haematuria, increased urinary frequency	Ultrasound, biopsy	Surgery, radiation therapy and chemotherapy	Do not smoke tobacco, avoid exposure to industrial chemicals	Occurs more frequently in adults over the age of 65 years
Head and neck cancer	Tobacco smoking and excessive alcohol consumption	Oral pain, bleeding, difficulty opening the mouth, chewing, swallowing and talking, pain in the neck	Endoscopic examination, biopsy	Surgery, radiation therapy and chemotherapy	Do not smoke tobacco, limit consumption of alcohol	Occurs more commonly in males aged 65 years or older
Lymphoma						
Hodgkin's disease	Infection with Epstein-Barr virus, human immunodeficiency virus	Painless swelling of the lymph nodes in the neck, armpit or groin	Microscopic examination of lymph tissue, presence of Reed-Sternberg cells, X-ray, CT scan, MRI, bone marrow sampling and lymphograms	Chemotherapy, radiation, bone marrow transplantation	Treatment of Epstein-Barr virus, safe sex practices to prevent infection with human immunodeficiency virus	Often occurs in young adults
Non-Hodgkin's lymphoma	HIV/AIDS viral infections with HTLV1 and EBV	Painless swelling of the lymph nodes in the neck, armpit or groin	Microscopic examination of lymph tissue, X-ray, CT scan, MRI, bone marrow sampling and lymphograms	Chemotherapy, radiation, bone marrow transplantation	Safe sex to prevent infection with HIV	Often occurs in young adults
Leukaemia	Unknown	Fatigue, weight loss, repeated infections, fever, easy bruising, nosebleeds and haemorrhages	Blood tests, bone marrow biopsy	Chemotherapy, bone marrow transplantation	Unknown	Diagnosed 10 times more often in adults; also occurs in children
Pancreatic cancer	Tobacco smoke, diet low in fibre, high in consumption of red meat	Weight loss, nausea, diarrhoea, weakness, jaundice and upper abdominal pain	Ultrasound, CT scanning, biopsy	Surgery and chemotherapy	Do not smoke tobacco	Common in individuals older than 65 years of age
Melanoma	Fair skin, sensitivity to sunlight, exposure to industrial chemicals	Appearance of a mole-like growth that increases in size and changes in colour	Skin examination, biopsy	Surgery, radiation therapy	Use of sunscreen, avoidance exposure to sunlight in susceptible individuals	Can occur at any age
Thyroid cancer	Exposure to radiation, iodine deficiency, radioactive iodine exposure	Palpable thyroid nodule, hoarseness, dyspepsia, dysphagia	Physical examination, biopsy	Surgery, radiation therapy and chemotherapy	Eat salt fortified with iodine, regular examinations following high radiation exposure	Can occur at any age

DISEASES AT A GLANCE Cancer (continued)

DISEASE	AETIOLOGY	SIGNS AND SYMPTOMS	DIAGNOSIS	TREATMENT	PREVENTION	LIFESPAN
Kidney cancer						
Renal carcinoma	Cigarette smoking, obesity, greater risk among dry cleaning workers, leather tanner and shoe workers, exposure to asbestos	Haematuria, lower back pain, palpable kidney mass, hypertension, fever, anaemia or erythrocytosis	Urine test, intravenous pyelogram, ultrasound, CT scan, biopsy	Surgery, radiation therapy, chemotherapy, immune modifiers	Do not smoke tobacco, physical examination for high risk individuals	Renal carcinoma occurs primarily in adults; Wilms' tumour occurs primarily in children
Wilms' tumour	Unknown	Swelling, palpable mass, moderate to severe pain	Urine test, intravenous pyelogram, ultrasound, CT scan, biopsy	Surgery, radiation therapy, chemotherapy, immune modifiers	Unknown	Paediatric cancer occurs between the ages of birth and 14 years
Cancer of the central nervous system						
Malignant glioma	Radiation therapy, prior history of leukaemia	Paresis, speech disturbance, seizures, headaches	CT scan, MRI, EEG, biopsy	Surgery, radiation therapy, chemotherapy, corticosteroid medication	Unknown	Incidence peaks between ages 60 and 70 years of age
Medulloblastoma	Defects in cell cycle control originating in fetal development	Headache, nausea, vomiting, blurred vision, dizziness, difficulty handling objects	CT scan, MRI, EEG, biopsy	Surgery, radiation therapy, chemotherapy, corticosteroid medication	Unknown	Incidence peaks between 3 and 12 years of age
Cancer of the sympathetic nervous system						
Neuroblastoma	Unknown	Lump or swelling of the abdomen	CT scan, biopsy	Surgery, radiation therapy and chemotherapy	Unknown	Paediatric cancer occurs between the ages of birth and 14 years
Sarcoma						
Rhabdomyosarcoma	Unknown	Tumour of red muscle, pain in the area of the tumour	CT scan, biopsy	Surgery, chemotherapy and radiation therapy	Unknown	Paediatric cancer occurs prior to the age of 20 years
Osteosarcoma	Unknown	Bone pain	CT scan, biopsy	Surgery, chemotherapy and radiation therapy	Unknown	Paediatric cancer occurs prior to the age of 20 years
Ewing sarcoma	Unknown	Bone pain commonly felt in the extremities	CT scan, biopsy	Surgery, chemotherapy and radiation therapy	Unknown	Paediatric cancer occurs prior to the age of 20 years

INTERACTIVE EXERCISES

Cases for critical thinking

1. A 45-year-old man presents to his GP with a persistent productive cough. He has recently missed a week of work due to fever, weakness and hoarseness. What diagnostic procedures should be used to rule out lung cancer? What type of historical information is needed to diagnose lung cancer?

2. A 30-year-old woman has recently noticed a lump in her breast. She has never been pregnant, and she has noticed a discharge from her left nipple. Describe some of the risk factors and diagnostic tests for breast cancer. What are the most definitive tests for the diagnosis of breast cancer?

Multiple choice

1. Which of the following does not control cell growth?

a. growth inhibitors   b. cell cycle proteins
c. mutation   d. apoptosis

2. _____ are(is) responsible for repairing errors in DNA replication.

a. oncogenes
b. tumour suppressor gene
c. DNA repair genes
d. apoptosis

3. _____ is(are) the major cause of lung cancer worldwide.

a. tobacco use
b. industrial chemicals
c. radiation
d. chronic infections

4. Inherited mutations, including familial adenomatous polyposis and hereditary non-polyposis, are non-modifiable risk factors for _____ cancer.

a. lung   b. liver
c. stomach   d. colorectal

5. Molecular and epidemiological studies have linked the human papilloma virus to _____ cancer.

a. breast   b. cervical
c. uterine   d. ovarian

6. The most important risk factor for the development of prostate cancer is

_____

a. diet high in saturated fat
b. age (greater than 65 years)
c. hormones
d. enlargement of the prostate

7. Malignant tumours in the testes originate from _____ cells.

a. seminoma   b. epithelial
c. squamous   d. germ

8. The most important risk factor for bladder cancer is _____

a. human papillomavirus
b. infection
c. cigarette smoking
d. exposure to environmental chemicals

9. Hodgkin's disease is distinguished from non-Hodgkin's lymphoma by the presence of _____ cells.

a. squamous   b. Reed–Sternberg
c. epithelial   d. lymphoid

10. Leukaemia is diagnosed _____ times more often in children than in adults.

a. 2   b. 4
c. 8   d. 10

True or false

_____ **1.** Lymphoma is characterised by massive proliferation of white blood cells in plasma.

_____ **2.** The diagnosis of pancreatic cancer is rarely made during early stages of the disease.

_____ **3.** Risk factors for the development of melanoma include sensitivity to sunlight, extent of sun exposure and exposure to industrial chemicals.

_____ **4.** Kidney cancer is more common in cigarette smokers than in non-smokers.

_____ **5.** Wilms' tumour is a malignant tumour that occurs in childhood.

_____ **6.** Neuroblastoma is a central nervous system tumour.

_____ **7.** Cancer is primarily a genetic disease.

_____ **8.** A mutation is an inherited form of a normal gene.

_____ **9.** Oncogenes normally regulate cell growth, differentiation and cell death.

_____ **10.** Exposure to asbestos increases the risk for mesothelioma.

Fill-ins

1. _____ is the most significant source of ultraviolet radiation.

2. Chronic infections with _____ and _____ viral infections have been linked to liver cancer.

3. Solid tumours can often be removed with _____.

4. The infectious bacterium _____ is a risk factor for stomach cancer.

5. _____ carcinoma accounts for more than 80% of all primary cancers in the liver.

6. Precancerous lesions on the cervix can be readily detected by the _____ test.

7. Neoplasms of lymphoid tissue are referred to as _____ .

8. A melanoma is a proliferation of _____ or pigment-producing cells.

9. Iodine deficiency is a risk factor for _____ cancer.

10. The majority of adult tumours in the central nervous system are derived from _____ cells.

Labelling exercise

Use the blank lines below to label the following photos.

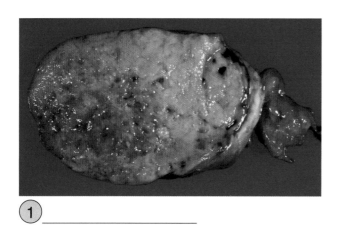

1 _____

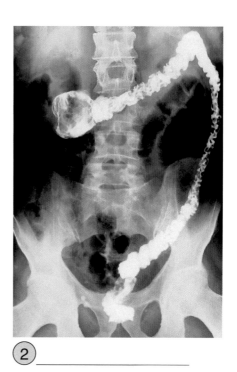

2 _____

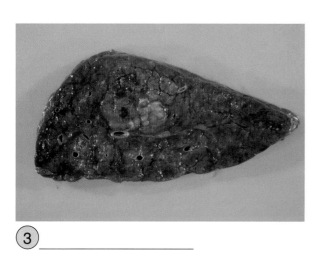

3 _____

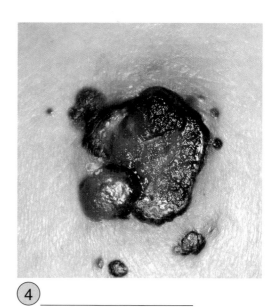

4 _____

5 GENETICS AND DISEASE

Spleen tissue in sickle cell anaemia.
(Courtesy of C. James Sung/BioMed Pathology and
Laboratory Medicine, Brown University)

Fact or fiction ?

Familial hypercholesterolaemia,
a disorder in which a person has
very high blood cholesterol, can
be inherited.

Fact: Five types of hypercholesterolaemia are known and all
can be inherited; a common form is
an autosomal dominant disorder.

Learning objectives

After studying this chapter, you should be able to:

✚ Describe DNA's unique composition and its role in heredity

✚ Describe mechanisms of transmission of hereditary diseases and give examples

✚ Explain genetic diseases based on abnormal chromosome construction

✚ Describe genetic diseases involving anomalies and numbers in the sex chromosomes

✚ Compare and contrast congenital diseases and hereditary disorders

✚ Discuss the concept of gene therapy

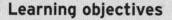

Disease chronicle

Then and now: Marfan syndrome

Some say that President Abraham Lincoln had a hereditary disease called Marfan syndrome, which today affects 1 in 10 000 people. President Lincoln exhibited key traits associated with Marfan, including a tall stature with a slender skeleton, long fingers, and a long, narrow face. Marfan also causes an abnormally shaped chest, loose joints and weak ligaments, which results in abnormal curvature of the spine. Weakened connective tissue in the walls of large arteries leads to aortic aneurysms. With ageing, or in demanding situations, the heart and other organs fail.

INTRODUCTION

DNA, which stands for **deoxyribonucleic acid**, is the blueprint for directing all cell activities and especially protein synthesis within the cell. DNA is a double helix similar in shape to a spiral staircase. It is made of four chemical bases, pairs of which form the 'rungs' of the DNA molecule. All **genes** are made from segments of these four bases, arranged in different orders and in different lengths (Figure 5.1).

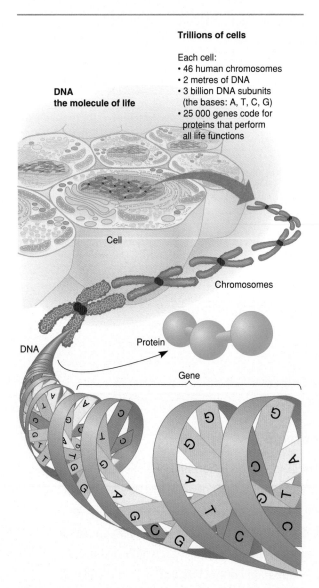

Figure 5.1 Each cell nucleus throughout the body contains the genes, DNA and chromosomes that make up the majority of an individual's genome.

Within the nucleus of cells, the DNA is assembled into stranded units called **chromosomes**, which must be copied during cell division and distributed to the resulting daughter cells. DNA has the unique ability to replicate itself and code for its partner RNA (ribonucleic acid). The coordination of these two allies will direct the programme for hereditary and metabolic activities. Within each primary sex organ (ovary or testis), 'parent' sex cells contain 46 chromosomes and divide by a process called meiosis (Figure 5.2) to produce gametes (egg and sperm) that contain 23 chromosomes each. Egg and sperm unite during fertilisation; therefore, each human cell contains 46 chromosomes in 23 pairs.

The chromosomes contain thousands of genes, each of which is responsible for the synthesis of a particular protein. Forty-four of the chromosomes are called **autosomes**. These are paired and numbered 1–22 and they are referred to by the chromosome number. The remaining two are called the X and Y (or sex) chromosomes. A male has a combination of one X and one Y chromosome, and a female has two X chromosomes. The complete chromosomal composition of the nucleus is called the **karyotype** of the cell. The karyotype can be visualised by extracting the chromosomes from the nucleus and photographing them under a microscope. In this way, abnormalities in number or structure of the chromosomes can be detected (Figure 5.3).

The Human Genome Project (HGP) goals were to identify all of the approximately 30 000 genes in human DNA, determine the sequences of the 3 billion chemical base pairs that make up human DNA, and store this information in databases.

The full DNA sequence was completed and published in April 2003. Upon publication of the majority of the genome in February 2001, Francis Collins, the director of the National Human Genome Research Institute, noted that the genome could be thought of in terms of a book with multiple uses. 'It's a history book – a narrative of the journey of our species through time. It's a shop manual, with an incredibly detailed blueprint for building every human cell. And it's a transformative textbook of medicine, with insights that will give health-care providers immense new powers to treat, prevent,

(3) Meiosis II

(2) Meiosis I

(1) Interphase

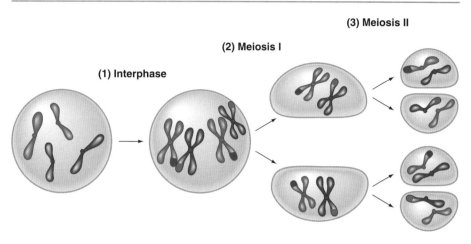

Figure 5.2 Meiosis involves two complete divisional operations forming four potential sex cells.

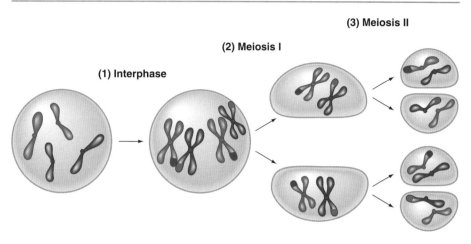

Figure 5.3 Human karyotype.
(© Custom Medical Stock Photo)

and cure diseases.' Genes, chromosomes and other causes for selected hereditary diseases have been located and are listed in the Diseases at a Glance table at the end of the chapter; a complete list can be found at *www.ncbi.nlm.nih.gov*.

The genes for a particular trait, such as eye colour, hair colour and hair type, occupy a particular site on a chromosome. Each person has two sites or two copies of each gene, one copy from each parent. **Alleles** are alternative forms of a gene. If the pair of alleles is similar (hh, HH), the person is **homozygous** for that trait. If the alleles are different (Hh), one for dark and one for light hair, for example, the person is **heterozygous**. Some alleles always produce their trait when inherited and are said to be **dominant**. The result of the dominant allele is the same whether a person is homozygous or heterozygous. The allele for brown eyes, for example, is dominant to that for blue eyes. Other alleles are **recessive** and only manifest themselves when the person is homozygous for the trait. This combination is significant in many hereditary diseases.

Certain factors may cause a deviation from the basic principles of inheritance that have been described. Some alleles are co-dominant, so that when both are inherited, both traits are expressed. An example of co-dominant alleles is found in blood type AB. The allele for the A factor is inherited from one parent and that for the B factor from the other, but both alleles are expressed. At times, a dominant allele is not fully expressed, a condition known as *reduced penetrance*. Various factors modify the expression of genes, including other genes, environmental conditions and gender. One example of a reduced penetrance trait is syndactly, which results in varying degrees of webbing in fingers or toes. Polydactyly is another dominant trait that will be described later in the chapter.

TRANSMISSION OF HEREDITARY DISEASES

Many of the diseases described throughout this book are called *hereditary* or *familial diseases*. Hereditary diseases or disorders are generally the result of metabolic breakdown caused by a lack of direction from a missing or compromised gene or chromosomal segment. Often the gene responsible for the production of a particular protein (e.g. enzyme or structural protein) is missing or defective, and that interrupts the chain of events required to ensure proper metabolic activities. For example, haemochromatosis is more common in Caucasian populations, occurring in 1 in 300 to 1 in 400 people. This defect is a recessive trait and stems from the body's unusual ability to absorb extra iron.

Further explanation of the mechanism of transmission will now be explored. Some diseases are caused by inheriting a single autosomal dominant allele. One such defective gene on chromosome 4 causes Huntington's disease, a disease described in Chapter 13, and another causes polydactyly, explained in the next section. Other diseases are caused by inherited autosomal recessive alleles. In this case, expression of the disease occurs only when that particular allele is inherited from each parent, making the person homozygous for that trait. Cystic fibrosis, described later in this chapter, is such a disease. A third type of inheritance is sex-linked, in which the defective allele is located on the X chromosome. Red–green colour blindness and haemophilia are examples of sex-linked inherited diseases and are explained later in this chapter. Sometimes a genetic disorder may be caused by several different genes, which is known as polygenic inheritance; for example, in polycystic kidney disease. Some genetic diseases may vary in their pattern of inheritance across the lifespan; for example, they could be inherited recessively or dominantly. Sometimes genetics may not be the only cause of a disease; for example, only 5–10% of cases of breast cancer run in families with a genetic predisposition. The remaining cases are linked to lifestyle and the causes are referred to as environmental factors.

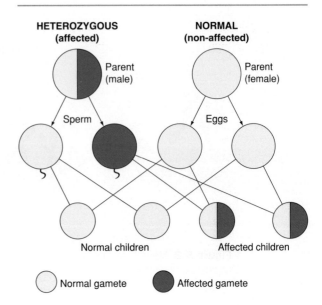

Figure 5.4 Transmission of autosomal dominant disorders (50% chance for an affected child).

Autosomal dominant

A defective dominant allele is usually transmitted from a parent who is heterozygous for the trait. If the other parent is normal for the particular condition, each child has a 50% chance of being affected and manifesting the genetic defect. This is illustrated in Figure 5.4. The disease appears in every generation, with males and females being equally affected. Exceptions to the rule are few.

Polydactyly (extra fingers or toes) is an example of an autosomal dominant disorder, or it may occur on its own. A boy or girl inheriting the defective allele from either parent will have the abnormality. Polydactyly is apparent at birth but is not a major disorder and may be surgically corrected; however, it may occur in conjunction with other genetic disorders.

Achondroplasia is another disorder resulting from one defective dominant allele (Figure 5.5). In this disease, cartilage formation in the fetus is abnormal. Normally, the fetal skeleton first forms as cartilage and is gradually replaced by bone in a process known as ossification. In achondroplasia, the defective cartilage formation results in improper bone development and **achondroplastic dwarfism**.

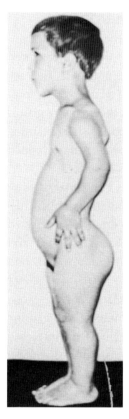 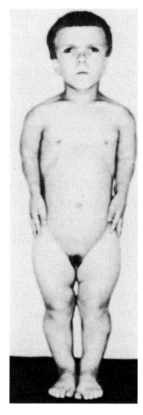

Figure 5.5 A 12-year-old achondroplastic dwarf. (Note the disproportion of the limbs to the trunk, the curvature of the spine and the prominent buttocks.)

The long bones of the arms and legs are short, the trunk of the body is normal in size, the head is large and the forehead is very prominent. The person has normal intelligence, develops sexually, and is muscular and agile.

Marfan syndrome results from the dysfunction of the gene that normally codes for the connective tissue protein fibrillin. Fibrillin is essential for the maintenance of connective tissue in various organs, including tendons, heart valves and blood vessels. Tendons and blood vessel walls with abnormal connective tissue become loose and cannot support normal body functions. As connective tissue is widespread in the body, Marfan syndrome is a multi-systemic disease affecting about 1 in 10 000 people. Blood tests support the diagnosis, by finding a lack of fibrillin. This protein deficiency causes skeletal changes, dilatation of the aorta, floppy heart valves

and ocular changes, including lens displacement, retinal detachment and blindness.

There is no cure for Marfan syndrome; treatment is supportive, aiming to detect changes early to allow treatment to occur sooner rather than later. Annual visual examination, plus echocardiograms and heart valve or vessel replacement, are standard procedures. Usually the disease onset is by age 20, and death is most often caused by heart failure or ruptured aortic aneurysm (vessel weakness).

Familial hypercholesterolaemia (FH) affects 1 in 500 of the population and is a common cause of cardiovascular disease in this country. Frequently, familial hypercholesterolaemia is caused by a mutation in the gene encoding the receptor for low density lipoprotein (LDL). Blood screening confirms the increase of LDLs, which transport approximately 70% of the total blood cholesterol and are the principal carriers for the removal of cholesterol from the blood. The receptor deficiency in patients with familial hypercholesterolaemia causes LDL cholesterol to be removed by a less efficient receptor-independent mechanism. Inefficient cholesterol removal results in hypercholesterolaemia and the deposition of lipids in the arteries. This inefficiency results in accelerated atherosclerosis (plaque build-up) and increased incidence of coronary heart disease. In this case, the progression of familial hypercholesterolaemia can be slowed by exercise, a low fat diet and drugs (statins) that block uptake of cholesterol in blood vessels.

As this disease is actually caused by an **incomplete dominant** gene activity, it results in different outcomes. If the genes are both mutated (homozygous) in favour of hypercholesterol, then the person succumbs as a child. If one gene is normal and one mutated (heterozygous), then death could occur later as a young or middle-aged adult, depending upon lifestyle and other risk factors.

Autosomal recessive

Autosomal recessive diseases manifest themselves only when a person is homozygous for the defective allele. Two parents who are both carriers of the recessive allele are themselves heterozygous for the trait

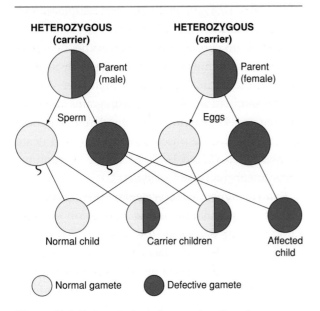

HETEROZYGOUS
(carrier)

HETEROZYGOUS
(carrier)

Parent
(male)

Parent
(female)

Sperm

Eggs

Normal child

Carrier children

Affected
child

○ Normal gamete ● Defective gamete

Figure 5.6 Transmission of recessive disorders (25% chance for an affected child).

but do not have the disease. Each of their children has a 25% chance of inheriting two recessive alleles and the disease. This potential probability is shown in Figure 5.6. The chance for inheriting two recessive alleles increases in close intermarriage. Cystic fibrosis is a single gene autosomal recessive disease affecting the respiratory and digestive systems. The **exocrine glands** of the body secrete a viscous type of mucus excessively which blocks gland ducts and prevents the glands from delivering their products. Exocrine glands are common glands that secrete mucus, wax, perspiration and digestive enzymes.

The most serious manifestation of cystic fibrosis is in the respiratory system. The trachea and bronchi secrete thick mucus that accumulates and blocks the airway. Symptoms of cystic fibrosis are **dyspnoea** (laboured breathing), wheezing, persistent cough and thick sputum. The abnormally thick mucosal surface increases susceptibility to recurrent bacterial infections. Bronchiectasis (weakened and dilated bronchial tubing) is a common complication of cystic fibrosis. Bronchiectasis is not a disease but a sequela or residual effect of chronic inflammation and congestion. Lung collapse can result from the inability to inflate the lungs, and most deaths caused by CF involve younger adults and occur as a result of

respiratory failure. Table 8.2 (see page 163) describes the complications of cystic fibrosis.

Excessive mucus also blocks the ducts of the pancreas, preventing the release of digestive enzymes, resulting in weight loss and malnutrition. The lack of proper fat digestion results in a large, bulky, foul-smelling stool. In the pancreas, the secretory glands become dilated and develop into cysts containing thick mucus. Fibrous tissue then develops, which explains how cystic fibrosis gets its name.

Cystic fibrosis is recognised as a hereditary disease that first manifests in young children. Before the disease was understood, the mortality rate in affected children was extremely high. Early diagnosis and treatment has greatly improved the prognosis and longevity.

In cystic fibrosis, the sweat glands excrete excessive perspiration and large amounts of salt, causing susceptibility to heat exhaustion. This increased excretion of salt in sweat is the basis for a 'sweat test' that helps to confirm cystic fibrosis.

Basic treatment includes pancreatic enzyme supplements that can be given with food. Antibiotic treatment reduces the incidence of respiratory tract infection, and regular respiratory physiotherapy and medications relieves congestion in the respiratory tract.

Phenylketonuria (PKU) is an inborn error of metabolism caused by an autosomal recessive allele. Persons with PKU lack a specific enzyme that converts one amino acid, phenylalanine, to another, tyrosine. This mechanism is illustrated in Figure 5.7. As a result, high levels of phenylalanine and its derivatives build up in the blood and are toxic to the brain, interfering with normal brain development. PKU must be diagnosed and treated very early or severe learning difficulties results. Physical development proceeds normally, but the child is very light in colour, somewhat similar to albinism. Production of the pigment melanin is impaired because of inadequate tyrosine, a result of the missing enzyme. The child may manifest disorders of the nervous system, such as a lack of balance, tremors and hyperactivity, and may suffer fits. PKU frequency varies widely around the globe. In Europe it occurs in about 1 in 10 000 people.

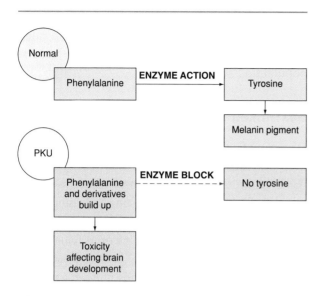

Figure 5.7 Enzyme block in phenylketonuria (PKU).

To prevent the serious learning difficulties that accompany PKU, newborn babies are screened by a blood test using a heel prick or Guthrie test for the defective gene or metabolic pathway. When the trait is found, a synthetic diet is prescribed that greatly reduces or eliminates phenylalanine. Good results have been achieved with this treatment. However, the diet is unpleasant and controversy exists as to the length of time for which the diet must be maintained. Beginning treatment immediately and continuing during the earliest years of life seems to be the most critical factor in preventing learning difficulties. Some soft drink and food labels alert consumers to the presence or lack of phenylalanine.

Sickle cell anaemia is a severe anaemia generally confined to the Afro-Caribbean population, who carry the sickle cell trait at a ratio of 1 per 12 individuals. Sickle cell anaemia is an autosomal recessive disorder in which the haemoglobin (a protein molecule) is abnormal, resulting in deformed red blood cells. The improperly formed cells may become lodged in capillaries and block circulation, causing infarcts, pain and necrosis (death of tissues). The sickle-shaped red blood cells rupture easily and are primarily removed from the circulation by the spleen. The depletion of red blood cells results in severe anaemia.

The person with sickle cell anaemia is homozygous, having inherited one altered allele from each parent. A person who is heterozygous has both normal and abnormal haemoglobin and possesses the **sickle cell trait**. The heterozygous person is mildly anaemic, but the one defective allele provides an advantage because sickle cell trait confers increased resistance to malaria, which kills about 2 million persons per year, many of whom are children. See Chapter 7 for more information on this disease.

Thalassaemia is a condition which is more common in the Mediterranean, Middle East and some Asian populations. It is an autosomal recessive condition in which the globin chains in haemoglobin are either absent or produced in reduced amounts. α-Thalassaemia is associated with absent or reduced production of α-globin chains. When there are no chains produced, death occurs in utero or soon after in a condition known as hydrops fetalis. Those with reduced chains suffer from a varying degree of anaemia as the erythrocytes undergo haemolysis. In contrast, those with β-thalassaemia have deficiency of the β chains; this is more common in the Greek and Cypriot populations. More severe deficiency is referred to as thalassaemia major, which presents with early anaemia that requires treatment with blood transfusion. Due to hyperplasia of the bone marrow, the bones of those affected can lead to altered appearance, particularly in the face, which has a more prominent forehead. Those with thalassaemia minor are heterozygotes, and are sometimes referred to as having thalassaemia trait. Although they lack symptoms, they may still suffer from a milder anaemia. Screening for thalassaemia is possible during pregnancy to detect if the baby will be born with this disease.

Tay-Sachs is an autosomal recessive condition that primarily affects families of Eastern Jewish origin; occurrence is approximately 1 in 3600 of the affected Ashkenazi (Jewish) community. Tay–Sachs is caused by the absence of the enzyme hexosaminidase A (Hex-A). Without Hex-A, a lipid called GM2 ganglioside accumulates in cells, especially nerve cells of the brain. The result is progressive learning difficulties and physical regression. Symptoms appear by 6 months of age when no new skills are learned, fits occur and blindness develops. A cherry-red spot may be seen on each retina. Children usually die between 2 and 4 years of age. No cure exists, and treatment is aimed at relieving symptoms. Prevention may require genetic counselling and testing.

There are two tests available to determine if someone is a carrier of Tay–Sachs. The initial test uses an enzyme assay to measure the level of Hex-A in blood: a lower Hex-A quantity would indicate a carrier status, as carriers have less Hex-A than non-carriers. Next, a DNA-based carrier test looks for specific mutations in the gene that codes for Hex-A. Some carriers may not be identified by DNA analysis alone because not all known mutations in the Hex-A gene are detected by the test. Other mutations responsible for the disease have yet to be identified.

Albinism is an autosomal recessive disorder that is easily recognised. There are two types of albinism, oculocutaneous albinism which affects the skin, hair and eyes, and ocular albinism, which affects the eyes only. People with albinism have an increased risk for skin cancer and exhibit visual problems such as nearsightedness and abnormally high sensitivity to light. Even on cloudy or overcast days, albinos may wear sunglasses, wide-brimmed hats and full-length clothing or use umbrellas to reduce exposure. The occurrence of albinism is rare in the general population.

Sex-linked inheritance

Diseases of sex-linked inheritance generally result from defective genes on the X chromosome, because the Y chromosome is small and carries very few genes. Because a male has only one X chromosome, if he inherits a defective recessive gene found on the X chromosome, that trait is expressed. A female may be heterozygous for the gene, having a defective recessive allele on one X chromosome but a normal allele on the other X. In that case, the female carries the disease and she has a 50% chance of transmitting the allele to her sons and daughters. A male transmits the disease only to his daughters. His sons are unaffected, because the Y chromosome is normal and fathers contribute only the Y chromosome to males. This linkage is illustrated in Figure 5.8. Thus, the abnormalities of **sex-linked inheritance** tend to occur more frequently in males, but are transmitted

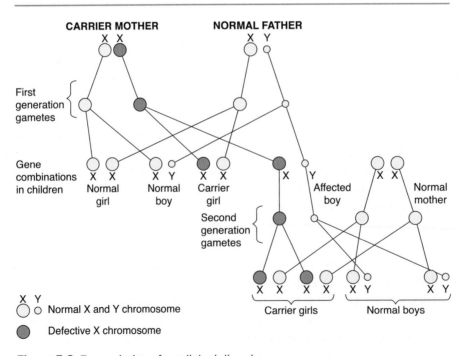

Figure 5.8 Transmission of sex-linked disorders.

by females. It is far less common for a female to inherit a sex-linked disease because she must inherit two defective X chromosomes. Duchenne's muscular dystrophy is an X-linked recessive disease that is discussed in Chapter 15.

Colour blindness Red–green colour blindness, the inability to distinguish between certain colours, is a disorder of sex-linked inheritance. The defect that causes colour blindness is apparently in certain specialised receptors of the retina called *cones*. Three types of receptors are stimulated by wavelengths of the primary colours: red, green and blue. Impulses are then sent to the brain and interpreted. Diagnosis is made when the colour-blind person is most frequently unable to distinguish reds and greens. Corrective lenses are available that may offer some treatment for red–green colour blindness. This condition is rare in women but occurs in about 1 in 10 men.

Haemophilia People with haemophilia do not bleed more profusely or bleed faster than normal; they bleed for a longer period of time. Factor VIII, an intrinsic clotting factor, is usually inactive in people with haemophilia. Diagnosis results from suspected bleeding episodes or family history. Beyond treatment with clotting factors (VIII) and blood transfusions, there have been significant advances in treating haemophilia in the past decade. A new genetically engineered clotting protein is now used for treatment of some types of haemophilia. Research is also under way to develop gene therapy for the disease. The therapy will replace the missing or deficient gene with one that has the instructions for producing the clotting factor. Gene therapy has been successful in treating mice with haemophilia B, and a procedure for it will be described toward the end of this chapter.

Fragile X syndrome This is a genetic condition associated with learning difficulties. It is identified by thin, thread-like strands on the long arm of the X chromosome. This weakened area is more subject to breakage (thus the term *fragile* is used), and because this abnormality is associated with a sex chromosome, it is referred to as X-linked. Mothers are the carriers and their sons are at risk of being affected, whereas daughters are at risk of being carriers and are sometimes mildly affected. The prevalence of fragile X is approximately 1 in 1250 males (compared with 1 of 2500 females), and the prevalence of carriers in the population is 1 in 600. Fragile X is the most commonly inherited cause of learning difficulty known, accounting for up to 10% of cases. Fragile X is diagnosed by DNA testing, and the gene responsible for the condition has been identified as *FMR-1* (denoting fragile X mental retardation gene).

About 80% of boys with fragile X have mental impairment ranging from severe learning difficulties to low–normal intelligence. The majority of patients are mildly to moderately impaired. Men and boys with fragile X are usually socially engaging, but they have an unusual style of interacting. They tend to avoid direct eye contact during conversation, and hand-flapping or hand-biting is common. They may have an unusual speech pattern characterised by a fast and fluctuating rate of repetitions of sound, words or phrases. They may also have a decreased attention span, hyperactivity and motor delays. Girls are much less affected because they have two X chromosomes, and estimates are that about 30% with the condition have some degree of learning difficulty. The physical features, including a long, narrow face and protruding ears, are much more subtle in females.

There is no cure for fragile X syndrome, but medical intervention can improve the problems related to attention and hyperactivity. A variety of medications can treat attention span, hyperactivity and other behaviour problems. In addition, speech and physiotherapy as well as vocational training can be beneficial.

Familial diseases Some diseases appear in families, but the means of inheritance is not understood. Examples of diseases with a higher incidence in certain families are epilepsy, diabetes, cardiovascular problems and allergies. The cause of these diseases does not seem to be a single gene but the effect of several genes working together, known as a **multifactorial** trait. In fact, some familial diseases may not be inherited at all but instead result from unique environmental conditions or behaviours that are shared by family members.

ABNORMAL CHROMOSOME DISEASES

The hereditary diseases described to this point result from a defective gene. Abnormalities in the chromosomes, either in their number or structure, also cause disorders. At times, chromosomes fail to separate properly during cell division, causing one daughter cell to be deficient and one to have an extra chromosome. The loss of an autosomal chromosome is usually incompatible with life because each autosome contains a large number of essential genes. A fetus affected by this condition is generally spontaneously aborted. The loss of a sex chromosome or the presence of an extra one is less serious, but many abnormalities accompany the condition.

Down's syndrome

Down's syndrome is an example of a disorder caused by the presence of an extra autosomal chromosome. Chromosome 21 is inherited in triplicate, a condition called **trisomy 21**. The extra chromosome results from a **non-disjunction**, or the failure of two chromosomes to separate as the gametes, either the egg or the sperm, are being formed. Therefore, when an egg or sperm with a double chromosome 21 is fused with its counterpart at the time of fertilisation, a trisomy chromosome is formed. The incidence of Down's syndrome is about 1 in 1000 and is higher among children born to mothers over age 35. There are estimated to be approximately 60 000 individuals in the UK who have Down's syndrome.

The Down's syndrome child has a characteristic appearance (Figure 5.9). The eyes appear slanted because of an extra fold of skin at the upper, medial corner of the eye; the tongue is coarse and often protrudes; and the nose is short and flat. The child is usually of short stature and the sex organs are

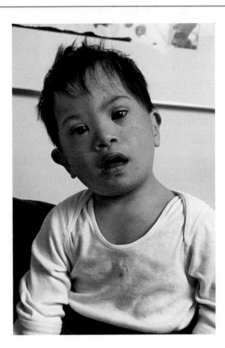

Figure 5.9 Boy with Down's syndrome.

underdeveloped. A straight crease extends across the palm of the hand, and the little finger is often shorter than normal.

The life expectancy of a child with Down's syndrome can be relatively short because of complications that may accompany the condition, such as congenital heart disease; however, the average life expectancy is between 50 and 60 years of age. In addition, there is a greater susceptibility to respiratory tract infections, including pneumonia, and a higher incidence of leukaemia among those with Down's syndrome.

The Down's syndrome child has learning difficulties to some degree. The excessive enzyme production from the extra genes may cause a toxic effect on the brain. The child can be taught simple tasks and is generally very affectionate. Today, compared to past years, the Down's syndrome individual may receive more exposure to special education and cooperative work opportunities.

Testing for Down's syndrome in pregnancy involves a test for four substances in the blood and is known as the quadruple test. If the test is positive for Down's syndrome, some women may choose to terminate the pregnancy.

Cri du chat syndrome

Cri du chat syndrome, or cat cry syndrome, is caused by a deletion of part of the short arm of chromosome 5 (5p15.2). The occurrence for this trait is 1 in 37 000 to 1 in 50 000. Infants with cri du chat syndrome have an abnormally small head with a deficiency in cerebral brain tissue. Those who are born alive have a weak, cat-like cry. The eyes are spaced far apart, and children with cri du chat syndrome exhibit learning difficulties. Treatment is supportive until the infant dies, usually in the first 5 or 6 years. Parents may seek genetic counselling and request a karyotype test to determine if one or both parents have a rearranged chromosome 5.

SEX ANOMALIES

Turner syndrome

One of the sex chromosomes is missing in **Turner syndrome**, resulting in a karyotype of 45 chromosomes, with only one X chromosome present. This is referred to as XO. The person appears to be female, but the ovaries do not develop; thus, there is neither ovulation nor menstruation, and the person is sterile. In physical appearance, the mammary nipples are widely spaced, the breasts do not develop and the person is short of stature and has a stocky build. Congenital heart disease, particularly coarctation of the aorta (described in Chapter 6), frequently accompanies Turner syndrome. Facial deformities are often present. Figure 5.10 shows a Turner syndrome karyotype. The occurrence for Turner syndrome is about 1 in 2000 live births.

Klinefelter's syndrome

An extra sex chromosome is present in **Klinefelter's syndrome**, resulting in a karyotype of 47XXY, indicating the presence of 47 chromosomes, including two X and one Y chromosomes. A fairly simple chromosome check will reveal the condition. The occurrence is about 1 in 500 to 1 in 1000 males. This person appears to be a male but has small testes that fail to mature and that produce no sperm.

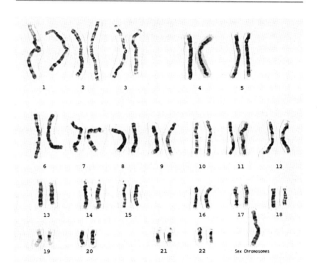

Figure 5.10 Karyotype for Turner syndrome (45XO). (Catherine G. Palmer, Indiana University)

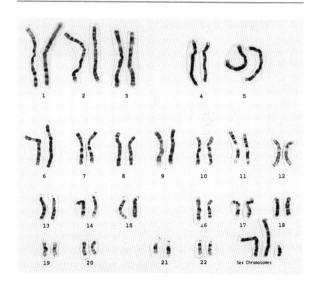

Figure 5.11 Karyotype for Klinefelter's syndrome (47XXY). (Catherine G. Palmer, Indiana University)

At puberty, with the development of secondary sex characteristics, the breasts enlarge and female distribution of hair develops. There is little facial hair, and the general appearance is that of an immature young adult. The person is tall and slender (with abnormally long legs), may have learning difficulties and is sterile (Figure 5.11).

Hermaphrodites

The number of true **hermaphrodites** who have both testes and ovaries is small. **Pseudohermaphrodites** do develop, and they have either testes or ovaries, usually non-functional, but the remainder of the anatomy is mixed. This condition is referred to as *sex reversal*, in which the chromosomal sex is different from the anatomical sex. Sex reversal occurs during fetal life. The sex glands are neutral during the first few weeks after conception, until the male gonads differentiate at about the sixth week under the influence of the male sex hormone (testosterone). In the absence of an adequate amount of this hormone, ovaries develop and the individual develops to be anatomically female but chromosomally male (XY).

Some cases of pseudohermaphroditism result from excessive production of sex hormones from the adrenal cortex. An affected female develops male secondary sexual characteristics at a very early age. The external genitalia of pseudohermaphrodites are ambiguous, resembling that of both males and females.

GENETIC COUNSELLING

A genetic counsellor usually begins with a complete family history of both prospective parents. A complete, detailed family history is called a *pedigree*. Pedigrees are used to determine the pattern of inheritance of a genetic disease within a family. When the pedigree is complete, the genetic counsellor can inform prospective parents of the possibility of having genetically abnormal offspring, and the parents can make an informed decision.

Diagnosis of genetic diseases

Early diagnosis is critical to prevention and treatment of genetic diseases. During **amniocentesis**, a small amount of amniotic fluid is withdrawn after the fourteenth week of pregnancy. Fetal cells in the amniotic fluid are removed, the chromosomes are examined and the amniotic fluid is analysed for biochemical abnormalities. Test results in amniocentesis are available approximately 2 weeks after the procedure. Amniocentesis can detect approximately 200 genetic diseases before birth.

Chorionic villi are projections of the membrane that surrounds the embryo in early pregnancy. **Chorionic villus sampling** involves removing cells from the villi through the cervix. Samples may be taken between 8 and 10 weeks of pregnancy. The chromosomes of the cells obtained can be analysed immediately. Chorionic villus sampling gives embryonic or fetal results (gender and chromosomal information) sooner within the pregnancy, allowing time for options, including termination of pregnancy or preparation for a child with special needs.

Gene therapy for genetic diseases

Gene therapy is a procedure that involves identification, manipulation and transference of genetic segments into a host to replace defective genes and to perform desired genetic activities. The genetic material used is compatible with human DNA that may be cultured in a microbe and delivered in a viral package or by injection. This sophisticated procedure is also referred to as genetic engineering.

Gene therapy has certain risks, but with continued improvement in techniques the future appears

 Prevention PLUS!

Spontaneous mutation

With spontaneous mutation, genetic diseases may not be preventable (e.g. Queen Victoria and the royal family lineage of haemophilia). However, with pedigree and DNA analysis and proper immunisations, many genetic disorders can be prevented.

brighter. So far, treatment for genetic diseases has progressed in three stages:

1. Donors supply deficient or defective proteins, because genes are responsible for making the necessary protein products required by all cells; in this case, the defective genes could be circumvented.
2. New DNA is made by recombinant manipulation (multiple contributors) to produce pure protein agents.
3. New/replacement genes are inserted into the proper (deficient or defective) location for corrective measures.

Gene therapy requires specific guidelines or protocols to be followed to qualify for clinical trials. Basically, clinical trials determine the future prospects of most new therapy agents. Development, funding and resources are necessary to ensure a successful research project.

A common form of gene delivery for gene therapy is the use of 'tamed' viruses in a carrier called a **vector**. The original virus is stripped of its deleterious impact and its shell is used as a biological vehicle to deliver the prescribed genetic material into the selected site.

Other applications use various physical and chemical means, such as microinjection with or without liposomes (fat bodies) to slip DNA, encased in fat, through the fat-soluble membrane. DNA is unable to penetrate or be absorbed through a cell membrane on its own.

A new approach for the future is called **picoarray gene synthesis**. This uses artificial genes synthesised on microchips and this advancement may pave the way for quicker and less costly genetic procedures. As stem cell research expands, so too will the new ways of treatment and prevention of many genetic conditions.

CONGENITAL DISEASES

Congenital diseases are those appearing at birth or shortly after, but they are not caused by genetic or chromosomal abnormalities. Congenital defects usually result from some failure in development during the embryonic stage (the first 2 months of pregnancy). *Therefore, congenital diseases cannot be transmitted to offspring.* The systems chapters in Part II of this book provide further discussion of selected congenital conditions.

Various factors – inadequate oxygen, maternal infection, drugs, malnutrition and radiation – can interfere with normal development. Rubella (German measles) contracted by the mother during the first trimester of pregnancy can produce serious birth defects. The rubella virus can cross the placental barrier and affect the central nervous system of the embryo, causing learning difficulties, blindness and deafness. Cerebral palsy and hydrocephalus can develop as a result of a viral infection. Cerebral palsy and learning difficulty may be the result of oxygen deprivation, such as when the umbilical cord gets squeezed or contorted and slows or shuts down blood flow to the fetus. Low oxygen may also be a factor in very high altitude environments.

Syphilis can be transmitted to a developing fetus and cause multiple anomalies: structural deformities, blindness, deafness and paralysis. Children with congenital syphilis may have future mental health problems. Syphilitic infection of a fetus frequently results in spontaneous abortion or stillbirth. A mother with syphilis should be treated for it before the fifth month of pregnancy to prevent fetal infection. A child born with syphilis should be treated immediately with penicillin, but considerable irreversible damage may already have occurred. Syphilis is discussed further in Chapter 11.

The tragic effect of the drug thalidomide, introduced in the 1950s and used in early pregnancy until 1962, alerted the public to the danger of harmful drugs for the developing embryo. Within the first 2 months of pregnancy, some babies who had been exposed to thalidomide before birth were born without limbs or had flipper-like appendages. Thalidomide was subsequently banned and thus spared many parents the congenital outcome just described.

Many congenital defects result from improper development, such as failure of organ walls to form or close or failure of two parts to unite and fuse. The chambers and vessels of the heart are sites of such abnormalities, and congenital heart diseases are discussed in Chapter 6. Spina bifida is an improper union of the lateral ridges of the embryo to form the vertebral column, a primary example of a neural tube defect (NTD). Although the cause of NTD is unknown, folic acid intake prior to and through the first few weeks of pregnancy decreases the incidence. Since neural tube closure occurs at 28 days after conception and prior to the recognition of pregnancy by many women, NTD prevention is best achieved by adequate folic acid intake (400 micrograms per day) before a planned pregnancy and for up to 12 weeks into the pregnancy. In America, folic acid is added to flour with the aim of preventing spina bifida; there is no addition of folic acid to flour in the UK. Spina bifida is further explained in Chapter 13.

Cleft lip and cleft palate are common birth defects. One in 700 newborns is affected by cleft lip and/or cleft palate, which is a gap between the left and right halves of the lip or upper palate (roof of the mouth). In trisomy 13, about 60–80% of babies born have cleft lip and palate. The defects are due to failure of the two sides of the embryo to fuse during gestation and affect speech, respiration, feeding and physical appearance. Clefts can be corrected with surgery.

A variety of types of congenital defects occur in the alimentary tract. The absence of a normal opening in an organ is called **atresia**. The lack of an opening from the oesophagus to the stomach is oesophageal atresia; it is frequently accompanied by an abnormal opening between the oesophagus and the trachea, known as a tracheal oesophageal fistula (TOF).

Intestinal atresia is a complete obstruction of the intestine, resulting in vomiting, dehydration, scanty stool production and distension of the abdomen.

Another congenital obstruction of the intestinal tract is pyloric stenosis, in which the pyloric sphincter hypertrophies, closing the opening between the stomach and the beginning of the small intestine (duodenum). Symptoms include projectile vomiting, dehydration, constipation and weight loss. Corrective surgery has been very effective in removing these congenital obstructions of the intestinal tract, just as it has been for congenital heart disease.

The bile ducts are blocked in biliary atresia, causing severe jaundice to develop. In biliary atresia, the liver and spleen become greatly enlarged. Excess bile accumulation may cause jaundice and brain damage due to toxicity.

AGE-RELATED DISEASES

The DNA blueprint foretells the future and the past. Some genetic diseases are noticed on the day of birth or shortly thereafter. Disease onset may start at birth, such as with PKU and thalassaemia, or appear in a few months, as with Tay–Sachs. However, diseases such as haemochromatosis may appear from age 30 to 40, and Parkinson's disease often exhibits the first noticeable symptoms in middle age.

Resources

The National Health Service Genetics education: *www.geneticseducation.nhs.uk*

http://www.albinism.org.uk

http://www.downs-syndrome.org.uk/

http://www.criduchat.org.uk/

http://www.tss.org.uk/ (Turner Syndrome)

The National Marfan Foundation: *www.marfan.org*

DISEASES AT A GLANCE Heredity*

DISEASE	AETIOLOGY	SIGNS AND SYMPTOMS	DIAGNOSIS	TREATMENT	PREVENTION	LIFESPAN
Autosomal dominant inheritance						
Achondroplasia	Chromosome 4, autosomal dominant, usually spontaneous	Short arms and legs, normal trunk, dwarfism, megalocephaly, lordosis; may depend on parent age	Present at birth, DNA tests before birth	Nothing definitive	Family history, genetic counselling	Because of appearance there may be some altered body image issues, but usually thrive well into adulthood
Marfan syndrome	Chromosome 15, autosomal dominant	Skeletal malformations, long facial appearance, aortic aneurysm, scoliosis, hypermobile joints, ocular lens defects	Onset varies, detection of protein fibrillin on skin, culture DNA tests	Depends on affected areas. Drugs to reduce aorta expansion (e.g. beta-blocker) or bone surgery	None without family history, genetic screening; one-third are sporadic cases	May die early owing to cardiovascular problems
Familial hypercholesterolaemia	Incomplete autosomal dominant	Atherosclerosis, coronary artery disease	Onset at birth, high LDLs	Exercise, low fat diet, statins	None, detect as early as possible	Relatively normal life if heterozygous with medication, diet and exercise; homozygous results in death as young adult
Autosomal recessive inheritance						
Fragile X syndrome	Constricted segment on long arm of X, *FMR1* gene mutation	Learning difficulty, large head, flat feet, prominent ears and forehead	DNA sequencing	Special education, physical and occupational therapy	None, perhaps counselling if aware	Symptoms throughout life, primarily affects males because of only one X chromosome
Haemochromatosis	Autosomal recessive, more males	Early: abdominal pain, arthritis; Later: diabetes, liver damage	Blood test for excess serum ferritin-iron, DNA test for *HFE* mutation, liver biopsy	Phlebotomy, blood donation	DNA test, genetic screening	Onset age 30–40, liver damage may be critical, continue blood transfusion throughout normal life expectancy
Galactosemia	Autosomal recessive, lack enzyme for lactose digestion	Enlarged liver, ascites, vomiting, diarrhoea, cataracts, learning difficulties, cerebral palsy	High blood galactose levels	Diet control, no lactose in food	Screened at birth	Normally do well with early diagnosis and controlled diet

*Exceptions or additions may be found in many of these cases; some diseases are covered further in system chapters.

DISEASES AT A GLANCE Heredity (continued)

DISEASE	AETIOLOGY	SIGNS AND SYMPTOMS	DIAGNOSIS	TREATMENT	PREVENTION	LIFESPAN
Phenylketonuria	Chromosome 12, autosomal recessive	Light skin tone, blue eye, learning difficulty if not corrected	Blood and urine levels of phenylalanine	Restricted diet within day of birth	Enzyme assay, strict diet, along with family history	If untreated within 4 months, results in severe brain damage, learning difficulties and social abnormalities. With early detection and diet restriction, life is basically normal
Tay-Sachs	Mutant Hex-A gene on chromosome 15	Learning difficulties, very dependent	Genetic blood screening	Genetic counselling	Genetic blood screening for parental traits, family history	Die by age 3-4 years
Change in chromosomal structure						
Cri du chat	Part of chromosome 5 missing	Severe learning difficulty, petite, wide space between eyes, cat cry sound	At birth	Supportive until death	None	Most die within first year (rarely live beyond 5-6 years)
Change in chromosomal number						
Down's syndrome	Extra chromosome 21 due to non-disjunction	Learning difficulty, rounded face, protruding tongue, short stature	Observation, chromosomal screen	Supportive, special education	Mother age under 35	Usually die by mid-life; if beyond age 45, tend to have Alzheimer's disease
Klinefelter's syndrome	Extra X chromosome (47 chromosomes in total)	Tall and slender, long legs, sparse body hair, weak breast development, usually sterile, male	Genetic screen	Counselling, family supported	None, chance occurrence	Varies, may have rather normal life with strong support and live to mid-life
Turner syndrome	Missing X chromosome (45 chromosomes in total)	Short stature female, broad flat breast, malformed elbows, sterile, hearing problems	May not be known until puberty, lack physical development	May need growth hormone and other supplements	None, mostly miscarried and die at fetal stage	May live relatively normal life to age 50-55 years

INTERACTIVE EXERCISES

Cases for critical thinking

1. What is the reason that Turner and Klinefelter's syndromes can occur as a result of non-disjunction in either the sperm or the egg but XYY can occur only as a result of non-disjunction in the sperm?

2. Marfan syndrome is an autosomal dominant disease. What is the probability that a child with a parent with Marfan syndrome will have Marfan syndrome?

3. If a mother is a carrier for the X-linked disease haemophilia A, what is the probability that her male child will have haemophilia A? Her female child?

4. A 36-year-old father of three with a new job thought stress had brought on abdominal pain and joint pain. He had noticed a darkening of his complexion and consulted a doctor, who found excess ferritin levels in his blood. What problem seems evident, and what treatment would help this individual?

Multiple choice

1. What do polydactyly and achondroplasia have in common?

   a. Both are autosomal recessive
   b. Both are sex-linked
   c. Both are congenital defects
   d. Both are autosomal dominant traits

2. Except for sperm and ova, how many chromosomes do human cells each have?

   a. 23   b. 46
   c. 96   d. 21

3. What combination of alleles manifest themselves only when the person is homozygous for the trait?

   a. recessive   b. dominant
   c. homozygous   d. heterozygous

4. Why do sex-linked diseases affect men more than women?

   a. Men have two X chromosomes
   b. Men have two Y chromosomes
   c. Men have one X chromosome
   d. Men have no Y chromosome

5. Colour-blind people most frequently can't distinguish which colours?

   a. red and yellow   b. green and blue
   c. red and green   d. blue and yellow

6. What type of disorder is thalassaemia?

   a. autosomal dominant
   b. autosomal recessive
   c. sex-linked
   d. congenital

7. If a female is a carrier of a sex-linked disease, what is the percentage chance of transmitting the allele to her children?

   a. 25   b. 50
   c. 75   d. 100

8. If both parents are carriers of an autosomal recessive disease, what is the percentage chance of each of their children inheriting the disease?

   a. 0   b. 25
   c. 50   d. 100

9. If alleles are different for a trait, what would be the genotype for that individual?

   a. homozygous   b. recessive
   c. heterozygous   d. dominant

10. Forty-four of our chromosomes (22 pairs) of the 46 total are called _____

    a. sex chromosomes   b. genes
    c. autosomes   d. alleles

True or false

_____ 1. DNA contains genetic information.

_____ 2. The incidence of Down's syndrome increases with the mother's age.

_____ 3. Fragile X syndrome is found equally in men and women.

_____ 4. A patient with Turner syndrome has an extra sex chromosome.

_____ 5. Tay-Sachs is an autosomal dominant disease.

_____ 6. Marfan syndrome is caused by an extra sex chromosome.

_____ 7. Albinism is a sex-linked disease.

_____ 8. Homozygous traits lead to carriers

_____ 9. If one parent is heterozygous for an autosomal dominant disease and the other parent is normal, a child has a 50% chance of getting the disease.

_____ 10. Fragile X syndrome is more demonstrative in girls than boys.

Fill-ins

1. _____ diseases are those appearing at birth or shortly after, but they are not caused by genetic or chromosomal abnormalities.

2. _____ have both functional testes and ovaries.

3. _____ alleles manifest themselves when the person is heterozygous for that trait.

4. _____ encode information for the synthesis of proteins.

5. _____ are alternative forms of a gene.

6. _____ is the condition of extra fingers or toes.

7. _____ is the failure of two chromosomes to separate as the gametes are being formed.

8. Sex cells contain _____ chromosomes.

9. A recessive genetic disease which can be controlled by diet is _____.

10. Replacement of genetic material by recombinant application is called _____ .

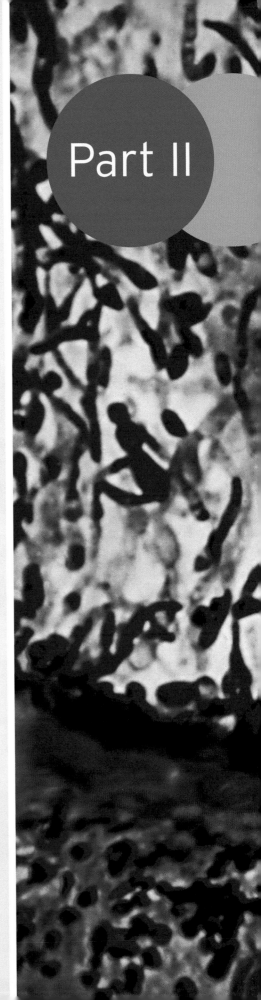

DISEASES OF
THE SYSTEMS

Part II presents diseases of the body's systems. Each chapter reviews the normal structure and function of a body system, and then discusses diseases associated with that system. Signs, symptoms, aetiology, diagnosis, treatment and prevention are described for each disease.

Chapters

6 Diseases of the cardiovascular system
 7 Diseases of the blood
 8 Diseases of the respiratory system
 9 Diseases of the gastrointestinal system
10 Diseases of the renal and urinary systems
11 Diseases and disorders of the reproductive system
12 Diseases of the endocrine system
13 Diseases of the nervous system and the special senses
14 Mental illness and cognitive disorders
15 Diseases of the musculoskeletal system
16 Diseases of the integumentary system

6 DISEASES OF THE CARDIOVASCULAR SYSTEM

This photomicrograph reveals histopathological changes indicative of endocarditis caused by the fungus *Candida albicans*.

(Courtesy of the CDC/Sherry Brinkman, 1963)

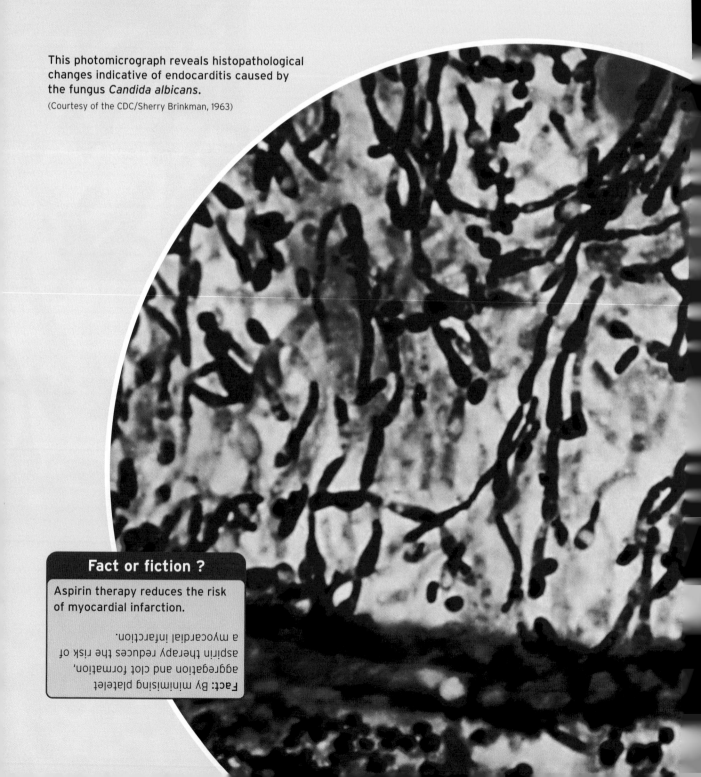

Fact or fiction ?

Aspirin therapy reduces the risk of myocardial infarction.

Fact: By minimising platelet aggregation and clot formation, aspirin therapy reduces the risk of a myocardial infarction.

Learning objectives

After studying this chapter, you should be able to:

+ Describe the normal structure and function of the heart and blood vessels
+ Describe the key characteristics of the diseases of the arterial circulation and heart
+ Explain the association between arteriosclerosis and atherosclerosis
+ Identify the role of hyperlipidaemia in atherosclerosis
+ Describe the aetiology, signs and risks associated with arterial hypertension
+ Compare and contrast pulmonary hypertension and arterial hypertension
+ Describe the role of varicose veins in peripheral vascular disease
+ Understand the risks associated with venous thrombosis
+ Differentiate between endocardial and myocardial diseases of the heart
+ Understand the distinguishing features of heart valve stenosis and heart valve regurgitation
+ Explain the different types of atrial and ventricular arrhythmias
  + Name the aetiologies of shock
    + Describe normal fetal circulation
      + Describe the epidemiology, symptoms, aetiology, diagnosis and treatment of congenital heart abnormalities
        + Review and understand the differences between cyanotic and non-cyanotic congenital heart disease
          + Review the risks and pathological changes associated with heart disease in older adults

Disease chronicle

Dr Christiaan Barnard

Dr Christiaan Barnard performed the first human heart transplant in 1967. In the Union of South Africa, Dr Barnard performed this famous surgery on a 53-year-old dentist named Louis Washkansky. The dentist received the donated heart of a 25-year-old car accident victim named Denise Davall. Although the surgery was a technical triumph and a beacon of hope for many with terminal heart disease, Washkansky died 18 days later from infection. Still risky today, heart transplants owe their successes to the generosity of Denise Davall, the courage of Louis Washkansky, and the brilliance of Dr Barnard, who died of a heart attack in 2001.

THE CIRCULATORY SYSTEM

The main function of the circulatory system, which includes the heart and blood vessels, is transport. The circulatory system delivers oxygen and nutrients needed for metabolism to the tissues; carries waste products from cellular metabolism to the kidneys and other excretory organs for elimination; and circulates electrolytes and hormones needed to regulate various bodily functions. The circulatory system is divided into two parts: the systemic and the pulmonary circulation. The heart pumps blood, and the blood vessels serve as tubes through which blood flows. The arterial system carries blood from the heart to the tissues, and the veins carry it back to the heart.

Structure and function of the heart

The heart is a hollow muscular organ located in the centre of the chest. The heart consists of four chambers: a right and left atrium and a right and left ventricle. The chamber walls consist of cardiac muscle, known as **myocardium**, and their internal lining, which consists of a smooth, delicate membrane called the **endocardium**. The **pericardium**, a double-layered membrane, encloses the heart (Figure 6.1).

The right and left sides of the heart have an upper atrium that collects blood from the body and the lungs, respectively, and a lower ventricle that ejects blood throughout the body and the lungs, respectively.

Valves between the atria and the ventricles, the atrioventricular (AV) valves, permit one-way blood flow from atria to ventricles. The **mitral valve**, between the left atrium and left ventricle, has two flaps called cusps that meet when the valve is closed. The **tricuspid valve**, between the right atrium and right ventricle, is named for its three cusps. Figure 6.2 shows these valves in the closed position.

The pulmonary semilunar valve permits one-way blood flow from the right ventricle to the pulmonary artery, while the aortic semilunar valve controls blood flow from the left ventricle to the aorta.

During every heartbeat cycle (the cardiac cycle), each heart chamber relaxes as it fills, and then contracts as it pumps blood. This filling period is

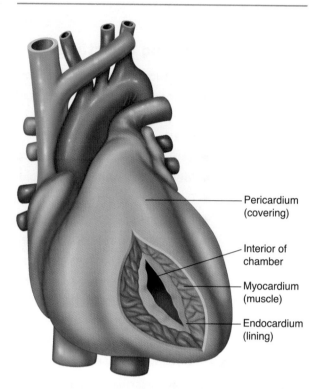

Figure 6.1 Heart covering and layer of the heart.

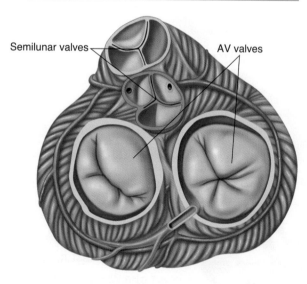

Figure 6.2 Heart valves in closed position viewed from the top.

diastole, or the diastolic phase, while the contracting phase of each chamber is **systole**, or systolic phase. The alternate contraction and relaxation of atria and ventricles comprises the **cardiac cycle**, which takes

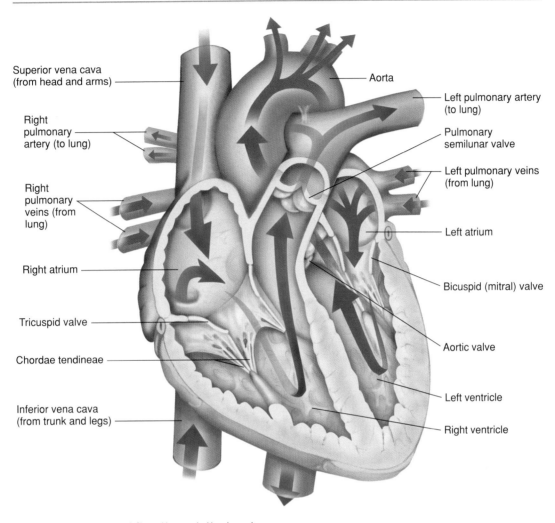

Superior vena cava
(from head and arms)

Aorta

Left pulmonary artery
(to lung)

Right
pulmonary
artery (to lung)

Pulmonary
semilunar valve

Left pulmonary veins
(from lung)

Right
pulmonary
veins (from
lung)

Left atrium

Right atrium

Bicuspid (mitral) valve

Tricuspid valve

Aortic valve

Chordae tendineae

Left ventricle

Inferior vena cava
(from trunk and legs)

Right ventricle

Figure 6.3 The blood flow through the heart.

about 0.8 of a second. The flow of blood through the heart chambers, vessels and lungs is reviewed in Figure 6.3.

Coronary arteries provide the heart muscle (myocardium) with a reliable blood supply. The left coronary artery begins at the aorta on the front of the heart and divides within an inch into the anterior interventricular coronary artery and the circumflex artery, which continues left around the back of the heart. The right coronary artery also branches from the front of the aorta and sends divisions to the right side and back of the heart (Figure 6.4).

Unlike skeletal muscle, cardiac muscle contracts continuously and rhythmically without conscious effort. A small patch of tissue, the **sinoatrial node**

(SA node), acts as the pacemaker of the heart. The impulse for contraction initiates at the SA node and spreads over the atria, then passes to the ventricles via conductive tissue called the atrioventricular (AV) node. The impulse continues along left and right bundle branches and terminates in the **Purkinje fibres**, which further branch throughout the ventricle walls. This conduction system is illustrated in Figure 6.5.

Heart muscle does not depend on nerve stimulation for contraction, but is influenced by the autonomic nervous system and hormones such as adrenaline (epinephrine). Two sets of nerves work antagonistically, one slowing the heart and the other accelerating it. The vagus nerve slows the heart

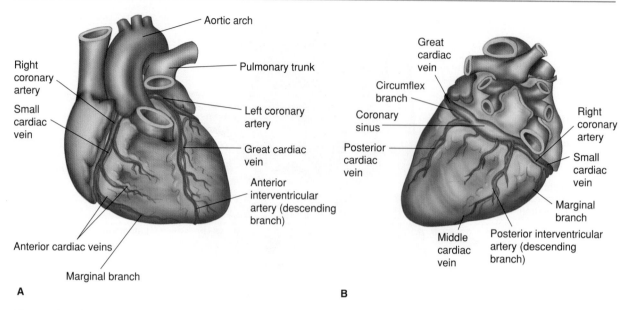

Figure 6.4 Coronary arteries and major vessels.

rate during rest and sleep by means of a chemical it secretes, acetylcholine. The excitatory portion of the autonomic nervous system increases heart rate during periods of stress, strenuous physical activity and excitement. This excitation is brought about by the release of adrenaline and noradrenaline (norepinephrine), which stimulate the heart's pacemaker.

Blood flows through two circulatory routes: the systemic circulation and the pulmonary circulation. The systemic circulation distributes oxygen-rich

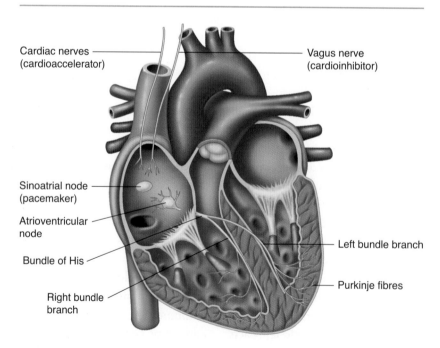

Figure 6.5 Conducting system of the heart.

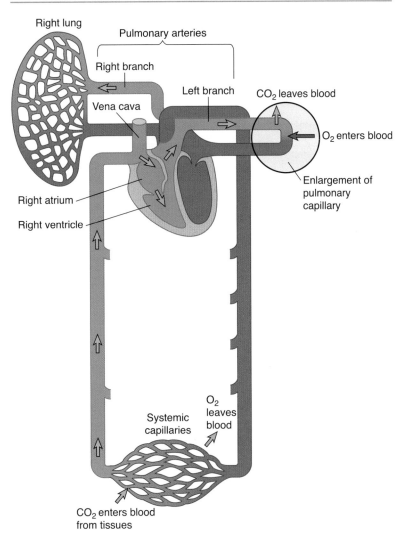

Figure 6.6 Venous return to the heart and blood flow to the lungs (red = oxygenated blood, blue = deoxygenated blood).

blood from the left ventricle, beginning at the **aorta** (large artery of the systemic arterial system) and continuing through arteries to all parts of the body, and returns oxygen-poor blood by veins to the right atrium. The pulmonary circulation carries oxygen-poor blood from the right ventricle, beginning at the pulmonary trunk and continuing through smaller arteries to the lungs to be oxygenated, and returns the blood through pulmonary veins to the left atrium. Partitions called the interatrial septum and interventricular septum separate oxygen-rich from oxygen-poor blood in the atria and ventricles, respectively (Figures 6.6 and 6.7).

Branches of the aorta carry blood to the head, upper extremities, chest, abdomen, pelvis and lower extremities. These arteries continue to divide into smaller and smaller arteries, and eventually into vessels called **arterioles**, the smallest arteries. Arterioles lead into **capillaries**, the connecting links between arteries and veins. Capillaries deliver oxygen and nutrients to tissues. Blood continues into **venules**, the smallest veins, and then into larger veins. Veins from the upper body empty blood into the superior vena cava, and veins of the lower body carry blood to the inferior vena cava. The superior and inferior **venae cavae** deliver systemic blood to the right atrium.

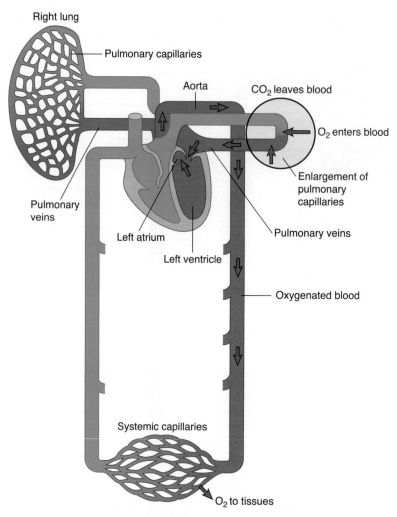

Figure 6.7 Return of oxygenated blood to heart and entry into aorta (red = oxygenated blood, blue = deoxygenated blood).

Structure and function of the blood vessels

The walls of arteries are muscular, thick and strong, with considerable elastic tissue, and are lined with endothelium. Arterioles have a smaller diameter than arteries, with thinner walls consisting mostly of smooth muscle fibres arranged circularly and a lining consisting of endothelium. Arterioles can change their diameter by constricting or dilating, which alters blood flow to the tissues. Capillaries are minute vessels about 0.5–1.0 mm long with a lumen as wide as a red blood cell. Their wall consists only of a layer of endothelium. Vein walls are much thinner than companion arteries, but their lumens are considerably larger. With less muscle and elasticity in their walls, veins tend to collapse when empty. Veins, particularly those of the legs, contain valves that help return blood upward to the heart against gravity.

DIAGNOSTIC TESTS AND PROCEDURES FOR CARDIAC DISORDERS

Many techniques for diagnosing and treating heart problems exist. **Auscultation**, listening through a stethoscope for abnormal sounds, and the electrocardiogram (ECG) provide valuable information regarding heart condition. The **electrocardiogram** is an electrical recording of heart action and aids in the diagnosis of coronary artery disease, myocardial infarction, valve disorders and some congenital heart diseases. It is also useful in diagnosing arrhythmias and heart block. **Echocardiography** (ultrasound cardiography) is also a non-invasive procedure that utilises high frequency sound waves to examine the size, shape and motion of heart structures. It gives a time–motion study of the heart, which permits direct recordings of heart valve movement, measurements of the heart chambers and changes that occur in the heart chambers during the cardiac cycle. Colour **Doppler echocardiography** explores blood flow patterns and changes in velocity of blood flow within the heart and great vessels. It enables the cardiologist to evaluate valve stenosis or insufficiency.

An exercise tolerance test is used to diagnose coronary artery disease and other heart disorders. This test monitors the ECG and blood pressure during exercise. Problems that normally do not occur at rest are revealed.

Cardiac catheterisation is a procedure in which a catheter is passed into the heart through blood vessels to sample the blood in each chamber for oxygen content and pressure. The findings can indicate valve disorders or abnormal shunting of blood and aid in determining cardiac output.

X-rays of the heart and great vessels, the aorta and the pulmonary artery, in conjunction with **angiocardiography**, in which a contrast indicator (dye) is injected into the cardiovascular system, can detect blockage in vessels. **Coronary arteriography** employs a selective injection of contrast material into coronary arteries for a film recording of blood vessel action.

CARDIOVASCULAR DISEASE

Cardiovascular disease includes a range of diseases that affect the heart and the blood vessels. Globally, mortality from cardiovascular disease is expected to reach 23.6 million by 2030 (WHO, 2009). Heart disease is the leading cause of death and a major cause of disability in the UK, with 16% of all female deaths and 20.2% of all male deaths caused by cardiovascular disease.

Disorders of blood flow and pressure and disorders of cardiac function are directly and indirectly responsible for many of the diseases that affect the pulmonary and systemic circulation. Disorders of blood flow and pressure include the diseases of the arterial circulation and the venous circulation. Disorders of cardiac function consist of diseases of the pericardium, coronary heart disease, myocardial and endocardial diseases, heart valve disease, cardiac conduction disturbance, heart failure and heart disease in infants and children.

Diseases of the arterial circulation

Hyperlipidaemia Hyperlipidaemia is a general term used to describe an elevation of lipids or fats in the blood. Lipids include cholesterol, phospholipids and triglycerides. Cholesterol is a soft waxy substance that is important in the formation of cell membranes and various hormones. Cholesterol is made by the liver and is also introduced to the body through food. It is transported throughout the systemic circulation by transport proteins called **lipoproteins**.

Low density lipoprotein (LDL) is the major cholesterol carrier in the blood. LDL transports cholesterol to the tissues of the body. LDL is also known as the 'bad' cholesterol because accumulations of LDL form a **plaque** or thick hard deposit that narrows the arteries and impedes blood flow. LDL cholesterol enters cells via binding with LDL receptors (on the cell surface) that then causes entry via endocytosis. **High density lipoprotein (HDL)** carries about one-quarter to one-third of the cholesterol. Known as the 'good' cholesterol, HDL carries cholesterol away from the arteries and to the liver, where it is eliminated from the body as a component of bile. **Phospholipids** are a type of lipid that are also important for the synthesis of cell membranes.

Triglycerides are another form of fat that is stored in fat cells in the human body. An increase in triglycerides is linked to coronary artery disease.

Prevention PLUS!

Trans fat

Trans fats are made by the process of hydrogenation (hydrogen is added to vegetable oil) and are found in many processed foods as they help to extend shelf life. Trans fats are not essential to health and high amounts of these fats in the diet can increase the risk of heart disease as they contribute to the increase in the blood levels of LDL cholesterol. In the UK, the addition of trans fats to food was stopped by many of the major food manufacturers by 2007.

Hypercholesterolaemia Hypercholesterolaemia can be classified as primary, in which the condition develops independent of other causes, and secondary, in which it is associated with other health problems or lifestyle.

Many types of primary cholesterolaemia have a genetic basis. For example, the LDL receptor is deficient or defective in the autosomal dominant genetic disorder known as *familial hypercholesterolaemia*. In this case, cholesterol cannot be taken up by cells and high levels of LDL are seen in the blood. Secondary causes of hypercholesterolaemia include obesity and diabetes mellitus. High-calorie diets increase the production of LDL and cholesterol. Diets that are high in triglycerides and saturated fat increase cholesterol synthesis and suppress LDL receptor activity.

Arteriosclerosis Arteriosclerosis and atherosclerosis are diseases of the arteries. Because these diseases significantly contribute to the development of many other diseases in the cardiovascular system, most notably heart disease, they are discussed first.

In **arteriosclerosis**, artery walls thicken and become hard and inflexible, partly due to calcium deposition. 'Hardening of the arteries' aptly describes this condition, because affected arteries are unable to stretch and rebound in response to the pressure of blood as it is forced through them by contraction of the heart. As a result, arteriosclerosis leads to hypertension. The most common cause of arteriosclerosis is atherosclerosis (discussed next), in which fatty material accumulates within the walls of the artery (Figure 6.8). Arteriosclerosis is also associated with the aging process.

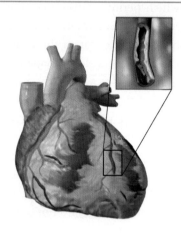

Figure 6.8 An atherosclerotic artery.

Atherosclerosis **Atheroslerosis**, or a hardening of the arteries, is a multifaceted disease that results from a number of insults that damage the vasculature, and is specifically related to the development of an atheromatous plaque. Hypercholesterolaemia, smoking, hypertension and diabetes mellitus are the key risk factors that initiate the atherosclerotic process. The lesions associated with atherosclerosis are of three types:

- the fatty streak;
- the fibrous atheromatous plaque;
- the complicated lesion.

Fatty streaks are thin, flat discolorations in the vasculature that progressively enlarge and become thicker as they grow in length. Fatty streaks are present in children and increase in number until about the age of 20 years, and then they either remain static or regress.

The **fibrous atheromatous plaque** is the basic lesion of clinical atherosclerosis. It is characterised by the accumulation of intracellular and extracellular lipids and the formation of scar tissue. The lesion begins as a whitish grey lesion thickening of the vessel intima (inner coat of the vessel) that contains a lipid core covered by a fibrous plaque. There is usually disruption of the underlying tunica media with an increase in the number of smooth muscle cells. As the lesion increases in size, the lesion may begin to occlude a vessel, causing a reduction of blood flow (Figure 6.9).

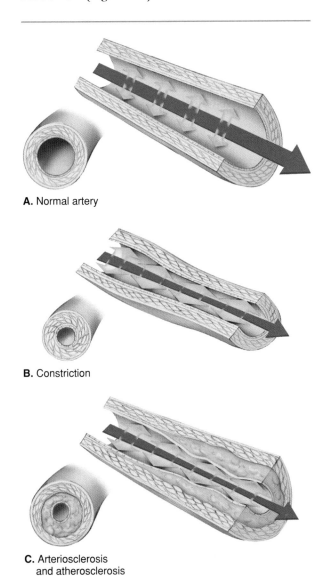

A. Normal artery

B. Constriction

C. Arteriosclerosis
and atherosclerosis

Figure 6.9 Blood vessels: (A) normal artery; (B) constriction; (C) arteriosclerosis and atherosclerosis.

The more advanced or **complicated lesions** are characterised by haemorrhage, ulceration and scar tissue deposits. **Thrombosis**, or a clot within a blood vessel, is formed by turbulent blood flow in the region of the plaque and ulceration of the plaque.

Males and people with a history of cardiovascular disease have an increased risk for atherosclerosis. Modifiable risk factors such as hypercholesterolaemia, high blood pressure, diabetes, obesity, physical inactivity, untreated or under-treated hypertension and smoking can be controlled to reduce the risk for atherosclerosis.

A variety of tests are available to confirm the diagnosis of atherosclerosis. The electrocardiogram measures normal and abnormal electrical activity of the heart that may result from atherosclerotic disease. Coronary angiography is a test that is used to visualise the coronary arteries with the use of a contrast media. A CT scan or computerised tomography scan sends X-rays through the body at various angles. The CT scan can directly visualise the heart arteries and measure the amount of calcium deposits in the arteries.

Atherosclerosis is not usually associated with symptoms until the interior of the artery is extensively occluded. Symptoms depend on the location and the severity of the occluded artery. Occlusion of the coronary arteries may result in chest pain and shortness of breath. Blockage of the **carotid arteries** can reduce blood supply to the brain, causing a stroke. A hardening of the arteries in the legs, or **peripheral vascular disease**, leads to pain in the muscles of the leg, especially when walking; however, in severe cases ulceration or **gangrene** of the extremities may result.

Control of blood pressure, reduction of cholesterol and lifestyle changes contribute significantly to the treatment and prevention of consequences that can result from atherosclerosis. Medications commonly prescribed in the treatment of atherosclerosis include antihypertensive and cholesterol lowering medications. Numerous controlled clinical trials confirm the beneficial effects of controlling blood cholesterol levels. Treatment of hypertension reduces the potential for further injury and insult to the arteries.

Peripheral arterial disease Diseases that affect peripheral arteries are similar to those affecting the coronary (heart) or carotid (brain) arteries in that they produce **ischaemia**, a lack of blood and consequently oxygen. Pain, impaired function, infarction and tissue necrosis may then follow. Atherosclerosis is an important cause of peripheral arterial disease. The most commonly affected arteries are the femoral (leg) or popliteal arteries. The disease is seen most commonly in men aged 70–80 years. The risk factors for this disease are the same as those for atherosclerosis, namely heredity and environmental risks.

Inspection of the limbs for signs of ischaemia, such as subcutaneous atrophy, pallor, coolness and absent pulses, provides a preliminary diagnosis. Doppler ultrasound, ultrasound imaging, radionuclide imaging and contrast angiography may also be used to confirm the diagnosis.

The primary symptom of chronic obstructive peripheral artery disease is **intermittent claudication**, or pain with walking. Other signs include a thinning of the skin and subcutaneous tissues of the lower leg. The foot may feel cool to the touch and a lower leg pulse may be faint or absent. When blood flow is significantly reduced, the oxygen and nutritional needs may not be met, and ischaemic pain at rest, ulceration and gangrene may result.

Treatment of peripheral vascular disease is aimed at prevention of further complications in the affected tissues. Walking slowly is usually encouraged because it increases circulation around the clots. Avoidance of injury is important because extremities affected by atherosclerosis are easily injured and slow to heal. Blood thinning agents are used to prevent additional clots from forming. In severe cases, surgical bypass around the clot may be indicated. Removal of the clot may also be considered if the section of the diseased vessel is short.

Raynaud's disease Raynaud's disease is a functional disorder of the arteries caused by **vasospasms**, or intense spasms of the arteries and arterioles in the fingers and toes. Raynaud's disease usually occurs in healthy young women. It is often precipitated by exposure to cold or emotional stress and is usually limited to the fingers (Figure 6.10). The causes

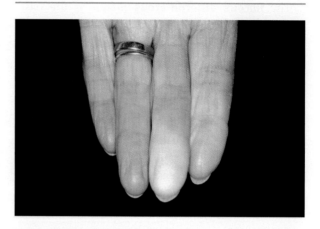

Figure 6.10 Raynaud's disease
(Science Photo Library Ltd/Dr P. Marazzi)

of vessel spasms are unknown, although hyperactivity of the sympathetic nervous system has been suggested.

Symptoms of vasospasm include changes in skin colour, from pallor to cyanosis, accompanied by a sensation of cold, numbness or tingling. The colour changes are most noticeable in the tips of the fingers, later moving to the more distant parts of the fingers and hands. In severe progressive disease, the nails may become brittle and the skin over the affected fingers may thicken. Deprivation of oxygen and nutrients in the affected area may give rise to arthritis, ulceration or, rarely, gangrene of the fingers.

Treatment of Raynaud's disease is aimed at reducing triggers for the symptoms and protecting the hands from trauma. Abstinence from smoking, protection of the hands from cold and avoidance of emotional stress are important. Medications that prevent vasospasm may be used in individuals with frequent symptoms.

Aortic aneurysm Aortic aneurysm refers to dilatation of the aortic lumen. Aneurysms are usually described by their location, size, **morphology** (configuration and structure), and origin. The morphology of an aortic aneurysm is either **fusiform** or **saccular** (Figure 6.11). A **fusiform** aneurysm has a uniform shape, with symmetrical dilatation that involves the circumference of the aortic wall.

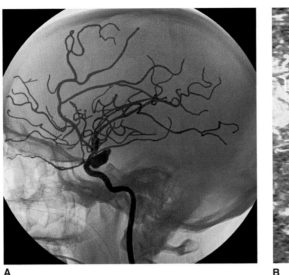
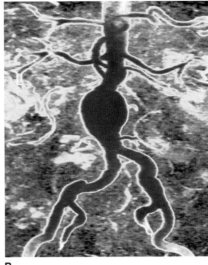

A   B

Figure 6.11 Aneurysms: (A) saccular (Simon Fraser/RNC, Newcastle/Photo Researchers, Inc); and (B) fusiform (Zephyr/Photo Researchers, Inc.).

Saccular aneurysms, on the other hand, appear as an out-pouching of only a portion of the aortic wall.

Ultrasound imaging, echocardiography, computed tomography (CT) and magnetic resonance imaging (MRI) scans are often used to diagnose and monitor the progression of an aneurysm.

Aneurysms usually occur in the abdomen below the kidneys (**abdominal aortic aneurysm**) or in the chest cavity (**thoracic aneurysm**). **Cerebral** or brain **aneurysm** is diagnosed less frequently. Regardless of location, the danger of an aneurysm is the tendency to increase in size and rupture, resulting in haemorrhage, possibly in a vital organ such as the heart, brain or abdomen.

Aortic aneurysms typically produce no symptoms and usually develop after age 50 and occur more frequently in men than in women. Atherosclerosis is the most common cause of abdominal aneurysms. Other causes of aortic aneurysms include connective tissue diseases and conditions that cause inflammation of the vessels such as trauma or infections.

Depending on the size and rate of expansion, surgical repair of an aneurysm is at times indicated to prevent rupture. The diseased area of the vessel is removed and replaced with an artificial graft or segment of another blood vessel.

Disorders of arterial pressure

Arterial hypertension Arterial blood pressure is a measure of the force of blood against the arterial walls. In healthy adults, the highest pressure, called the **systolic** pressure, is ideally less than 120 mmHg, and the lowest pressure, called the **diastolic** pressure, is less than 80 mmHg. Blood pressure normally varies throughout the day, increasing with activity and decreasing with rest (Table 6.1).

Hypertension is broadly defined as an arterial pressure greater than 140/90 mmHg in adults on at least three consecutive measures.

Table 6.1 Adult blood pressure guidelines.

Category	Systolic	Diastolic
Optimal	<120	<80
Normal	120–129	80–84
High normal	130–139	85–89
Grade 1 hypertension (mild)	140–159	90–99
Grade 2 hypertension (moderate)	160–179	100–109
Grade 3 hypertension (severe)	≥180	≥110
Isolated systolic hypertension	≥140	<90

Source: European Society of Hypertension & European Society of Cardiology (2003).

Table 6.2 Risk of stroke and heart disease increase with increasing blood pressure.

Blood pressure (mmHg)	Risk
115/75	Normal
135/85	2 times normal
155/95	4 times normal
175/105	8 times normal

Advancing age, sedentary lifestyle, excess weight and excessive dietary salt and alcohol consumption are risk factors for the development of hypertension. Family history of hypertension and African ancestry are also observed risk factors for developing high blood pressure.

Hypertension is the most common cardiovascular disorder and affects about 20% of the adult population worldwide. It is considered one of the major risk factors for heart disease, stroke and kidney disease (Table 6.2). Because of the asymptomatic nature of hypertension, it remains untreated or under-treated in the majority of affected individuals.

Blood pressure measurements obtained by using a sphygmomanometer and stethoscope are important in the diagnosis and follow-up treatment for hypertension. The diagnosis of hypertension using this method is based on the average of at least two or more blood pressure readings taken on at least two separate occasions.

The aetiology of hypertension is divided into two categories: primary and secondary hypertension. Primary hypertension is also called **essential** hypertension; this chronic increase in systolic and diastolic blood pressure occurs without evidence of other disease. Approximately 90–95% of hypertension is classified as primary or essential. In **secondary hypertension**, the elevation in blood pressure results from some other disease, such as kidney disease, or may be related to an endocrine disorder such as a phaeochromocytoma (tumour of the adrenal gland).

Primary hypertension typically does not cause symptoms. When symptoms do occur, they are usually related to the long-term effects of hypertension on the organ systems of the body, including the kidneys, heart, eyes and blood vessels. Hypertension is a major risk factor for the development of atherosclerosis, cardiovascular disease (including heart failure), coronary artery disease, peripheral vascular disease, and cerebrovascular diseases and stroke.

Treatment of primary and secondary hypertension is aimed at reducing blood pressure to less than 140/90 mmHg and preventing organ damage. For individuals with secondary hypertension, control of the disease causing the hypertension may often be curative. Lifestyle modifications such as weight loss, exercise and reduction of salt intake enhance the effectiveness of medication therapy and help reduce further disease risks. The type of medication selected to treat hypertension depends on the stage of hypertension, age, other conditions and patient-specific risk factors.

Pulmonary arterial hypertension Pulmonary arterial hypertension (PAH) is a condition of high blood pressure in the pulmonary artery. The average normal pressure in the pulmonary artery is about 14 mmHg at rest. In PAH, pressures in the pulmonary artery are greater than 25 mmHg at rest and greater than 30 mmHg during exercise.

A number of tests are used to diagnose and assess the severity of PAH. Echocardiography provides information about the severity of the pulmonary hypertension, estimated pulmonary artery pressure and potential causes. An electrocardiogram provides information on cardiac abnormalities. Pulmonary function tests, lung scans and blood tests are useful for identifying secondary causes. Cardiac catheterisation provides a precise measure of the blood pressure in the pulmonary artery.

There are both idiopathic and secondary causes of PAH that cause three general changes in the pulmonary arteries: vasoconstriction, endothelial and/or smooth muscle proliferation, and intimal fibrosis and thrombosis of the pulmonary capillaries or arterioles. **Vasoconstriction** results in a narrowing of the walls of the arteries, which makes the lumen of arteries narrower. As the endothelial cells and smooth muscles proliferate, the walls of the pulmonary artery thicken. Scar tissue forms on

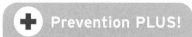

the walls of the arteries, causing the lumen to narrow. Intimal fibrosis and thrombosis involves the formation of blood clots, causing blockages.

Symptoms of pulmonary arterial hypertension include **dyspnoea** (shortness of breath), fatigue and **syncope** (loss of consciousness, or fainting). As the disease advances, the pumping ability of the heart weakens and symptoms occur at rest.

Without treatment, the prognosis of PAH is poor, with a median survival of less than 3 years. Patients with severe symptoms require aggressive treatment to remove the underlying cause, reduce symptoms and improve quality of life, slow endothelial proliferation and the development of further narrowing of the lumen, and increase the supply of blood and oxygen to the heart. Treatments include medications, oxygen therapy and lung transplantation.

Diseases of the venous circulation

Venous circulation of the lower extremities

The venous systems in the lower extremities consist of the superficial (saphenous) veins and the deep venous channels. Blood from the skin and the subcutaneous tissue accumulates in the superficial veins and is then transported into the deeper venous channels for return to the heart. Venous valves are located along the veins and prevent backflow of blood into the venous system. The leg muscles also assist in moving venous blood from the lower extremities to the heart.

Varicose veins Varicose veins are dilated, distorted veins that usually develop in the superficial veins of the leg, such as the greater saphenous vein. The veins become swollen and painful and appear knotty under the skin. Varicose veins are caused by blood pooling within the veins because of decreased, stagnated blood flow (Figure 6.12).

Varicose veins can be an occupational hazard related to long periods of sitting or standing. Normally, the leg muscle movement moves blood up within the vein from one valve to the next. In the absence of this 'milking action' of the muscles, the blood exerts pressure on the closed valves and thin walls of the veins. The veins dilate to the extent that the valves are no longer competent. The blood collects and becomes stagnant, and the veins become more swollen and painful.

Pregnancy or a tumour in the uterus can also cause varicose veins because pressure on veins causes resistance to blood flow. Heredity and obesity are also associated with varicose veins.

Complications of varicose veins include ulcers and infection, owing to poor circulation, and haemorrhage, caused by weakened vein walls.

Treatment depends on the severity of the symptoms. An elastic bandage or support hose may

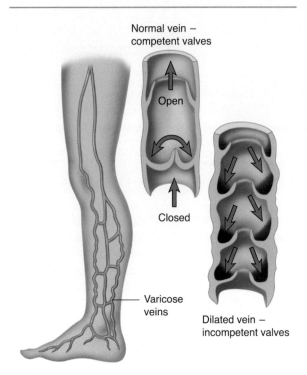

Figure 6.12 Development of varicose veins.

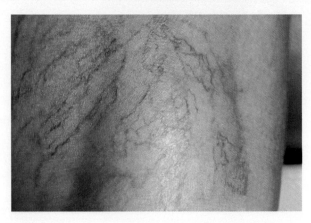

Figure 6.13 Spider veins.
(Courtesy of Jason L. Smith MD)

increase circulation and provide relief from discomfort. Symptoms can be relieved by walking, elevating the legs when seated, and losing weight. A surgical procedure called surgical vein stripping is very successful and involves removing the veins and tying off the remaining open ends. Collateral circulation tends to develop to compensate for the loss of the vein segment.

Spider veins are small, dense networks of veins that appear as red or blue discolorations on the skin. The cause of spider veins is unknown, though there appears to be a genetic link. Spider veins appear in both men and women, but more frequently in women. Female hormones may play a role in their development; puberty, birth control pills, pregnancy or hormone replacement therapy may contribute to them. Spider veins can be treated with laser. The light heats and scars the tiny superficial veins, which closes them off to blood flow (Figure 6.13). Another treatment is **compression sclerotherapy**, in which a strong saline solution is injected into specific sites of the varicose veins. The irritation causes scarring of the inner lining and fuses the veins shut. The

procedure is followed by uninterrupted compression for several weeks to prevent re-entry of blood. A daily walking programme during the recovery period is required to activate leg muscle venous pumps.

Chronic venous insufficiency Chronic venous insufficiency (CVI) is a condition of poor venous blood return to the heart. The most common cause of CVI is deep vein **thrombosis**, incompetence of the venous valves and muscles that aid in venous return.

Similar to other diseases, diagnostic screening consists of assessment of medical history, such as smoking, obesity, family history, pregnancy and history of sedentary lifestyle. Additional tests include plethysmography studies and Doppler imaging studies. Outflow plethysmography is a simple tourniquet procedure that requires placing and releasing a tourniquet on the lower extremities. Upon release of the tourniquet, the vein should return to baseline. Doppler imaging studies are used to assess venous flow and the presence of a thrombus.

Signs and symptoms associated with poor blood flow include tissue congestion, oedema, necrosis or skin atrophy and pain upon walking. In advanced disease, venous stasis ulcers may develop.

Risk factors for CVI include advancing age, family history of deep vein thrombosis, sedentary lifestyle, obesity and smoking. The peak incidence of CVI occurs in women aged 40–49 years and men aged 70–79 years.

The treatment of CVI depends on the severity of the disease. Mild cases can be managed with controlled diet and exercise and the use of compression stockings. Compression stockings squeeze the leg and prevent excess blood from flowing backward. Surgical repair of the veins includes repairing the valves, bypassing the incompetent veins and vein stripping (surgical procedure in which the diseased vein is removed). An incision is made below the vein, a flexible instrument is threaded up the vein, and the vein is grasped and removed.

Venous thrombosis A clot, or **venous thrombosis**, can develop in the superficial or the deep veins of the lower extremities. Venous thrombosis is accompanied by an inflammatory response to the vessel wall that results from venous blood stasis, vessel wall injury and increased blood coagulation.

Risk factors for venous thrombosis include conditions that cause venous stasis, hypercoagulability and vascular trauma. Older adults and postsurgical patients are at increased risk for venous thrombosis as immobilisation results in decreased blood flow and venous pooling in the lower extremities.

Venous thrombosis is not associated with symptoms in about 50% of patients. Signs and symptoms of inflammation, such as pain, swelling and deep muscle tenderness, are indications of venous thrombosis.

Early detection and prevention of venous thrombosis is vital to prevent potentially fatal complications such as **emboli**, or distant clots to vital organs such as the lung. Early ambulation after surgery or childbirth, exercising the legs and use of compression stockings are measures that decrease the risk for thrombus formation. Blood thinners are beneficial for patients at high risk. Surgery is performed to remove the thrombus or embolism.

Disorders of cardiac function

Coronary heart disease The coronary circulation supplies the heart with oxygen and nutrients to maintain cardiac function and thus supply the remainder of the body with blood. The body's metabolic needs change rapidly and widely, often requiring rapid adaptation of cardiac function and coronary blood flow. An imbalance in cardiac oxygen demand and supply can cause myocardial ischaemia, cardiac contractile dysfunction, arrhythmias, infarction and death.

A preliminary diagnosis of coronary heart disease (CHD) requires a physical examination, patient medical history and an electrocardiogram (ECG). A patient's medical history is used to identify hereditary and lifestyle risk factors for the disease. The ECG records the heart's electrical activity and can aid in identifying abnormalities in heart rate and rhythm as well as areas of damaged heart tissue. Additional diagnostic tests include echocardiograms, stress tests, nuclear imaging and angiography.

CHD is a disease of reduced coronary blood flow most often due to atherosclerosis. More than 90% of persons with CHD have coronary atherosclerosis. Atherosclerosis can affect the major coronary arteries and their branches. Risk factor categories define major, emerging and underlying conditions that influence the development of atherosclerotic CHD (Table 6.3).

CHD is the leading cause of death worldwide. Approximately 3.8 million men and 3.4 million women worldwide die each year from CHD. The aging world population will have major implications for CHD. By the year 2025, more than 60% of all CHD deaths will be among persons over 65 years

Table 6.3 Risk factor categories for atherosclerotic cardiovascular disease.

Major risk factors	Emerging risk factors
Cigarette smoking	Prothrombotic state
Elevated blood pressure	Proinflammatory state
Elevated LDL cholesterol	Insulin resistance
Low HDL cholesterol	**Underlying risk factors**
Diabetes mellitus	High fat diet
Metabolic syndrome	Obesity
	Physical inactivity
	Family history

Source: Adapted from Grundy, S.M. (2007) Cardiovascular and metabolic risk factors: how can we improve outcomes in the high-risk patient. *The American Journal of Medicine*, **120**(9A): S3-S9.

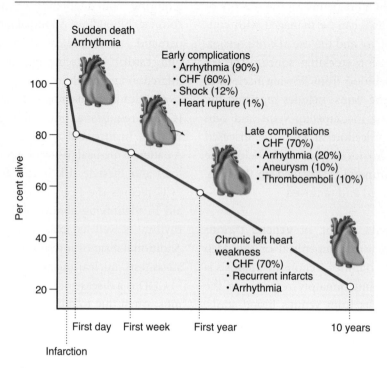

Figure 6.14 Outcome of myocardial infarction. Of 1-week survivors, 40% have late complications resulting in death; 10-year survival is about 25%. CHF, Congestive heart failure.

of age and more than 40% among persons over 75 years of age.

Symptoms of CHD include chest pain, or **angina pectoris**, which is pain and pressure felt in the chest that results from ischaemia; **palpitations**, or a sensation of a rapid pounding heartbeat; dizziness or fainting; weakness upon exertion or at rest; and shortness of breath. The most devastating sign of CHD is a heart attack, also known as a **myocardial infarction** (Figure 6.14). Crushing pain in the chest, shortness of breath, nausea, pallor, weakness and faintness are among the symptoms of a myocardial infarction.

Treatment of CHD depends on the severity of the disease as well as patient risk factors that may contribute to additional morbidity and mortality. Medications used to treat CHD include blood pressure lowering agents, blood thinners, diuretics (medication that increases excretion of water via the urine), nitrates such as nitroglycerin to stop chest pain and lipid lowering medication. Lifestyle changes, such as a healthy low salt diet and exercise,

are important to prevent further progression of disease.

Angioplasty is a procedure used to open a partly occluded artery (Figure 6.15). The procedure involves inserting a balloon-tipped catheter into the femoral artery, guiding it to the heart and into the narrowed coronary artery. The balloon is expanded to press against the vessel walls and open the lumen. A stent, which is a cylindrical wire mesh of stainless steel or other alloy, surrounds the balloon. Expansion of the balloon forces the mesh into the lining of the vessel, which physically holds the lumen open. Because the vessels commonly become occluded again (re-stenosis) within months or a year, stents are coated with drugs that prevent re-stenosis.

In cases of severe blockage of the coronary arteries, coronary artery bypass surgery may be needed. Coronary artery bypass surgery reroutes blood flow around the clogged arteries to improve blood flow and oxygen supply to the heart. A segment of a healthy blood vessel from another part of the body is attached or grafted from the aorta to the coronary

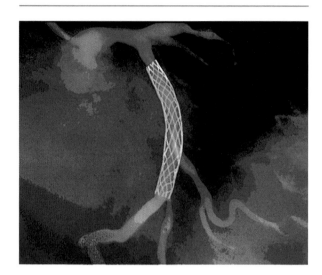

Figure 6.15 Angioplasty procedure. Note stent.
(ISM/Phototake NYC)

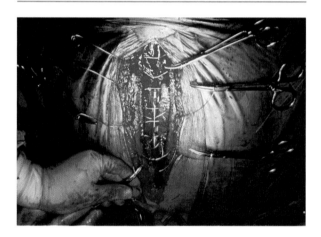

Figure 6.16 Bypass surgery of blocked coronary arteries.
(Antonia Reeve/Photo Researchers, Inc.)

artery below the blocked area. Depending on the number of blocked arteries, one or more grafts may be surgically placed (Figure 6.16).

Myocardial and endocardial diseases

Myocarditis Myocarditis is an inflammatory disease of the heart muscle. Viruses such as the Coxsackie virus, adenovirus and echovirus are the most common infecting viruses. Other potential aetiologies include infections with the human immune deficiency virus (HIV) and various bacterial infections.

Diagnosis of myocarditis can be suggested by clinical symptoms of the disease. An ECG recording provides evidence for conduction disturbances, and echocardiography may show an enlargement or inflammation of the heart muscle. Blood culture tests provide evidence for an infection. Elevations in certain heart muscle enzymes validate evidence for myocardial cell damage.

Myocarditis is often an asymptomatic condition. Patients usually have a history of viral illnesses, fever, chest pain that may feel like a heart attack, shortness of breath and tachycardia, or a rapid heartbeat.

The goal for treatment of myocarditis is prevention of further myocardial damage through patient supportive measures. Bed rest and activity restriction help decrease myocardial work. Antibiotics may be prescribed in cases where an infectious organism has been identified.

Cardiomyopathy Cardiomyopathy is a functional disease of the myocardium. There are three types of myocardial functional impairment: dilated, hypertrophic and restrictive cardiomyopathy (Figure 6.17). **Dilated cardiomyopathy** is the most common form and is characterised by dilatation of the ventricle, contractile dysfunction and symptoms of congestive heart failure. Ventricular hypertrophy is the

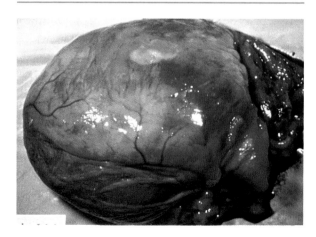

Figure 6.17 Cardiomyopathy.

dominant feature of **hypertrophic cardiomyopathy**. **Restrictive cardiomyopathy** is the least common form and is associated with reduced heart filling pressures and endocardial scarring in the ventricle.

Dilated cardiomyopathy may result from infections, myocarditis, toxic agents, metabolic disorders, genetic disorders and immune disorders. Often the cause is designated as **idiopathic dilated cardiomyopathy** as the aetiology is unknown. The symptoms of dilated cardiomyopathy include dyspnoea on exertion, orthopnoea, weakness, fatigue, ascites (accumulation of fluid in the abdomen) and peripheral oedema. Treatment is aimed at relieving the symptoms with medications, rest and surgical transplantation in severe cases.

Evidence for excessive ventricular growth is diagnostic for hypertrophic cardiomyopathy. Hypertrophic cardiomyopathy is a disease of young adulthood and is the most common cause of sudden cardiac death in the young. The aetiology is often unknown, although genetic mutations are identified in a small number of cases. The treatment of hypertrophic cardiomyopathy includes medications and surgery. The goal of medication therapy is to decrease symptoms of the disorder and to prevent sudden cardiac death. Surgery consists of incision to the ventricular septum and removal of parts of the diseased tissue.

Restrictive cardiomyopathy is distinguished by restricted ventricular filling owing to excessive rigidity of the ventricular walls. This condition is endemic in parts of Africa, India, South and Central America and Asia. The most common cause is a condition called **amyloidosis**, a group of diseases in which one or more organ systems in the body accumulate deposits of abnormal proteins. Symptoms of restrictive cardiomyopathy include dyspnoea, orthopnoea, peripheral oedema, ascites, weakness and fatigue.

Diseases of the endocardium

Infective endocarditis Infective endocarditis is a microbial infection that affects the endocardial endothelium and the heart valves. It occurs in adults and children with predisposing conditions. Rheumatic heart disease, valvular disease, degenerative heart

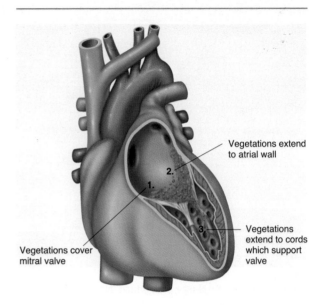

Figure 6.18 Bacterial endocarditis.

disease, congenital heart disease and intravenous drug abuse increase the risk for endocarditis.

Many species of bacteria and fungi cause the majority of cases of infectious endocarditis. Acute forms of this disease involve the formation of nodules or **vegetations** that consist of the infectious organisms and cellular debris enmeshed in a fibrous clot. Typical lesions of endocarditis are shown in Figure 6.18. As fragments of the vegetations break apart, they enter the bloodstream to form emboli which can travel to the brain, kidney, lung or other vital organs, causing a variety of symptoms. The emboli can lodge in small blood vessels of the skin or other organs and cause the blood vessels to rupture.

Symptoms of infective endocarditis include fever, chills, a change in the sound or character of an existing heart murmur and evidence for embolisation of the vegetative lesions. A blood culture test provides a definitive diagnosis of the causative organism and directs antimicrobial treatment. Echocardiograms are useful to detect any underlying valve disease and vegetations.

Immediate and extensive antimicrobial treatment is necessary to eliminate the causative microorganism. Surgical interventions are indicated in cases where the heart is severely damaged by the infection.

Rheumatic heart disease Rheumatic heart disease is a sequela of infection by group A haemolytic streptococci of skin, throat or ear, although the organisms are no longer present when the disease presents itself. Approximately 2 weeks after the streptococcal infection, rheumatic fever develops, characterised by fever, inflamed and painful joints, and sometimes a rash.

Rheumatic fever is an **autoimmune disease** that results from a reaction between streptococcal antigens and the patient's own antibodies against them. All parts of the heart may be affected, and this frequently includes the mitral valve. Blood clots deposit on the inflamed valves, forming nodular structures called vegetations along the edge of the cusps. The normally flexible cusps thicken and adhere to each other. Later, fibrous tissue develops, which has a tendency to contract.

If the adhesions of the cusps seriously narrow the valve opening, the mitral valve becomes stenotic. If sufficiently damaged, the cusps may not be able to meet properly, resulting in stenosis of the heart valves.

The incidence of rheumatic fever is highest among children and young adults. Prompt treatment of the streptococcal infection with antibiotics can prevent rheumatic fever and its complications. One consequence of rheumatic fever is the need for mitral valve surgery later in life.

Valvular heart disease

Valves maintain unidirectional flow of blood through the heart. Valve disorders include stenosis and valvular insufficiency. **Stenosis** refers to a narrowing of the valves opening and failure of the valve to open normally. **Valvular insufficiency** or **regurgitation** refers to a valve that allows backward flow of blood within the heart. Stenotic valves produce distension of the heart chamber that empties blood through the diseased valve and impaired filling of the chamber that receives the blood. Incompetent valves produce distension and strain the chamber ejecting blood through the diseased valve.

Mitral stenosis In **mitral stenosis**, the mitral valve opening is narrow, and the cusps that form the valve, normally flexible flaps, become rigid and fuse together. A deep funnel shape develops, increasing resistance to blood flow from the left atrium to the left ventricle. As back-pressure develops in the left atrium, the left atrial wall hypertrophies. The right side of the heart is also affected (Figure 6.19). Pressure within the heart makes it difficult for the pulmonary veins to deliver blood to the left atrium, leading to increased pressure within the veins. As the congestion increases in the veins, fluid from the blood leaks out into the tissue spaces of the lungs, causing pulmonary oedema. Poor circulation causes cyanosis because an inadequate amount of oxygen is reaching the tissues. The back-up of blood and congestion cause the heart to become exhausted and may lead to congestive heart failure. Another complication of a valve defect is the increased risk for a thrombus (blood clot) to form on the valve. If the thrombus becomes detached, it travels as an embolism and may occlude a blood vessel supplying the brain, kidney or other vital organ.

The predominant cause of mitral stenosis is rheumatic fever, which can cause inflammation of the valve leaflets. The leaflets may further stick together and/or form rigid scar tissue. Rheumatic fever most often occurs in children aged 5–15 years; however, symptoms of mitral stenosis may not be seen for a number of years.

Stenotic valves may be widened to restore blood flow with valvuloplasty, a surgical technique similar to angioplasty. A complication of the surgery may be a leaky valve, in which case the valve may be surgically replaced with metal alloy or pig valve.

Mitral regurgitation In mitral insufficiency, also called mitral regurgitation, the valve is unable to close completely, which allows blood to leak back into the atrium each time the ventricle contracts. As the volume of blood and pressure in the left atrium increases, blood pressure increases in other vessels, including the vessels (pulmonary veins) leading from the lungs to the heart, resulting in lung congestion. The insufficiency is exacerbated by sclerosis and retraction of the valve cusps.

Another cause of regurgitation is the failure of specialised valve muscles in the ventricle, called

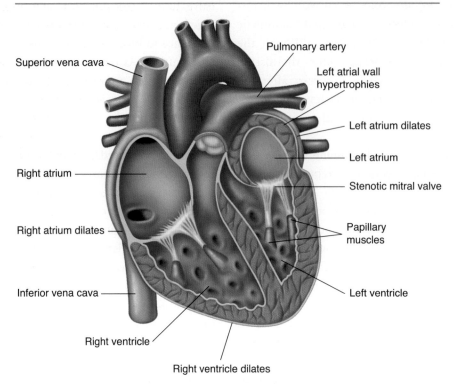

Figure 6.19 Effect of mitral valve stenosis on the heart.

papillary muscles. These muscles attach to the under-side of the cusps by means of small cords (chordae tendinae) that normally prevent the cusps from flipping up into the atria when the ventricles contract. If the papillary muscles fail to contract, the cusps open upward toward the atria under the force of expelled ventricular blood. This failure is commonly called mitral valve prolapse (MVP).

Most individuals with MVP are asymptomatic and lead normal lives. Those who have moderate or more severe cases of MVP take antibiotics such as amoxicillin to prevent bacteria from colonising the defective valves. If the prolapse becomes severe, it may be corrected with surgical reconstruction or replacement.

Aortic stenosis **Aortic stenosis**, the narrowing of the valve leading into the aorta, occurs more often in men than in women and most frequently in men over 50 years old. It may result from rheumatic fever, a congenital defect or arteriosclerosis. Aortic stenosis is characterised by rigid cusps that adhere together and deposits of hard, calcified material

which give a warty appearance to the valve. Because the left ventricle pumps blood through this narrowed valve into the aorta, this chamber hypertrophies. Even with enlarged ventricles, inadequate blood flow to the brain persists and can cause **syncope** (fainting). This valve defect, like others, can be corrected surgically.

Aortic regurgitation In aortic regurgitation, the valve does not close properly. With each relaxation of the left ventricle, blood flows back in from the aorta. Backflow of blood causes the ventricle to dilate, become exhausted and eventually fail. This condition can result from inflammation within the heart, endocarditis or a dilated aorta.

Symptoms of aortic regurgitation have a gradual onset. As the valve disease progresses, backflow of blood in the left ventricle increases, diastolic blood pressure falls, and the left ventricle enlarges. Most persons with aortic regurgitation remain asymptomatic for a number of years. The only sign for a number of years is a heart murmur. With advanced disease, symptoms of heart failure, such as dyspnoea, or shortness of breath, on exertion and at rest, occur.

Valvular defects are usually detected through cardiac auscultation (heart sound) heard via a stethoscope. Diagnosis is confirmed by a number of tests, including echocardiography, cardiac catheterisation, or phonocardiogram. A phonocardiogram is a device that records heart sounds. An ECG tracing is usually collected simultaneously to correlate the sounds to ventricular and atrial contractions.

Cardiac conduction disorders

Cardiac arrhythmias Abnormal heart rhythms, or **arrhythmias**, develop from irregularity in impulse generation and impulse conduction. Electrical impulses from the heart's pacemakers stimulate contraction of the atria and the ventricles. Many forms of heart disease can disrupt the normal contraction and relaxation cycle of the atria and ventricles.

Cardiac arrhythmias are commonly divided into two categories: supraventricular and ventricular. The **supraventricular arrhythmias** include those that are generated by electrical abnormalities in the sinoatrial (SA) node, atria, atrioventricular (AV) node and junctional tissue in the heart. The **ventricular arrhythmias** include those that are generated in the ventricular conduction system and in the ventricle. Because the ventricles are the pumping chambers of the heart, ventricular arrhythmias are the most serious as they can be life-threatening.

Disorders of cardiac rhythm can range from a sustained rapid heart rate of greater than 100 beats per minute, or **tachycardia**, to an abnormally slow heart rate of less than 50 beats per minute, or **bradycardia**. An interruption of the flow of impulses through the conduction system of the heart can lead to **heart block**. Heart block results when impulses are blocked, causing the atria and ventricles to contract independently of one another. The most serious effect of some forms of heart block is a slowing of the heart rate to the extent that circulation to vital organs such as the brain is blocked. An **ectopic pacemaker** is an excitable focus outside of the normally functioning pacemaker of the heart. Ectopic foci can cause additional beats (observed as

premature contractions) or take over the normal pacemaker activity of the SA node.

Fibrillation is the result of disorganised current flow within the atria, called **atrial fibrillation**, or ventricles, called **ventricular fibrillation**. Fibrillation interrupts the normal contraction of the atria or the ventricles. In ventricular fibrillation, the ventricle quivers and does not contract and carry out effective coordinated contractions. Because no blood is pumped from the heart, ventricular fibrillation is a form of cardiac arrest. Immediate attempts at resuscitation must be made, or death will result.

Cardiac rhythm disturbances cause a wide variety of symptoms, including palpitations, **syncope** or light-headedness, oedema or shortness of breath. The aetiologies of arrhythmias are numerous and include a history of coronary heart disease, heart valve disease, myocardial infarction, hypertension, atherosclerosis, metabolic diseases, smoking and drug abuse.

Medical therapy for the treatment of cardiac arrhythmias includes medications, electrocardioversion and catheter ablation. Antiarrhythmic medications alter the physiological properties of the heart's conduction system. Electrocardioversion is accomplished using an external device or a surgically placed internal pacemaker. A machine called an automated external defibrillator (AED) delivers electrical shocks and is used to re-establish normal heart rhythm (Figure 6.20). Defibrillators are implanted under the skin of the shoulder to resynchronise the heart on a daily basis, similar to a pacemaker device. Catheter ablation is a non-surgical procedure in which a catheter is inserted into the

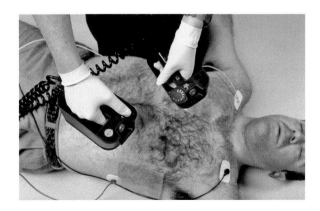

Figure 6.20 Electrocardioversion paddles.

diseased area of the heart. A machine directs energy through the catheter to small areas of the heart that cause the abnormal heart rhythm. This energy severs the connecting pathway of the abnormal rhythm.

CONGESTIVE HEART FAILURE

Congestive heart failure is a condition in which the heart cannot pump enough blood to meet the blood and oxygen needs of other body organs. It is a complication of most forms of heart disease, including coronary and peripheral atherosclerosis. There are nearly 23 million people living with heart failure worldwide.

Diagnostic methods for the diagnosis of heart failure include history and physical examination, laboratory studies, electrocardiography, chest radiography and echocardiography. The patient history includes collecting information on symptoms related to shortness of breath, fatigue and oedema. A complete physical examination includes assessment of heart sounds, heart rate and blood pressure; examination of the neck veins for congestion; and examination of the extremities for oedema. Laboratory tests are used to diagnose anaemia, blood disorders or signs of liver congestion. Echocardiography is useful in assessing the anatomical and functional abnormalities of heart failure, and electrocardiographic studies are useful in diagnosing underlying disorders of cardiac conduction and rhythm. Chest X-rays provide information on the size and shape of the heart and surrounding vasculature. They can also be used to determine the severity of heart failure by revealing the presence of pulmonary oedema.

The manifestations of heart failure depend on the extent of cardiac dysfunction, patient age, concurrent medical illnesses and the extent and rate at which cardiac performance becomes impaired. The severity of impairment ranges from mild, in which symptoms manifest clinically only during stress, to the most advanced form, in which the heart is unable to sustain life without external support. Mild symptoms of heart failure include ankle swelling and shortness of breath with exertion. Severe signs and symptoms include shortness of breath at rest, fatigue and limb weakness, neck vein swelling, rales (wet, crackly lung noises), pulmonary oedema (fluid in the lungs), cyanosis and abnormal heart sounds.

The goals of treatment for heart failure are aimed at relieving the symptoms, improving quality of life and halting the progression of cardiac dysfunction. Treatment includes correction of the underlying causes, medications, restriction of salt and water intake and modification of activities and lifestyle that are consistent with the functional limitations of the patient. Medication management of heart failure is complex and includes diuretics, medications that improve cardiac output, antihypertensives, anti-arrhythmics and medications that slow the heart rate and allow the heart muscle to relax and fill with blood. In severe cases, restriction of activity with bed rest often facilitates temporary improvement of heart function.

SHOCK

Shock is a life-threatening condition in which blood pressure drops too low to sustain life. Any condition that reduces the heart's ability to pump effectively or decreases venous return can cause shock. This low blood pressure results in an inadequate blood supply to the cells of the body. The cells can be quickly and irreversibly damaged and die. Major causes of shock include cardiogenic, hypovolaemic, anaphylactic, septic and neurogenic shock. See Table 6.4 for types and aetiology.

Table 6.4 Types of shock and aetiology.

Type of shock	Aetiology
Cardiogenic	Cardiac arrhythmias Myocardial infarction
Hypovolaemic	Haemorrhage Trauma Surgery Extensive burns
Anaphylactic	Allergic reaction
Septic	Toxins released by a bacterial infection
Neurogenic	Damage to the central nervous system

Untreated shock is usually fatal. The prognosis depends on the underlying cause, pre-existing illnesses, the time between onset and diagnosis, and rapidity of response to therapy.

HEART DISEASE IN INFANTS AND CHILDREN

Fetal and perinatal circulation

Fetal circulation is anatomically different from postnatal circulation (Figure 6.21). Before birth, oxygenated blood flows through the placenta from the umbilical vein. The fetal lungs are entirely bypassed either by direct passage from the inferior vena cava to the right atrium through the foramen ovale to the left atrium, or from the right ventricle through the pulmonary artery through the ductus arteriosus to the aorta.

The umbilical vein connects to the fetal venous system, which returns blood to the fetal right atrium via the inferior vena cava. From the inferior vena cava, blood flows into the right atrium and then moves through the foramen ovale into the left atrium. It then passes into the left ventricle and is pumped into the ascending aorta to perfuse the heart and upper extremities. At the same time, venous blood from the heart and upper extremities returns to the right side of the heart by way of the superior vena cava, moves into the right ventricle and is pumped into the pulmonary artery. Blood that is ejected into the pulmonary artery is diverted through the ductus arteriosus into the descending aorta. This blood perfuses the lower extremities.

When a baby takes its first breath after birth, the newly expanded lungs initiate a switch from placental to pulmonary oxygenation of the blood. Cord clamping and removal of the placental circulation cause an increase in left ventricular pressure. The decrease in right atrial pressure and decrease in left atrial pressure produce a closure of the foramen ovale. The newly expanded lungs favour the flow from the right heart via the pulmonary artery to the lungs as opposed to the ductus arteriosus. Closure of both the foramen ovale and the ductus arteriosus leads to the establishment of the postnatal circulation.

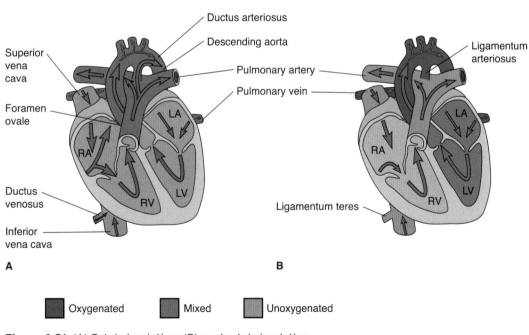

Figure 6.21 (A) Fetal circulation; (B) postnatal circulation.

Congenital heart disease

The embryological development of the heart is complex, and many errors can occur during development. Genetic, environmental and chromosomal changes may alter the development of the heart. Infants born to parents with a history of congenital heart disease are at a higher risk. Infants born with chromosomal abnormalities such as Down's syndrome or Turner syndrome have an increased risk for congenital heart disease. Maternal diabetes, congenital rubella, maternal alcoholism and treatment with anticonvulsant drugs are also associated with congenital heart disease.

Approximately 6 babies in 1000 births in the UK have some form of congenital heart disease. Owing to advances in technology and early recognition of congenital heart disease, approximately 85% of infants born with congenital heart disease can be expected to survive into adulthood. Congenital defects can affect almost any of the cardiac structures or circulatory blood vessels.

Congenital heart disease is divided into aetiologies that cause cyanosis, or blue babies, and those that do not cause cyanosis. For cyanosis to occur, deoxygenated blood must bypass the lungs and enter the systemic circulation.

Cyanotic heart disease

Tetralogy of Fallot Tetralogy of Fallot is one of the most serious of the congenital heart defects and consists of four abnormalities: (1) ventricular septal defect; (2) narrowing of the pulmonary outflow channel, including pulmonary valve stenosis, or a decrease in the size of the pulmonary trunk; (3) misplaced aorta that crosses the interventricular septum; and (4) hypertrophy of the right ventricle (Figure 6.22).

Maternal factors during pregnancy that are associated with tetralogy of Fallot include a history of rubella, poor nutrition, overuse of alcohol, history of diabetes and maternal age over 40. Heredity may also play a role, as parents with a history of tetralogy of Fallot have a greater risk of having a child with this disease. Children with genetic disorders such as Down's syndrome often have congenital heart defects, including tetralogy of Fallot.

Symptoms of this condition include difficulty feeding, failure to gain weight, poor development, cyanosis that becomes more pronounced during feeding, crying or defaecation, fainting, sudden death, clubbing of the fingers and squatting during episodes of cyanosis.

Surgical repair is often advised for all children born with this defect. More than one surgical procedure is required to increase blood flow to the lungs, patch the ventricular septal defect, open the narrowed pulmonary valve, and close any abnormal connections between the aorta and pulmonary artery.

Transposition of the great arteries In this condition, the aorta and the pulmonary artery connect

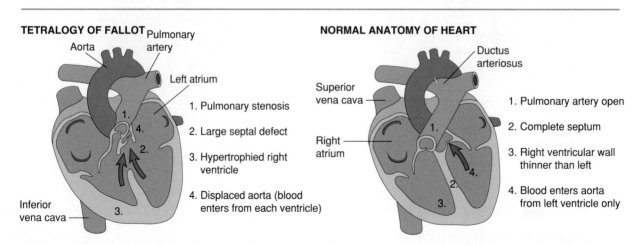

Figure 6.22 (A) Tetralogy of Fallot; (B) normal anatomy.

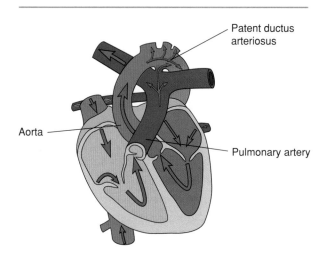

Figure 6.23 Transposition of the great arteries.

to the wrong ventricle. The pulmonary artery is attached to the left ventricle, and the aorta is attached to the right ventricle; thus blood flow in the lungs and in the body occurs independently. Deoxygenated blood returns to the right heart and is pumped to the aorta, which pumps blood to the

systemic circulation. The left heart receives blood from the lungs and then pumps the blood back to the lungs (Figure 6.23).

Symptoms include cyanosis, shortness of breath, poor feeding and clubbing of the fingers. If diagnosed prior to birth, prostaglandins are administered to maintain a patent ductus arteriosus and allow mixing of oxygenated and deoxygenated blood to occur. Corrective surgery within the first 2–3 weeks of life is essential for long-term survival. An arterial switch procedure corrects both systemic and pulmonary blood flow.

Non-cyanotic congenital heart disease

Septal defects Septal defects may occur between the two atria, an atrial septal defect (ASD), or between the ventricles, a ventricular septal defect (VSD). Often these defects can be detected by the presence of a heart murmur on physical examination. In both conditions, blood in the right heart will be a mixture of deoxygenated blood and oxygenated blood that has traversed the left side of the heart (Figure 6.24).

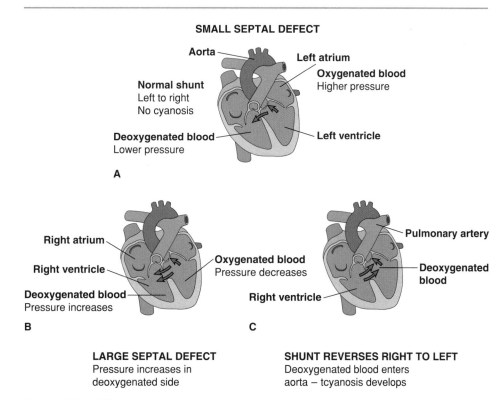

Figure 6.24 Effects of septal defects: (A) normal shunt; no cyanosis; (B) increased pressure in right ventricle; (C) shunt reversal; cyanosis develops.

Small ASDs may not cause any symptoms. Large ASDs can lead to significant overload and enlargement of the right ventricle. Large ASDs require surgical repair.

A VSD causes increased blood flow to the lungs, which can eventually cause severe pulmonary hypertension. In this condition, oxygenated blood is shunted from the left ventricle to the right ventricle, which contains deoxygenated blood. This results in increased pressures in the lungs. As pressure continues to build, the right ventricle shunts unoxygenated blood to the left ventricle, leading to cyanosis. Large VSDs require surgical correction.

Patent ductus arteriosus (PDA) The ductus arteriosus serves as a fetal connection between the pulmonary artery and the aorta. In the fetal circulation, this allows blood to bypass the non-functional fetal lungs. At birth the ductus arteriosus normally closes. If the ductus remains open, blood intended for the body flows from the aorta to the lungs, overloading the pulmonary artery. Persistent increases in pulmonary arterial pressures can result in heart failure (Figure 6.25).

It is more common in premature infants but does occur in full-term infants. Premature babies with PDA are more vulnerable to its effects. PDA is twice as common in girls as in boys.

A patent ductus can be treated medically with anti-inflammatory medications to close the PDA and with antibiotics to prevent endocarditis. If medication therapy fails, a transcatheter device procedure or surgery may be performed to close the PDA.

Coarctation of the aorta Coarctation of the aorta is a congenital narrowing of the aorta that can occur anywhere along its length (Figure 6.26). Most commonly it occurs near the ductus arteriosus. A severe coarctation causes increases in resistance to the left ventricle and can eventually lead to heart failure.

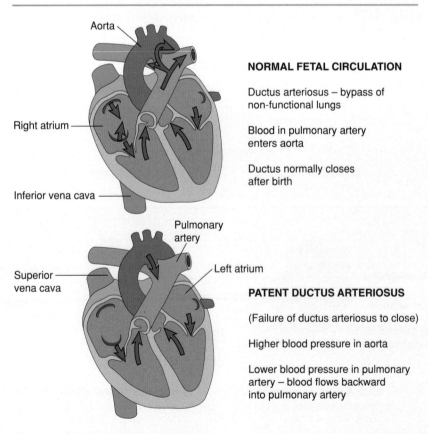

Aorta

Right atrium

Inferior vena cava

NORMAL FETAL CIRCULATION

Ductus arteriosus – bypass of non-functional lungs

Blood in pulmonary artery enters aorta

Ductus normally closes after birth

Pulmonary artery

Superior vena cava

Left atrium

PATENT DUCTUS ARTERIOSUS

(Failure of ductus arteriosus to close)

Higher blood pressure in aorta

Lower blood pressure in pulmonary artery – blood flows backward into pulmonary artery

Figure 6.25 Patent ductus arteriosus.

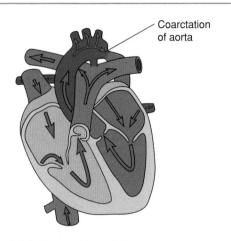

Figure 6.26 Coarctation of the aorta.

Aortic coarctation occurs in approximately 1 out of 10 000 live births. It is often diagnosed in childhood, especially in cases where the narrowing is severe.

In severe cases, symptoms are observed in infancy and include dizziness, shortness of breath and cold legs. A harsh murmur heard on the back with the stethoscope along with X-ray scans, echocardiography and Doppler ultrasound provide a definitive diagnosis for this condition.

Surgery is often recommended to enlarge the narrowing of the aorta. The coarctation of the aorta is surgically corrected by cutting the narrowed segment of the aorta and rejoining the healthy ends.

AGE-RELATED DISEASE

Worldwide, the population of individuals older than 65 years is projected to increase to 973 million (12%) by the year 2030 and comprise about 20% of the population in 2050.

Cardiovascular disease is the most frequent diagnosis in older adults and the leading cause of death in both men and women older than 65 years. In older adults, cardiovascular disease differs from that in younger people. With age, systolic blood pressure and left ventricular mass progressively increase, and ventricular filling, heart rate and cardiac output, exercise capacity and reflex responses of heart rate decrease. Cellular, enzymatic and molecular changes in the arterial vessels lead to arterial dilatation, thickening of the arterial intima and vascular stiffness. With age, the cardiovascular system is less able to respond to increases in workload and stress; therefore, thresholds for symptoms of cardiovascular disease become more common with age.

Resources

Centers for Disease Control: *www.cdc.gov*

World Health Organization: *www.who.int/mediacentre/factsheets/fs317/en/index.html*

American Heart Association: *www.americanheart.org*

National Institutes of Health: *www.nhlbi.nih.gov.guidelines/cholesterol/atglance.htm*

DISEASES AT A GLANCE Cardiac system

DISEASE	AETIOLOGY	SIGNS AND SYMPTOMS	DIAGNOSIS	TREATMENT	PREVENTION	LIFESPAN
Hypercholestero-laemia	Genetic, lifestyle, obesity and diabetes, diet high in saturated fat	Elevated serum cholesterol	Blood test	Change in dietary habits, low fat diet, cholesterol lowering medication	Healthy lifestyle, diet and exercise, weight loss, low fat diet	Can occur at any age
Atherosclerosis	Genetic, lifestyle, obesity and diabetes, diet high in saturated fat	Occlusion of an artery. Symptoms depend on location of occlusion	ECG, coronary angiography, blood tests, CT scan	Weight loss, exercise, control blood pressure with antihypertensives, reduce cholesterol with cholesterol lowering medication	Healthy lifestyle, diet and exercise, weight loss, low fat diet	Occurs in adults, older adults
Peripheral artery disease	Genetic, lifestyle, obesity and diabetes, diet high in saturated fat	Intermittent claudication, thinning of the skin of the lower leg, ulceration of the skin, gangrene can occur in advanced stages of this disease	Physical examination for ischaemia, skin atrophy, pallor, absent pulses, Doppler ultrasound	Weight loss, exercise, control blood pressure with antihypertensives, reduce cholesterol with cholesterol lowering medication	Healthy lifestyle, diet and exercise, weight loss, low fat diet	Occurs in adults, older adults
Raynaud's disease	Unknown	Changes in skin colour from pallor to cyanosis, sensation of cold, numbness, or tingling	Physical examination	Abstinence from cigarette smoking, protection of the hands from cold, medications that prevent vasospasm	Abstinence from cigarette smoking, protection of the hands from cold, medications that prevent vasospasm	Most often occurs in healthy young women
Aortic aneurysm	Atherosclerosis, connective tissue disease, infections, trauma, inflammation	Usually asymptomatic until rupture	Physical examination, ultrasound, echocardiography, CT scan, MRI	Surgery to repair aneurysm, control of blood pressure and atherosclerosis	Healthy lifestyle; control of hypertension, diabetes and hypercholesterolaemia	Usually develops after the age of 50 years
Arterial hypertension	Older age, sedentary lifestyle, overweight, excessive dietary salt intake, family history	Elevated blood pressure	Blood pressure measurement via sphygmomanometer	Blood pressure lowering medication, diet, weight loss and exercise	Healthy lifestyle with proper diet and exercise; control of diabetes, hypercholesterolaemia, weight loss	Incidence of high blood pressure increases with age
Pulmonary arterial hypertension	Aetiology unknown in many cases, ventricular septal defect, patent ductus arteriosus	Asymptomatic	Echocardiography, pulmonary function test, lung scan, cardiac catheterisation	Medications to lower pressure, oxygen, lung transplant	Unknown as aetiology often unknown, surgical correction of ventricular septal defect and patent ductus arteriosus	Can occur at any age
Varicose veins	Long periods of standing, pregnancy	Swollen veins of the legs, knotty appearance under the skin	Physical examination of the legs	Elastic bandages, support hose, walking, elevating the legs, surgical vein stripping, compression sclerotherapy	Weight loss, walking, elevation of the legs after long periods of standing	Occurs mostly in adults

DISEASES AT A GLANCE Cardiac system (continued)

DISEASE	AETIOLOGY	SIGNS AND SYMPTOMS	DIAGNOSIS	TREATMENT	PREVENTION	LIFESPAN
Chronic venous insufficiency	Deep vein thrombosis, obesity, smoking, pregnancy, sedentary lifestyle	Tissue congestion, oedema, necrosis or skin atrophy, pain with walking	Outflow plethysmography, Doppler imaging studies	Diet, exercise, compression stockings, surgical bypass procedure	Weight loss, control of atherosclerosis and hypercholesterolaemia, diabetes, exercise, healthy eating	Peak incidence is between the ages of 40 and 49 years in women and 70 and 79 years in men
Venous thrombosis	Hypercoagulability, vascular trauma, surgery, immobilisation	No symptoms in about 50% of individuals. Symptoms of inflammation such as pain, swelling, deep muscle tenderness	Doppler imaging, physical examination	Blood thinning medication, surgery to remove the thrombus	Early ambulation following surgery or childbirth, compression stockings	Can occur at any age, more common in adults and older adults
Coronary heart disease	Atherosclerosis, high blood pressure, diabetes, obesity, inactivity	Angina pectoris, palpitations, myocardial infarction	Physical examination, ECG, stress test, nuclear imaging, angiography	Angioplasty, coronary artery bypass surgery, blood pressure lowering medication, blood thinners, diuretics, nitrates to stop chest pain, cholesterol lowering medication, diet, exercise	Control of atherosclerosis; diet, exercise, weight loss if overweight or obese	Occurs in adults and older adults
Myocarditis	Coxsackie virus, adenovirus, echovirus, HIV	Fever, chest pain, shortness of breath, tachycardia	Echocardiography, ECG, physical examination	Bed rest to prevent further myocardial damage, treatment of the viral infection	Unknown	Can occur at any age
Dilated cardiomyopathy	Infections, myocarditis, metabolic disorders, genetic disorders, immune disorders	Dyspnoea, orthopnoea, weakness, fatigue, ascites and peripheral oedema	Echocardiography, ECG, physical examination	Medications to treat symptoms, rest, heart transplant if severe	Unknown	Can occur at any age
Hypertrophic (A) cardiomyopathy	Unknown	Excessive ventricular growth	Echocardiography, ECG, physical examination	Medications to treat symptoms and prevent sudden cardiac death	Unknown	Usually a disease of young adulthood. Most common cause of sudden cardiac death in the young
Restrictive cardiomyopathy	Endemic in parts of Africa, India, South and Central America and Asia; amyloidosis	Dyspnoea, orthopnoea, peripheral oedema, weakness, fatigue	Echocardiography, ECG, physical examination	Medications to treat symptoms	Unknown	Can occur at any age

DISEASES AT A GLANCE Cardiac system (continued)

DISEASE	AETIOLOGY	SIGNS AND SYMPTOMS	DIAGNOSIS	TREATMENT	PREVENTION	LIFESPAN
Infective endocarditis	Rheumatic heart disease, valvular disease, degenerative heart disease, congenital heart disease, intravenous drug abuse, bacterial infections	Fever, chills, change in sound of an existing murmur, vegetative lesion on the heart valves	Blood cultures, echocardiography, ECG, body temperature, blood cultures to identify bacterium	Antimicrobial therapy, surgery in severe cases to remove vegetations	Prompt treatment of bacterial infections, prophylactic antimicrobial therapy	Can occur at any age
Rheumatic heart disease	Infection with group A haemolytic streptococci	Fever, inflammation of the joints, rash	Blood cultures, ECG, echocardiography	Antimicrobial therapy	Prompt treatment of bacterial infections, prophylactic antimicrobial therapy	Incidence is highest among children and young adults
Valvular heart disease						
Mitral stenosis	Rheumatic fever	Increased pressure in the heart, congestion of the veins, cyanosis, congestive heart failure	ECG, echocardiography, phonocardiogram, cardiac catheterisation	Valvuloplasty, surgical valve replacement	Prompt treatment of bacterial infections, prophylactic antimicrobial therapy, treatment of cardiac symptoms	Can occur at any age
Mitral regurgitation	Mitral valve prolapse	Usually no symptoms	ECG, echocardiography, phonocardiogram, cardiac catheterisation	Surgery to replace valve	Prophylactic antimicrobial therapy prevents bacteria from colonising defective valve	Can occur at any age
Aortic stenosis	Rheumatic fever, congenital defect, arteriosclerosis	Hypertrophy of the left ventricle, calcified deposits on the valve	ECG, echocardiography, phonocardiogram, cardiac catheterisation	Surgery to replace valve	Prophylactic antimicrobial therapy prevents bacteria from colonising defective valve	Occurs more frequently in men over 50 years of age than women
Aortic regurgitation	Endocarditis, dilated aorta	Dilatation of the ventricle. Backflow of blood into the left ventricle, decreased diastolic pressure, symptoms of heart failure	ECG, blood pressure check, echocardiography, phonocardiogram, cardiac catheterisation	Surgery to replace valve	Unknown	Can occur at any age

DISEASES AT A GLANCE Cardiac system (continued)

DISEASE	AETIOLOGY	SIGNS AND SYMPTOMS	DIAGNOSIS	TREATMENT	PREVENTION	LIFESPAN
Cardiac arrhythmias						
Supraventricular	Abnormalities in the SA node, AV node, and junctional tissue of the heart, myocardial infarction, hypertension, atherosclerosis, metabolic disease, smoking and drug abuse	Tachycardia, bradycardia, heart block, syncope, oedema, shortness of breath	ECG, blood pressure check, echocardiography, phonocardiogram, cardiac catheterisation	Antiarrhythmic medications	Prevention of heart disease	Can occur at any age, most commonly occurs in adults and older adults as a consequence of heart disease
Ventricular	Generated by abnormalities in the ventricular conduction system and in the ventricle, myocardial infarction, hypertension, atherosclerosis, metabolic disease, smoking and drug abuse	Tachycardia, bradycardia, heart block, syncope, oedema, shortness of breath	ECG, blood pressure check, echocardiography, phonocardiogram, cardiac catheterisation	Antiarrhythmic medications	Prevention of heart disease	Can occur at any age, most commonly occurs in adults and older adults as a consequence of heart disease
Congestive heart failure	Complication of most forms of heart disease	Shortness of breath, fatigue, oedema	Physical examination, ECG, X-ray, echocardiography, blood pressure	Medication therapy includes diuretics, antihypertensives, antiarrhythmic medications, medications that improve cardiac output, bed rest	Treatment of underlying heart disease	Can occur at any age; most commonly occurs in adults and older adults
Shock	Heart disease, haemorrhage, trauma, surgery, allergic reaction, release of bacterial toxins, damage to the central nervous system	Drop in blood pressure too low to sustain life	Physical examination, medical history	Rapid administration of fluids to increase blood pressure, medication to increase heart rate	Fluid replacement during surgery, prompt treatment of severe bacterial infections, prompt treatment of allergic reactions, blood transfusion in cases of severe blood loss	Can occur at any age
Congenital heart disease						
Tetralogy of Fallot	Maternal history of rubella, overuse of alcohol, maternal history of diabetes or poor prenatal nutrition. Infants born with Down's syndrome	Difficulty feeding, failure to gain weight, poor development, cyanosis, fainting, sudden death	ECG, blood pressure check, echocardiography, phonocardiogram, cardiac catheterisation	Corrective surgery	Unknown	Occurs in infants

DISEASES AT A GLANCE Cardiac system (continued)

DISEASE	AETIOLOGY	SIGNS AND SYMPTOMS	DIAGNOSIS	TREATMENT	PREVENTION	LIFESPAN
Transposition of the great arteries	Unknown	Cyanosis, shortness of breath, poor feeding	ECG, blood pressure check, echocardiography, phonocardiogram, cardiac catheterisation	Administration of prostaglandins at birth to maintain patent ductus arteriosus until corrective surgery can be achieved	Unknown	Occurs in infants
Septal defects	Unknown	Heart murmur, a ventriculoseptal defect causes increased blood flow to the lungs	ECG, blood pressure check, echocardiography, phonocardiogram, cardiac catheterisation	Large defects require surgical correction	Unknown	Occurs in infants; small defects may persist unnoticed through adulthood
Patent ductus arteriosus	Unknown	Initially asymptomatic; increased pressure in the lungs can lead to pulmonary hypertension	ECG, blood pressure check, echocardiography, phonocardiogram, cardiac catheterisation	Antibiotics to prevent endocarditis, anti-inflammatory medication to close the patent ductus	Unknown	More common in premature infants
Coarctation of the aorta	Unknown	Increased pressure in the left ventricle, symptoms of heart failure in severe narrowing	ECG, blood pressure check, echocardiography, phonocardiogram, cardiac catheterisation, Doppler ultrasound	Surgical correction	Unknown	Diagnosed and corrected in infancy

INTERACTIVE EXERCISES

Cases for critical thinking

1. The paramedics are called to a 59-year-old male who is experiencing severe chest pain while playing golf. What type(s) of heart or vascular disease should be considered in this patient?

2. A 65-year-old female goes to her GP with shortness of breath, feeling of faintness, dizziness and productive cough, all of which have persisted over the past 2 months. Upon examination, the GP records a blood pressure of 90/50 mmHg, congestion in the lungs and abnormal heart sounds. What type of heart diseases should be considered in this patient?

3. A 30-year-old obese female complains of pain with walking. The patient has a history of smoking cigarettes and is a 'borderline diabetic'. Explain the role of cardiovascular risk factors for cardiovascular diseases for this patient.

Multiple choice

1. Syncope is _____
   a. hypertension   b. shortness of breath
   c. light-headedness   d. fluid retention

2. Diastole is the _____
   a. filling phase of the heart
   b. contracting phase of the heart
   c. alternation between relaxation and excitation of the heart
   d. impulse of the heart

3. The major cholesterol carrier in the blood is _____
   a. HDL   b. triglycerides
   c. blood   d. LDL

4. Blockage of the _____ can reduce blood supply to the brain, causing a stroke.
   a. pulmonary artery   b. carotid artery
   c. aorta   d. coronary artery

5. The most common cause of an aortic aneurysm is _____
   a. atherosclerosis   b. hypertension
   c. enlarged artery   d. embolism

6. A procedure involving insertion of a balloon-tipped catheter into the femoral artery to the heart is called a(n)_____
   a. defibrillator
   b. angioplasty

   c. transcatheter procedure
   d. echocardiography

7. The mitral valve is located _____
   a. between the right atrium and the right ventricle
   b. between the left atrium and the left ventricle
   c. in the atria
   d. in the ventricle

8. The pacemaker of the heart is the _____
   a. atrioventricular valve
   b. His-Purkinje fibres
   c. ventricle
   d. sinoatrial node

9. An inflammatory disease of the heart muscle is _____
   a. myocarditis
   b. pericardial disease
   c. cardiomyopathy
   d. coronary heart disease

10. Rheumatic heart disease is also known as a(n) _____ disease because it results from a reaction between bacterial antigens and the patient's antibodies.
   a. haemolytic   b. vegetative
   c. autoimmune   d. tricuspid valve

True or false

_____ **1.** Infants born with chromosomal abnormalities have a higher risk for congenital heart disease.

_____ **2.** Salt and water restriction is one form of treatment for congestive heart failure.

_____ **3.** An interruption of the flow of impulses through the conduction system is called bradycardia.

_____ **4.** In ventricular fibrillation, the heart quivers and is unable to maintain cardiac output.

_____ **5.** In mitral valve stenosis, delivery of blood via the pulmonary veins to the left atrium is impaired.

_____ **6.** Cardiomyopathy is a structural disease of the heart.

_____ **7.** The most common cause of infective endocarditis is a bacterial infection.

_____ **8.** The basic lesion of clinical atherosclerosis is a fatty streak.

_____ **9.** Intact aortic aneurysms typically cause symptoms.

_____ **10.** Hypertension is broadly defined as an arterial pressure greater than 120/80 mmHg.

Fill-ins

1. The most common cause of chronic venous insufficiency is deep vein _____.

2. More than 90% of patients with coronary heart disease have _____.

3. _____ is associated with reduced heart filling pressure and endocardial scarring.

4. _____ refers to a narrowing of the valves.

5. The predominant cause of mitral stenosis is _____.

6. Backflow of blood in aortic regurgitation causes the _____ to dilate.

7. An _____ is an excitable focus outside of the normally functioning pacemaker of the heart.

8. A machine called an _____ delivers electrical shocks and is used to re-establish normal heart rhythm.

9. Two forms of cyanotic congenital heart disease are _____ and _____.

10. The _____ arteries provide the heart muscle with blood and oxygen.

Labelling exercise

Use the blank lines below to label the following image.

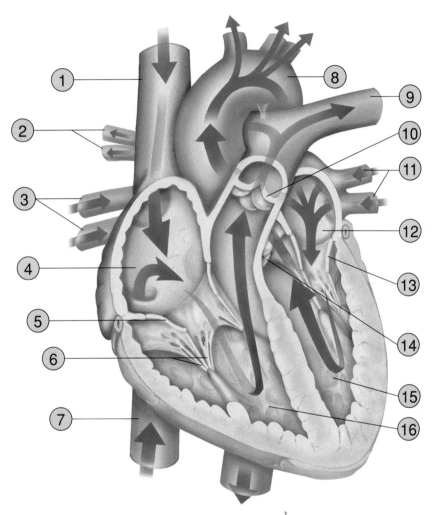

1. Superior vena cava
2. Pulmonary artery
3. R Pulmonary Veins
4. R Atrium
5. Tricuspid valve
6. _____
7. Inferior Vena Cava
8. aorta
9. L Pulmonary artery
10. Pulmonary semi lunar valve
11. Pulmonary veins
12. L Atrium
13. Bicuspid (mitral valve)
14. Aortic valve
15. L Ventricle
16. R Ventricle

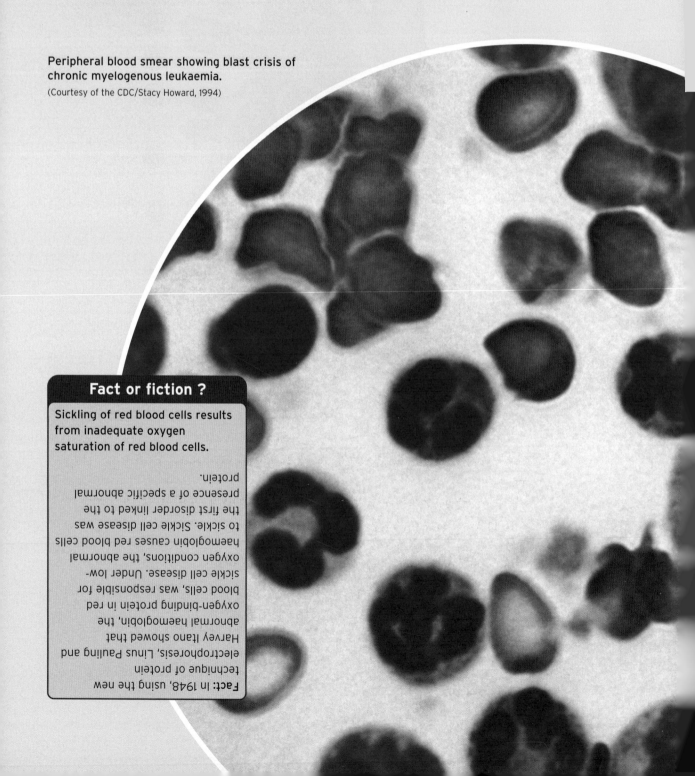

7 DISEASES OF THE BLOOD

Peripheral blood smear showing blast crisis of chronic myelogenous leukaemia.

(Courtesy of the CDC/Stacy Howard, 1994)

Fact or fiction ?

Sickling of red blood cells results from inadequate oxygen saturation of red blood cells.

Fact: In 1948, using the new technique of protein electrophoresis, Linus Pauling and Harvey Itano showed that abnormal haemoglobin, the oxygen-binding protein in red blood cells, was responsible for sickle cell disease. Under low-oxygen conditions, the abnormal haemoglobin causes red blood cells to sickle. Sickle cell disease was the first disorder linked to the presence of a specific abnormal protein.

Learning objectives

After studying this chapter, you should be able to:

✚ Distinguish between plasma and formed elements of the blood

✚ Delineate the function of red blood cells, white blood cells and platelets

✚ Identify the aetiology, signs and symptoms, diagnostic tests and treatment for selected diseases of the blood

Disease chronicle

Clinical use of leeches

The first clinical use of medicinal leeches (*Hirudo medicinalis*) occurred approximately 2500 years ago. They were thought to release 'bad blood' because they release substances that allow continued bleeding up to 10 hours after the animal has detached, thereby curing everything from headaches and gout to depression. However, today these small invertebrates are being rediscovered as a valuable aid in healthcare. In plastic surgery – for instance reconstructive surgery following traumatic amputation – it is relatively easy to re-join the severed edges of the arteries but not the more delicate edges of the veins. This means that the blood flows to the affected area, but cannot drain away, and so the limb becomes congested and the blood clots. A leech attached to the wound releases substances including an anticoagulant, a local vasodilator and local anaesthetic. This allows both a good flow of blood to the injured tissue and the means of escape for the blood. After a few days the venous drainage is usually restored and the leech's job is done. So a leech will not cure your headache, but it may save your limb.

INTRODUCTION

Blood is the medium for transporting oxygen, carbon dioxide, water, nutrients, proteins, hormones and heat where needed throughout the body and waste products to the excretory organs. The cellular components of the blood include the red blood cells, or erythrocytes, white blood cells, or leucocytes, and platelets or thrombocytes. These cells travel through the circulatory system suspended in the fluid portion of the blood called **plasma**.

Red blood cells

Erythrocytes, or red blood cells (RBCs), make up nearly half of the blood's volume. Red blood cells are the most abundant cells in the human body. Erythrocytes normally number about 5 million/mm^3 in males and about 4.5 million/mm^3 in females.

Red blood cells are highly specialised cells. They are biconcave sacs filled with an iron-rich oxygen-carrying protein called **haemoglobin**, the most important component of the cells. It is composed of a protein called **globulin** and a **haem** molecule which binds to iron.

In the oxygen-rich environment of the lungs, haem binds to oxygen in exchange for carbon dioxide. The oxygenated red blood cells are then transported to the oxygen-poor tissues, where the haemoglobin releases the oxygen in exchange for carbon dioxide. The less oxygen in the environment of the tissues, the more readily this occurs. The average lifespan of a red blood cell is 120 days, after which they are removed from the body by the liver and the spleen.

Erythrocytes do not contain a nucleus, so are unable to replicate and are produced from immature stem cells in the red marrow of the bones such as the vertebrae and the body of the sternum. The process of red blood cell formation, called **erythropoiesis**, is regulated by the hormone **erythropoietin**, from the kidney. Erythrocyte synthesis begins with large nucleated stem cells that progress through many stages before emerging as mature red blood cells. In the process, haemoglobin accumulates within the cytoplasm and the nucleus disappears. Mature red blood cells emerge from the bone marrow as reticulocytes.

DIAGNOSTIC TESTS FOR DISEASES OF THE BLOOD

Blood tests are diagnostic for systemic diseases as well as for specific blood disorders. Blood analysis measures total blood counts (red blood cells, white blood cells and platelets), haemoglobin, haematocrit, serum chemistry and enzyme and hormone levels within the body. Differential blood analysis provides information such as size, shape and ratio of one cell type to another.

A bone marrow sample is used to diagnose malignant blood disorders and increases or decreases in blood counts without any apparent cause. The samples are obtained by needle aspiration of the bone marrow from the bone marrow cavity. Analysis then provides information on the function of the bone marrow and the qualitative characteristics of stem cells that give rise to all blood cells.

ANAEMIA

Anaemia is a condition of reduced numbers of red blood cells. Causes include haemorrhage, excessive destruction of red blood cells and nutritional deficiency. These decrease the number of red blood cells and oxygen delivery to the cells and tissues.

The clinical diagnosis of anaemia requires a microscopic examination and analysis of red blood cells. A detailed medical history, including information on dietary habits, family history of anaemia and information regarding the patient's concurrent medical problems provides data for the potential aetiology of the anaemia.

Anaemia leads to tissue **hypoxia**, or lack of oxygen. Most patients develop anaemia slowly and have few symptoms, but acute haemorrhage results in rapid appearance of symptoms and, if severe, may result in shock. Usual complaints are fatigue, decreased tolerance for exercise, dyspnoea and palpitations. Upon examination, the major sign of

Anaemia

For a half a billion women in developing countries worldwide, anaemia is a lifelong burden that affects them, their infants and young children. Controlling anaemia in these vulnerable groups could significantly reduce maternal and infant morbidity. It would also enhance intellectual and work capacity, thereby improving family, community and national socioeconomic development.

Despite international efforts led by the United Nations, the global prevalence of anaemia has failed to decline. The reasons for this lack of improvement include the failure to identify the aetiology of the anaemia, underfunding and poor healthcare with inadequate nutritional supplementation.

Source: From WHO, 2007, 'Iron Deficiency Anaemia, Assessment Prevention, and Control. A Guide for Programme Managers.'

anaemia is pallor. Jaundice and enlargement of the spleen occurs with anaemia caused by **haemolysis**, or red blood cell death. Cardiac signs of anaemia include tachycardia, or rapid heartbeat, and heart murmurs.

Iron deficiency anaemia

Iron balance in the body is tightly controlled and designed to conserve iron for re-use. There is no excretory pathway for iron, and the only means of iron loss from the body is blood loss and the loss of epidermal cells from the skin and the gut. Iron should be replaced by sufficient dietary intake or from medicinal supplementation.

Women of childbearing years are advised to take 14.8 mg of iron a day; men and older women should take 8.7 mg a day. However, in the UK the average intake is 10 mg a day for women and 13.2 mg per day for men, and in both cases younger people tend to take less. Iron absorption takes place in the small intestine and is a carefully regulated process.

Iron deficiency anaemia is the condition in which there is anaemia with evidence of iron deficiency. The first stage in the development of iron deficiency anaemia is a negative iron balance, in which the demands for iron exceed the body's ability to absorb iron from the diet. This stage can result from a number of physiological problems, including blood loss, pregnancy, rapid growth spurts in children and adolescents, and inadequate dietary intake. During

pregnancy, the demands for red blood cell production by the fetus exceed the mother's ability to provide iron. During the first stage of iron deficiency, anaemia may not be present.

The second stage of iron deficiency anaemia occurs when the iron stores of the body become depleted. At this point the synthesis of haemoglobin becomes impaired. With progression of iron deficiency, the red blood cells lose their shape and appear as cigar- or pencil-shaped forms upon microscopic analysis of a peripheral blood smear (Figure 7.1).

Iron deficiency is the leading cause of anaemia worldwide. The prevalence of iron deficiency

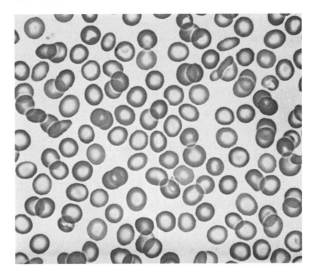

Figure 7.1 Iron-deficient red blood cells.
(Science Photo Library Ltd/Joaquin Carrillo Farga)

anaemia is greatest among preschool children and adolescent and adult females. In developing countries approximately 52% of pregnant women have iron deficiency anaemia, as have approximately 23% of pregnant women in developed countries. The prevalence of iron deficiency anaemia among preschool children ranges from 20% in developed countries to 39% in developing countries.

The most frequent cause of iron deficiency in men and postmenopausal women is gastrointestinal bleeding. In premenopausal women, iron deficiency occurs most frequently secondary to loss of iron with menstruation and during pregnancy. Dietary deficiency of iron most commonly seen in young children occurs when intake of iron does not keep pace with rapid growth and development.

Decreases in iron absorption occur with malabsorption syndromes and chronic disease. Iron absorption requires an intact gastrointestinal tract with healthy intestinal mucosal cells. Chronic disease, removal of the stomach and bowel disorders limit the absorption of iron.

Iron deficiency anaemia is associated with weakness and fatigue. Mild to moderate iron deficiency can affect cognitive performance, behaviour and impede growth in children. Iron deficiency during pregnancy increases overall infant mortality or death.

The best treatment for iron deficiency anaemia is dietary, including plenty of red meat, baked beans, eggs and leafy green vegetables. If necessary, oral iron supplements are readily available and injectable iron supplements are available for individuals with malabsorption or those who cannot tolerate oral supplements.

Anaemia of chronic disease

Anaemia often occurs in patients with chronic inflammatory, infectious and autoimmune diseases. The aetiology of anaemia of chronic disease most often is a defect in the synthesis of red blood cells, or erythropoiesis.

The severity of the anaemia of chronic disease depends on the primary condition. For example, patients with chronic disease such as rheumatoid arthritis or chronic infections with tuberculosis may have severe anaemia owing to depletion of iron stores. Moderate anaemia is associated with cardiac conditions such as angina pectoris and exercise intolerance. The anaemia of chronic disease may resolve if the underlying disease is treated.

Anaemia of renal disease

Chronic kidney or **renal failure** is associated with moderate to severe anaemia; the level of anaemia correlates with the severity of renal disease. This type of anaemia is caused by a failure to produce adequate amounts of erythropoietin and a reduction in red blood cell survival. Erythropoietin is now available in tablet form. Assessment of iron status provides information to distinguish the anaemia of renal disease from iron deficiency anaemia. Patients with anaemia of renal disease usually have normal serum iron; however, individuals on long-term haemodialysis may also develop iron deficiency from blood loss through the dialysis procedure.

Megaloblastic anaemia

The megaloblastic anaemias are disorders caused by impaired DNA synthesis. Megaloblastic red blood cells tend to be large and contain an increased ratio of RNA to DNA. The number of red blood cells produced is decreased by ineffective erythropoiesis. Most megaloblastic anaemias are caused by a deficiency in vitamin B_{12} and/or folic acid.

Vitamin B_{12} deficiency anaemia

Vitamin B_{12} is a complex compound that cannot be synthesised by the human body and must be supplied by the diet. The minimum daily requirement for vitamin B_{12} is about 2.5 micrograms. Normally about 2 milligrams of vitamin B_{12} are stored in the liver and another 2 milligrams are stored elsewhere in the body. It would take approximately 3–6 years for a normal individual to become deficient in vitamin B_{12} if absorption were to cease abruptly.

Vitamin B_{12} deficiency anaemia, or **pernicious anaemia**, is caused by inadequate intake or absorption of vitamin B_{12}. **Intrinsic factor** is produced in the stomach and is essential for the absorption of vitamin B_{12} from the small intestine. Without vitamin B_{12} and intrinsic factor, the membranes of immature red blood cells rupture easily within the chemical environment of the bloodstream. The result is fewer than normal red blood cells and consequently a reduced oxygen-carrying capacity.

Causes of pernicious anaemia include inadequate diet, inadequate absorption, inadequate utilisation, increased requirements and increased excretion of vitamin B_{12}. This vitamin is abundant in meat, fish and dairy products. Strict vegetarians (vegans) who omit all animal products develop pernicious anaemia without vitamin B_{12} supplements. Abnormal bacterial growth in the small intestine and bowel disorders induce pathological changes that either impair absorption and/or enhance elimination of vitamin B_{12}. Removal of the stomach or the upper bowel impairs availability of intrinsic factor and limits absorption of vitamin B_{12}.

Symptoms of pernicious anaemia include abdominal distress, such as nausea and vomiting, and burning of the tongue. Neurological disturbances include numbness, weakness and changes in sight, smell and taste, and ultimately personality and intellectual changes ('megaloblastic madness').

Vitamin B_{12} supplementation effectively reverses the effects of pernicious anaemia. In the absence of intrinsic factor, vitamin B_{12} may need to be replaced by injection. Vitamin B_{12} supplementation is required for life for strict vegetarians and for those with chronic bowel disorders or individuals who have had their stomach or bowel partially or fully removed.

Folic acid deficiency anaemia

Folic acid is synthesised by many different types of plants and bacteria. Fruits and vegetables – particularly dark green, leafy vegetables – constitute the primary dietary source of folic acid. The minimum daily requirement is normally about 50 micrograms, but this may be increased during periods of enhanced metabolic demand such as pregnancy.

Normal individuals have about 5–20 micrograms of folic acid in various body stores, half of which is in the liver. This is quite small and folic acid deficiency can occur within months if dietary intake or intestinal absorption is decreased.

Folic acid deficiency anaemia is common in the western world, where consumption of raw fruits and vegetables is low. Inflammation of the bowel, as in Crohn's disease, and adverse effects of certain drugs impair absorption of folic acid. Pregnant and lactating women, alcohol abusers and individuals with kidney disease are especially susceptible to folic acid deficiency anaemia owing to increased metabolic demands. A lack of folic acid very early in pregnancy is also associated with the development of neural tube defects (e.g. spina bifida), and pregnant women, or those planning to become pregnant, are often encouraged to take supplements.

Measurement of serum folic acid levels is conclusive for folic acid deficiency anaemia. Oral folic acid supplementation is effective in replacing folic acid and meeting increased requirements for those with increased metabolic demands.

Haemolytic anaemia

Red blood cells normally survive 90–120 days in the circulation. The lifespan of the red blood cells may be shortened by a number of disorders, often resulting in anaemia if the body is not able to replenish the prematurely destroyed red blood cells.

Haemolytic anaemia is a reduction in circulating red blood cells that is caused by pathological conditions that accelerate destruction of red blood cells. Inherited abnormalities such as defects in the haemoglobin, enzymes or membranes impair intrinsic physical properties that are needed for optimal red blood cell survival. Infectious agents, certain drugs and immune disorders may also reduce red blood cell survival.

Significant red blood cell destruction produces symptoms similar to those of other anaemias. Unlike other anaemias, haemolytic anaemia produces increased serum levels of **bilirubin** that result from the degradation of haem in destroyed red blood cells. Accumulation of bilirubin causes a jaundiced or yellow–orange appearance in the tissues, urine and faeces.

Treatment of haemolytic anaemia depends on the underlying aetiology. **Splenectomy**, or removal of the spleen, may be recommended in cases of inherited causes of haemolytic anaemia. This decreases the risk of gallstones, haemolytic crises and pathological changes to the bone marrow. Blood transfusions are recommended in cases of severe blood loss such as trauma. Infectious causes can be adequately treated with appropriate antibiotics and other supportive therapies. Similarly, immune disorders can be treated with various immune suppressive therapies. Offending medications are discontinued and rarely restarted in patients who develop haemolytic anaemia.

Haemoglobinopathies

Haemoglobin is critical for normal oxygen delivery to the tissues. **Haemoglobinopathies** are disorders affecting the structure, function or synthesis of haemoglobin. These conditions are usually inherited and vary in the severity of symptoms.

Haemoglobinopathies are mutations that result from the synthesis of abnormal haemoglobin. The most common haemoglobinopathies are sickle cell disease and the thalassaemias.

Sickle cell disease Sickle cell disease (sometimes called sickle cell anaemia) is a genetically transmitted disorder marked by severe haemolytic anaemia, episodes of painful crisis and increased susceptibility to infections. In the UK, approximately 10 000 people have sickle cell disease. It is more common in people whose origins are African, Afro-Caribbean, Asian or Mediterranean. It is rare in people of North European origin. On average, 1 in 2400 babies born in England have sickle cell disease, but rates are much higher in some urban areas and amongst those populations affected by the disease.

Those with the disease are homozygous or have inherited two genes (one from each parent). Those who are heterozygous for the disease are described as having sickle cell trait and experience a very mild form of the disease.

In sickle cell disease, red blood cells contain an abnormal form of haemoglobin, or haemoglobin S.

As the red blood cell deoxygenates, haemoglobin S forms cross-links with other haemoglobin S molecules, and long crystals develop. Crystals continue to form as oxygen is released; eventually, when a large amount of the haemoglobin has crystallised, the red cells assume a sickled shape.

Sickled red blood cells are inflexible and rigid and cause mechanical obstruction of small arterioles and capillaries, leading to pain and ischaemia. Sickled cells are also more fragile than normal, leading to **haemolysis** and haemolytic anaemia. Tissue death secondary to ischaemia causes painful crises that progress to organ failure with repeated occlusive episodes.

Sickle cell disease is diagnosed on the basis of symptoms and by blood examinations. It was also the first disease that could be diagnosed antenatally. Genetic counselling is recommended for individuals planning parenthood who have the disease or have trait status.

Sickle cell disease cannot be cured and patients require continuous management. Treatment is aimed at preventing sickle cell crisis, controlling the anaemia and relieving painful symptoms. Painful crises are adequately managed with narcotic analgesics. Blood transfusions and fluid replacement expand blood volume and oxygen exchange needed for reperfusion of occluded vessels.

Thalassaemia The **thalassaemias** are a group of inherited blood disorders in which there is deficient synthesis of one of the globin chains required for the haemoglobin molecule. Several different categories of thalassaemia produce mild to severe symptoms.

Thalassaemias are the most common genetic disorders in the world. About 5% of the world's population have the disease or the trait; however, this varies with the ethnic background: up to one in seven people from Cyprus carry one or two copies of the disease, as do one in twelve people from Greece. The most severe forms of thalassaemia produce serious, life-threatening anaemia, bone marrow hyperactivity, enlargement of the spleen, growth retardation and bone deformities. Blood transfusions are required to sustain life, but life expectancy is still reduced.

In the UK, all pregnant women with newborn babies are routinely offered screening for sickle

SIDE by SIDE Sickle cell anaemia

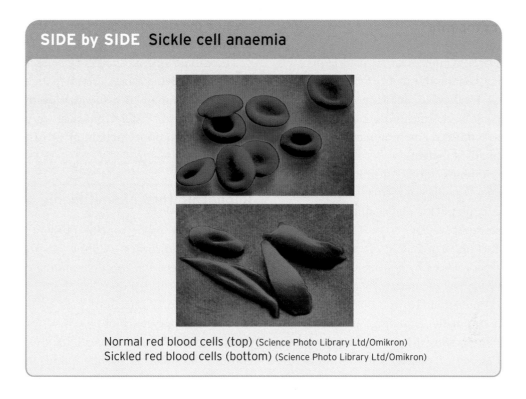

Normal red blood cells (top) (Science Photo Library Ltd/Omikron)
Sickled red blood cells (bottom) (Science Photo Library Ltd/Omikron)

cell and thalassaemia, which is achieved through a maternal or fetal blood sample.

Polycythaemia vera

Polycythaemia describes a condition in which too many red blood cells are present. Secondary polycythaemia can occur as a result of other physical or environmental stresses, such as dehydration or living at high altitude. Polycythaemia vera occurs when too many red blood cells are manufactured by the bone marrow. Other types of blood cell may also be affected. It is most commonly seen in men between the ages of 40 and 65 years. The aetiology of this disease is unknown, although chromosomal abnormalities have been documented in some cases.

The person may have no symptoms and any present are caused by increased viscosity of the blood as a result of the high cell count. They include neurological symptoms such as dizziness, headaches and visual disturbances. Hypertension accompanies increases in red blood cell mass. Patients may experience itching and pain in the fingers and toes. Thromboembolism may occur in severe undiagnosed cases of polycythaemia vera.

Treatment of polycythaemia vera is aimed at decreasing the thickness of the blood. This can be done by intravenously removing blood to reduce red blood cell volume. Chemotherapeutic agents may help suppress the production of all blood cells by the bone marrow. The symptoms of the disease can be managed with administration of analgesia, and antihistamines can help relieve the discomfort associated with itching.

DISORDERS OF HAEMOSTASIS

Disorders of **haemostasis**, commonly known as bleeding disorders, include a range of medical problems that lead to poor blood clotting and uncontrolled bleeding. Bleeding disorders result from platelet dysfunction or deficiency, vitamin K deficiency and clotting factor deficiencies. **Platelets** (or **thrombocytes**) are blood elements produced in the bone marrow that are essential for blood clotting in response to immediate injury and for the mobilisation of clotting factors. Clotting factors are formed in the liver and released in response to injury and platelet fragments to form insoluble fibrin clots. Vitamin K is required for the synthesis of the prothrombin and thrombin clotting factors. Platelets, prothrombin, thrombin, vitamin K and calcium are essential for haemostasis, or the arrest of bleeding.

Thrombocytopenia

An abnormally low number of circulating platelets, or **thrombocytopenia**, results from conditions that either impair production, increase destruction or cause sequestration (destruction) of platelets. Thrombocytopenia is the most common bleeding problem among hospitalised patients.

Microscopic examination of the blood is essential in diagnosing thrombocytopenia. Bone marrow examination is useful for diagnosing impairments in the synthesis of platelets.

The production of platelets can be suppressed by malignant diseases or by destruction of the bone marrow, most often secondary to cancer chemotherapies and radiation. Up to 30% of circulating platelets are normally contained in the spleen. Conditions that increase the size of the spleen cause increased trapping of platelets. Autoimmune disorders may increase platelet destruction or impair platelet function. Massive blood transfusions dilute circulating platelets and decrease platelet viability.

Shortage of platelets can lead to prolonged bleeding following minor trauma, and spontaneous haemorrhages are often visible on the skin, looking like purple discoloration. Small ones, under 1 cm in diameter, are called **petechiae**, and larger ones are called **ecchymosis** (Figure 7.2). They may also occur in the mucous membranes of the mouth and internal organs.

Thrombocytopenia should be corrected by treating the underlying cause, and the patient is advised to be extra careful to avoid trauma until platelet counts increase. Platelet transfusions are reserved for severe thrombocytopenia or in cases of severe bleeding.

Idiopathic thrombocytopenic purpura

Idiopathic thrombocytopenic purpura (ITP) is an autoimmune disorder resulting in excess destruction of platelets. ITP most commonly occurs as an acute problem in children less than 5 years of age following a viral infection. It is characterised by the sudden appearance of petechiae. Most children recover in a few weeks. In adults, this disorder is chronic and does not usually follow an acute viral infection.

The diagnosis of ITP is based on the appearance of severe thrombocytopenia. In patients with a suspected immune disorder, analysis of the blood for the presence of antibodies or phagocytic cells is helpful.

The treatment of ITP depends on the age of the patient and the severity of the illness. Haemorrhage in patients with either acute or chronic ITP can

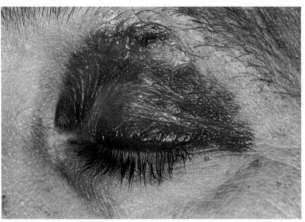
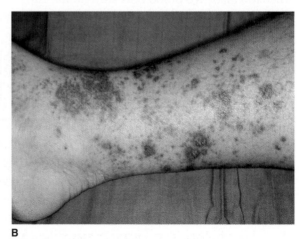

A   B

Figure 7.2 (A) Ecchymosis (Science Photo Library Ltd/Scott Camazine); and (B) petechiae (© ISM/Phototake USA).

usually be controlled by administration of corticosteroid drugs. Removal of the spleen is reserved for patients who do not respond to treatment or for those who are severely ill.

Coagulation defects

Blood clotting or coagulation is a complex process that involves many different plasma proteins in the control of bleeding. Coagulation is a tightly controlled cascade of biochemical events that results in the formation of a blood clot, or a **thrombus**, that prevents further blood loss. Coagulation disorders can result from deficiencies or impairment of one or more of the clotting factors. Deficiencies can arise because of defective synthesis, inherited disease or increased breakdown of clotting factors. Minor bleeds may be controlled by the local vascular reflexes and the formation of a platelet plug, and this can be achieved even by people suffering from coagulation disorders.

Impaired synthesis of coagulation factors

Certain coagulation factors are synthesised in the liver and in liver disease, synthesis of these clotting factors is reduced and bleeding may result. Coagulation factors VII, IX, X and prothrombin all require the presence of vitamin K for normal activity. In vitamin K deficiency, the liver produces an inactive form of the clotting factors. Vitamin K is a fat-soluble vitamin that is synthesised by intestinal bacteria; a mixed diet only yields about half of our vitamin K requirements. Deficiencies occur when intestinal synthesis of vitamin K is interrupted or absorption of vitamin K is impaired. Vitamin K deficiency can occur in newborns before the development of intestinal flora required for the synthesis of vitamins occurs. Neonates are now routinely given one or more doses of vitamin K.

HEREDITARY DISORDERS

The most common inherited bleeding disorders are haemophilia and the von Willebrand disease. There are about 6000 people in the UK affected by haemophilia, and von Willebrand disease may affect more than 1 in every 1000.

Haemophilia

Haemophilia is a deficiency of a clotting factor. The factor affected is usually factor VIII, in which case the disease is called haemophilia A. Haemophilia B is where the factor affected is factor IX. The disease is an X-linked recessive disorder that primarily affects males. The severity of the disease depends on how the genetic defect affects the activity of the clotting factor. In mild to moderate forms of the disease, bleeding usually does not occur unless there is a local lesion or trauma such as surgery or dental procedures. In severe haemophilia, bleeding can be spontaneous and severe, and can occur up to several times per month.

Bleeding often occurs in the gastrointestinal tract and in the joints of the hip, knee, elbow and ankle. The bleeding causes inflammation with acute pain and swelling. Without proper treatment, chronic bleeding and inflammation cause joint fibrosis that can progress to major disability. Intracranial haemorrhage is an important cause of death in severe haemophilia.

Treatment of haemophilia involves long-term replacement of factor VIII, with additional doses administered during phases of acute bleeding. Patients with mild haemophilia A can sometimes be treated with a synthetic hormone called desmopressin. Desmopressin stimulates the release of the carrier for factor VIII, thus causing increases in blood concentration of factor VIII.

Von Willebrand disease

Von Willebrand disease is an inherited bleeding disorder that is most often diagnosed in adulthood. There are many forms of this disease that cause a defect in the adhesion of platelets. Because von Willebrand factor (vWF) carries factor VIII, its deficiency may also be accompanied by reduced levels of factor VIII, contributing to impaired clotting.

Mild symptoms of von Willebrand disease include frequent bruises from minor bumps, frequent nosebleeds, extended bleeding following dental procedures, heavy menstrual bleeds and heavy bleeding following surgery. In severe cases, life-threatening gastrointestinal or joint haemorrhage may resemble symptoms of haemophilia.

Mild forms of von Willebrand disease are often diagnosed following a severe bleeding episode. Examination of the blood for antigens, vWF activity and examination of the structure of the vWF provides information on the type of defect as well as the severity of the defects. Examination of the platelets provides information on how well the platelets are functioning.

Treatment of von Willebrand disease includes medications and lifestyle changes to minimise trauma. Medications are used to increase the release of von Willebrand factor into the blood, replace von Willebrand factor, prevent the breakdown of clots and control heavy menstrual bleeding in women.

Disseminated intravascular coagulation

Disseminated intravascular coagulation (DIC) is a potentially life-threatening condition that involves destruction of the platelets and the consumption of clotting factors. DIC occurs in a variety of disorders, such as sepsis or blood infection, endothelial damage as in states of shock, obstetric complications and various cancers.

The pathogenesis of DIC involves the release of thrombin into the systemic circulation, causing systemic coagulation and suppression of normal physiological anticoagulation mechanisms. Extensive clotting produces diffuse tissue ischaemia, organ damage and depletion of platelets and clotting factors. The depletion of platelets and clotting factors (also known as **consumptive coagulopathy**) ironically results in extensive bleeding.

The diagnosis of DIC is based on the presence of clinical signs of bleeding in a patient with a clinical condition known to be associated with DIC. Clinically, DIC is usually diagnosed on the basis of the underlying disease, observed low platelet counts on a peripheral blood test, increases in bleeding times and the presence of degradation products in the blood plasma.

Treatment of the underlying disorder is the cornerstone of therapy for DIC. Supportive medical treatments include platelet transfusions, administration of concentrates of coagulation inhibitors and administration of an intravenous anticoagulant where appropriate.

WHITE BLOOD CELLS

Leucocytes, or white blood cells, include **neutrophils**, **eosinophils**, **basophils**, **monocytes** and **lymphocytes** (Figure 7.3). White blood cells are synthesised in the bone marrow from their respective stem cells. The primary function of leucocytes is to defend tissues against infections and foreign substances. Quantitative abnormalities, inherited acquired defects and neoplastic alterations result in disease and disability.

Disorders of white blood cells

Neutropenia A reduction of circulating neutrophils increases the risk of bacterial and fungal infections. Because neutrophils are responsible for most clinical findings during an acute infection, the classic signs of infection may be diminished or absent in a severely neutropenic individual.

Neutropenia is a frequent complication of drugs used for cancer chemotherapy or for immune

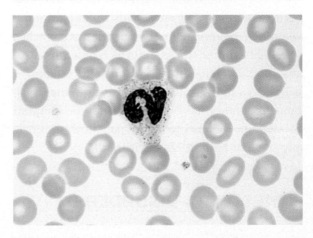

Figure 7.3 Neutrophils or white blood cells.
(Science Photo Library Ltd/Dr Gladden Willis/Visuals Unlimited)

suppression. These drugs suppress cellular proliferation within the bone marrow. Infectious complications depend on the severity of neutropenia and are often profound and severe in cancer patients.

Immune destruction of neutrophils occurs with rheumatoid arthritis or as a primary condition with unknown causes. Neutropenia may be either mild or severe, and infectious complications are variable. Chronic and severe cases require treatment with medicines that increase neutrophil proliferation or suppress immune function.

Patients with longstanding neutropenia may experience chronic infections. Acute and severe neutropenia may be associated with fever, skin inflammation, liver abscesses and septicaemia, or infection in the blood.

Diagnosis of neutropenia is based on assessment of a complete blood count. Examination of the bone marrow is useful to diagnose bone marrow failure syndromes that may be causing the neutropenia.

The treatment of neutropenia depends on its cause and severity; it may resolve without treatment and mild cases generally have no symptoms and may not need treatment. People with severe neutropenia are at risk of high fevers and serious infections. Hospitalisation with isolation and intravenous antibiotic therapy is needed for the severely neutropenic patient.

Growth factors, called colony-stimulating factors, which stimulate the production of white blood cells, are especially helpful for patients who develop neutropenia secondary to cancer treatment. Corticosteroids may help if the neutropenia is caused by an autoimmune reaction.

Abnormalities of eosinophils

Idiopathic hypereosinophilic syndrome The onset of **idiopathic hypereosinophilic syndrome** occurs between the ages of 20 and 50 years, and there is a strong male predominance. Persistent increases in blood eosinophils and associated involvement of the heart and nervous system are responsible for the most important clinical symptoms. Cardiac involvement produces congestive heart failure, valvular dysfunction, conduction defects and myocarditis.

Congestive heart failure is a frequent cause of death. Neurological findings may include altered behaviour and cognitive function, spasticity and ataxia.

Prognosis for the idiopathic hypereosinophilic syndrome historically has been poor, with median survival of approximately 1 year. However, chemotherapy has recently been reported to produce 70% survival at 10 years.

Eosinophilia-myalgia syndrome A recently described disorder, **eosinophilia-myalgia syndrome**, is a chronic, multisystem disease with a spectrum of clinical symptoms ranging from self-limited myalgias, or muscle pain, and fatigue to a progressive and potentially fatal illness characterised by skin changes, nervous system abnormalities and pulmonary hypertension. Elevation of circulating levels of eosinophils is a universal feature of this disorder, and the illness has been related to ingestion of the contaminated dietary supplement L-tryptophan. L-Tryptophan may be taken to treat migraine, depression and anxiety.

AGE-RELATED DISEASES

Anaemia is the most common blood disorder in persons greater than 75 years of age. The causes of anaemia in older adults are blood loss and nutritional deficiencies, chronic illness and chronic renal failure. Decreased physical performance, mental status changes and an increase in mortality are among the consequences of untreated anaemia in older adults. White blood cell disorders, platelet disorders and immune deficiency are often due to malignant disease. Neutropenia, thrombocytopenia and nutritional anaemias develop secondary to malignancy and cancer treatments.

Resources

Sickle cell society: *www.sicklecellsociety.org*
Haemophilia society: *www.haemophilia.org.uk*
World Health Organization: *www.who.int/nutrition/publications/anaemia_iron_pub/en*

DISEASES AT A GLANCE Blood

DISEASE	AETIOLOGY	SIGNS AND SYMPTOMS	DIAGNOSIS	TREATMENT	PREVENTION	LIFESPAN
Iron deficiency anaemia	Iron loss	Fatigue, decreased exercise tolerance, shortness of breath	Blood test	Iron replacement	Iron fortified diet, iron replacement in high-risk individuals	Can occur at any age
Anaemia of chronic disease and renal disease	Defect in erythropoiesis	Fatigue, decreased exercise tolerance, shortness of breath	Blood test, evidence for primary disease	Administration of injectable erythropoietin and iron	Treatment of the underlying disease	Can occur at any age
Vitamin B_{12} deficiency anaemia	Impaired intake or absorption of vitamin B_{12}	Abdominal distress, nausea, vomiting and burning of the tongue	Blood test, health history	Replacement of vitamin B_{12}. Administration of intrinsic factor	Treatment of underlying condition impairing vitamin B_{12} absorption	Can occur at any age
Folic acid deficiency anaemia	Impaired intake, depletion of body stores	Fatigue, decreased exercise tolerance, shortness of breath	Blood test	Replacement of folic acid	Folic acid fortified diet	Can occur at any age
Sickle cell anaemia	Genetic: results in formation of abnormal haemoglobin	Pallor, fatigue, shortness of breath, painful sickle cell crisis	Genetic testing, blood test	Prevention of sickle cell crisis; supportive therapy during crisis; blood transfusion	Cannot prevent sickle cell disease	Diagnosed in infancy and persists throughout life
Thalassaemia	Genetic: results in unbalanced globin chain production and defective haemoglobin	Pallor, fatigue, shortness of breath	Genetic testing, blood test	Supportive care; blood transfusion if anaemia is severe; treatment of iron overload from frequent blood transfusions	Cannot prevent thalassaemia	Diagnosed in childhood and persists throughout life
Polycythaemia vera	Idiopathic, unknown	Dizziness, headaches and visual disturbances	Blood test	Chemotherapeutic agents, blood letting	Unknown	Can occur at any age
Idiopathic thrombocytopenic purpura	Viral infection in children. Unknown in adults	Bleeding	Blood test	Corticosteroid medications, splenectomy	Unknown	Can occur at any age; more common in adulthood
Haemophilia A	Genetic: results in deficiency of clotting factor VIII	Bleeding, particularly into tissues	Genetic test, blood test	Replacement of factor VIII	Cannot prevent haemophilia	Diagnosed in infancy and persists throughout life
Von Willebrand disease	Genetic: results in decreased platelet adhesion	Bleeding	Genetic test, blood test	Desmopressin; lifestyle changes to prevent trauma and bleeding	Cannot prevent von Willebrand disease	Can occur at any age
Disseminated intravascular coagulation	Sepsis, endothelial damage, shock	Bleeding	Blood test; clinical signs and symptoms in high-risk patients	Supportive; treatment of the underlying condition; platelet transfusions	Cannot prevent this condition; difficult to predict when this will occur	Can occur at any age

DISEASES AT A GLANCE Blood (continued)

DISEASE	AETIOLOGY	SIGNS AND SYMPTOMS	DIAGNOSIS	TREATMENT	PREVENTION	LIFESPAN
Neutropenia	Drugs, cancer, chemotherapy, immune disorders	Infection, fever, skin inflammation	Blood test	Administration of medications to increase neutrophil count; antibiotics to prevent infections	Cannot prevent	Can occur at any age
Idiopathic hypereosinophilic syndrome	Unknown	Cardiac symptoms can lead to congestive heart failure	Blood test	Chemotherapy agents	Unknown	Can occur at any age
Eosinophilia-myalgia syndrome	Ingestion of contaminated L-tryptophan	Skin changes, nervous system abnormalities, pulmonary hypertension	Blood test	Discontinue use of the offending agent	Unknown as contaminants can be present without notice	Can occur at any age

INTERACTIVE EXERCISES

Cases for critical thinking

1. Emily is a 42-year-old female who has been 'worn out' for the past few months. The onset of her illness was poorly defined, and aside from a lack of energy she has no other complaints. She reported being easily short of breath when climbing the stairs or walking for any prolonged distance. She told her doctor that she had recently experienced a slight weight loss following the loss of her mother. What diseases or conditions should be considered in this patient? What additional information do you need to make a correct diagnosis?

2. Brian is a 65-year-old male admitted to the hospital for surgery. Brian had been on blood thinners (warfarin) in the past for the treatment of a clotting disorder. He is fearful of going to the hospital, because last time he had a severe bleeding episode. What conditions should Brian's doctors be concerned about? What are some of the symptoms and diagnostic tests that should be considered for this patient?

Multiple choice

1. The most important component of red blood cells is _____
   a. vitamin B_{12}
   b. folic acid
   c. erythropoietin
   d. haemoglobin

2. In anaemia of chronic disease and anaemia of chronic renal failure, the defect in the synthesis of red blood cells is caused by a lack of _____
   a. erythropoiesis
   b. iron
   c. haemoglobin
   d. folic acid

3. Pernicious anaemia is caused by inadequate absorption of _____
   a. vitamin B_{12} b. folic acid
   c. erythropoietin   d. haemoglobin

4. The minimum daily requirement of folic acid is about _____ micrograms.
   a. 200   b. 150
   c. 100   d. 50

5. Disorders affecting the structure and function or production of haemoglobin are classified as _____
   a. haemolytic anaemia
   b. iron deficiency anaemia
   c. haemoglobinopathy
   d. folic acid deficiency anaemia

6. Deficient synthesis of one of the globin chains of the haemoglobin molecule is characteristic of _____
   a. haemolytic anaemia
   b. thalassaemia
   c. sickle cell anaemia
   d. iron deficiency

7. A disease of increased viscosity of the blood with associated neurological symptoms is known as _____
   a. polycythaemia vera
   b. disseminated intravascular coagulation
   c. sickle cell anaemia
   d. thalassaemia

8. _____ is an autoimmune disorder resulting in destruction of platelets.
   a. Disseminated intravascular coagulation
   b. Polycythaemia vera
   c. Haemophilia A
   d. Idiopathic thrombocytopenic purpura

9. _____ is an X-linked recessive disorder that primarily affects males and results in a deficiency of clotting factor VIII.
   a. Disseminated intravascular coagulation
   b. Polycythaemia vera
   c. Haemophilia A
   d. Idiopathic thrombocytopenic purpura

10. _____ is a reduction in circulating red blood cells that increases the risk for severe bacterial and fungal infections.
   a. Haemophilia   b. Neutropenia
   c. Thrombocytopenia   d. Coagulopathy

True or false

_____ 1. Chemotherapy increases survival in patients with idiopathic hypereosinophilic syndrome.

_____ 2. Haemoglobin is the most important component of white blood cells.

_____ 3. The production of red blood cells is regulated by a kidney hormone, erythropoietin.

_____ 4. The symptoms of neutropenia are due to hypoxia.

_____ 5. The clinical diagnosis of blood disorders requires careful microscopic examination of blood in a peripheral blood smear.

_____ 6. Vitamin K is required for the synthesis of clotting factors.

_____ 7. Von Willebrand disease is a hereditary deficiency of vitamin K.

_____ 8. The depletion of platelets in disseminated intravascular coagulation is also known as a consumptive coagulopathy.

_____ 9. Enlargement of the spleen occurs in anaemia caused by haemolysis.

_____ 10. Women of childbearing years are advised to take 14.8 mg of iron a day.

Fill-ins

1. White blood cells are called _____.

2. Mature red blood cells are called _____.

3. Sickle cell disease causes formation of _____ that forms cross-links and sickling of red blood cells.

4. Thrombocytopenia is a disease of the circulating levels of _____.

5. The most severe, life-threatening forms of thalassaemia are _____ and _____.

6. The leading cause of anaemia worldwide is _____.

7. Vitamin B_{12} and folic acid deficiency anaemia are also called _____.

8. Red blood cells normally survive in the circulation for about _____ days.

9. A rise in red blood cell mass accompanied by an increase in white blood cells and platelets is known as _____.

10. The pathogenesis of disseminated intravascular coagulation involves the release of _____ into the circulation, causing extensive coagulation followed by consumption of platelets and clotting factors.

Labelling exercise

Use the blank lines below to label the following photos.

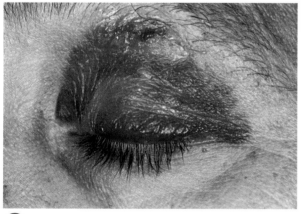

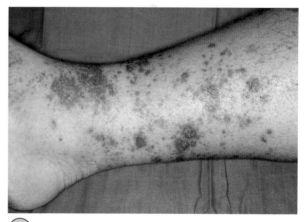

1. _____

2. _____

8

DISEASES OF THE RESPIRATORY SYSTEM

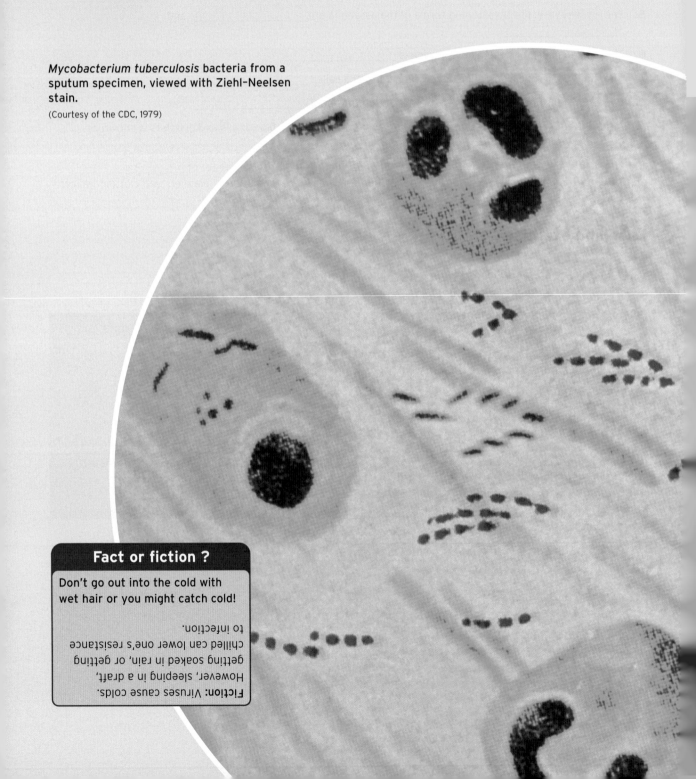

Mycobacterium tuberculosis bacteria from a sputum specimen, viewed with Ziehl–Neelsen stain.

(Courtesy of the CDC, 1979)

Fact or fiction ?

Don't go out into the cold with wet hair or you might catch cold!

Fiction: Viruses cause colds. However, sleeping in a draft, getting soaked in rain, or getting chilled can lower one's resistance to infection.

Learning objectives

After studying this chapter, you should be able to:

+ Describe the normal structure and function of the respiratory organs
+ Compare and contrast upper and lower respiratory tract infections
+ Differentiate between influenza, the common cold and allergies
+ Describe causes, symptoms, diagnosis and treatments of sleep apnoea
+ Compare acute bronchitis with chronic bronchitis
+ Discuss causes and treatments of emphysema
+ Discuss chronic pulmonary conditions, name examples, causes and treatments
+ Describe the various forms of pneumonia and manifestations, causes and treatments
+ Explain pneumothorax and atelectasis in trauma, disease and treatment
+ Define pleurisy and describe primary causes, symptoms and treatments
+ Describe the signs, symptoms, diagnosis, treatment and prevention of tuberculosis
+ Understand the conditions and factors that bring challenges for future respiratory diseases

Disease chronicle

Respiratory disease old and new

Respiratory diseases are a major cause of illness and death throughout the world. Unlike diseases related to other body systems, nearly everybody will have had respiratory tract infections such as the common cold or influenza at some time during their life and are aware how debilitating these conditions can be. Some respiratory diseases have been around for thousands of years – a condition such as tuberculosis (TB) has been associated with illness and death as long ago as the time of the pharaohs. However, other respiratory diseases appear newer in origin, being initiated by environmental factors and lifestyle choices, e.g. damage caused by cigarette smoking and asbestos. Respiratory diseases can be divided into upper and lower respiratory tract conditions, and thus a knowledge of the normal structure and function of the respiratory organs is important in understanding these pathologies.

STRUCTURE AND FUNCTION OF THE RESPIRATORY SYSTEM

The primary function of the respiratory system is to obtain oxygen from the air and deliver it to the lungs for exchange with carbon dioxide and then to the blood for distribution. In addition, respiratory structures in the nasal cavity filter, warm and moisten inhaled air for entry into the lungs. Secondary functions of the respiratory system include coughing, sneezing, talking and singing, none of which is required for oxygen delivery or carbon dioxide exchange.

Air enters the nasal cavity, or oral cavity, and passes back through the **pharynx**, or throat, and then down through the **larynx** to the **trachea**. Inferiorly the trachea branches into two primary **bronchi**, one going to each lung. The trachea and bronchi are continually kept open by ring structures called tracheal cartilages. The branching continues further into smaller and smaller tubules called **bronchioles**, which lack cartilaginous rings. The branching tubules resemble an inverted tree and are often referred to as the bronchial tree. The bronchioles terminate in the lungs as small air sacs called the **alveoli**. Figure 8.1 illustrates the respiratory system.

The alveoli are thin-walled sacs surrounded by blood capillaries and are the site of gaseous exchange (oxygen–carbon dioxide). With a moist surface, the alveoli tend to stick together, and therefore an oily lubricant called **surfactant** bathes the inner surfaces to reduce the surface tension. Without the

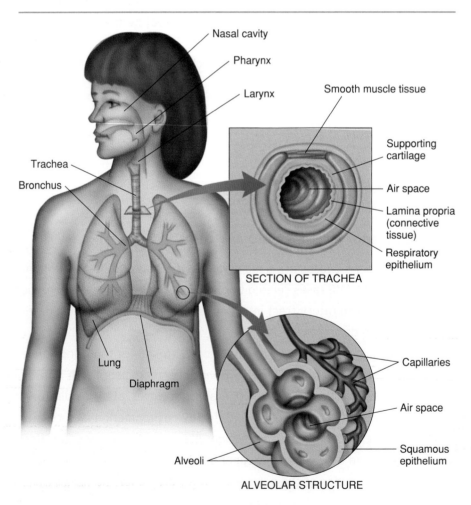

Figure 8.1 The respiratory system.

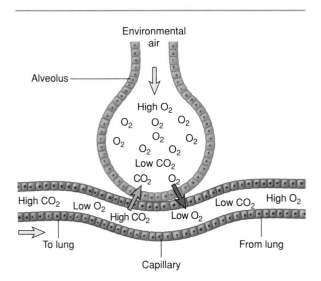

Figure 8.2 Exchange of gases between lungs and blood. High concentration of CO_2 in blood capillary entering the lung diffuses into alveolus. High concentration of O_2 in alveolus diffuses into blood capillary leaving lung.

surfactant, the resistance to opening the balloon structures is felt in a distress situation such as that found in premature newborns. Oxygen that is inspired, or inhaled, diffuses from the alveoli into the blood capillaries. The haemoglobin molecules of the red blood cells become saturated with oxygen. Carbon dioxide, a waste product of cellular metabolism, diffuses from the blood capillaries into the alveoli to be expired, or exhaled. This exchange of gases is illustrated in Figure 8.2.

To deliver oxygen to the alveoli, air must be inspired into the lungs. The **diaphragm** and the muscles between the ribs (called the external intercostals) are the main muscles of inspiration, or inhalation. Contraction of these muscles increases the volume of the chest cavity, which results in an increase in the volume of the lungs. The increased volume in the lungs decreases the pressure within the lungs, which allows air to rush in. When the same muscles relax, the volume of the chest cavity decreases, the volume of the lungs also decreases, and thus the pressure within the lungs increases and air is pushed out. Other muscles that assist exhalation include abdominal and internal intercostal

muscles, which are utilised during times of exertion; for example, running.

The lungs are encased by a double membrane consisting of two layers called **pleura**. One layer of this membrane covers the lungs, and the other lines the inner chest wall, or thoracic cavity. In between the pleura is the **pleural cavity**, which contains a small amount of fluid. This fluid lubricates the lung surfaces, reducing friction as the lungs expand and contract. The fluid also reduces surface tension, which helps to keep the lungs expanded. The airtight space between the lungs and the chest wall has a pressure slightly less than the pressure within the lungs. This difference is called the **intrapleural pressure**, and acts as a vacuum and prevents the lungs from collapsing.

The entire respiratory tract is lined with a mucous membrane, the **respiratory epithelium**. Numerous hair-like projections called **cilia** line the surface of this mucosa. The cilia exert a sweeping action, preventing dust and foreign particles from reaching the lungs. The breakdown of this mucous membrane paves the way for infection. The mucous membrane also protects the lungs by moistening and warming inhaled air, starting in the nasal cavity.

COMMON SYMPTOMS OF RESPIRATORY DISEASE

Respiratory diseases are common and many share similar signs and symptoms, including the following.

- Breathing irregularities, including **dyspnoea** (laboured breathing), **tachypnoea** (rapid breathing) and wheezing
- Coughs – dry, productive (produces mucus), **haemoptysis** (coughing blood)
- Cyanosis (blue colour in skin and nails)
- Fever
- Fatigue, owing to laboured breathing and less sleep
- Pain, especially sinuses, throat and chest
- Sinus and nasal drainage
- Weakness of muscles and voice.

DIAGNOSTIC PROCEDURES FOR RESPIRATORY DISEASES

The total lung volume for most individuals is about 6000 millilitres, or 6 litres. To have a baseline of pulmonary efficiency, the ventilation levels may be evaluated in two procedures. A vital capacity measurement is done using a spirometer. For this test, as much air as possible is drawn in and then expelled, with the volume expelled recorded. Normal vital capacity volumes range from about 2250 to 4500 millilitres. The vital capacity volume depends on age, gender, height and general health. By comparing the spirometry test volume to a standard index volume, the test will demonstrate if the person is within normal range or deficient. This quick test will show lung conditions at the time and may well reflect current problems or some conditions from the past or chronic cases.

A second examination procedure is the one-second-forced-expiratory volume (FEV_1). This test reveals the maximum volume of air that can be expelled in 1 second. Any impedance of air flow within the tubule system within the bronchial tree, such as spasms, excess mucus or tubule constriction, will tend to reduce the FEV_1.

Peak expiratory flow rate (commonly referred to as peak flow) is the maximum flow rate of air a person can rapidly expel following the deepest possible breath. It is a measure of speed and is therefore measured in litres per minute. It is also used as an indication of the degree that air flow is impeded.

Spirometry and peak flow recordings require a person to understand and be able to cooperate with the procedure; therefore, with children under 5 these tests are difficult and unreliable. Another test has been developed – **oscillometry** – which is available to those as young as 2 years old. This test allows the patient to breathe normally (20–30 times per minute) and then it shoots sound waves into the air passageways and, depending on how the waves echo back, measures the airway opening. Oscillometry helps the clinician to distinguish patients who have persistently narrowed airways versus a confirmed diagnosis of asthma. Asthma patients are more at risk of developing damage to their lungs as they grow, and early diagnosis may allow these individuals a chance to improve their outcomes over the course of time.

In chronic pulmonary deficiencies especially, arterial blood gases (ABGs) are used to analyse and evaluate gas levels of oxygen and carbon dioxide plus blood pH, which is a key indicator of respiratory function. Because of congestion, such as a thick respiratory membrane due to pneumonia or alveolar destruction and scar tissue from emphysema, less surface area is available for diffusing gases. ABGs normally show oxygen levels of 98–100%, while carbon dioxide levels are normally 35–45 mmHg (4.7–5.9 kPa) at rest. This procedure is somewhat invasive because it requires an arterial puncture to draw blood samples.

Sputum examination is helpful in the evaluation of pneumonia, TB and malignancies. Gram-stained smears and cultures are useful in identifying causative organisms, determining proper antibiotic treatment and diagnosing tuberculosis and fungal lung infections.

Several important imaging procedures include bronchoscopy, chest X-rays and **fluoroscopy**, which permits visualisation of the lungs and diaphragm during respiration. Computerised tomography, or CT scans, augment chest X-rays.

UPPER RESPIRATORY DISEASES

Upper respiratory diseases are typically infections, allergic reactions or conditions like nasal polyps that occur within the head and inflame the sinuses, nose and throat. Many upper respiratory diseases recur depending on current health status, immune sensitivity and season.

The common cold

The common cold is familiar to everyone. Why is it so common? More than 200 strains of viruses, including adenoviruses, rhinoviruses and a type of paramyxovirus, are capable of causing colds. Unlike many other diseases, infection provides no immunity because so many strains of virus exist.

A relatively contagious disease, a cold is an acute inflammation of the mucous membrane lining the upper respiratory tract. The virus infection triggers swelling of the nasal mucous membrane and mucous secretion, causing nasal congestion. There is no cure for the common cold, but symptoms can be treated. An analgesic is advised if a patient has a headache, muscle pain or fever. Decongestants and cough medicines may have some benefit in relieving symptoms. Occasionally, secondary infections of sinuses occur and, if they become bacterial, these infections may be treated with antibiotics (e.g. amoxicillin). Simple home remedies like hot soup and rest can be soothing.

Sinusitis

This is a fairly common condition. In the UK approximately 1–5% of adults are diagnosed with acute sinusitis each year. The sinuses are air-filled spaces that reduce the weight of the skull and contribute resonance to the voice. The cavities are referred to

as paranasal sinuses because they all are connected to, and drain their mucus secretions into, the nasal cavity. The sinuses are named for the skull bone in which they are found: frontal, ethmoid, maxillary and sphenoid.

In sinusitis, there is inflammation of the mucous membrane linings which causes pressure, pain and often a headache. Children tend to have ethmoid sinus inflammation more commonly than do adults (Figure 8.3).

Sinusitis is caused by viruses, bacteria and allergens. Environmental conditions such as changes in barometric pressure, airplane flights, swimming and diving activities may precipitate sinusitis. Inflammation may also follow a tooth extraction or dental work. Nasal congestion may accompany the common cold and can reduce or block sinus drainage and thus cause sinusitis.

Sinusitis may be diagnosed using physical examination, patient history, X-ray and endoscopic sinoscopy. Nasal discharge may be sent to the laboratory to confirm or rule out bacterial infections.

Over-the-counter drugs like decongestants and analgesics are common, inexpensive measures for

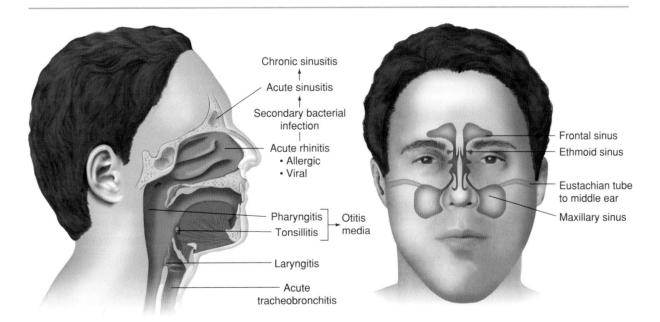

Figure 8.3 Paranasal sinuses are part of the upper respiratory system. From here, infections may spread via the nasopharynx to the middle ear or inferiorly to the bronchi.

treating sinusitis. If pressure becomes chronic and painful, the sinuses may be drained with a sinus tap under local anaesthesia.

Chronic sinusitis is sinusitis that lasts for more than 12 weeks and results in painful headaches, along with facial swelling, and requires a host of antibiotics and steroid regimens. Some medications lose their effectiveness with increased frequency and may be inadequate to resolve the issue because of re-infection and deeper sinuses that are unable to be cleared properly. There are surgical options if the medical treatments fail and the aim is to improve sinus drainage. The most common operation is functional endoscopic sinus surgery (FESS), where an endoscope is inserted into the nose and any blockage to sinus drainage removed. A relatively newer procedure is **balloon sinuplasty** (similar to angioplasty used for cardiac patients) where a balloon device is inserted into the natural sinus space to restore the normal drainage process.

Nasal polyps

Nasal polyps are non-cancerous growths within the nasal or sinus passageway. The exact cause of these growths is unknown. Possible triggers are an allergy or a bacterial or viral infection. Between 1 and 20 out of every 1000 people will be subject to these growths, more commonly in men than women and over the age of 40. Individuals with asthma and chronic rhinitis (nasal inflammation) are susceptible, as are children with cystic fibrosis. Large polyps cause nasal drainage, interfere with smell capability and may occasionally be linked to obstructive sleep apnoea.

Treatment may include steroid-based nasal sprays that can reduce the inflammation and the size of the polyps, and surgery if the polyps are troublesome. However, even if surgery clears the passageway, it may not prevent the recurrence of the polyps.

Snoring and obstructive sleep apnoea

Snoring is usually the production of exaggerated breathing sounds while sleeping and is caused by nasal congestion, postnasal drip or inflamed sinuses. When the congested areas are cleared, the snoring

sounds may be resolved. Heavy snoring on a more consistent basis is often a symptom that accompanies a more serious problem called **obstructive sleep apnoea (OSA)**, the most common sleep disorder.

Interruption or hesitation of the normal breathing cycle during the sleep period is called **apnoea**. The blood oxygen levels fall to a point that alerts the system to the need for a new breathing cycle with such a jolt that a snore results. Some individuals may actually wake themselves up or annoy a spouse or others in the immediate vicinity. On the surface, snoring individuals may appear to be getting a good, sound sleep when in fact they are not.

Sleep apnoea is caused by various blockage areas within the air passageways (thus the name *obstructive sleep apnoea*). The primary sites that are blocked are found within the nasal cavity, like a deviated septum or nasal polyps; the base of the tongue; and soft tissue like the soft palate and enhanced uvula. Obstructive sleep apnoea causes heavy, long and loud snoring and snorting. Four or five episodes of sleep apnoea per sleep hour significantly affect the quality of life, while 20 episodes per hour are severe. Extreme cases reach 100–500 apnoeic episodes in a single night. Without proper sleep, individuals awake tired and feel drowsy most of the day while functioning at a low capacity. It is estimated that in 75% of the cases, there is a decreased blood flow to the brain during these episodes. Therefore, the potential for cerebral stroke is increased, especially in moderate and severe apnoea cases, which is another factor in seeking quick medical attention. Some studies dispute these findings, but most agree that obstructive sleep apnoea is not a healthy situation, and corrective measures are warranted. The incidence of sleep apnoea is highest among middle-aged overweight males, but anyone may have this condition.

Those suspected of having obstructive sleep apnoea undergo a test known as a **polysomnography**. One test method is performed in a clinical setting to monitor brain waves, respiratory and auditory activities, and blood oxygen levels. Another test method allows the patient to be hooked up in an office and then take a computerised polysomnography programme home to record happenings through the night; data are returned the next day.

Treatment depends on the cause or severity and ranges from behavioural therapy to mechanical or physical procedures (most common) or surgery. Issues with alcohol and tobacco may need to be addressed and, if being overweight is a problem, counselling and lifestyle changes are suggested. As little as a 10% decrease in weight may offer a 25% reduction in apnoea episodes.

Mechanical or physical therapy tends to involve a mask placed over the nose to apply pressurised air into the nasal passages. Moderate and severe levels of obstructive sleep apnoea are typically treated using a continuous positive airway pressure (CPAP) device. This procedure keeps the airways open and clear of any minor obstructive material. Some machines have variable pressure mechanisms to adjust pressure during inhaling and exhaling (Figure 8.4). The mask arrangement is somewhat uncomfortable, and about half of all patients eventually stop using the apparatus.

If sinuses or nasal cavities are mis-shaped or blocked, they need repair. Some patients find more relief with uvulopalatopharyngoplasty (UPPP), the trimming of the uvula (including laser treatment) to prevent blockage of the breathing passageway.

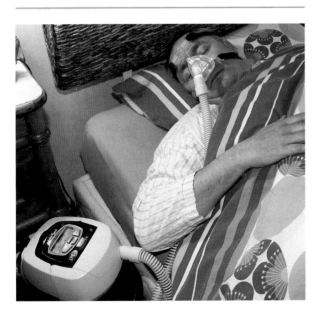

Figure 8.4 Continuous positive airway pressure apparatus.
(Science Photo Library Ltd/Patrick Dumas/Look At Sciences)

Other control measures to consider when dealing with sleep apnoea include avoiding or limiting alcohol indulgence, avoiding tranquillisers or sleeping pills, avoiding lying on the back, treating allergies or irritants promptly, and getting a full quota of sleep whenever possible.

Hay fever (seasonal allergic rhinitis)

Hay fever, also called seasonal allergic rhinitis, is caused by a sensitivity to airborne allergens, especially pollens of ragweed and grasses. Allergens trigger respiratory mucosa to secrete excessive mucus, causing a runny nose and congestion. Mucosal surfaces of the eyes react to the allergens, causing redness, tearing and itching. Hay fever is a very common condition, affecting about 20% of the population, and is most prevalent in adolescents.

Because the release of histamine causes these signs and symptoms, treatment includes antihistamine medications both in tablet form and nasal spray. These medications may have side effects, such as drowsiness, dizziness or muscular weakness. Steroid nasal sprays and drops are effective treatments.

Many hay fever sufferers take allergy injections to **desensitise** them to pollen or other allergens. Desensitising works by administering small doses of antigen and gradually increasing the dosage, allowing the person to produce antibodies against it. These antibodies can inactivate the pollen before it interacts with the nasal mucosa and thus prevent the hay fever reaction.

Tonsillitis, pharyngitis, laryngitis

The tonsils, pharynx and larynx can be irritated or infected with bacteria, viruses or other pathogens. Infections of these tissues lead to difficulty swallowing and redness and pain in the throat (pharynx) area.

The palatine tonsils are masses of lymphatic tissue embedded into the lateral mucous membranes of the midsection of the throat (oropharynx) (Figure 8.5). When infected, the tonsils may swell and become painful, making swallowing very difficult. If infections are severe and recurrent, the tonsils may be surgically removed (tonsillectomy). Surgery usually includes removal of the **adenoids** (pharyngeal tonsils) as well.

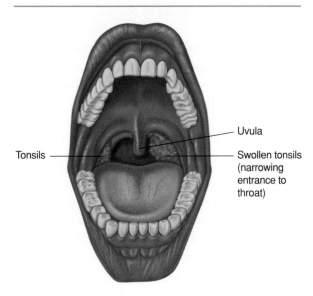

Tonsils

Uvula

Swollen tonsils (narrowing entrance to throat)

Figure 8.5 Tonsils; normal and enlarged.

Pharyngitis, an inflammation of the pharynx, is characterised by pain in the throat. Foreign objects, hot liquids or spicy foods may contribute to short-term pharyngitis. Breathing through the mouth because of nasal congestion or falling asleep with an open mouth dries the throat and can cause temporary discomfort. Strep throat is caused by strepto-cocci bacteria and is characterised by a red, purulent sore throat. A throat swab may be taken for laboratory analysis as will blood tests. Treatment includes analgesics to relieve pain and fever, and antibiotics, if appropriate.

Laryngitis, an inflammation of the larynx or voice box, is characterised by hoarseness or lost voice (**aphonia**). Bacteria, viruses, allergies, overuse of the voice or exposure to caustic chemicals and smoke may cause a 'lost voice'. Antibiotics are used for bacterial infections. A viral infection called **croup** causes laryngitis, especially in young children. Symptoms of croup or other laryngitis forms can be alleviated by resting the voice, drinking fluids and using steam inhalations and air humidifiers. If symptoms such as recurrent fever and continued lethargy do not improve rapidly, other respiratory conditions like pneumonia should be considered.

Influenza

Influenza is a viral infection of the upper respiratory system. Many different strains of viruses cause influenza. Unfortunately, immunity for one strain does not protect against another strain.

The symptoms of flu are common and familiar. The onset is sudden, and within 2 days of exposure to the virus, symptoms develop, including chills, fever, cough, sore throat, runny nose, chest pain, muscle aches and gastrointestinal disorders. The severity of flu cases varies from mild to severe, with pneumonia chief among the complications. The virus destroys the respiratory epithelial lining, and with the loss of this protection, the lungs become susceptible to a host of agents like pneumococci, streptococci and staphylococci. All of these pathogens can cause pneumonia. Influenza is particularly serious in the elderly and chronically ill, as well as in young children.

No medication cures influenza. Treatments are symptomatic and include rest, fluids and analgesics to reduce pain and fever. Antibiotics are prescribed to treat secondary bacterial infections. Flu vaccines are available before the onset of the season, typically in October and November, and are recommended for those considered at high risk. Unfortunately, these flu inoculations do not give immunity for all strains of the influenza virus.

Allergy, influenza and cold share some characteristics but actually are quite distinct (Table 8.1).

LOWER RESPIRATORY DISEASES

Chronic pulmonary conditions

Chronic obstructive pulmonary disease (COPD) is a term for conditions in which there is air flow obstruction; this includes chronic bronchitis and emphysema. It is estimated that around 1.5 million people have COPD in the UK. The average age of diagnosis is about 67 and the condition is more common in men, although the prevalence in women is increasing. Asthma, cystic fibrosis and

Table 8.1 Comparison of allergy, cold and influenza.

Symptom/sign	Allergy	Cold	Flu
Onset	Response to allergen	Slow	Fast
Duration	>1 week	1 week	1-3 weeks
Season	Spring/summer	Autumn/winter	Autumn/winter
Fever	None	Rare, <37.8°C	38-40°C; lasts 3-4 days
Fatigue, weakness	Mild; varies	Quite mild	May last 2-3 weeks
Extreme exhaustion	Rare	Never	Early and prominent
General aches, pains	Varies	Slight	Usual; often severe
Headache	Usual	Rare	Prominent
Sneezing	Usual	Usual	Varies
Sore throat	Varies	Common	Varies
Stuffy nose	Common	Common	Varies
Nasal discharge	Clear	Yellow/greenish	Varies
Chest discomfort	Sometimes	Mild to moderate	Common; can be severe
Cough	None; dry	Yes	Yes; dry hacking
Vomit and/or diarrhoea	Rare; varies	Rare	Common

pneumoconiosis are also long-term lung conditions that result in lung damage.

Bronchitis **Bronchitis** is an inflammation of the bronchi that can be acute or chronic. The mucous membrane lining the bronchi becomes swollen and red, the typical inflammatory response. Irritants such as cigarette smoke, industrial fumes, automobile exhaust, viruses and bacteria can cause acute bronchitis.

Acute bronchitis is most serious in small children, the chronically ill and the elderly. The small bronchioles of children can become easily obstructed. The elderly or chronically ill are likely to develop a secondary infection, such as pneumonia. Acute bronchitis is characterised by a hacking cough, chest pains, **dyspnoea**, fever and sometimes chills. The sputum may contain pus. Depending on the cause, antibiotics may be administered; however, viruses do not respond to antibiotics. Analgesics may be taken to relieve fever and pain, although some medications are not recommended for those with asthma or for use by children. Over-the-counter cough medicines may be taken for relief; however,

 Prevention PLUS!

Influenza vaccination

Why do we hear about the influenza vaccine every year? Who should get the flu vaccine? Complications of influenza can be serious or fatal; in the UK, about 600 people a year die from seasonal flu. A seasonal flu vaccine is available free for people considered at risk, those over 65 years of age, and those that have a serious medical condition or live in a residential home. It is also recommended for healthcare and social care staff directly involved in patient care to reduce the risk of transmission to those who are vulnerable. The vaccine formula is different every year because the virus strains are different. The viruses are capable of continual mutation; therefore, the immunity level an individual has in one year may not protect against a different strain that emerges the following year.

there is little medical evidence to support their effectiveness. Smoking should be discouraged as it aggravates acute bronchitis and could facilitate the development of chronic bronchitis.

Chronic bronchitis is indicated by repeated attacks of acute bronchitis and coughing with sputum production lasting for at least 3 months for 2 consecutive years. The symptoms of chronic bronchitis are the same as in acute bronchitis, but they persist. In chronic bronchitis, there is an excessive secretion of mucus from the mucous glands of the bronchial mucosa (lining). The mucous glands hypertrophy, and the mucosa itself is thickened and inflamed. The interference in the air passageway caused by the swelling and mucus reduces the person's ability to attain a proper blood oxygen level efficiently. **Hypoxia**, an insufficient oxygenation of the tissues, results. Poor drainage of the mucus sets the stage for bacterial infection. Parts of the respiratory tract can become necrotic, and fibrous scarring follows.

Chronic bronchitis may be a complication of another respiratory infection. It can result from long-term exposure to air pollutants or cigarette smoking. Respiratory diseases such as the flu or a common cold exacerbate chronic bronchitis. There is no cure for chronic bronchitis. However, the symptoms can be treated with antibiotics. Smoking cessation should be encouraged and clean air environments sought out at all times. When necessary, protective respiratory masks and respiratory therapy may be beneficial.

Emphysema Emphysema is a disabling and debilitating disease caused by a restriction or obstruction resulting in the destruction of lung and vascular tissue. In emphysema, the alveolar walls break down, adjacent alveoli fuse, and the lungs lose their elasticity. Air cannot be adequately exhaled to allow oxygen to enter, and the lungs become filled with air that is high in carbon dioxide. Symptoms include a suffocating feeling and great distress caused by the inability to breathe unimpeded (Figure 8.6). Intense pain accompanies the difficulty in breathing. To compensate for the reduced gas exchange, breathing becomes faster and deeper than normal. With the breakdown of alveolar walls,

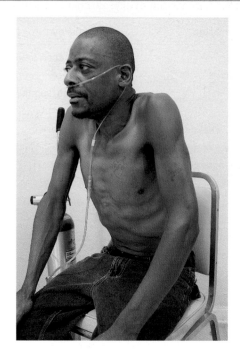

Figure 8.6 Typical appearance of emphysema patient. (Ray Kemp/911 Imaging)

surrounding blood capillaries are damaged or lost, and this causes obstruction of the pulmonary artery. The large weak air sacs, formed by the fusion of the alveoli, tend to rupture. Air flows into the pleural cavity, the thin space between the lungs and the chest wall, causing a condition called a **pneumothorax**. Air in this space causes an increased intrapleural pressure and the lung is subject to collapse, called **atelectasis**.

The cause of emphysema is not known, but it is strongly associated with heavy cigarette smoking. An inherited form involves a genetic deficiency in alpha-1-antitrypsin, which leaves the lungs susceptible to alveolar destruction. Other causes may include air pollution, long-term exposure to chemical irritants and chronic bronchitis.

The most significant diagnostic test for emphysema uses a simple instrument, a **spirometer**, to measure the movement and volume of air in and out of the lungs. X-rays do not show emphysema in the early stages. Gradually, over time a physical examination reveals a chest wall permanently expanded, producing a characteristic 'barrel' chest.

A stethoscope placed on the chest detects abnormal respiratory sounds called **rales**. In addition, the right side of the heart becomes weak because of pulmonary resistance. Therefore, the blood is less saturated with oxygen (hypoxia) and that causes a blue–grey appearance of the skin called **cyanosis**.

Progression of the disease can be controlled by quitting smoking and avoiding polluted air containing smoke, fumes, irritating dust and ozone, especially on days when the ozone level is high. Medications that clear mucus from the lungs help prevent infection. Emphysema cannot be cured, but some medications relieve difficult breathing. Physical therapy teaches the patient how to use more muscle groups for respiration from the abdomen and chest wall. Prognosis for emphysema depends on age, severity and general health. Like other chronic conditions, this disease is manageable by close monitoring.

Asthma Following the common cold, asthma is one of the most common chronic conditions worldwide. The Greek derivation for *asthma* is 'breathlessness or panting'; both features accurately describe a typical asthma attack. **Bronchial asthma** is the chronic inflammation of the bronchi and bronchioles that has ramifications throughout the lung tissue and denotes a location for the disease. Other types of asthma are known by virtue of timing, like nocturnal, exercise-induced or occupational by work environment.

The incidence of asthma has increased dramatically in the UK. It is estimated that 5.2 million people receive treatment for asthma: 1 in 10 children and 1 in 12 adults. The UK has one of the highest levels of asthma, with a peak prevalence occurring between 5 and 15 years old (more commonly in boys than girls) and then later in life between the ages of 55 and 64. Between those ages the prevalence then falls. Approximately 1000 people die annually from asthma. The cause of the rise in asthma cases has not been determined and may result from a complex set of factors dealing with environment, such as congested urban areas, processed foods, plus heredity and individual sensitivities.

Bronchial asthma is characterised by hypersensitivity to various allergens, like dust, mould, pollen, animal dander and various foods. In large urban areas even cockroach remains may act as a trigger for asthma attacks. Eighty per cent of asthmatic children and 50% of adult asthmatics have allergies.

Constriction of smooth muscle in the walls of the bronchi and bronchioles narrows the lumen of the tubes. Recall the lack of cartilaginous rings in the bronchioles; this structural change allows spasms to occur. The spasm is caused by a sustained or intermittent contraction of the smooth musculature, making breathing, particularly expiration, very difficult. Figure 8.7 shows the narrowed bronchi resulting from muscular contraction. The mucous membrane becomes swollen with fluid, and that also narrows the lumen. Excessive secretion of mucus enhances the obstruction. A characteristic **wheezing** sound results from air passing through the narrowed

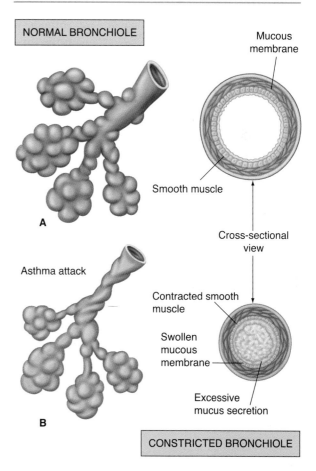

Figure 8.7 Normal bronchiole (A) and one constricted in asthma attack (B).

tubes. Stale air becomes trapped, which decreases the amount of fresh air that can enter the lungs.

Allergens typically trigger asthma symptoms because most asthma sufferers are prone to allergies. Non-allergenic causes include anxiety, overexertion, infection, bronchitis and exposure to some aerosol sprays and perfumes. It is important to avoid the responsible allergens and other known triggers. Athletes should warm up before an event to prevent asthma responses caused by sudden overexertion. Asthma attacks tend to lead to fatigue, and a cough that continues to drain away vigour or vitality from an individual may progress to lung infection.

There is no definitive test for asthma, even though a simple instrument, the **spirometer**, can make a relative measurement in a rapid manner (Figure 8.8). Children under age 5 are not able to perform this test well and need a more sophisticated test, while children aged 7–8 may not express or communicate their condition as fully as needed. Also, some tests are inconclusive if symptoms are absent at the time of testing. Therefore, in making their diagnosis, doctors rely more on family histories and thorough questioning about symptoms and allergen exposure.

The growing incidence of obesity has made asthma diagnosis more difficult. More children coming into healthcare facilities being diagnosed for asthma are found to be obese. Therefore, when a child has a longstanding cough, shortness of breath or wheezing, the parent and doctor should take particular notice.

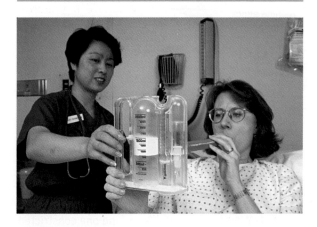

Figure 8.8 Incentive spirometer.

Skin tests can show which allergens are responsible. Medication and allergy injections can reduce the incidence or severity of asthma attacks. There are British Thoracic Society (BTS) guidelines for the management of asthma, which use a 'step' approach. As symptoms worsen, then treatment moves up a step and, if symptoms get better, they move down. Treatment involves both relieving symptoms and preventing them from occurring. Bronchodilators such as beta-2 agonists are used to relieve the symptoms of asthma by bronchodilatation and decreasing the amount of mucus. Aerosol sprays delivered by a **nebuliser** are effective for acute attacks because they can emit a suspension of very small liquid droplets directly into the deeper bronchiole for immediate relief with few side effects (Figure 8.9).

Inhaled glucocorticoids are mainly used for long-term prophylaxis of asthma, while oral glucocorticoids are used for short-term therapy of severe, acute asthma. Generally, oral medications are given at higher dosage and take longer to act; they are primarily used to help control or prevent attack onset.

Steroid drugs may be used for prevention and to reduce inflammation, but long-term use is associated with negative side effects. All medications used in the treatment of asthma must be carefully controlled and administered under close supervision. Drugs are used to prevent asthmatic attacks or to terminate an acute attack.

The most severe form of asthma attack, called **status asthmaticus**, is a life-threatening condition and requires urgent medical intervention. If not treated, this condition may end in respiratory failure and death.

There is no cure for asthma, although attacks may become less frequent or severe after age 18 and older. By learning the trigger for attacks and using proper medical aides, many patients do well to avoid asthma suffering. In older adults, asthma symptoms may return occasionally or be induced by medications and other respiratory ailments. Asthma attacks and symptoms may be caused by environmental occurrences like volcano dust or the particulates experienced by many survivors at ground zero in New York City on 9/11.

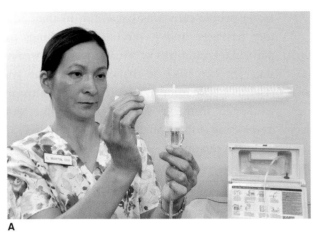
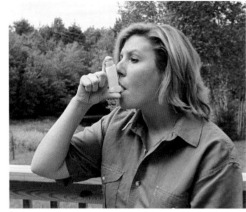

A   B

Figure 8.9 Nebuliser (A) and inhaler medication (B) delivery devices for asthma.

Cystic fibrosis Cystic fibrosis (CF) is an inherited disease that affects the **exocrine glands** of the body, causing them to secrete a viscous type of mucus excessively which blocks gland ducts and prevents the glands from delivering their products. Exocrine glands are common glands that secrete mucus, wax, perspiration and digestive enzymes.

The most serious manifestation of cystic fibrosis is in the respiratory system. The trachea and bronchi secrete thick mucus that accumulates and blocks the air passageways. Symptoms of cystic fibrosis are dyspnoea, wheezing, persistent cough and thick sputum. The abnormally thick mucosal surface increases susceptibility to recurrent bacterial infections. Bronchiectasis (weakened and dilated bronchial tubing) is a common complication of cystic fibrosis. Bronchiectasis is a sequela or residual effect of chronic inflammation and congestion. Lung collapse can result from the inability to inflate the lungs, and most deaths caused by this condition involve younger adults and occur as a result of respiratory failure. Table 8.2 describes complications of cystic fibrosis.

Excessive mucus also blocks the ducts of the pancreas, preventing the release of digestive enzymes and resulting in weight loss and malnutrition. The lack of proper fat digestion results in a large, bulky, foul-smelling stool. In the pancreas, the secretory glands become dilated and develop into cysts

Table 8.2 Complications of cystic fibrosis.

Malnutrition	Blockage of pancreatic duct prevents secretion of digestive enzymes and inability to digest and absorb nutrients
Dyspnoea, lung collapse	Blocked airways, bronchiectasis (weakened airways)
Recurrent respiratory infections	Abnormal mucosal lining Inability to clear thick mucus
Electrolyte imbalance	Abnormal salt excretion

containing thick mucus. Fibrous tissue then develops, which explains how cystic fibrosis gets its name.

Cystic fibrosis is recognised as a hereditary disease that first manifests in young children. It is transmitted through a recessive gene carried by each parent (see Chapter 5). Before the disease was understood, the mortality rate in children was extremely high. Early diagnosis and treatment has greatly improved the prognosis and longevity.

In cystic fibrosis, the sweat glands excrete excessive perspiration and large amounts of salt, causing susceptibility to heat exhaustion. This increased excretion of salt in sweat is the basis for a 'sweat test' that helps to confirm cystic fibrosis.

Basic treatment includes pancreatic enzyme supplements that can be given with food. Antibiotic treatment reduces the incidence of respiratory tract infection, and regular physiotherapy relieves congestion in the respiratory tract.

Pneumoconiosis **Pneumoconiosis** refers to a group of lung diseases (including silicosis and asbestosis) caused by dust particles that seem to infiltrate or embed into lung tissue. As a result of incomplete filtering by the normal action within the air passageways and because of overload, the individual accumulates 'grit' in the lungs, which causes shortness of breath, some wheezing and low physical endurance. The dust is usually the result of industrial mining of coal and stone or milling of grains or environmental activity like asbestos or volcanoes, and as a result there is usually a long delay between exposure and the clinical onset of the disease. Following respiratory testing by X-ray, spirometry and exercise, individuals gain some relief with bronchodilators to ease breathing and corticosteroid medications to reduce inflammation. There are about 200 pneumoconiosis-related deaths per year in the UK.

Pneumonia

Pneumonia is an acute inflammation of the lungs in which air spaces in the lungs become filled with an inflammatory exudate (fluid). Pneumonia can be caused by a variety of micro-organisms and therefore can be classified on the basis of its cause. Pneumonia can also affect different areas within the lungs, and can thus be classified on its anatomical position. Aside from the ill and the vulnerable elderly, pneumonia typically runs in seasonal or cyclical patterns, and is more common during the autumn and winter, somewhat like the flu. In general, pneumonia affects up to 11 in 1000 adults per year in the UK.

Symptoms include dyspnoea, fever, chest pain and a productive cough. Listening to lung activity, a chest X-ray and analysis of sputum can diagnose pneumonia and determine its cause.

Lobar pneumonia **Lobar pneumonia** is inflammation of a section, often an entire lobe, of the lung. Lobar pneumonia is usually caused by the

pneumococcus bacterium *Streptococcus pneumoniae*. Many people carry this bacterium in their respiratory passages, and it can infect the lungs under particular conditions or situations, like a weakened state (broken hip) or challenged immune system (Figure 8.10). Influenza, chronic bronchitis and a weakened immune system increase the risk of developing lobar pneumonia. Antibiotics are a common treatment.

Bronchopneumonia **Bronchopneumonia** is a form of pneumonia focused in small bronchi. Infection and inadvertent aspiration of gastric contents or vomit are common causes. Because many foci (sites) of infection develop in the various bronchi, the chest X-ray will show a diffuse pattern of inflammation. This type of pneumonia is more common in debilitated patients who are less mobile or bedridden from other diseases. Major factors that increase the risk for bronchopneumonia include:

● Chronic bronchitis
● Measles or whooping cough
● Bronchiectasis
● Old age
● Cancer.

Primary atypical pneumonia Also known as 'walking pneumonia,' **primary atypical pneumonia** is caused by a variety of pathogens, including viruses and atypical bacteria like *Mycoplasma pneumoniae*. Interstitial pneumonia, common in viral pneumonia, is a descriptive term denoting the diffuse pattern of the disease spread within the lungs on the X-ray. This disease is more common among adolescents and young adults because of crowded conditions in schools and contacts made by sharing of facilities and contaminated items. Initially, flu-like symptoms prevail, such as fatigue, fever, general weakness, headache, sore throat and stomach and intestinal distress. This disease may not require a visit to a healthcare provider for otherwise healthy individuals who continue to go to school or work and keep up a basic routine. However, children and overstressed or more severely impacted individuals may suffer from pneumonia and other respiratory

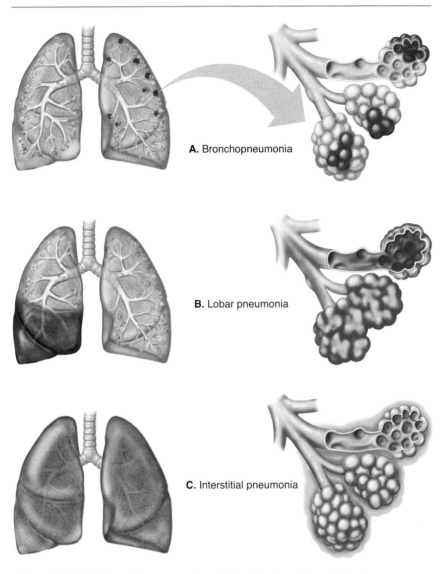

A. Bronchopneumonia

B. Lobar pneumonia

C. Interstitial pneumonia

Figure 8.10 (A) Bronchopneumonia with localised pattern. (B) Lobar pneumonia with a diffuse pattern within the lung lobe. (C) Interstitial pneumonia is typically diffuse and bilateral.

complications that require immediate attention to prevent hospitalisation or home care. Advanced cases of pneumonia may be more common and serious for those with diabetes, cirrhosis, sickle cell disease or cancer. Hospitalisation may be required along with rest and a medication schedule to treat and clear the lungs of the fluid build-up and congestion.

The presence of the signs and symptoms of pneumonia in an individual not in the hospital environment has been defined by the British Thoracic Society as community-acquired pneumonia.

Secondary pneumonia Pneumonia can develop as a secondary disorder from other diseases that weaken the lungs or the body's immune system. Graft recipients and immunocompromised subjects, especially HIV/AIDS patients, are susceptible to pneumonia caused by unusual infectious agents like the fungi *Pneumocystis carini* and *Cryptococcus* *neoformans*. Postoperative patients, bedridden patients and those with chronic respiratory illness may lack the ability to clear their lungs effectively and thus are at risk for developing pneumonia.

Perhaps the most dangerous **secondary pneumonia** is the one acquired as a complication of influenza. It was responsible for most of the estimated 20 million deaths worldwide in the influenza epidemic of 1918–1919. This devastating disease apparently started in the United States. It was carried to (and from) Europe by the huge influx of American troops and support personnel and always precipitated into double pneumonia (both lungs). Today, influenza still causes many cases of pneumonia; therefore, the flu vaccine is strongly recommended for persons at risk to prevent or reduce flu symptoms.

Legionnaire's disease This lung infection is caused by the bacterium *Legionella pneumophila*. The disease is predominantly acquired by inhaling small droplets contaminated with the bacteria from large air conditioning cooling systems, humidifiers, hot tubs and other equipment or environmental conditions that produce contaminated aerosol water droplets. It is accompanied by flu-like symptoms, which sets it apart from other pneumonias, like lobar, and therefore suggests another atypical form of pneumonia. Because this is a serious and potentially fatal disease, it is important to differentiate it from other forms of pneumonia using sputum cultures and chest X-rays. The antibiotic erythromycin is the treatment of choice.

Residual effects of pneumonia, regardless of its form, occur in many victims and lead to long-term problems like fatigue, coughing, shortness of breath and neuromuscular impairments. Complications from pneumonia range from lung abscesses to lung collapse and respiratory failure.

Pleurisy (pleuritis)

Pleurisy is an inflammation of the pleural membranes that occurs as a complication of various lung diseases, such as pneumonia or tuberculosis. It may also develop from an infection, trauma injury or tumour formation. In addition to a cough, fever and chills, pleurisy is extremely painful, with a sharp, stabbing pain accompanying each inspiration. The pain may stem from an excess or deficiency of pleural fluid, or from pus or blood in the pleural space. It is treated with antibiotics, heat applications and bed rest.

Pulmonary tuberculosis

Pulmonary tuberculosis (TB) is a chronic infectious disease characterised by necrosis of vital lung tissue. Although TB most commonly attacks the respiratory system, it can secondarily attack, in similar fashion, other body systems as well (e.g. bone).

TB is caused by the bacterium *Mycobacterium tuberculosis* and related bacteria. These bacteria are most commonly transmitted in contaminated sputum expelled in the coughs of infected persons, although TB can also be caused by contaminated milk from infected cattle. Expelled sputum may dry and settle in dust that can contain infective bacteria for a long time. Close quarters or contacts promote the spread of TB owing to its contagious properties. Crowded campuses, cities or planes are potential sites of TB exposure and outbreaks.

The inhaled bacteria infect the lungs and induce a chronic inflammatory response that leads to necrosis. The tissue in this site becomes soft and cheeselike, which is why it is described as a **caseous** lesion. The tissue heals with fibrosis and calcification, walling off the bacteria into pockets for months or many years. These lesions are called **tubercles**. During this period, a person may have no symptoms. A secondary infection occurs when the person is infected again or when the bacteria escape the walled-off lesions in the lungs. The bacteria may spread this way when resistance is reduced because of stress, infection, malnutrition or immunodeficiency. During the secondary infection, leucocytes now recognise the bacteria and mount an attack that leads to greater necrosis and destruction of lung tissue. Necrotic tissue, blood and bacteria may be coughed up. The bacteria may spread to other organs like the brain, kidney and bones. Those in the secondary stage of the disease also lose weight and become cachectic (wasting away); this is the basis for the classic name for TB, *consumption*.

Screening for TB involves the Mantoux skin test, in which antigens from the bacteria are injected beneath the skin. If previously exposed to TB, the skin swells with slight elevation at the injection site. A positive skin test should be followed up with a sputum culture and a chest X-ray to determine if there is an active infection. Active infections are dangerous because they put others at risk for TB infection.

Antibiotics specially designed for *Mycobacterium* species include rifampin, isoniazid and ethambutol. The drugs must be taken over an extended period of time, perhaps as long as 18 months, to ensure that the bacteria are killed or eliminated. This waxy coated bacterium is resilient and difficult to treat generally because it can be sealed in lung tissue (tubercles) or may be antibiotic-resistant.

TB was relatively common in the nineteenth century, but the incidence fell owing to better living conditions, treatment regimens and vaccinations; however, it has re-emerged, with its incidence increasing since the 1980s and 1990s. The evolution of antibiotic-resistant bacteria and the increased numbers of HIV-infected people, homeless people and immigrants contribute to this increase (Table 8.3).

Worldwide, however, the incidence of TB is rising rapidly, especially in Asia, Russia and parts of Africa. In fact, TB remains the largest cause of death due to infectious disease, killing 3000 people per day worldwide, and is a major cause of death among people infected with HIV. More than one-third of the world's population has been exposed to *Mycobacterium tuberculosis*.

Thoracic trauma and pulmonary distress

Pneumothorax This literally suggests 'air in chest'. This condition involves the accumulation of air that

Table 8.3 Summary of tuberculosis increase in the United States

Primary cause	Secondary/support causes for TB spread
Drug-resistant bacteria	More infections that cannot be treated with a single drug
	More infections resistant to multiple drugs
	Infections last longer and expose more people
Homeless/refugees/ poverty	Reduced access to healthcare, screening and treatment
	Living conditions, malnutrition and other infections increase susceptibility
Immigration	Infected immigrants from areas where the disease is endemic, prevalent, drug-resistant and where there is little healthcare
HIV/AIDS	Reduced resistance and increased susceptibility to disease

escapes its normal entrapment within the lung, or outside air that enters from a breach in the chest wall (e.g. stab wound or gun shot). When the internal chest (intrapleural) pressure exceeds the internal lung pressure, then the lung will collapse, an event known as **atelectasis**. This term may also apply to lungs that fail to inflate in premature infants. Because these two events often occur together, they are considered to be the same thing.

Pneumothorax most commonly occurs in cases involving newborns that have a stiff or inflexible lung and results in **infant respiratory distress syndrome (IRDS)**. Other cases involve ventilators or continuous positive airway pressure (CPAP) devices that may cause air to seep into the thorax. Acute atelectasis may compound the situation, and cause a reduced blood pressure because the relatively higher (internal) chest pressure slows blood flow to the heart. Therefore, with a circulatory deficiency, immediate medical attention is required. A needle and syringe are used to syphon air within the thorax to let the air pressure subside and allow the lung and chest membranes to adhere and re-establish their bond. A tube for ventilation may be left in place for a day or two to ensure complete adjustment.

If the internal pressure is slight or symptoms are not apparent, a healthcare provider may discover the problem when listening to each lung and noticing a lower sound quality to the air entering and leaving the lung on the side where the pneumothorax exists. Premature infants may receive a fibreoptic examination that provides a transillumination effect and makes the defect more visible. In these cases the infant may be placed in an oxygen hood to assist breathing efforts.

Atelectasis may involve the whole lung or a partial lung that becomes airless or contracts. The primary reason the collapse comes about is an obstruction of a major bronchus. Blockage may be excess internal mucus forming a plug, a foreign object inadvertently inhaled, or a tumour or excessive fluid build-up in the pleural space. Accidental or acute atelectasis may result from a car accident involving chest compression or a fall onto a hard surface or object. Symptoms include shortness of breath, increased heart rate and cyanotic appearance because the blood oxygen levels are low owing to lack of respiratory function.

Diagnosis requires a physical examination and possibly a chest X-ray or CT scan. If obstruction is suspected, a bronchoscope may pinpoint the occluded site and assist removal. Antibiotics may be prescribed to reduce potential or anticipated infection that frequently develops in traumatised or inflamed tissues. If a chronic atelectasis situation ensues due to (slow) tumour development, residual excess fluid from unresolved pneumonia, or scarred areas, ventilation and antibiotics may be in order.

Adult respiratory distress syndrome (ARDS)

This may develop because of aspiration or inhalation of food or vomit material into the respiratory pathways. Heavy smoke from a burning structure or toxic fumes may scar the respiratory linings of the tubules and cause them to become less able to function. Oxygen assistance and physiotherapy, along with antibiotics and rest, help resolve most

cases. Chronic bronchitis or asthma symptoms may become considerations in advanced cases.

Bronchogenic carcinoma Bronchogenic carcinoma is the most common type of lung cancer, causing 18% of all cancer deaths worldwide, making it the leading cause of death from cancer among both men and women. *Bronchogenic* implies that the cancer originated in the bronchi of the lung versus another site. In addition to primary carcinoma of the lungs, the lungs are a frequent site of metastases from the breast, gastrointestinal tract, female reproductive system and kidneys.

The great danger in bronchogenic carcinoma is blockage of the airway by the malignant tumour as it grows into the lumen of a bronchus, causing collapse of the affected part of the lung. Few symptoms or signs accompany early stage lung cancer, but symptoms of later stages include a persistent cough and haemoptysis. The blood in the sputum results from the erosion of blood vessels by the growing malignancy. Anorexia, weight loss and weakness accompany the disease, caused partly by poor oxygenation of the blood. Other symptoms include difficulty in breathing caused by airway obstruction due to compression and body fluids such as mucus and blood. Because these symptoms develop late in the disease, when metastasis is likely to have occurred, immediate and aggressive treatment is in order. Prevention or early detection is preferred but is not always achievable. At present, however, the average age for diagnosis is 60, and it is likely that many of these cancers began years earlier.

Approximately 80% of lung cancer is related to cigarette smoking, and it is 10 times more common in smokers than in non-smokers. Other related causes include inhalation of carcinogens from second-hand smoke that kills 3000+ non-smokers per year. Second-hand smoke increases the risk of developing lung cancer by 20–30%. Occupational hazards among workers also increase the probability of lung cancer because of a constant exposure to air pollution from exhaust gases and industrial fumes.

Diagnosis of lung cancer is made using X-ray, a biopsy of the tumour, detection of cancer cells

SIDE by SIDE Lung cancer

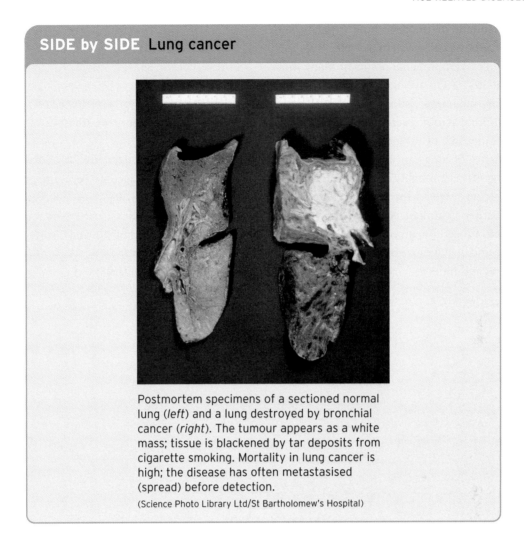

Postmortem specimens of a sectioned normal lung (*left*) and a lung destroyed by bronchial cancer (*right*). The tumour appears as a white mass; tissue is blackened by tar deposits from cigarette smoking. Mortality in lung cancer is high; the disease has often metastasised (spread) before detection.

(Science Photo Library Ltd/St Bartholomew's Hospital)

in the sputum or washings from the bronchoscopy examination. Coughing up blood is a major sign of lung cancer.

Treatment includes surgery that does not cure cancer but reduces a central source and mass, which allows other treatments to work. Where possible, radiation and/or chemotherapy are common approaches depending on the particular circumstance of tumour size, location and general health.

AGE-RELATED DISEASES

Because respiratory infections are generally highly contagious, they are common among infants and children. Historically, children have suffered a high mortality rate from diphtheria, pertussis, measles and other contagious respiratory diseases. Vaccinations for these and other respiratory diseases have significantly reduced mortality in the UK. However, around the world where vaccines are unavailable, these diseases continue to kill many children.

The onset of asthma may be early or later in life and, while some cases of early-onset asthma may resolve, later-onset asthma generally tends to persist, but with less frequent attacks and at a reduced impact. Untreated sleep apnoea tends to get worse with advancing years.

In the elderly, elastic tissue of the lungs deteriorates and reduces lung capacity in normal situations. This condition is exacerbated by weakening of respiratory muscles and arthritis in joints of the ribs and vertebrae. Prescribed exercises performed regularly can help maintain or improve lung capacity and benefit the cardiovascular system as well.

Some degree of emphysema occurs in many individuals aged 50–70. On average, one square foot of the respiratory membrane is lost each year after age 30. Again, routine aerobic exercise or walking helps to keep the lungs in a healthier state.

The incidence of lung cancer increases with age. However, the cancer probably begins earlier in life, and this incidence reflects the relatively late age at diagnosis. Earlier treatment is crucial for a better life. Even with cancer, pneumonia will likely be the final disease and actual cause of death in the elderly who are weak and frail.

Resources

British Thoracic Society: *www.brit-thoracic.org.uk*

Centers for Disease Control and Prevention: *www.cdc.gov/nchs/fastats/asthma.htm*

www.cdc.gov/tobacco/data_statistics/factsheets/health_effects.htm

Clinical Knowledge Summaries: *www.cks.nhs.uk*

Health and Safety Executive: *www.hse.gov.uk*

National Heart, Lung, and Blood Institute: *www.nhlbi.nih.gov*

National Institute for Health and Clinical Excellence: *www.nice.org.uk*

National Institutes of Health: *www.nlm.nih.gov/medlineplus*

World Health Organization: *www.who.org*

DISEASES AT A GLANCE Respiratory system

DISEASE	AETIOLOGY	SIGNS AND SYMPTOMS	DIAGNOSIS	TREATMENT	PREVENTION	LIFESPAN
Upper respiratory						
Pharyngitis	Bacteria, viruses, irritants	Red, sore throat; pus; dysphagia	Physical examination, throat culture	If bacterial, antibiotics	Maintain good health and hygiene; do not smoke or eat or drink spicy foods	Occurs at all ages
Tonsillitis	Bacteria, viruses, irritants	Sore throat, swollen tonsils, dysphagia	Physical examination, throat culture	Antibiotics if bacterial infections	Maintain good health and hygiene; treat common cold	Typically in children, but also adults
Laryngitis	Bacteria, viruses, irritants	Sore throat, difficulty speaking	Physical examination	Resting voice, steam inhalations, higher fluid intake	Maintain good health and hygiene; reduce voice usage	Occurs at any age
Common cold	Paramyxoviruses	Nasal congestion, cough, sore throat	Physical examination	Analgesic Decongestant	Reduce exposure, but difficult to prevent	Any and all ages
Seasonal allergic rhinitis (hay fever)	Airborne allergens, pollens	Nasal and sinus congestion; watery, itchy eyes	Physical examination, allergy tests	Antihistamines	Reduce exposure, take medication as needed	Some are more susceptible
Influenza	Viruses	Fever, headache, weakness, body aches	Physical examination	Bed rest, fluids, analgesics to reduce pain and fever	Difficult, especially in 'flu' season, reduce exposure, vaccine for those with compromised health	Especially very young, compromised adolescents, elderly
Lower respiratory						
Asthma	Allergies, fumes, heavy exertion, cockroaches	Dyspnoea, difficulty exhaling, wheezing	Spirometry, physical examination, family history	Beta-2 agonists, corticosteroids	With hereditary markers and/or environmental inducements may not be preventable, do not smoke	Children, and middle aged to older adults
Bronchogenic carcinoma (lung cancer)	Smoking, fumes, air pollution	Obstruction of airways and associated complications, weight loss, weakness	Bronchoscopy, X-ray, CT scan, biopsy, sputum evaluation	Radiation, chemotherapy, surgery	Do not smoke, limit exposure in work environment if possible	Usually adults
Chronic bronchitis	Fumes, bacteria, viruses, smoking	Chest pains, dyspnoea, chronic productive cough	Patient history, physical examination	Cough medicine; if bacterial, antibiotics	Avoid toxic areas or wear respiratory protection, do not smoke	Usually middle aged to older adults
Cystic fibrosis	Genetic, chromosome 7, recessive	Recurrent lung infections, dyspnoea, coughing and lung obstruction, weight loss owing to poor absorption of fats and vitamin D	Sweat test for excess salt	Physiotherapy, antibiotics, pancreatic enzyme supplements	Heredity	At birth and throughout life

DISEASES AT A GLANCE Respiratory system (continued)

DISEASE	AETIOLOGY	SIGNS AND SYMPTOMS	DIAGNOSIS	TREATMENT	PREVENTION	LIFESPAN
Emphysema	Cigarette smoking, fumes, genetic	Difficulty exhaling, cyanosis, fatigue, barrel chest, pneumonia as complication	Spirometry, physical examination	Elimination of inhaled irritants, mucus-thinning drugs	Do not smoke and limit exposure to aerial toxins. With genetic input, may not be preventable	Generally early to mid-adulthood, not curable
Pneumonia	Bacteria, viruses, fungi	Chest pain, fluid in lungs on X-ray, fever, productive cough	Chest X-ray, sputum analysis	If bacterial, antibiotics	Uncertain, good health, try to avoid exposure (e.g. hospitals)	Any age; may kill the young and many older patients
Pulmonary tuberculosis	Mycobacterium	Primary may be asymptomatic, secondary with fever, weakness, weight loss/cachexia, cough producing blood, tissue, bacteria	Chest X-ray, skin test, sputum analysis	Antibiotics such as isoniazid and rifampicin	Good health, but may not know of contagious source, thus unpreventable. Avoid known contact sources, reduce exposure to crowds	Any age, especially in areas of high exposure

INTERACTIVE EXERCISES

Cases for critical thinking

1. A young man has chest pain, cough, difficulty breathing and a fever. Obviously, these symptoms could be caused by a variety of diseases. What diagnostic procedures would be helpful in diagnosing the man's disease?

2. At age 62, Harry decided to retire from the grain factory where he had worked for 40 years. He was walking much more slowly and felt weaker even though he was walking less. He had enjoyed his cigarette breaks and lunches with the lads, but now he had difficulty getting his breath, while his breathing rate had increased and his chest seemed inflated. What disease seems apparent here, and how may it be addressed?

3. Sara loved to run. She watched sports day at school. An asthmatic, she occasionally had to use an inhaler, but she seemed determined to be an athlete. Should Sara be discouraged from pursuing her goal? Why or why not?

Multiple choice

1. What COPD is primarily caused by smoking, may have a genetic link and has no cure?
   a. bronchitis   b. diphtheria
   c. tuberculosis   d. emphysema ✓

2. Inflammation of bronchial membranes, destruction of cilia and excess thick mucus production are characteristics of which disease?
   a. emphysema
   b. chronic bronchitis
   c. asthma ✓
   d. tuberculosis

3. Which of the following diseases is typically *not* treated with antibiotics?
   a. pneumonia
   b. emphysema ✓
   c. Legionnaire's disease
   d. pharyngitis

4. What disease was formerly known as 'consumption?'
   a. pneumonia   b. asthma
   c. tuberculosis ✓ d. lung cancer

5. What disease of the young or old may be triggered by allergies and emotions or heavy exercise?
   a. bronchitis   b. sinusitis
   c. asthma ✓   d. pharyngitis

6. Which of the following tends to be caused by streptococci?
   a. pneumonia ✓
   b. tuberculosis
   c. Legionnaire's disease
   d. influenza

7. A 'barrel chest' is often indicative of what respiratory disease?
   a. pneumonia   b. emphysema ✓
   c. cancer   d. bronchitis

8. Legionnaire's disease is caused by what condition or organism?
   a. fungi
   b. viruses
   c. low-humidity climates
   d. bacteria ✓

9. What disease is characterised by a lack of alveolar surfactant that typically happens to premature infants?
   a. asthma
   b. infant respiratory distress syndrome (IRDS) ✓
   c. TB
   d. pneumonia

10. Excess or deficient pulmonary fluid results in what painful disease?
    a. pulmonitis   b. pneumonia
    c. pleurisy ✓   d. cystic fibrosis

True or false

_T_ 1. The flu can be prevented by vaccine.
_F_ 2. The common cold is easily treated with antibiotics.
_F_ 3. Laryngitis may be treated by removal of the tonsils.
_T_ 4. The lungs are a common site for metastatic cancer.
_F_ 5. Incidences of asthma and tuberculosis are declining because of new potent antibiotics.
_F_ 6. Dyspnoea is the coughing of blood.
_F_ 7. Bronchiectasis is a collapse of lobes of the lung.
_T_ 8. Pneumothorax simply means 'air in the chest cavity'.
_F_ 9. COPD means 'COntagious Pulmonary Disorder'.
_F_ 10. Pharyngitis is usually outgrown by age 15.

Fill-ins

1. The _____ test is used to screen for tuberculosis.

2. A lung collapse regardless of aetiology is called _____.

3. The main cause of lung cancer is _____.

4. A simple breathing test for pulmonary function is _____.

5. The common cold, influenza and atypical pneumonia are caused by _____.

6. Painful swelling of the membranes surrounding the lungs is called _____.

7. The most common form of pneumonia is _____.

8. Wheezing and difficulty in exhaling are symptoms of _____.

9. Mucus secretion is thick and excessive in the inherited disease called _____.

Labelling exercise

Use the blank lines below to label the following images.

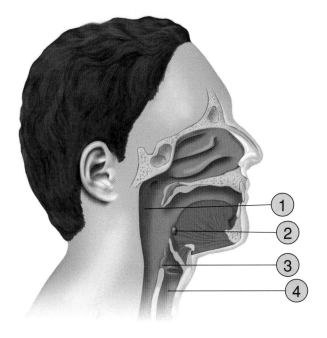

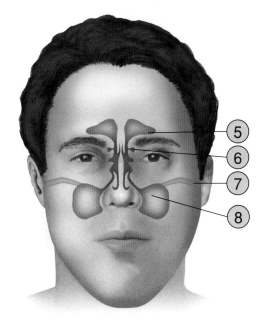

1 _____

2 _____

3 _____

4 _____

5 _____

6 _____

7 _____

8 _____

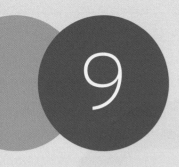

9

DISEASES OF THE GASTROINTESTINAL SYSTEM

C. difficile is a major cause of pseudo-membranous colitis and antibiotic-associated diarrhoea.
(Courtesy of the CDC/Dr Gilda Jones, 1980)

Fact or fiction ?

Cancer of the colon or rectum is the second leading cause of cancer-related death in the UK.

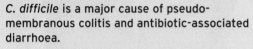

only to lung cancer.
colorectal cancer in the UK, second
approximately 16 000 people die of
estimates that each year
Fact: Cancer Research UK

Learning objectives

After studying this chapter, you should be able to:

+ Describe the normal structure and function of the digestive tract
+ Describe the key characteristics of major diseases of the digestive tract
+ Name the diagnostic tests for diseases of the digestive tract
+ Explain the aetiology of gastrointestinal diseases
+ Describe the treatment options for diseases of the digestive tract
+ Describe the normal structure and function of the liver, gallbladder and pancreas
+ Describe the key characteristics of major diseases of the liver, gallbladder and pancreas
+ Name the diagnostic tests for diseases of the liver, gallbladder and pancreas
+ Explain the aetiology of liver, gallbladder and pancreas diseases
+ Describe the treatment options for diseases of the liver, gallbladder and pancreas
+ Describe age-related diseases of the digestive system

Disease chronicle

Dysentery

Diseases of the digestive system include common ailments familiar to nearly everyone. Some are a minor inconvenience; others are serious, life-threatening diseases. The impact of digestive system diseases is undeniable: during the Crimean War, injured soldiers were sent to Scutari hospital, where Florence Nightingale made her name. But while less than one-sixth of the mortalities were due to battle injuries, half were due to dysentery. Despite modern medical diagnosis and treatment, cancer of the pancreas, colon and liver remain deadly and, worldwide, dysentery remains a leading cause of death among children.

THE GASTROINTESTINAL SYSTEM

The digestive system consists of a digestive tract through which food passes, and accessory organs that assist the digestive process. The digestive tract begins at the mouth and includes the pharynx, oesophagus, stomach, small intestine and large intestine. The accessory organs include the liver, gallbladder and pancreas (Figure 9.1).

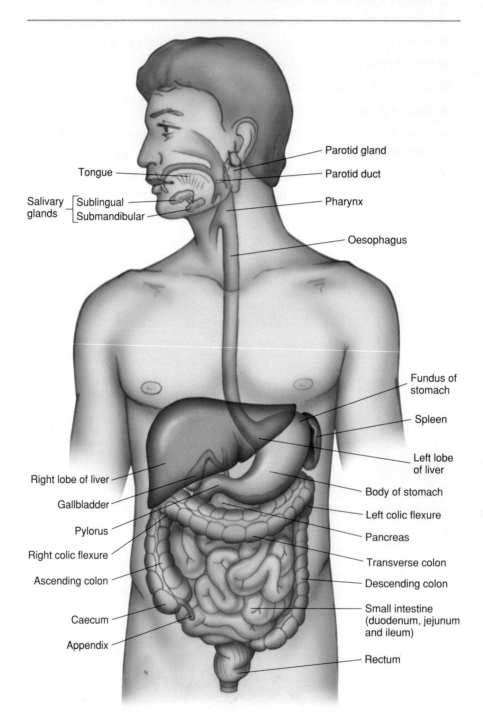

Figure 9.1 The gastrointestinal system.

Digestion begins in the mouth with chewing, or mastication, the mechanical breakdown of food. Salivation, the secretion of saliva, moistens the food and provides an enzyme for initial digestion of starch. The food is then swallowed and passes through the pharynx, or throat, and into the oesophagus.

The moistened food moves down the oesophagus to the stomach. A sphincter muscle at the juncture of the oesophagus and stomach prevents regurgitation while digestion continues. The stomach secretes gastric juice that contains enzymes, biological catalysts that act on protein. Gastric juice also contains hydrochloric acid, which activates these enzymes. The acidic gastric contents would be irritating to the stomach lining if the lining were not protected by a thick covering of mucus. A great deal of moistening and mixing occurs within the stomach. The moistened, mixed and acidic food is called chyme.

Chyme passes from the stomach into the small intestine through a sphincter muscle, the **pyloric sphincter**. This sphincter is closed until it receives nerve and hormonal signals to relax and open. Chyme is propelled along its course by rhythmical, smooth muscle contractions of the intestinal wall called **peristalsis**.

Most digestion occurs in the first part of the small intestine, the **duodenum**. Intestinal secretions contain mucus and digestive enzymes, which enter by means of the pancreatic duct from the pancreas. The pancreas secretes enzymes that digest proteins, lipids and carbohydrates. It also secretes an alkaline solution to neutralise the acid carried into the small intestine from the stomach.

Bile, secreted by the liver and stored in the gallbladder, enters the duodenum through the common bile duct. Bile is not an enzyme but an emulsifier, a substance that reduces large fat droplets into much smaller fat droplets, called micelles, which provide a large surface area for the enzymes to digest fat into molecules small enough to be absorbed.

When digestion is complete, nutrients such as simple carbohydrates, fatty acids and amino acids are absorbed into blood capillaries and lymph vessels in the intestinal wall. The inner surface of the small intestine is arranged to provide the greatest surface area possible for digestion and absorption. This mucosal surface contains numerous finger-like projections called villi, each of which contains capillaries and lymph vessels for absorption (Figure 9.2).

Material not digested passes into the large intestine, or colon. The first part of the colon is the caecum, to which the appendix, a finger-like mass of lymphatic tissue, is attached. Water and minerals are absorbed from the large intestine, and the remaining matter is excreted as faeces.

In this chapter, the diseases of each part of the digestive system are described. These include diseases of the mouth, oesophagus, stomach, small and large intestines, pancreas, liver and gallbladder.

GENERAL DISORDERS OF THE DIGESTIVE TRACT

Pathologies within the digestive system can cause discomforts such as vomiting, diarrhoea, constipation and haemorrhoids. These common disorders are signs and symptoms and could indicate the presence of any number of different diseases. The physiological basis and significance of each disorder is described briefly.

Vomiting

Vomiting, or emesis, is a protective mechanism, a response to the presence of an irritant, infection, distension or blockage. These conditions stimulate sensory nerve fibres, and the message is conveyed to the vomiting centre in the medulla of the brain. Motor impulses then stimulate the diaphragm and abdominal muscles; contraction of these muscles squeezes the stomach. The sphincter at the base of the oesophagus is opened, and the gastric contents are **regurgitated**. A feeling of nausea often precedes vomiting. The cause of the nausea may be factors other than a gastric or intestinal irritant; for instance, motion sickness. An extremely unpleasant smell or sight can cause nausea with possible subsequent vomiting.

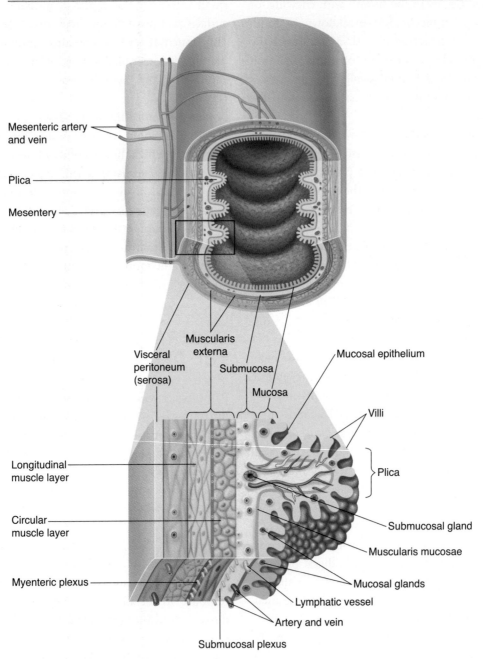

Figure 9.2 Mucosal surface of the small intestine.

Diarrhoea

Diarrhoea is the frequent passage of watery stools and results when the contents of the bowel intestine are rushed through the large intestine. It was stated earlier that the main function of the large intestine is to reabsorb water and minerals. In an episode of diarrhoea, peristalsis is so vigorous that there is no time to reabsorb water and the resultant stool is loose and watery. Anxiety and stress can trigger this increased motility of the large intestine. Intestinal infections and food poisoning can also increase intestinal motility or impair water absorption by mucosal cells.

Constipation

Constipation is the presence of stools that are hard and dry. It occurs when material remains within the large bowel for an excessive amount of time, and too much water is absorbed. The resultant hard, dry stool is difficult and uncomfortable to pass. Poor habits of elimination, dehydration and low fibre diets may cause constipation. Defaecation should be allowed to occur when the defaecation reflexes are strong; otherwise faeces remain in the colon and additional water reabsorption occurs. A diet containing adequate amounts of fibre aids elimination by encouraging osmosis of water into the bowel and so provide bulk, which stimulates intestinal motility. Fibre is obtained from fresh fruits, vegetables and cereals. This chapter will discuss several disorders and diseases of the digestive system that cause constipation.

Haemorrhoids

Haemorrhoids are varicose veins in the lining of the rectum near the anus. Haemorrhoids may be internal or external. A physician can observe internal haemorrhoids with a **proctoscope**, a hollow tube with a lighted end. External haemorrhoids can be seen with a hand-held mirror and appear blue because of decreased circulation; they can become red and tender if inflamed. Causes of haemorrhoids include heredity, poor dietary habit and inadequate fibre, overuse of laxatives and lack of exercise. Straining to have a bowel movement can cause bleeding or cause the haemorrhoid to **prolapse**, or come through the anal opening. Haemorrhoids frequently develop during pregnancy because of pressure from an enlarged uterus. Treatment includes adding fibre and water to the diet and stool softeners to reduce straining and subsequent inflammation. Medicinal suppositories and anorectal creams relieve pain and reduce inflammation.

DISEASES OF THE MOUTH

Complete coverage of diseases of the mouth is beyond the scope of this book. This chapter focuses instead on the major oral inflammatory diseases and neoplasms. Diseases of the mouth can adversely affect the ability to taste, chew, moisten and swallow food.

Oral inflammation

Oral inflammation, or **stomatitis**, refers to a widespread inflammation of oral tissue. Depending on the cause, stomatitis may appear as patches, ulcers, redness, bleeding or necrosis. Stomatitis can be caused by local infection of the mouth with bacteria, viruses or fungi, or it may be a sign of a systemic infection.

Streptococci, spread in salivary and respiratory droplets, are a common cause of oral and throat bacterial infections, resulting in red, swollen mucosa. Bacteria also cause canker sores, small circular lesions with a red border. These painful lesions heal without scars after a week. *Neisseria gonorrhoea*, the cause of the sexually transmitted disease gonorrhoea, causes painful ulcerations in the mouth and throat. Also sexually transmitted, *Treponema pallidum* causes syphilis, which causes oral chancres and ulcerations. These bacterial infections are treated with antibiotics.

Herpes simplex is a common cause of oral virus infections. Transmitted by oral–genital contact, herpes simplex type 2 causes vesicles that rupture to form ulcers. These lesions can appear inside and outside the mouth. Herpes simplex type 1 can also be acquired from salivary droplets. Pain makes eating, drinking and swallowing difficult. The symptoms typically subside within 2 weeks when the viruses move from the area to nerve tissue known as ganglia. The infection can be reactivated following stressful events or suppression of immune function. Treatment is aimed at reducing inflammation and pain with systemic anti-inflammatory and analgesic drugs or topical anaesthetics.

The fungus *Candida albicans* is normally present in the mouth in low levels, but can grow excessively in healthy neonates and those with immune deficiencies or following long courses of antibiotic or corticosteroid treatment. The fungal overgrowth, called candidiasis (or thrush), forms painless white patches that resemble cheese curds. Removing the white patches leaves a raw, damaged mucosal surface. Candidiasis of the oesophagus causes throat pain and difficulty swallowing. Antibiotics and antiviral drugs are ineffective for fungal infections (see Chapter 3). Oral candidiasis is treated with the oral antifungal agents fluconazole, nystatin or clotrimazole.

Cancer of the mouth

The most common form of oral cancer is squamous cell carcinoma. Most of these cancers appear on the floor of the mouth, tongue and lower lip. An aggressive form of the cancer occurs on the upper lip. Mouth and throat cancer ranks eleventh among the leading causes of cancer death worldwide. While the causes remain unknown, it is clear that tobacco – chewed or smoked – and alcohol use are major risk factors, and it appears that use of alcohol and tobacco in combination increases the risk. Treatment for lip and tongue cancer includes surgical removal. Radiation therapy may be used to treat local cancers on the floor of the mouth. See Chapter 4 for oral cancer specifics.

DISEASES OF THE OESOPHAGUS

The function of the oesophagus is the controlled passage of food to the stomach. Oesophageal disease manifests itself as **dysphagia**, difficult or painful swallowing.

Cancer of the oesophagus

Cancer of the oesophagus occurs most commonly in men over 60 and is often fatal. The disease ranks sixth among leading causes of cancer death worldwide but is most common in Japan, China, the Middle East and parts of South Africa. Like mouth cancer, tobacco and alcohol use are major risk factors. The cancer narrows the oesophageal lumen, causing the principal symptom, dysphagia. The obstruction causes vomiting, a bad taste in the

mouth and bad breath. Oesophageal cancer is accompanied by weight loss because of the inability to eat. Diagnosis includes X-ray with barium swallow to study motility and functional defects. The cancer frequently metastasises into adjacent organs, often the lungs and liver, and to remote sites through the lymph vessels before it is detected. Because of early metastasis and nutritional complications, the prognosis for oesophageal cancer is poor. See Chapter 4 for further information on oesophageal cancer.

Oesophageal varices

Varicose veins that develop in the oesophagus are called **oesophageal varices**. Cirrhosis of the liver is the chief cause of oesophageal varices. Cirrhosis impairs blood flow through the liver, which elevates pressure in the veins of the abdomen and elsewhere, including the oesophagus. The increased venous pressure causes the oesophageal veins to dilate and become knotty. The most serious danger in oesophageal varices is haemorrhage. Bleeding oesophageal varices require emergency treatment. Diagnosis usually requires endoscopy. Infusion of vasopressin may reduce bleeding, or bleeding can be stopped with pressure on the varices by inserting a Minnesota or Sengstaken–Blakemore tube. These are temporary measures: surgical bypass of the portal vein to systemic circulation may reduce pressure in the veins and thus stop bleeding, but it will not repair liver damage and ultimately will not improve the prognosis.

Oesophagitis and GORD

Oesophagitis, inflammation of the oesophagus, causes burning chest pains, 'heartburn', which can resemble the pain of heart disease. The pain may follow eating or drinking, and some vomiting of blood may occur. The most common trigger of oesophagitis is a **reflux**, a backflow of the acid contents of the stomach. The condition is known as **gastro-oesophageal reflux disease**, or **GORD**. GORD may be caused by an incompetent **lower oesophageal sphincter**, which normally prevents stomach contents from ascending into the oesophagus. Other causes include hiatus hernia and drugs that compromise the sphincter or induce excess acid secretion. The incidence of GORD increases with age, which suggests that age-related changes occur in the sphincter. Whatever the cause, regurgitated stomach acid irritates the lining of the oesophagus and stimulates an inflammatory response. Diagnosis is based on history, signs, symptoms, as well as barium fluoroscopy, measure of oesophageal pH, or endoscopy. Risk factors for GORD include old age, obesity and pregnancy. Treatment includes choosing a bland diet, antacids and acid-reducing drugs. Frequent, small meals are recommended. Painful symptoms frequently occur at night while the body lies prone and relaxed; thus patients are advised to sleep with the head raised and to avoid eating 2–3 hours before sleeping. Alcohol is an irritant to the inflamed mucosal lining and should be avoided.

Hiatus hernia

A hernia is the protrusion of part of an organ through a muscular wall or body opening. A **hiatus hernia** is the protrusion of part of the stomach through the diaphragm at the point where the oesophagus joins the stomach. The condition is caused either by a congenital defect in the diaphragm or by increased intra-abdominal pressure associated with obesity. Figure 9.3 shows this condition. Indigestion and heartburn may occur after eating; shortness of breath may also occur. Diagnosis is based on a chest X-ray that may show air behind the heart, or a barium X-ray that can show a bulge at the lower oesophagus, or endoscopy to visualise the hernia and rule out cancer or varices. The aim of treatment is to reduce symptoms. The most effective treatment is cholinergic drugs, which strengthen the lower oesophageal sphincter and reduce reflux after eating. Patients should avoid irritants such as spicy foods and caffeine, and should take frequent small meals, and obese patients should lose weight. Surgery may be required to correct the structural defect, but it is difficult surgery and hiatus hernias tend to recur.

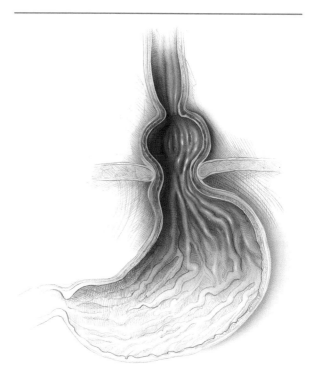

Figure 9.3 Hiatus hernia.
(Science Photo Library Ltd/Molly Borman)

DISEASES OF THE STOMACH

The stomach is well adapted for storing and mixing food with acid and enzymes. Alterations in the stomach lining or malignancies can cause painful and sometimes serious disease.

Gastritis

Acute **gastritis** is an inflammation of the stomach frequently accompanied by vomiting of blood. Irritants such as aspirin, excessive coffee, tobacco, alcohol or infection cause acute gastritis. Acute alcoholism is a major cause of haemorrhagic gastritis. Chronic alcohol use stimulates acid secretion, which irritates the mucosa. **Gastroscopy** and biopsy is extremely valuable in diagnosing this disease. A camera may be attached to the gastroscope, and the entire inner stomach is photographed. Treatment includes avoiding the aforementioned irritants and treating infections. Medical treatment includes cimetidine, which blocks gastric secretion. If bleeding is involved, surgery may be required.

Chronic atrophic gastritis

Chronic atrophic gastritis is a degenerative condition in which the stomach lining does not secrete intrinsic factor and hydrochloric acid. Intrinsic factor is required for absorption of vitamin B_{12}, and hydrochloric acid aids protein digestion. Chronic atrophic gastritis may be caused by stomach cancer, chronic alcoholism or chronic exposure to certain irritants such as alcohol, aspirin and certain foods, and colonisation by *Helicobacter pylori*. Any underlying disease or infection should be treated, but often there is little can be done to treat this disease.

Peptic ulcers

Ulcers are lesions of any body surface where necrotic tissue forms as a result of inflammation and is sloughed off, leaving a lesion. Ulcers of the stomach and small intestine are termed **peptic ulcers**. Ulcers of the stomach are called **gastric ulcers**, and those of the small intestine are called **duodenal ulcers**. Approximately 80% of peptic ulcers are duodenal ulcers and occur most frequently in men between ages 20 and 50 years. Figure 9.4 shows common sites of peptic ulcers.

Peptic ulcers have three main causes: infection with *Helicobacter pylori*, use of non-steroidal anti-inflammatory drugs, and acid hypersecretion, which can be an inherited disorder. Because hydrochloric

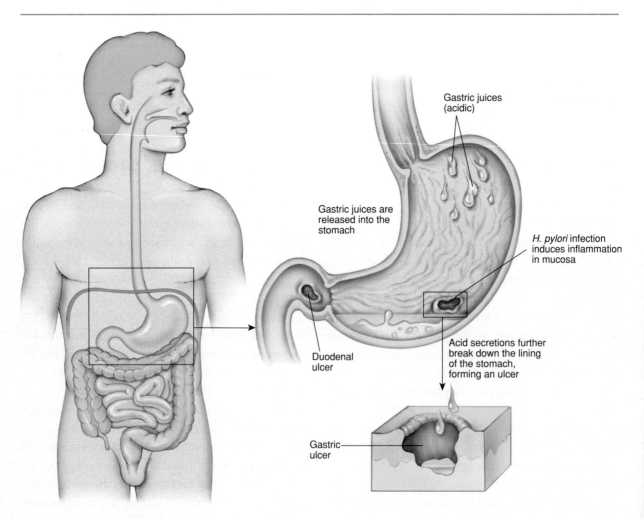

Figure 9.4 Peptic ulcer disease.

SIDE by SIDE Gastric ulcer

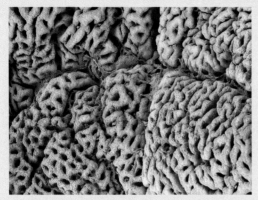

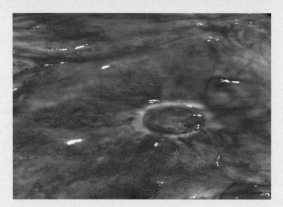

Normal mucosa showing openings of gastric glands.

(Science Photo Library Ltd/Steve Gschmeissner)

Superficial gastric ulcer in the stomach lining.

acid secretion is under nerve and hormonal control, stressful situations can trigger or exacerbate ulcers. Gastric contents contribute to ulcer formation in all cases. The ulcers are caused, in part, by pepsin, a proteolytic enzyme secreted by the stomach. Hydrochloric acid within the stomach and intestinal juice (including bile), regurgitated through the pyloric sphincter, irritate the gastric mucosa. Irritated and inflamed mucous membrane may become necrotic, leaving a lesion.

Heartburn and indigestion are frequently the first signs of an ulcer. The ulcer pain is caused by the action of hydrochloric acid on the exposed surface of the lesion. The muscular contractions of peristalsis also intensify the pain. Symptoms of gastric ulcer include nausea, vomiting, abdominal pain and, occasionally, massive gastrointestinal bleeding.

A potential complication of any ulcer is haemorrhage; severe haemorrhage may lead to shock. It is possible for a large artery at the base of the ulcer to rupture as the lesion erodes deeper into underlying tissues. Bleeding from the ulcer may appear as **haematemesis** or bloody vomiting, or the blood may appear in stools, where it gives the stools a dark, tarry appearance, referred to as **melaena**. A serious ulcer complication is **perforation**. If an ulcer perforates – that is, breaks through the intestinal or

gastric wall – there is sudden and intense abdominal pain. **Peritonitis**, inflammation of the lining of the abdominal cavity, usually results when the digestive contents enter the cavity, because this material contains numerous bacteria. Surgical repair of the perforation is required immediately. Obstruction of the gastrointestinal tract can result from an ulcer and the scar tissue surrounding it. Obstruction occurs most frequently in a narrow area of the stomach, near the pyloric sphincter. Ulcer pain can cause the sphincter to go into spasm, also resulting in obstruction.

Diagnosis is based on an upper gastrointestinal barium swallow, an X-ray, detection of blood in stools, blood tests to determine elevated levels of white blood cells and gastric content analysis. The main objectives of treatment for peptic ulcer disease are to promote healing, prevent complications and recurrences, and provide pain relief. Acid reducers, such as omeprazole or ranitidine, are more effective for peptic ulcers than are antacids and mucosal barriers such as sucralfate. However, antibiotic therapy in combination with acid reducers is required to eradicate *H. pylori* and to reduce the rate of ulcer relapse. If the ulcer is stress- or tension-related, certain changes in lifestyle or approach to stress might be beneficial.

Gastroenteritis and food poisoning

Gastroenteritis is an inflammation of the stomach and intestines. Symptoms include anorexia, nausea, vomiting and diarrhoea. The onset may be abrupt, with rapid loss of fluid and electrolytes. Possible causes are bacterial or viral infection, chemical toxins, lactose intolerance or other food allergy, although the actual cause is not always clear. Treatment replaces fluid and nutritional requirements, including the lost salts. Antispasmodic drugs can control the vomiting and diarrhoea.

Contaminated food, perhaps from human or animal faeces, carries micro-organisms that cause gastroenteritis and food poisonig. *Escherichia coli* are a normal inhabitant of human or animal large bowel; that is to say, it is a **commensal**. Certain strains, or commensals in a different location – perhaps higher up the gastrointestinal tract – may cause disease, including haemolytic uraemic syndrome, in which toxins cause potentially fatal shutdown of the kidneys. To prevent infection, cook meat thoroughly and practise good hygiene in the kitchen.

One of the common forms of food poisoning is caused by the bacterium *Salmonella*. These bacteria invade the intestinal mucosa and cause sudden, colicky abdominal pain, nausea and vomiting, and sometimes bloody diarrhoea and fever that begins approximately 6–48 hours after eating contaminated food and lasts up to 2 weeks. A stool culture can identify the bacteria. *Salmonella* food poisoning (salmonellosis) is associated with contaminated eggs and poultry, but almost any food may harbour the bacteria. Treatment usually consists of replenishing water, electrolytes and nutrients. Elderly individuals, young children and immunocompromised people are particularly at risk of developing serious infection, and they may require further intervention, including a short course of antibiotics and anti-diarrhoeal drugs.

Cancer of the stomach

Cancer of the stomach may be a large mass projecting into the lumen of the stomach, or it may invade the stomach wall, causing it to thicken. As the tumour grows, the lumen is narrowed to the point of obstruction. The remainder of the stomach becomes extremely dilated due to the blockage, and pain results from pressure on nerve endings. Infection frequently accompanies cancer, which causes additional pain. Because pain is not an early sign, carcinoma of the stomach may be very advanced before it is detected. It may even have spread to the liver and surrounding organs through the lymph and blood vessels. Early symptoms are vague and include loss of appetite, heartburn and general stomach distress. Blood may be vomited or appear in the faeces. Pernicious anaemia generally accompanies cancer of the stomach, because the gastric mucosa fails to secrete intrinsic factor. The aetiology of this malignancy is not known, but current research suggests an association with the consumption of preserved, salted, cured foods and a diet low in fresh fruits and vegetables. The incidence of stomach cancer in the UK has been falling since the 1930s, probably due to refrigeration making the use of food preservative less common. However, it remains the eighth most commonly diagnosed cancer, and represents 3% of all cancer diagnoses, with approximately 8000 per year.

Gastric analysis by means of a stomach tube demonstrates the absence of hydrochloric acid, or **achlorhydria**. Biopsy of any lesions seen through the gastroscope is an essential diagnostic procedure for carcinoma of the stomach.

H. pylori infection appears to increase the risk for stomach cancer, probably through its damaging effects on the mucosal cells. Good prognosis for this disease depends on early detection and treatment. See Chapter 4 for more information.

DISEASES OF THE SMALL AND LARGE INTESTINES

The small intestine is the site of most of the digestion and absorption that occurs in the digestive tract, while the large intestine absorbs remaining water and stores and concentrates the faeces. Diseases in these areas may manifest themselves as diarrhoea, constipation, changes in stool characteristics or secondary diseases that arise as a result of poor nutrition.

Appendicitis

Appendicitis is an acute and painful inflammation of the appendix. Appendicitis can occur at any age, but it is more common for males before puberty to age 25. The wormlike shape of the appendix and its location on the caecum make it a trap for faecal material, which contains bacteria, particularly *Escherichia coli*. Figure 9.5 illustrates this potential site of infection. Obstruction with faecal material and infections cause the appendix to become swollen, red and covered with an inflammatory exudate. Because the swelling interferes with circulation to the appendix, it is possible for **gangrene** to develop. The appendix then becomes green and black. The wall of the appendix can become thin and rupture, spilling faecal material into the peritoneal cavity, causing **peritonitis**. Before antibiotic treatment, peritonitis was usually fatal. Rupture of the appendix tends to give relief from the pain, which is very misleading.

Diagnosis depends on physical examination. The pain of appendicitis often begins in the middle of the abdomen and shifts to the lower right quadrant. Patients may walk or lie bent over and draw the right leg up to the abdomen to seek pain relief.

Other diagnostic signs and symptoms include nausea, vomiting, fever up to 39° and elevated white blood cell count. Appendicitis is serious and treatment must commence before rupture occurs.

Malabsorption syndrome

The inability to absorb fat or some other substance from the small intestine is known as **malabsorption syndrome**. Signs and symptoms of malnutrition occur, including lack of energy and inability to maintain weight. Because fat cannot be absorbed from the intestine, it passes into the faeces, and the result is unformed, fatty, pale stools that have a foul odour. The fat content causes the stools to float.

Many disorders can result in secondary malabsorption syndrome. A diseased pancreas or blocked pancreatic duct deprives the small intestine of **lipase**. In the absence of lipase, fat is not digested and cannot be absorbed. Inadequate bile secretion, owing to liver disease or a blocked bile duct, also inhibits lipid digestion and causes secondary malabsorption. One of the complications of the malabsorption syndrome is a bleeding tendency. Vitamin K, a fat-soluble vitamin that is essential to the blood-clotting mechanism, cannot be absorbed. Treatment for malabsorption syndrome depends on its cause, and diet is carefully controlled. Supplements are administered, such as the fat-soluble vitamins A, D, E and K.

Coeliac disease

Coeliac disease is associated with intolerance to gluten, a protein found in flour, and is characterised by poor nutrient absorption. Signs and symptoms include recurrent diarrhoea, wind, abdominal cramps and systemic signs of malnutrition owing to low caloric intake and poor absorption of vitamins. Onset is usually in the first year of life, when wheat products are first consumed. Coeliac disease often runs in families, and may involve an inherited immune dysfunction. It affects females and males in approximately equal numbers, about 1% of the European population. It is unusual in the non-white population. Coeliac disease is diagnosed by

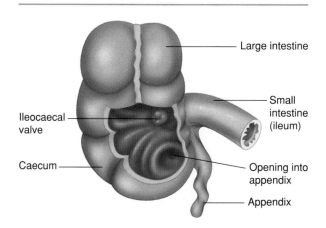

Figure 9.5 Appendix attached to caecum into which the small intestine empties.

Large intestine

Small intestine (ileum)

Ileocaecal valve

Caecum

Opening into appendix

Appendix

Prevention PLUS!

Bacteria, coolers and food poisoning

Refrigeration and freezing do not kill bacteria. The cold temperature inhibits their growth, which can resume at warmer temperatures. Bacteria can multiply rapidly; under optimum conditions, they may double their numbers every 30 minutes. A contaminated potato salad may be safe to eat right out of the refrigerator, but it may become the source of a serious infection if brought to a picnic and left to stand at air temperature for a couple of hours. So it is a good idea to keep the potato salad in the cool bag while you are playing frisbee at your next picnic!

the signs and symptoms as well as by biopsy of the small intestine, which reveals atrophy and flattening of intestinal villi. Treatment involves elimination of gluten from the diet, fluid replacement and vitamin supplements.

Diverticular disease

Diverticulae are little pouches or sacs formed when the mucosal lining pushes through the underlying muscle layer of the intestinal wall. This condition is called **diverticulosis** and may cause no harm in itself, but **diverticulitis** is an inflammation of the diverticulae, which occurs when the sacs become impacted with faecal material and bacteria. The patient experiences low, colicky pain, usually on the left side of the abdomen. As inflammation spreads,

the lumen of the intestine narrows, an obstruction can develop and abscesses frequently form. Diverticular disease is most prevalent in western industrialised nations where fibre consumption is lowest. About 50% of adults over the age of 50 years develop diverticulosis, but of these 75% will not experience any symptoms. Diverticular disease is diagnosed with a barium enema. Antibiotic therapy, together with diet, is usually effective. Figure 9.6 shows an example of diverticulitis.

Inflammatory bowel disease

This is a complex and diverse group of disorders that has major implications for the patients' lifestyle and wellbeing. There are two major manifestations of the disease.

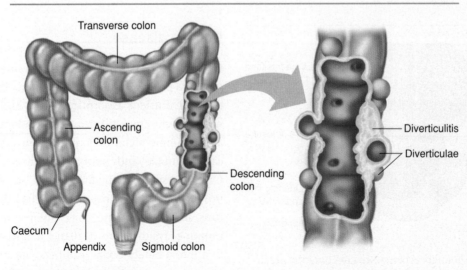

Figure 9.6 Diverticulitis.

Crohn's disease **Crohn's** is an inflammatory disease of the bowel. Any part of the bowel can be affected but it most frequently affects the upper colon and sometimes the distal end of the ileum. Crohn's disease is most prevalent in adults aged 20–40, is two to three times more common among Jewish populations, and is least common in blacks. Possible causes include inheritance, allergies and immune disorders, but the exact cause remains unknown. As inflammation progresses, the intestinal walls become thick and rigid. With thickening, the lumen narrows and chronic obstruction develops. The pain resembles that of appendicitis, occurring in the lower right quadrant of the abdomen, where a tender mass may be felt. Diarrhoea alternating with constipation and **melaena** (dark stools containing blood pigments) are common. Severe diarrhoea can cause an electrolyte imbalance because of the large amount of water and salt lost in the stools. **Anorexia**, nausea and vomiting lead to weight loss. Periods of exacerbation, remission and relapse are common; during flare-ups, the inflammation can also manifest as rheumatoid arthritis. Severe cases entail a risk for haemorrhage or perforation. Crohn's disease is diagnosed by elevated levels of white blood cells; low levels of potassium, calcium and magnesium; and by sigmoidoscopy or colonoscopy. Biopsy confirms the diagnosis. Crohn's disease is usually treated with anti-inflammatory drugs such as corticosteroids and aminosalicylates; immunosuppressive agents such as azathioprine, sulfasalazine and olsalazine; and with antispasmodics. Surgery is performed to correct complications such as obstruction, perforation or massive haemorrhage. Ileostomy is necessary if the large intestine has been severely damaged.

Ulcerative colitis **Ulcerative colitis** is a serious inflammation of the colon characterised by extensive ulceration of the colon and rectum. Around 100 000 people in the UK have ulcerative colitis, but the majority of these have their symptoms well controlled. Ulcerative colitis occurs primarily in young adults, especially women, and usually begins between ages 15 and 20. No known causes have been found; however, ulcerative colitis may be related to autoimmunity, *E. coli* infection or hypersensitivity to certain foods.

Typical symptoms include diarrhoea with pus, blood and mucus in the stools, and cramp-like pain in the lower abdomen. Periods of remission and exacerbation are common in ulcerative colitis. Anaemia may accompany ulcerative colitis because of the chronic blood loss through the rectum. Increased risk for colon malignancy is associated with longstanding ulcerative colitis.

Diagnosis is based on colonoscopy and a barium X-ray in which the colon has a characteristic appearance; the normal pouch-like markings of the colon are lacking, and the colon appears straight and rigid, a '**pipe stem colon**'.

Treatment is aimed at reducing symptoms, correcting the patient's nutritional status and their electrolytes and urea levels, stopping blood loss and preventing complications. The symptoms may be alleviated by reducing stress, eliminating foods found to trigger symptoms, and taking adrenal corticosteroids such as prednisone and hydrocortisone to control autoimmunity. If these treatments are not effective, surgery may be necessary, occasionally requiring a colostomy. A **colostomy** is an artificial opening in the abdominal wall with a segment of the large intestine attached. Faecal waste is evacuated through this opening and collected in a bag. A colostomy may be temporary or permanent depending on the nature of the surgery.

Colorectal cancer

Cancer of the colon and rectum is a leading cause of death from cancer in the UK and is the third leading cause of cancer (after breast and lung). The incidence in men and women is roughly equal, with approximately 36 700 cases diagnosed each year; 14 000 of these are diagnosed with rectal cancer; the remainder have colonic cancer.

The symptoms vary according to the site of the malignancy. A change in bowel habits, diarrhoea or constipation is symptomatic. As the tumour grows, there may be abdominal discomfort and pressure. Blood often appears in the stools, and continuous blood loss from the malignant tumour causes anaemia. The mass can partially or completely obstruct the **lumen** of the colon. As the tumour invades underlying tissue, the cancer cells spread through the lymph vessels and veins. Colorectal cancer is diagnosed with a digital rectal examination, sigmoidoscopy, colonoscopy and biopsy.

Two diseases increase the risk for cancer of the colon: longstanding ulcerative colitis and familial polyposis of the colon. **Familial polyposis** is a hereditary disease in which numerous polyps, benign lumps of mucosal material, develop in the intestinal tract. The polyps are usually asymptomatic unless a malignancy develops. Another factor associated with risk for colon cancer is a diet high in red meat and low in food sources of fibre, such as vegetables, legumes and whole-grain cereals.

Colorectal cancer grows slowly, tends to remain localised and is thus potentially curable with early diagnosis. As in all cancers, early detection and treatment are essential to prevent its spread. Most malignancies of the large intestine are in the rectum or the sigmoid colon, which makes their detection and removal easier than malignant tumours in other areas of the digestive tract. Men and women aged 60–75 years are now offered screening every 2 years, as are those known to be at special risk. The screening is based on the presence of occult blood in their stools, followed by endoscopy for those found to have blood present. Treatment is by surgery, possibly with chemotherapy if the tumour has metastasised, or if residual masses remain inoperable (see Chapter 4). If sections of the colon are removed, a colostomy may be necessary.

Intestinal obstructions

An obstruction can occur anywhere along the intestinal tract, preventing contents within the tract from moving forward. Obstructions are classed as **organic** when there is some material blockage, or **functional**, which is where the function, or peristalsis, of the gut decreases, preventing the propulsion of intestinal contents.

Tumours and hernias, both hiatus and inguinal, can cause organic obstructions. The intestine may be twisted on itself, a condition known as **volvulus** that may be unwound surgically (Figure 9.7). The intestine may be kinked, allowing nothing to pass. **Adhesions**, the linking of two surfaces normally separate, can distort the tract. Abdominal adhesions sometimes follow surgery, when scar tissue grows

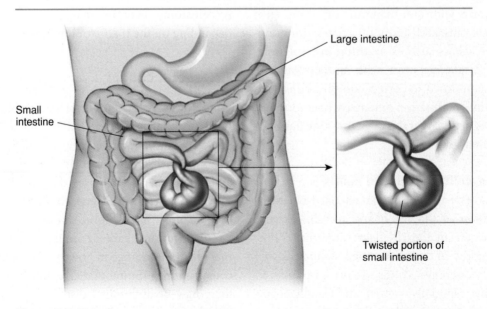

Figure 9.7 Volvulus.

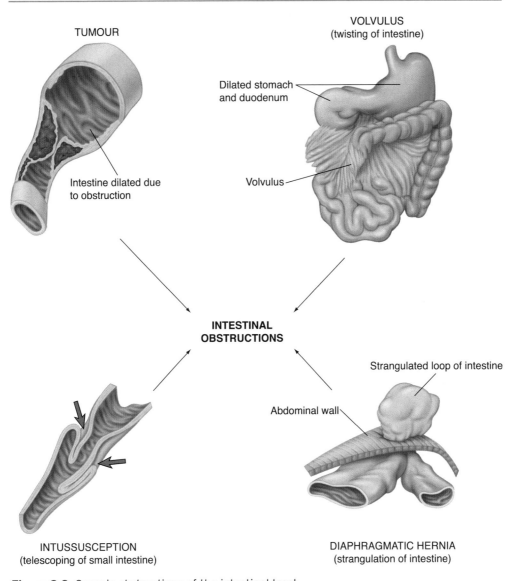

Figure 9.8 Organic obstructions of the intestinal tract.

around the incision. Adhesions also develop as a result of inflammation. Another type of organic obstruction is **intussusception**, in which a segment of intestine telescopes into the part forward of it. This occurs more often in children than in adults. Figure 9.8 shows various types of organic obstructions. An acute organic obstruction causes severe pain. The abdomen is distended and vomiting occurs. There is complete constipation; not even wind, or **flatus**, is passed. Sometimes the obstruction can be relieved by means of a suction tube, but frequently surgery is required. If the obstruction is a strangulated hernia, a protrusion of intestine through the abdominal wall, surgery is required because the blood supply is cut off to the strangulated segment, and it can become gangrenous.

A functional obstruction can result from peritonitis. If a loop of small intestine is surrounded by pus from the infection, the smooth muscle of the intestinal wall cannot contract. Sphincters can go into spasm and fail to open as a result of intense pain.

Irritable bowel syndrome

Irritable bowel syndrome (or **spastic colon**) is relatively common, occurring in 10% of the UK population at any one time, although the actual figure may be higher, as many people may manage without assistance from a healthcare professional. It affects twice as many women as men, particularly young adults. Irritable bowel is marked by diarrhoea or constipation, abdominal pain and wind. The difference between an **irritable colon** and the diseases already discussed is that the irritable colon has no discernible lesion, tumour or ulceration. It is a functional disorder of motility, the movement of the colon. The pain is probably caused by muscle spasms in the wall of the intestine.

Abuse of laxatives and consumption of certain foods and beverages, particularly caffeine, alcohol, spicy foods, fatty foods and concentrated orange juice, can irritate the bowel. Foods such as beans and cabbage, which contain carbohydrates which are fermented by colon bacteria, promote gas production and should be avoided. Laxatives should be avoided as well. Adding fibre to the diet helps to prevent constipation. Emotional stress has an adverse effect on the digestive system, because the nerves of the autonomic nervous system affect digestion. If stressful situations can be alleviated, the colon will function more normally. Tension-relieving activities such as sports, hobbies or regular exercise may help.

Dysentery

Dysentery is an acute inflammation of the colon. The major symptom of dysentery is diarrhoea containing pus, blood and mucus accompanied by severe abdominal pain. Bacteria, parasitic worms and other micro-organisms can cause dysentery. The protozoan *Entamoeba histolytica*, which is transmitted in food and water contaminated by faeces, causes amoebic dysentery. Amoebic dysentery is uncommon in the United Kingdom and is usually found among travellers arriving from countries with poor water quality and sanitary procedures. British tourists can acquire amoebic dysentery when drinking contaminated water abroad. *E. histolytica* invade the wall of the colon and cause numerous ulcerations, which account for the pus and blood in the stools. Bacillary dysentery is caused by various species of Gram-negative bacteria of the genus *Shigella*. Antibiotics can be effective for bacillary dysentery, and amoebicides are used for amoebic dysentery.

DISEASES INDICATED BY STOOL CHARACTERISTICS

Microscopic examination of stool may identify the cause of food poisoning, gastroenteritis or dysentery. Other information can also be obtained from stool samples. Signs of several of the diseases discussed include blood in the stools. Blood appears differently, however, depending upon the site of bleeding.

If the blood in the stools is bright red, the bleeding originated from the distal end of the colon, the rectum. Streaks of red blood can indicate bleeding haemorrhoids. This symptom can also indicate cancer of the rectum. Dark blood may appear in the stools, giving them a dark, tarry appearance, the condition of **melaena**. This blood has been altered as it passed through the digestive tract, so it originated from the stomach or duodenum. A bleeding ulcer or cancer of the stomach may be indicated by melaena. Certain drugs (those containing iron, for instance) can also give this tarry appearance to the stools. Blood may not be apparent to the naked eye, but a chemical test can show its presence. This is referred to as **occult blood**. It can indicate bleeding ulcers or a malignancy in the digestive tract.

If the stools are large and pale, appear greasy and float on water, they contain fat. This is a symptom of malabsorption syndrome. It may also indicate a diseased liver, gallbladder or pancreas. Diseases of these organs are discussed next.

FUNCTIONS OF THE LIVER AND THE GALLBLADDER

The liver is located below the diaphragm, in the upper right quadrant of the abdominal region.

The liver is the largest glandular organ of the body, and it is unique in that it has great powers of regeneration; it can replace damaged or diseased cells. Nevertheless, chronic liver disease may cause irreversible damage and loss of function.

The liver has a dual blood supply. It receives oxygenated blood from the hepatic artery and blood rich in nutrients from the portal vein. The blood reaching the liver through the portal vein comes from the stomach, intestines, spleen and pancreas. Blood from the small intestine carries absorbed nutrients such as simple sugars and amino acids. One of the functions of the liver is to store any excess of these substances. The liver plays an important role in maintaining the proper level of glucose in the blood. It takes up excess glucose, storing it as **glycogen**. When the level of circulating glucose falls below normal, the liver converts glycogen into glucose, which is then released into the blood. The liver also stores iron and vitamins.

The liver synthesises various proteins, including the enzymes necessary for cellular activities. One means of evaluating liver function is to determine the level of these enzymes in the blood. The liver also synthesises plasma proteins. Albumin is a plasma protein that has a water-holding power within the blood vessels. If the albumin level is too low, plasma seeps out of the blood vessels and into the tissue spaces, causing oedema. Other essential plasma proteins synthesised by the liver are those required for blood clotting: fibrinogen and prothrombin. If the liver is seriously diseased or injured and cannot make these proteins, haemorrhage may occur.

The liver can detoxify various substances; that is, it can make poisonous substances harmless. Ammonia, which results from amino acid metabolism, is converted to urea by the liver. The urea then enters the bloodstream and is excreted by the kidneys. Certain drugs and chemicals are also detoxified by the liver. Specialised cells called **Kupffer cells** line the blood spaces within the liver. These cells engulf and digest bacteria and other foreign substances, thus cleansing the blood.

Bile, necessary for fat digestion, is secreted by the liver. Bile is an emulsifier, acting on fat in such a way that the lipid enzymes can digest it. The products

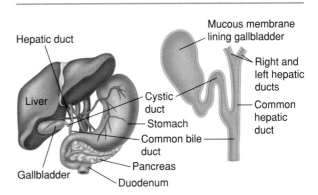

Figure 9.9 Bile duct system of the liver and gallbladder.

of lipid digestion are then absorbed by the walls of the small intestine. In the absence of bile, the fat-soluble vitamins A, D, E and K cannot be absorbed. Bile consists of water, bile salts, cholesterol and bilirubin, which is a coloured substance resulting from the breakdown of haemoglobin. It is bilirubin that gives bile its characteristic colour of yellow or orange.

The gallbladder is a small, sac-like structure underneath the liver. Bile is secreted continuously by the liver into the hepatic duct, which carries bile to the gallbladder for storage and concentration (Figure 9.9). The gallbladder releases the bile through the cystic duct to the common hepatic duct, which carries the bile to the duodenum. Release of bile is coordinated with the appearance of fats in the duodenum, and is controlled by the hormone **cholecystokinin**.

DISEASES OF THE LIVER

Liver disease manifests itself when chronic damage to liver cells cannot be repaired. When fibrous tissue replaces liver cells, the normal functions of the liver become impaired.

Jaundice

One sign frequently associated with liver disease is jaundice. **Jaundice** is a yellow or orange discoloration of the skin, tissues and the whites of the eyes.

It is caused by a build-up of bilirubin, a pigment that is normally secreted in the bile and removed from the body in the faeces.

Jaundice has several causes. The normal flow of bile from the gallbladder to the duodenum may be obstructed by a tumour, a gallstone in the duct system or a congenital defect. Because the bile cannot move forward, it leaks into the blood, with bilirubin colouring the plasma. When the blood reaches the kidneys, the bile appears in the urine, giving it a dark colour. Because bile is unable to reach the duodenum, the stools are light in colour. They are usually described as clay-coloured. Complications can result from this blockage to bile flow. Infection or inflammation of the gallbladder or bile ducts could occur. Lack of bile interferes with fat digestion and absorption, which means that the fat-soluble vitamins are not absorbed. In the absence of vitamin K, bleeding disorders may develop. The obstruction can also cause liver damage. Jaundice can also indicate liver disease, such as hepatitis or cirrhosis.

Haemolytic jaundice has an entirely different aetiology. This type of jaundice accompanies the haemolytic anaemias explained in Chapter 7. In these anaemias, the red blood cells haemolyse, and an excess of bilirubin results from the breakdown of released haemoglobin. Abnormal discoloration follows.

Viral hepatitis

Hepatitis, or inflammation of the liver, is caused by a number of factors, including several viruses. Important causes are hepatitis viruses A, B, C and D. Hepatitis E is uncommon in the United Kingdom.

Hepatitis virus A, formerly called *infectious hepatitis*, is the least serious form and can develop as an isolated case or in an epidemic. It is unusual in the UK, but can affect travellers from areas where standards of sanitation are poor, such as Africa, southern and eastern Europe, southern Asia and Central America. It is caused by eating food (perhaps raw fruit) contaminated with faecal material. Immunisation is available for people planning to travel in affected areas, but this needs to be done months before travel.

Immunoglobulin is a quick and cheap alternative, and offers effective short-term protection.

The incubation period, the time from exposure to the development of symptoms, is from 2 to 6 weeks. The symptoms include anorexia, nausea and mild fever. The urine becomes dark in colour, and jaundice appears in some cases. On examination, the liver may be found to be enlarged and tender. Contaminated water or food is the usual source of the infection, which spreads under conditions of poor sanitation. The virus is excreted in the stools and urine, infecting soil and water. Hepatitis virus type A is usually mild in children; it is sometimes more severe in adults. Prognosis is usually good, with no permanent liver damage resulting. Immunoglobulin injections provide temporary protection against hepatitis virus type A for people exposed to it. A vaccine now in use has proven to be effective. Exposure to hepatitis A gives lifelong immunity.

Hepatitis virus B, formerly called *serum hepatitis*, is a more serious and common disease. The symptoms are similar to those of hepatitis virus A, but develop more slowly. The incubation period is long, lasting from 2 to 6 months. The severity of the disease varies greatly. Those with poor nutritional status, for example, will be more adversely affected. Occasionally, a **fulminating** form of hepatitis virus B develops, and this is fatal. This form has a sudden onset and progresses rapidly. Delirium is followed by coma and death. Hepatitis virus B can be transmitted by donated blood or serum transfusions that contain the virus. It is also transmitted sexually and through contaminated needles or syringes used by drug addicts. Physical condition at the onset of the disease makes a difference in the seriousness of the infection. Blood and plasma donors are screened for hepatitis, as are the products themselves, but hospital personnel must still be well informed of the hazards that can lead to acquiring hepatitis. Precautions must be taken by nurses, laboratory technicians, dialysis workers and blood bank personnel to prevent becoming infected. Immunisation provides immunity to the virus, and it should be administered to personnel who handle or come in close contact with blood or other bodily fluids (see Chapter 3).

Hepatitis C infections appear to have reduced in number recently but remains the leading viral cause of chronic liver disease and cirrhosis and is now the most common reason for liver transplant. This is a long-term result of relatively high rates in the 1980s. The main route for HCV is through blood to blood transmission, and rates have fallen since the risk of developing from a blood transfusion has been almost eliminated in the UK. Rates of HCV are now relatively low in the UK compared to some parts of the world: it is estimated that about a quarter of a million people are currently infected in the UK, although many will not have been diagnosed. The initial symptoms are non-specific and similar to those of hepatitis A or B, but the disease persists for months, even years. About 20% of those infected develop cirrhosis, and a number of these cases can lead to end-stage liver disease. The virus is transmitted mostly through blood transfusions, although transmission has been traced to intravenous drug use, and epidemiological studies show a risk associated with sexual contact with someone with hepatitis and with having had more than one sex partner in a year. Treatments of hepatitis C include interferon injections and oral ribavirin. Treatment for end-stage cirrhosis may include liver transplant.

Hepatitis D virus is described as a defective virus because it cannot reproduce in a cell unless the cell is also infected with hepatitis B. The resulting disease is more serious and more frequently progresses to chronic liver disease. Rates of hepatitis D are not known because surveillance is not systematically conducted; however, hepatitis D is quite uncommon but its transmission is known to be similar to that of hepatitis B.

Hepatitis E is very rare in the United Kingdom, but worldwide it is the leading cause of epidemics of infectious hepatitis. Major epidemics occur in Africa, Asia and Mexico, where it is transmitted primarily through faecal-contaminated drinking water. Nearly every case in the United Kingdom occurs in travellers from areas where the disease is endemic. No effective treatment or vaccine exists. Fortunately, there is no evidence that type E progresses to chronic disease.

Cirrhosis of the liver

Cirrhosis is chronic destruction of liver cells and tissues with a nodular, bumpy regeneration. It affects 30 000 people at any one time, and 7000 are diagnosed in the UK each year. In 2001 it killed 14.1 men per 100 000 men and 7.7 women per 100 000 women in England, but the figures in Scotland are even worse, 34.4 and 16.1, respectively. The total death toll in the UK is 22 000 per year. This is becoming a particularly British problem, as other European countries appear to be reducing their alcohol intake while, for some groups within the UK population, it is spiralling out of control. Alcoholic cirrhosis, the most common type of cirrhosis, is described in detail. This disease is also called portal, Laennec or fatty nutritional cirrhosis (an accumulation of fat often develops within the liver). The exact effect of excessive alcohol on the liver is not known, but it may be related to the malnutrition that frequently accompanies chronic alcoholism, or the alcohol itself may be toxic. In the normal liver, there is a highly organised arrangement of cells, blood vessels and bile ducts. A cirrhotic liver loses this organisation and, as a result, the liver cannot function. Liver cells die and are replaced by fibrous connective tissue and scar tissue with none of the liver cell functions. At first, the liver is generally enlarged due to regeneration but it then becomes smaller as the fibrous connective tissue contracts. The surface acquires a nodular appearance. This is sometimes called a 'hobnailed' liver.

In cirrhosis, circulation through the liver is impaired. As a result, high pressure builds in vessels of the abdomen and in other areas. The oesophageal veins swell, forming oesophageal varices. Abdominal organs like the spleen, pancreas and stomach also swell. These organs and vessels may haemorrhage, causing haemorrhagic shock. Haemorrhage of vessels in the stomach or intestines may cause vomiting of blood, **haematemesis**. A characteristic symptom of cirrhosis is distension of the abdomen caused by the accumulation of fluid in the peritoneal cavity. This fluid is called **ascites** and develops as a result of liver failure. The pressure within the obstructed

SIDE by SIDE Cirrhosis

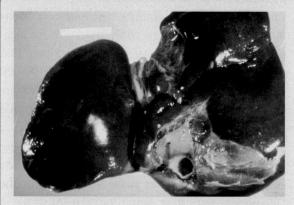

Normal human liver.

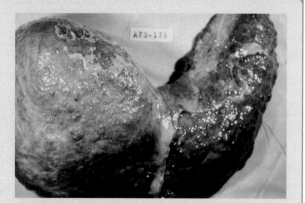

Cirrhosis of the liver from chronic alcoholism.

veins forces plasma into the abdominal cavity. This fluid often has to be drained. When the liver fails to produce adequate amounts of albumin, an albumin deficiency, **hypoalbuminaemia**, develops and fluid leaks out of the blood vessels, causing oedema. Because the necrotic cells of the cirrhotic patient fail to produce albumin, ascitic fluid develops, as does oedema, particularly in the ankles and legs.

Blockage of the bile ducts, like that of the blood vessels, follows the disorganisation of the liver. Bile accumulates in the blood, leading to jaundice and, because bile is not secreted into the duodenum, stools are clay-coloured. The excess of bile, carried by the blood to the kidneys, imparts a dark colour to urine.

Other signs are related to the fact that the diseased liver cannot perform its usual biochemical activities. Normally, the liver inactivates small amounts of female sex hormones secreted by the adrenal glands in both males and females. Oestrogens then have no effect on the male, but the cirrhotic liver does not inactivate oestrogens. They accumulate and have a feminising effect on males. The breasts enlarge, a condition known as **gynaecomastia**, and the palms of the hands become red because of the oestrogen level. Hair on the chest is lost, and a female-type distribution of hair develops. Atrophy of the testicles can also occur.

The damaged liver cells are unable to carry out their normal function of detoxification, so ammonia and other poisonous substances accumulate in

 Prevention PLUS!

Know your viruses

The more you know about how a virus is transmitted, the better prepared you can be to prevent infection. Hepatitis A is transmitted primarily through contaminated food and water. Workers in the food service industry must use hygienic procedures when handling food, including the simple task of washing their hands. You can protect yourself at home by thoroughly cooking meat and seafood, and by storing raw and cooked food separately. Hepatitis B and C are transmitted through blood transfusions, contaminated needles and syringes and sexual intercourse. Healthcare workers receive immunisation against hepatitis B, and blood is screened for contamination by hepatitis B and C.

the blood and affect the brain, causing various neurological disorders. Confusion and disorientation, even to the point of stupor, and a characteristic tremor or shaking develop. This shaking is called 'liver flap'. Somnolence or abnormal sleepiness are symptoms of cirrhosis, which can lead to **hepatic coma** and death.

Although chronic alcoholism is the leading cause of cirrhosis, other diseases can also cause cirrhosis. Severe chronic hepatitis, chronic inflammation of the bile ducts and certain drugs and toxins can cause necrosis of the liver cells, which is the first step in the development of cirrhosis.

There is no effective treatment for cirrhosis. Liver damage cannot be reversed, but further damage can be prevented by treating the underlying cause. Symptoms of cirrhosis may be treated. For example, oedema is treated with diuretics and portal hypertension is remedied with beta blockers to reduce blood pressure. Liver transplant is the only way to restore liver function.

Cancer of the liver

Hepatocarcinoma, or cancer of the liver, is a primary malignancy of the liver that is rare but has a high mortality rate. While liver cancer comprises 1% of all cancers in the UK, it accounts for 6% and 2% of cancer deaths in men and women, respectively. Just over 3000 cases are diagnosed annually. Liver cancer is most prevalent in men over age 60, and the incidence increases with age. In Africa and parts of Asia, where there is a high incidence of hepatitis B infection, liver cancer comprises 10–50% of all cancers. Most cancer found in the liver is secondary; that is, it results from metastasis from cancer in other organs, especially the colon, rectum, stomach, pancreas, oesophagus, lung or breast. Primary cancer of the liver is usually caused by viral hepatitis and cirrhosis. Other causes of liver cancer may include aflatoxin, a toxin from a mould that grows on peanuts and rice.

The symptoms of hepatocarcinoma vary according to the site of the tumour. If the tumour obstructs the portal vein, ascites develops in the abdominal cavity, as it does in cirrhosis. If the fluid contains blood, a malignancy is indicated. A tumour blocking the bile duct will cause jaundice. General symptoms may include loss of weight and an abdominal mass and pain in the upper right quadrant of the abdomen.

Diagnosis includes serum levels of enzymes that arise from diseased liver tissue, but correct diagnosis depends on liver biopsy, itself a hazardous procedure. Prognosis for cancer of the liver is poor because usually the malignancy has developed elsewhere and has spread to the liver.

DISEASES OF THE GALLBLADDER

The gallbladder stores and concentrates bile. Gallbladder disease impairs the storage and delivery of bile to the duodenum.

Gallstones (cholelithiasis)

Gallstones are precipitated bile components in the gallbladder and bile ducts. Gallstones and gallbladder disorders (cholecystitis, discussed in the following subsection) are common: about one-tenth of the population develop gallstones. Most remain symptom-free, with only 30% of those with stones experiencing problems with them. Nevertheless, gallstones remain the greatest cause for emergency hospital admission for people with abdominal pain. Gallstones affect twice as many women as men. The stones arise in the gallbladder when the bile composition changes or when gallbladder muscle activity reduces, as it may in pregnancy, use of oral contraceptives, diabetes mellitus, obesity, cirrhosis and pancreatitis. The stones consist principally of cholesterol, bilirubin and excess calcium. Gallstones, also called **biliary calculi**, may be present in the gallbladder and give no symptoms. There may be one gallstone present or several hundred, which can be large or small (Figure 9.10). Small stones, referred to as gravel, can enter the common bile duct and cause an obstruction, which is excruciatingly painful.

Gallstones can be diagnosed and located by ultrasound and X-ray. The usual treatment for gallstones

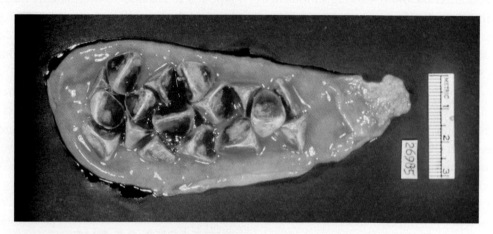

Figure 9.10 Gallbladder opening showing gallstones.
(Photolibrary.com/Martin Rotker)

is surgical removal of the gallbladder, a **cholecystectomy**. The cystic duct is ligated and the common bile duct examined for stones. Occasionally, undetected cholesterol stones are retained in the common bile duct after surgery. Administering a solubilising agent through a catheter into the bile duct may dissolve the remaining stones, preventing the necessity of repeated surgery.

Cholecystitis

Cholecystitis is an inflammation of the gallbladder usually associated with gallstones (cholelithiasis). Acute cholecystitis is most common in middle age. The gallbladder becomes extremely swollen, causing pain under the right rib cage that radiates to the right shoulder. At this point, the gallbladder can usually be palpated. Chills and fever, nausea and vomiting, belching and indigestion are symptoms; in chronic cholecystitis these symptoms occur especially after eating fatty foods. The presence of fat in the duodenum stimulates the gallbladder to contract and release bile, and the contraction of the inflamed gallbladder causes pain. Prolonged inflammation causes the gallbladder to lose its ability to concentrate bile. The walls of the gallbladder may thicken, making it impossible for the gallbladder to contract properly. Serious complications can result from cholecystitis. Lack of blood flow because of the obstruction brought about by the swelling can cause an infarction. With the death of the tissues, gangrene can set in. The acutely inflamed gallbladder, like an inflamed appendix, may rupture, causing peritonitis. A complication of chronic cholecystitis is that bile accumulates in the bile ducts of the liver. This causes necrosis and fibrosis of the liver cells lining the ducts. This is another form of cirrhosis, **biliary** (bile) **cirrhosis**.

STRUCTURE AND FUNCTION OF THE PANCREAS

The pancreas is a fish-shaped organ extending across the abdomen behind the stomach. The head fits into the curve of the duodenum, where the pancreatic duct empties digestive enzymes from the pancreas. These enzymes include amylase, which breaks down carbohydrates; trypsin and chymotrypsin, which digest protein; and lipase, which breaks down lipid or fat.

Diseases of the pancreas severely interfere with digestion and absorption of nutrients. Also, a diseased pancreas may release enzymes that can damage the pancreas and surrounding tissues. Figure 9.11 shows the structure of the pancreas, and Figure 9.12 shows the relationship between the pancreas and other digestive organs.

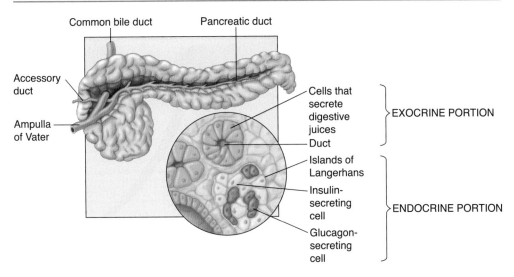

Figure 9.11 The pancreas: an endocrine and exocrine gland.

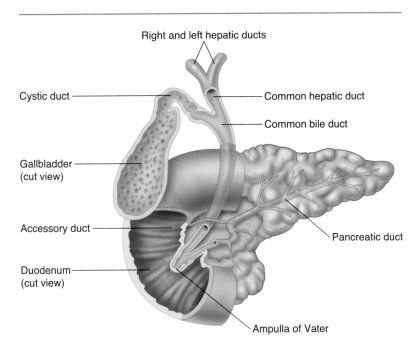

Figure 9.12 Relationship between the pancreas and the digestive system.

DISEASES OF THE PANCREAS

Pancreatitis

Acute **pancreatitis** is a serious, painful inflammation of the pancreas. Pancreatitis is more prevalent in women than in men and usually occurs after age 40. In men it is often associated with alcoholism or peptic ulcers. In women it is more commonly associated with gallbladder disease. The prognosis is good if pancreatitis is associated with gallbladder disease but is very poor if it is related to alcoholism.

Pancreatitis may be caused by local swelling, necrosis, haemorrhage or trauma.

Severe, steady abdominal pain of sudden onset is the first symptom. The intense pain radiates to the back and resembles the sharp pain of a perforated ulcer. Drawing up the knees or assuming a sitting position may provide some relief. There may also be nausea and vomiting. Jaundice sometimes develops if the swelling blocks the common bile duct. If a large area of the pancreas is affected, both endocrine and digestive functions of the gland become impaired. In the absence of lipases from the pancreas, fat cannot be digested, resulting in greasy stools with a foul odour. Secondary malabsorption syndrome develops because undigested fat cannot be absorbed. In pancreatitis, the protein- and lipid-digesting enzymes become activated within the pancreas and begin to digest the organ itself. Severe necrosis and oedema of the pancreas result. The digestion can extend into blood vessels, which causes severe internal bleeding and shock. When the condition becomes this severe, it is called acute haemorrhagic pancreatitis.

The most significant diagnostic procedures for pancreatitis are blood and urine tests for amylase. Treatment is aimed at maintaining circulation to the pancreas and surrounding tissues, maintaining blood and fluid volume, and reducing pain.

Cancer of the pancreas

Adenocarcinoma of the pancreas has a high mortality rate. It occurs more frequently in males than in females, is most prevalent in men between the ages of 35 and 70, and is most prevalent in Israel, the United States, Sweden and Canada. Pancreatic cancer is linked to cigarette smoking, high protein and fat diets, food additives and exposure to industrial chemicals like beta-naphthalene, benzidine and urea. Chronic alcohol abuse, chronic pancreatitis and diabetes mellitus increase the risk of developing pancreatic cancer.

A malignancy in the head of the pancreas can block the common bile duct (Figure 9.13), and symptoms are experienced earlier than those of cancer in the body or tail of the pancreas, which can

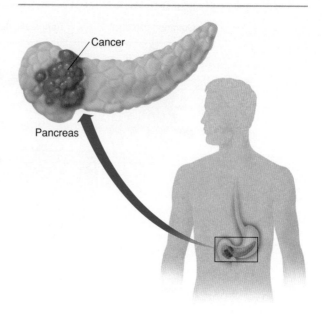

Figure 9.13 Pancreatic cancer. A common site of pancreatic cancer is in the head of the pancreas within the pancreatic ducts.

be very advanced before it is discovered. Obstruction of the bile duct causes jaundice and impairs digestion because the pancreatic enzymes and bile cannot enter the duodenum. This causes malabsorption of fat and clay-coloured stools; sufficient nutrients and calories cannot be absorbed, and weight loss occurs. Great pain is experienced as the tumour grows, and the cancer usually metastasises to the nearby duodenum, stomach and liver.

Diagnosis depends on laparoscopic biopsy and ultrasound. Prognosis for cancer of the pancreas is poor, and death occurs in a relatively short time. Treatment includes surgery, chemotherapy and radiation but is rarely successful.

AGE-RELATED DISEASES

Infants and young children are especially vulnerable to the effects of digestive system disorders because their developing bodies require substantial fluids, calories and nutrients. For example, unchecked vomiting and diarrhoea can cause dehydration and malnutrition more easily in children than in adults.

The digestive system functions fairly well in healthy elderly people, despite normal age-related changes like thinning mucosa and decreased muscle motility. However, some diseases occur with greater frequency with increasing age and thus significantly impact elderly populations.

Mouth and oesophagus

Dental caries (decay) is more prevalent in children than in adults. After adolescence, the incidence of caries reduces and the risk for gingivitis and periodontal (gum) disease increases. Periodontal disease and osteoporosis contribute to tooth loss in elderly people. The number of taste buds decreases and, together with decreased saliva secretion, this may lead to decreased appetite. Oesophageal cancer incidence is highest in those over age 60. As stated earlier, this cancer is closely linked with the use of alcohol and tobacco.

Gastrointestinal tract

Infectious diarrhoeal diseases are the leading cause of death in children worldwide. Children cannot tolerate the loss of enormous amounts of water, electrolytes and nutrients associated with diarrhoea. Hiatus hernia is a common disorder in elderly people. Peptic ulcers are no more common in elderly than in middle-aged people; however, the risk of haemorrhage is greater in old age. Colon cancer incidence increases after age 45, which emphasises the importance of regular screening and early diagnosis. Diverticulae are most common in the elderly, and therefore the incidence of diverticulitis rises. Diarrhoea poses a great risk of dehydration and malnutrition. Therefore, gastrointestinal infections like food poisoning and dysentery can be serious diseases. Overall, the function of the intestines remains fairly normal, although intestinal motility is slightly decreased. Thus, changes in diet or new drugs that affect intestinal motility can more easily lead to constipation or diarrhoea.

Liver and gallbladder

Disorders are uncommon in children. In adulthood, liver function diminishes with increasing age, which results in the persistence of high blood levels of drugs or toxins. In old age, levels of clotting factors decline, increasing the risk for haemorrhage. The incidence of cholelithiasis is highest in those over age 80.

Pancreas

Disorders in children are uncommon, although insulin-dependent diabetes does have its onset in childhood (see Chapter 12). The incidence of pancreatic cancer peaks in the seventh decade and is most common among older men. Acute pancreatitis is common in the elderly. In younger people, acute pancreatitis is associated with alcoholism, while in the elderly acute pancreatitis is more likely due to gallstones that block the pancreatic duct.

Resources

Cancer research UK:
http://www.cancerresearchuk.org/

NHS choices:
http://www.nhs.uk/Pages/HomePage.aspx

BBC: *http://www.bbc.co.uk/health/*

NHS direct: *http://www.nhsdirect.nhs.uk/*

British Liver Trust:
http://www.britishlivertrust.org.uk/home.aspx

DISEASES AT A GLANCE Digestive system

DISEASE	AETIOLOGY	SIGNS AND SYMPTOMS	DIAGNOSIS	TREATMENT	PREVENTION	LIFESPAN
Stomatitis	Bacteria, viruses, fungi	Redness, ulcers, patches, bleeding, depending on the cause	Physical examination, immunodiagnostic tests and pathogen culture	Antibiotics, antiviral or antifungal, depending on the pathogen	Good oral hygiene; do not use antibiotics unnecessarily or incorrectly	More common in infants, young children and older adults with weakened immune systems
Cancer of the mouth	Use of tobacco products, especially in conjunction with consuming alcohol	Abnormal growths, sores or lesions that don't heal	Physical examination, biopsy	Surgical excision of tumour, radiation	Avoid tobacco products; use alcohol only in moderation	Occurs in adults; incidence increases with age
Cancer of the oesophagus	Use of tobacco and alcohol	Dysphagia, vomiting, weight loss	Endoscopy and oesophageal washings	Surgery, radiation, chemotherapy	Avoid tobacco products; use alcohol only in moderation	Occurs in adults; incidence increases with age
Oesophagitis	Acid reflux owing to incompetent lower oesophageal sphincter	Burning chest pain (heartburn), especially after eating or while lying down	Physical examination	Non-irritating diet, antacids, acid-reducing drugs	Take small meals; avoid known irritants	Occurs in adults; incidence increases with age
Oesophageal varices	Increased venous pressure; accompanies advanced cirrhosis	Dilated oesophageal veins, haemorrhage	Endoscopy, physical examination, history of alcoholism	Haemorrhage requires infusion of vasopressin or insertion of inflatable tube to compress veins; surgical bypass of portal veins to reduce intravenous pressure	Treat underlying alcoholism or liver disease	Occurs in adults; incidence increases with age
Hiatus hernia	Stomach protrudes through weakened diaphragm	Indigestion, heartburn following meals, acid reflux and oesophagitis	X-ray	Avoid irritating foods, eat frequent small meals, surgery to repair diaphragm	Avoid spicy food, caffeine; eat small meals	Occurs in adults; incidence increases with age
Gastritis	Aspirin, coffee, tobacco, alcohol, infection	Stomach pain, haematemesis	Gastroscopy	Avoid irritants, drink ice water, take antacid drugs; surgery to control bleeding	Avoid known irritants	Occurs in adults; incidence increases with age
Atrophic gastritis	Degeneration of stomach mucosa results in no HCl secretion and no intrinsic factor secretion	Gastritis, poor digestion and absorption of nutrients, weight loss	Analysis of stomach content reveals low levels of HCl and intrinsic factor	Avoid stomach irritants, take vitamin B_{12} supplements	Avoid known irritants	Occurs in adults; incidence increases with age
Peptic ulcer	Infection with *H. pylori* and erosion of mucosa by stomach acid	Upper abdominal pain, haemorrhage, blood in stool	Gastroscopy, gastric washings, barium X-ray	Antibiotics	Reduce stress	Occurs in adults; incidence increases with age

DISEASES AT A GLANCE Digestive system (continued)

DISEASE	AETIOLOGY	SIGNS AND SYMPTOMS	DIAGNOSIS	TREATMENT	PREVENTION	LIFESPAN
Gastroenteritis	Food- and water-borne infection by bacteria, viruses, protozoa	Nausea, vomiting, diarrhoea, abdominal discomfort or pain, and possibly fever, depending on the pathogen	Stool culture, history	Fluid and electrolyte replacement; anti-diarrhoeal drugs; self-limiting in healthy people	Safe food handling, including correct storage, refrigeration and thorough cooking as needed	Occurs at all ages; especially debilitating in young children and older adults
Cancer of the stomach	Idiopathic; associated with salted, cured foods and diet low in vegetables and fruit; associated with prior infections with *H. pylori*	Appetite loss, stomach discomfort, haematemesis, blood in stool, late-stage pain	Gastroscopy, biopsy, gastric fluid analysis (low HCl), barium X-ray	Surgery, chemotherapy	Reduce intake of salt and cured meat	Occurs in adults; incidence increases with age
Appendicitis	Obstruction with faecal material leads to infection, inflammation and necrosis	Acute lower right quadrant abdominal pain, nausea, fever	Blood count, physical examination	Surgery	Maintain good bowel habits	Most prevalent at puberty and through 20s
Malabsorption syndrome	Congenitally abnormal intestinal mucosa or malabsorption secondary to diseases of pancreas or gallbladder	Malnutrition, failure to absorb fats and fat-soluble vitamins, failure to grow in children and weight loss in adults	Stool analysis and history	Manage diet and take vitamin supplements	Treat underlying diseases	Onset around age 1 as gluten introduced in solid meals
Diverticulitis	Diverticulae of colon become impacted with faecal material and infected or inflamed	Cramping and pain in lower abdomen	Endoscopy	Antibiotics, manage diet	Good bowel habits	Occurs in young adults; incidence increases with age
Crohn's disease	Idiopathic; possible link to autoimmune disease	Lower right pain, diarrhoea and constipation, emission and exacerbation, weight loss, melaena	Stool analysis, endoscopy, patchy thickening of intestinal wall	Corticosteroids, occasionally surgery	None known	Occurs in young adults; incidence increases with age
Ulcerative colitis	Idiopathic; may be autoimmune, stress-related, food allergy-related	Diarrhoea; pus, blood, mucus in stool; cramping in lower abdomen	Stool analysis, endoscopy, diffuse thickening of colon (pipestem colon)	Corticosteroids, stress reduction, diet management, colostomy	Reduce stress	Occurs in young adults; incidence increases with age
Cancer of colon and rectum	Genetic; associated with familial polyposis and chronic ulcerative colitis	Change in bowel habits, diarrhoea or constipation, blood in stool	Endoscopy, biopsy, barium X-ray, stool analysis	Surgery, radiation, chemotherapy	Regular screening to include endoscopy and biopsy if at risk	Occurs in adults; incidence increases with age
Irritable bowel syndrome	Abuse of laxatives, irritating foods, stress	Diarrhoea, pain, gas, constipation	History and physical examination; no lesions present	Avoid caffeine, alcohol, spicy food, fat; increase fibre in diet; reduce stress	Avoid laxatives	Occurs in young adults; incidence increases with age

DISEASES AT A GLANCE Digestive system (continued)

DISEASE	AETIOLOGY	SIGNS AND SYMPTOMS	DIAGNOSIS	TREATMENT	PREVENTION	LIFESPAN
Dysentery	Food- or water-borne intestinal infection by bacteria or protozoa	Abdominal pain, bloody diarrhoea with pus and mucus	Stool culture and history	Antibiotics if bacterial and amoebicides if caused by protozoa	Safe food and water handling	Occurs at all ages; especially debilitating for young children and older adults
Viral hepatitis A (infectious hepatitis)	Food- or water-borne infection with hepatitis A virus	Anorexia, nausea, mild fever, jaundice, enlarged tender liver	Physical examination, stool analysis, immunodiagnostics	Immunoglobulin injections for exposures and infections	Immunisation; safe food and water handling	Occurs at all ages; especially debilitating for young children and older adults
Hepatitis B (serum hepatitis)	Bloodborne or sexually transmitted infection with hepatitis B virus	2-6-month incubation period followed by anorexia, nausea, mild fever, jaundice, enlarged tender liver; may lead to chronic hepatitis and cirrhosis	Physical examination, stool analysis, immunodiagnostics	Immunoglobulin injections for exposures and infections, antiviral drugs, vaccine for prevention	Immunisation	Occurs at all ages; especially debilitating for young children and older adults
Hepatitis C	Bloodborne or sexually transmitted infection with hepatitis C virus	Symptoms as for hepatitis A and hepatitis B following incubation period of months to decades; commonly results in cirrhosis and end-stage liver disease	Physical examination, stool analysis, immunodiagnostics	Ribavarin, interferon, liver transplant	Safe sex, avoid sharing needles	Occurs at all ages; especially debilitating for young children and older adults
Hepatitis D	Rare bloodborne or sexually transmitted coinfection with hepatitis D virus and hepatitis B virus	Same as for hepatitis B; more serious and frequently progresses to chronic liver disease	Physical examination, stool analysis, immunodiagnostics	Immunoglobulin injections, antiviral drugs	Safe sex, avoid injection drug abuse	Occurs at all ages; especially debilitating for young children and older adults
Hepatitis E	Water-borne infection with hepatitis E virus; rare in United Kingdom	As for hepatitis A	Physical examination, stool analysis, immunodiagnostics	No treatment, no immunisation	Safe food and water handling	Occurs at all ages; especially debilitating for young children and older adults
Cirrhosis	Alcohol-induced damage to liver; hepatitis	Jaundice, abdominal distension, ascites, bleeding tendencies, oedema, malabsorption of fats, gynaecomastia, delirium tremens, hepatic coma	Patient history, physical examination, serum liver enzyme levels	No specific treatment; symptomatic treatment for oedema and portal hypertension or bleeding; improved diet, liver transplant	Treat underlying alcoholism or liver disease	Occurs in adults
Cancer of the liver	Primary carcinoma is complication of cirrhosis; more common is secondary or metastatic	Bile duct obstruction, jaundice, impaired clotting, ascites, weight loss	Ultrasound, CT scan, needle biopsy	Chemotherapy (prognosis poor)	None	Rare; occurs in adults and occasionally children

DISEASES AT A GLANCE Digestive system (continued)

DISEASE	AETIOLOGY	SIGNS AND SYMPTOMS	DIAGNOSIS	TREATMENT	PREVENTION	LIFESPAN
Cholecystitis	Obstruction by infection/ inflammation or by tumour	Upper right abdominal pain, especially following a meal of fatty food; nausea, indigestion, belching	Ultrasound, CT scan, faecal fat test	Cholecystectomy	None	Occurs in young adults and prevalence increases with age
Cholelithiasis	Related to obesity; higher incidence in pregnancy and among women	None, or upper right abdominal pain, especially following a meal	Ultrasound, CT scan, faecal fat test	Cholecystectomy, administration of solubilising agent into bile duct	Reduce weight	Occurs in young adults and prevalence increases with age
Pancreatitis	Idiopathic, commonly associated with excessive alcohol consumption or with gallstones	Acute, severe, sharp, radiating abdominal pain; risk of haemorrhage; jaundice; vomiting; malabsorption	Ultrasound, CT scan, serum pancreatic enzymes	No specific treatment; analgesics, fluid replacement, IV nutrients	Treat underlying alcoholism	Occurs in young adults and prevalence increases with age
Cancer of the pancreas	Linked to cigarette smoking, alcohol abuse, chemical carcinogens, chronic pancreatitis, diabetes mellitus	Malabsorption, jaundice, upper abdominal pain	Ultrasound, CT scan, needle biopsy	Chemotherapy (prognosis poor)	Stop tobacco use, alcohol abuse, treat underlying diabetes	Occurs in young adults and prevalence increases with age

INTERACTIVE EXERCISES

Cases for critical thinking

1. A 45-year-old woman experiences frequent heartburn, difficulty swallowing and sharp pains below her sternum. At night, she experiences gastric reflux, or a regurgitation of stomach acid into the oesophagus, a condition that is extremely painful. What could produce these symptoms? What diagnostic procedures could be used? How should she be treated?

2. Timothy experiences sharp pain in his upper right abdomen after eating high fat meals. Also, he has noted that his faeces are greyish-white instead of brown. What disease is the likely cause of his symptoms? Explain why each of these symptoms occurs with this disease.

3. Explain how cirrhosis leads to each of these signs and symptoms: jaundice, malnutrition, haemorrhage and oesophageal varices.

Multiple choice

1. Which of the following is a sign of gastritis?
   a. constipation
   b. inflammation of stomach mucosa
   c. achlorhydria
   d. diarrhoea

2. Recurrent bloody diarrhoea may be a symptom of
   _____
   a. gastric ulcer   b. ulcerative colitis
   c. hiatus hernia   d. oesophagitis

3. Which disease is characterised by the destruction of intestinal villi, leading to inability to absorb fats and other nutrients?
   a. ulcerative colitis
   b. coeliac disease/malabsorption syndrome
   c. Crohn's disease
   d. peptic ulcer

4. Small pouches of the large intestine become inflamed during which disease?
   a. Crohn's disease   b. gastritis
   c. haemorrhoids   d. diverticulitis

5. Which statement about pancreatic cancer is *false*?
   a. it is characterised by abdominal pain, weakness, weight loss
   b. it has a higher incidence with age
   c. most cancers are diagnosed after the cancer has metastasised
   d. the prognosis is good, with an 85% cure rate

6. Which statement about cirrhosis is *false*?
   a. irreversible degenerative changes occur in the liver
   b. the normal liver tissue is replaced with fibrous scar tissue
   c. it is most often caused by diabetes
   d. it is associated with oesophageal varices

7. Acute pancreatitis is most closely associated with
   _____
   a. hepatitis C virus infection
   b. chronic alcoholism
   c. bile duct obstruction
   d. complication of cirrhosis

8. Oesophageal varices arise in which disease?
   a. cirrhosis   b. pancreatic cancer
   c. cholecystitis   d. cholelithiasis

9. Oral thrush is caused by _____
   a. *Candida albicans*
   b. herpes simplex virus type 1
   c. *Treponema pallidum*
   d. *Streptococcus pyogenes* virus type 1

10. Pain in the upper right quadrant, especially after eating, could be a sign of _____
    a. appendicitis   b. pancreatitis
    c. cholecystitis   d. colitis

True or false

_____ 1. Haemorrhoids are caused by infection with *E. coli*.

_____ 2. Oral and oesophageal cancers are linked to tobacco and alcohol use.

_____ 3. Drinking too much water causes diarrhoea.

_____ 4. Dark stools are known as melaena.

_____ 5. Neurological disorders can accompany liver disease.

_____ 6. Hepatitis A is acquired through blood products.

_____ 7. Most cancer in the liver is primary liver cancer.

_____ 8. Gallstones are made of undigested food particles too large to pass.

_____ 9. There is no vaccine for hepatitis B.

_____ 10. Gastric ulcers are caused by infection with *Helicobacter pylori*.

Fill-ins

1. *Entamoeba histolytica* is the cause of _____ _____.

2. Thickened intestinal walls, leading to obstruction and abdominal pain, are found in _____ _____.

3. An abdominal _____ is protrusion of an organ through the abdominal wall muscles.

4. An instrument called a(n) _____ is used to view the lining of the oesophagus or other organs of the digestive tract.

5. Hepatitis type _____ is the major viral cause of cirrhosis.

6. Cholecystectomy is used to treat _____.

7. Biliary cirrhosis arises if there is obstruction of the _____ _____.

8. Accumulation of fluid in the abdomen is called _____.

9. Stomatitis refers to inflammation of the _____.

10. The primary function of the _____ _____ is to absorb water.

Labelling exercise

Use the blank lines below to label the following images.

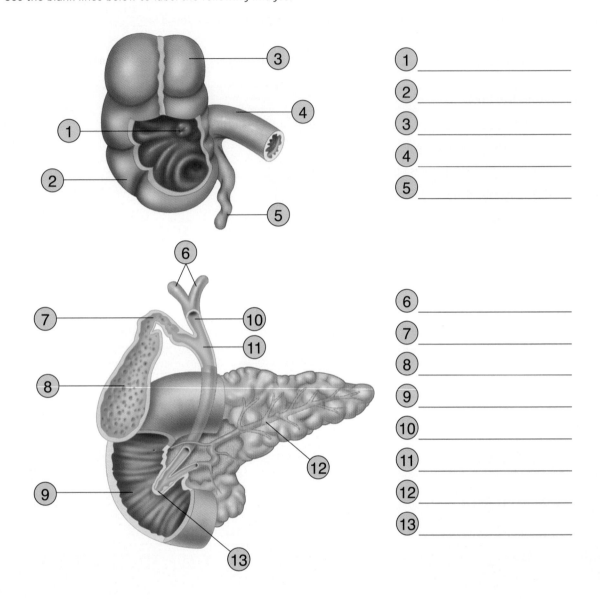

1 _____

2 _____

3 _____

4 _____

5 _____

6 _____

7 _____

8 _____

9 _____

10 _____

11 _____

12 _____

13 _____

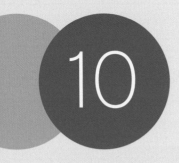

10 DISEASES OF THE RENAL AND URINARY SYSTEMS

Histopathology of kidney showing nodular glomerulosclerosis characteristic of diabetes mellitus.
(Courtesy of the CDC/Dr Edwin P. Ewing Jr, 1974)

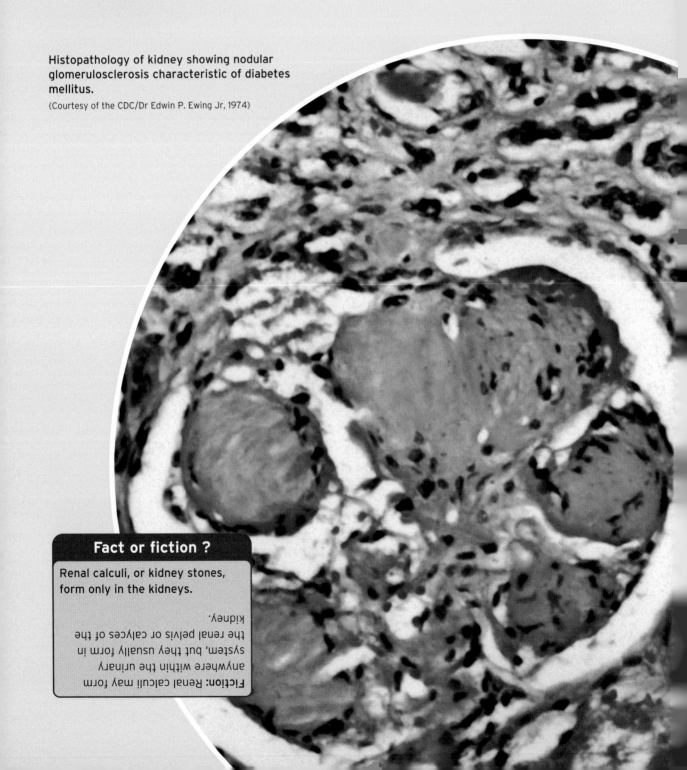

Fact or fiction ?

Renal calculi, or kidney stones, form only in the kidneys.

Fiction: Renal calculi may form anywhere within the urinary system, but they usually form in the renal pelvis or calyces of the kidney.

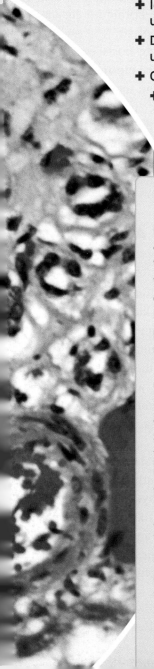

Learning objectives

After studying this chapter, you should be able to:

✚ Describe the primary functions of the major organs of the urinary system – the kidneys and the urinary bladder

✚ Identify the aetiology, signs and symptoms, diagnostic tests and treatment for selected diseases of the kidney

✚ Describe the aetiology, signs and symptoms, diagnostic tests and treatment of urinary tract infections (UTIs)

✚ Differentiate between ascending and descending modes of urinary tract infections

✚ Explain how urinary tract infections or dysfunctions affect other organ systems

✚ Distinguish among the various modes of kidney dialysis

✚ Identify the aetiology, signs and symptoms and treatments of various types of urinary stones (calculi)

✚ Describe causes and treatments of inflammation within the urinary bladder and urethra

✚ Contrast neurogenic bladder with stress and other forms of urinary incontinence

  ✚ Recognise the aetiology, signs and symptoms and treatment for bladder cancer

    ✚ Describe age-related changes of the urinary system

Disease chronicle

Kidney dialysis

In 1913, a pharmacologist at Johns Hopkins University named John Abel published an article about haemodialysis using animals. In the 1930s, Dr Willem Kolff, who at the time was struggling to develop an artificial kidney in the Netherlands, read the article and was curious about applying Abel's concepts to human dialysis. Even under the dark cloud of world war, Kolff and his associates managed to construct a dialyser in 1943. However, progress was slow. The crude dialyser failed to save the first 16 patients placed on it, and these patients suffered acute renal failure. In 1945, a woman in a uraemic coma survived and lived seven more years and the future looked bright.

However, when Dr Kolff moved to the United States following the war, he was not recognised or supported for his efforts. He struggled again for success. At Peter Bent Brigham Hospital in Boston, Kolff met George Thorn, who modified the dialyser with a stainless steel container and later called it the Kolff-Brigham kidney. This new machine saved many soldiers during the Korean War and paved the way for the first kidney transplant in 1954. Because machines were not thought to work as well over time as natural organs and puncture sites would be difficult to find after continual trauma, the dialyser was not promoted.

Dr Belding Scribner from the University of Washington formed a connection between an artery and a vein using plastic tubing and a shunt device with a new material called Teflon. By the 1960s, small portable units were made and haemodialysis could be performed at home. Dr Kolff, however, is considered the father of dialysis, and he was instrumental in developing the heart-lung machine and the artificial heart. In the past 60 years, incredible advancements have been made in kidney treatments. Dr Kolff died in 2009 aged 97.

FUNCTIONS OF THE KIDNEY

The kidneys filter the blood, producing approximately 1 millilitre of urine per minute. In fact, between 20% and 25% of the body's blood volume is contained within the kidneys at any given time. As they filter the blood (plasma), the kidneys maintain water and **electrolyte balance**, and they maintain pH levels. The kidneys also produce hormones like erythropoietin, which stimulates red blood cell production, and renin, which elevates blood pressure.

The nephron

The functional unit of the kidney is the **nephron**. Approximately 1 million nephrons reside in each kidney. As blood passes through the nephrons, metabolic waste products are filtered from the blood plasma. At the same time, most of the water (99%) is reabsorbed along with nutrients such as glucose and amino acids. Extra water, unwanted ions, some drugs and metabolic wastes are then excreted. The product at the end of the nephron is urine.

Each nephron consists of a pair of arterioles, a **glomerulus**, a glomerular capsule, a proximal convoluted tubule, a loop of Henlé and a distal convoluted tubule that leads to a collecting duct. The components of the nephron unit are shown in Figure 10.1.

Formation of urine

Blood in the renal arteries enters via the afferent arteriole a tuft of capillaries called the glomerulus, which is situated inside the Bowman's capsule. The capillary inside the Bowman's capsule is thin and porous (the pores are called fenestrations). Because the blood pressure is higher in the afferent arteriole, fluid can pass through the fenestrae into the Bowman's capsule. This blood filtrate is equivalent to protein-free plasma. In a healthy nephron, neither protein nor red blood cells pass through the filter into the capsular space and into the proximal convoluted tubule.

In the proximal convoluted tubule, most of the nutrients and a large amount of water are reabsorbed

and enter the peritubular capillary that surrounds the tubules. Salts, particularly sodium and chloride, are selectively reabsorbed according to the body's needs. Eventually, about 99% of the water is also reabsorbed along with the salts.

The nitrogen-containing waste products of protein metabolism, **urea** and **creatinine**, pass on through the tubules to be excreted in the urine. Those substances that are in excess in the body fluids, such as hydrogen ions when the fluid is too acidic, are secreted into the distal convoluted tubules to be excreted.

Aldosterone and **antidiuretic hormone (ADH)** play very important roles in the regulation of salt and water reabsorption. These hormones are discussed in detail in Chapter 12.

Urine from all the collecting ducts eventually empties into the **renal pelvis**, the juncture between the kidneys and the **ureters**, and moves down the ureters to be stored in the urinary bladder. Following the signals given by the **micturition** process, the bladder empties urine into the urethra, which leads outside the body. Figure 10.2 illustrates the urinary system.

DIAGNOSTIC TESTS AND PROCEDURES

Pain, **dysuria** (painful urination), blood or pus in urine, or oedema indicates kidney disease, but specific diagnostic tests are required to determine the nature of the disease. Oedema is caused by the loss of protein from the blood; these blood proteins have a water-holding power within the blood vessels. With their depletion, fluid moves out of the capillaries and into the tissues, causing swelling or oedema.

Significant information can be obtained by a simple diagnostic procedure, urinalysis, in which a urine specimen is studied physically, chemically and microscopically. Physical observation allows notation of urine colour, pH and specific gravity of a urine specimen. A centrifuged urine sample is examined microscopically for solids such as crystals, epithelial cells or blood cells.

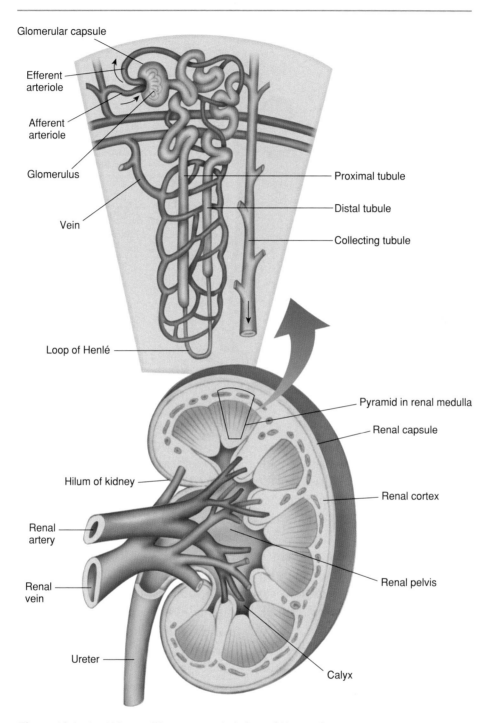

Figure 10.1 The kidney with an expanded view of the nephron.

Chemical tests (e.g. Chemstrip) reveal the presence of abnormal substances such as protein (specifically albumin), glucose and blood. Urine is normally yellow or amber, but haematuria (blood in the urine) can darken the colour to a reddish brown. The degree of colour depends on the amount of water the urine contains. Specific gravity (SG) is a measure of density. Distilled water has a

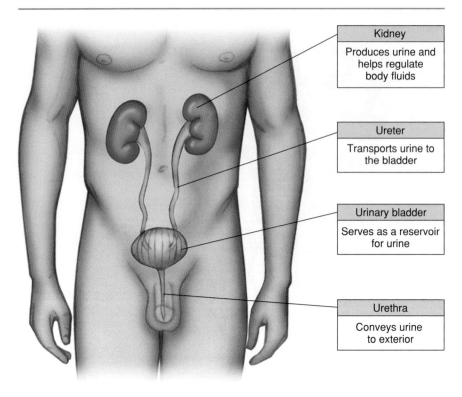

Kidney
Produces urine and helps regulate body fluids

Ureter
Transports urine to the bladder

Urinary bladder
Serves as a reservoir for urine

Urethra
Conveys urine to exterior

Figure 10.2 The urinary system.

SG of 1.000; urine contains particles that the body no longer needs or cannot absorb and therefore the SG of urine is within the range 1.001 (very dilute) to 1.035 (very concentrated). Urine is pale in the case of diabetics, whose water output is large because glucose acts as a diuretic. In longstanding kidney diseases, the ability of the tubules to concentrate the urine is lost. As a result, the urine is dilute and pale, and the specific gravity is low, as found in chronic glomerulonephritis.

The pH of urine has a broad range. The ability of the kidneys to excrete acidic or alkaline urine typically permits the kidney to regulate the pH of the blood within narrow limits. Urine specimens should be examined when fresh because they tend to become alkaline on standing owing to bacterial contamination. Urine from a cystitis patient tends to be alkaline for the same reason.

Albuminuria indicates inflammation of the urinary tract, particularly of the glomeruli. The inflammation increases the permeability of blood vessels, allowing protein and albumin to enter the nephrons

and appear in the urine. This continual protein loss reduces the level of water 'holding power' by the blood (plasma) and results in hypoproteinaemia, leading to a loss of fluids to the surrounding tissues and causing oedema. Microalbumin reagent strips can be used on an overnight sample when determining hypoalbuminaemia.

The presence of sugar (glucose) in the urine may indicate diabetes mellitus. This is not a sign of a disease of the kidneys, but of the pancreas. Diabetes over an extended period of time adversely affects the kidneys (see Chapter 12). Diabetes insipidus is another endocrine problem caused by the lack of ADH or reduced sensitivity of the kidney tubules to the hormone. In either case, the kidney loses its power to control water maintenance and the patient dehydrates owing to copious water loss. Treatment involves ADH-type medication such as Pitressin (vasopressin) that helps to resolve the occurrence of dehydration.

Haematuria may be obvious to the naked eye or require microscopic determination. Haematuria is associated with many serious diseases of the urinary tract, including glomerulonephritis, kidney, ureter, bladder or urethral stones, tuberculosis, cystitis and tumours. If the passage of urine is accompanied by pain, then a stone, an infection or potentially tuberculosis may be the cause. Painless haematuria can indicate the possibility of a malignant tumour in the urinary system.

Pyuria results from a suppurative inflammation caused by pyogenic bacteria that causes the urine to appear cloudy. Microscopic examination of the urine reveals numerous leucocytes. Diseases such as pyelonephritis, pyelitis, tuberculosis and cystitis show pus in the urine.

Casts are shaped like cylindrical rods because they form within kidney tubules. These cast structures consist of coagulated protein, a substance not normally present in kidney tubules. Casts can include various kinds of blood cells as well as epithelial cells from the lining of the urinary tract, and they always indicate inflammation.

Microscopic examination determines the presence or absence of bacteria. Bacteria are found in tuberculosis of the kidney, pyelonephritis and frequently in cystitis. For microscopic examinations, a urine sample may be removed from the bladder by catheterisation to ensure that no external contamination occurs.

A cystoscopic examination enables the healthcare provider to view the inside of the bladder and urethra. The cystoscope is a long, lighted instrument resembling a narrow hollow tube. Tumours, stones and inflammations may be identified with this device. Using an additional instrument, small tumours or polyps may be removed and biopsied. Stones in the bladder can be crushed or surgically removed via procedures such as litholapaxy.

The intravenous urogram (IVU) allows the visualisation of the urinary system by means of contrast media injected into the veins followed by X-ray examination. When these contrast media concentrate in the urinary system, it is possible to note tumours, obstructions and other deformities. A kidney is viewed by renal ultrasound, and the whole urinary system is surveyed by computed tomography (CT) or kidney, ureters, bladder (KUB) exams.

DISEASES OF THE KIDNEY

Glomerulonephritis

Glomerulonephritis is an inflammatory disease of the glomeruli. It is non-suppurative; that is, non-pus-forming, and therefore no bacteria are found in the urine when examined microscopically during a urinalysis procedure. Glomerulonephritis is typically caused by an antigen–antibody reaction that occurs approximately 1–4 weeks following a skin (e.g. impetigo) or throat infection by a haemolytic streptococcus bacterium. Antigens from the streptococci and the defensive antibodies form complexes in the bloodstream that become trapped within the glomeruli, causing an inflammatory response. Numerous neutrophils crowd into the inflamed glomeruli, and blood flow to the nephrons is reduced. The impeded blood flow causes a reduction in the filtration rate and results in decreased urine formation. Many glomeruli degenerate, and the remaining glomeruli become extremely permeable, allowing albumin (plasma protein) and red blood cells to appear in the urine (Figure 10.3). Primary signs of glomerulonephritis include proteinuria, haematuria, oedema and hypertension.

Additional causes include other infective agents (e.g. viruses), parasites (malaria), vasculitis (inflamed blood vessels or lymph vessels), systemic lupus erythematosus (SLE) and Goodpasture syndrome, described later in this chapter.

Acute glomerulonephritis is more common in young children, but it can occur at any age and usually follows a streptococcal infection from a prior sore throat or skin inflammation (e.g. erysipelas). The symptoms include chills and fever, loss of appetite and a general feeling of weakness. There may be oedema, or swelling, particularly in the face and ankles. Urinalysis shows **albuminuria**, the presence of the plasma protein albumin in the urine. **Haematuria**, blood in the urine, is also commonly found. **Casts**, which are the structural elements or moulds of kidney tubules consisting of coagulated protein and blood, are present. The signs and symptoms of acute glomerulonephritis are presented in Figure 10.4.

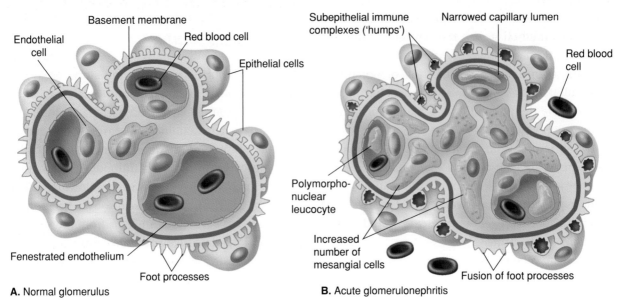

Figure 10.3 Normal glomerulus and acute glomerulonephritis.

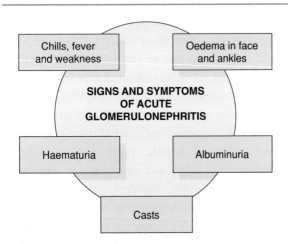

Figure 10.4 Signs and symptoms of acute glomerulonephritis.

The prognosis for acute glomerulonephritis is good. Normal kidney function is generally restored following bed rest and dietary restrictions (e.g. reduced intake of salt). Medications used for treatment include diuretics, calcium channel blockers and beta blockers.

Repeated attacks of acute glomerulonephritis can lead to weakened kidneys and a chronic condition.

Chronic glomerulonephritis

Chronic glomerulonephritis may persist for many years with periods of remission and relapse. Hypertension generally accompanies this disease. As more glomeruli are destroyed, blood filtration becomes increasingly impaired. Prevalence of glomerulonephritis is inconclusive, but the chronic cases are estimated at less than 1%.

Part of the urinalysis examination is a measure of specific gravity to determine the extent of kidney function. In advanced chronic glomerulonephritis, the specific gravity is low and fixed, indicating that the kidney tubules are unable to concentrate the urine. (See Appendix C for normal urine values.)

Chronic glomerulonephritis causes the kidneys to shrink, or atrophy, and cease to function. **Uraemia**, a build-up of metabolic toxins in the blood, results from kidney failure. Chief among these waste products is **urea**, a small, water-soluble nitrogenous molecule that easily penetrates red blood cells and causes their destruction (haemolysis). Therefore, uraemia is often associated with gastrointestinal, neuromuscular and cardiovascular insufficiencies.

Individuals suffering uraemic toxicity experience nausea, headache, dizziness and visual changes. Left unchecked, this condition may result in convulsions and coma. Dialysis treatment is quickly recommended to restore blood nitrogen and electrolyte balance, in order to reduce symptoms.

Goodpasture syndrome

Goodpasture syndrome is a rarely occurring renal problem considered to be an autoimmune disease. The precise cause of Goodpasture syndrome is not known, although it may be triggered by viral agents attacking the respiratory system or by inhaling hydrocarbon solvents. Therefore, the lungs and kidneys may be stressed together or individually. It develops in days to weeks, and once the body attacks the agents mentioned above, or unknown causes, it tends to attack itself. The primary 'glue' that the body uses for constructive support, a protein known as collagen, is somehow recognised as foreign and becomes the target of immune responses, which is similar to glomerulonephritis. Unfortunately, these autoantibodies are directed against the basement membranes of the glomerular capillaries; this disorder is also called *antiglomerular basement membrane glomerulonephritis*. In this case, the inflammatory disease results in scarring and fibrosis of the glomerular structure (see Figure 10.3). These same autoantibodies (anti-GBM antibodies) are found in Goodpasture syndrome and must be removed to improve the functional unit.

Symptoms of Goodposture syndrome vary and include foamy urine, weakness, nausea and vomiting. Signs include haematuria, **oliguria** (low urine production) and proteinuria. In addition, respiratory symptoms include haemoptysis, coughing, dyspnoea and chest pain. Diagnostics require physical examination, urinalysis and more refined chemical tests.

Treatment requires cleansing the plasma of antibodies, and this is accomplished by plasmaphoresis. This process cleans out the causative agents and replaces lost plasma with donor plasma and/or fluids and protein. Dialysis may be required in progressive cases or when permanent kidney damage is moderate; in advanced cases, a kidney transplant is recommended.

Preventative steps are to avoid solvent-type fumes, many of which are aromatic (sweet smelling) and dangerous (e.g. glue sniffing).

SYSTEMIC LUPUS ERYTHEMATOSUS OR LUPUS NEPHRITIS

Lupus nephritis results when autoantibodies collect in the glomeruli, which causes a major inflammation sufficient to create scars and reduce kidney functioning. Primary treatment involves two drugs in tandem; one to reduce inflammation, prednisolone, and one to suppress the immune system, cyclophosphamide or mycophenolate mofetil. Kidney function is vital, especially when the whole body is attacked by another (autoimmune) disease.

IGA NEPHROPATHY

In this disease, immunoglobulin A (IgA) forms deposits in the glomeruli, causing inflammation. The most common symptom is blood in the urine (haematuria), but it tends to go unnoticed and remain undetected for years. Even without exact numbers, IgA nephropathy is thought to be the most common cause of primary glomerulonephritis. This status, primary glomerulonephritis, excludes other causes like lupus or diabetes mellitus, which are systemic.

IgA nephropathy is more common in men and young people although it can affect all age groups. Because it takes years to become recognised and cause complications, younger people seldom display symptoms. No treatment is recommended for mild IgA nephropathy with normal blood pressure and proteinuria levels, but elevated blood pressure requires medications like angiotensin converting enzyme (ACE) inhibitors.

Renal failure

Ischaemia (reduced blood flow), haemorrhage, poisons and severe kidney diseases may cause renal failure. In renal failure, the kidneys are unable to clear the blood of urea and creatinine, which are nitrogen-containing waste products of protein metabolism. These metabolic products are toxic if they accumulate in the blood. Uraemia signifies the terminal stage of renal insufficiency.

The level of blood urea nitrogen, or BUN, reflects the degree of renal failure. Measurement of the glomerular filtration rate (GFR) can also assess the severity of renal disease or follow its progress. GFR is evaluated through tests designed to determine the ability of the kidney to clear the waste product creatinine. Serum creatinine level rises and creatinine clearance rate falls when the GFR is impaired. As may be expected, creatinine clearance levels decline in renal insufficiency and with aging. The test for creatinine is the most specific for kidney functioning and therefore a crucial diagnostic measurement.

Acute renal failure Acute renal failure may develop suddenly but has a better prognosis than chronic renal failure. Acute renal failure is caused by various factors such as decreased blood flow to the kidneys resulting from haemorrhage, including vasculogenic shock following an incompatible blood transfusion, or severe dehydration. Kidney disease, trauma or poisons from toxic fumes or heavy metals can also cause acute renal failure.

Significant signs of acute renal failure are characterised by a sudden drop in urine volume, called **oliguria**, or complete cessation of urine production, called **anuria**. Symptoms include headache, gastrointestinal distress and the odour of ammonia on the breath caused by accumulation in the blood of nitrogen-containing compounds. Of special concern is **hyperkalaemia**. This elevated blood potassium causes muscle weakness and can slow the heart to the point of cardiac arrest. Treatment includes restoration of the blood volume to normal, with necessary electrolytes, restricted dietary fluid intake and dialysis as needed.

Chronic renal failure Chronic renal failure is life-threatening and has a much poorer prognosis than acute renal failure. Chronic renal failure results from longstanding kidney disease such as chronic glomerulonephritis, hypertension and **diabetic nephropathy (DN)**, a kidney disease resulting from diabetes mellitus.

Diabetic nephropathy, as in glomerulonephritis, is caused by thickening of the glomerular apparatus that permits relatively high levels of protein (albumin) to escape into the urine. This glomerular change may be very slow, and routine urinalysis may not detect a small continual protein loss. Called microalbuminuria, it requires a more comprehensive or sensitive test to detect protein. Unless other factors (e.g. hypertension, family history) indicate the need for a more reliable test, the albumin continually goes undetected. Early-stage diabetic nephropathy has no symptoms, but as the condition advances it becomes more noticeable and debilitating.

Diabetics are particularly at risk if blood glucose remains uncontrolled and high blood pressure is pronounced. A host of symptoms becomes apparent as diabetic nephropathy evolves over a 5–10-year span. These symptoms include fatigue, headache, generalised itching, frothy urine, frequent hiccups and oedema, particularly in the legs. A renal biopsy is the confirming element of diagnosis, and it helps to determine the extent of the disease. However, if the protein loss is progressive or diabetic retinopathy is noted, the biopsy may be too risky.

Today, diabetic nephropathy is recognised as the most common cause of chronic kidney failure and end-stage renal disease (ESRD).

Chronic renal failure responds to diuretic intervention until alternative measures are warranted, such as kidney dialysis or transplant. Drugs such as furosemide will help reduce oedema and hypertension as well, because hypertension is a medical priority. Either separately or in combination, ACE inhibitors or angiotensin receptor blockers (ARBs) are utilised. Additionally, controlling weight, blood lipids and sugar levels and engaging in regular exercise are recommended. Common over-the-counter drugs like ibuprofen or aspirin tend to aggravate or weaken the kidney and should be discouraged. As the condition worsens and ESRD develops, in which kidney function declines to less than 10% of normal, the option of choice is kidney transplant or kidney–pancreas transplant when available. Even with a successful transplant, continued diligence is necessary, such as dietary considerations for restricting salt and fluid intake and monitoring for anaemia or infection.

The condition develops slowly, with urinary output reducing slowly over time. Metabolic wastes accumulate in the blood, with adverse effects on all body systems. For example, urea builds up to toxic levels, and some is converted to ammonia, which acts as an irritant in the gastrointestinal tract, producing nausea, vomiting and diarrhoea. Vision becomes dim, cognitive functions decrease, and convulsions or coma may ensue. Manifestations of chronic renal failure are summarised in Figure 10.5. These cases are now primarily considered end-stage kidney disease.

Renal failure is treated with kidney dialysis, a technique that removes toxic substances from the blood. Known as **haemodialysis**, blood is removed from the body, toxic substances are removed from the blood, and the blood is returned to the body (Figure 10.6). For haemodialysis, a patient must typically visit a clinic or hospital for dialysis and stay for 3–6 hours during the process. However, residential dialysis units are available that allow patients more convenient and private treatment. Small portable dialysis units have further reduced cost and have increased availability for treatment.

In **peritoneal dialysis (PD)**, dialysing fluid is introduced into the abdominal cavity, where the peritoneum (cavity lining) acts as a filtration membrane. The fluid draws toxic materials out of capillaries surrounding the body cavity, and after a suitable amount of time, the peritoneal fluid is removed, along with its dissolved toxins. A bag may be attached externally to collect the fluid, permitting the patient to remain mobile and providing more freedom and flexibility during treatment. Dialysis may be required for years but may not be sufficient in advanced chronic renal failure.

An alternative treatment for advanced kidney failure is kidney transplant. Advances in anti-rejection medications have reduced complications and allowed kidney transplants to prolong and save thousands of lives (Figure 10.7).

Prevention of ESRD requires early detection to halt chronic kidney failure, even though it may take many years (10–20) to develop. With advanced age, other ailments, or lack of attention, ESRD may not be preventable.

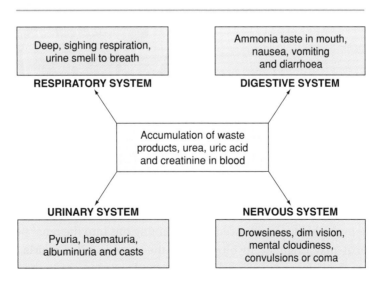

Figure 10.5 Manifestations of chronic renal failure.

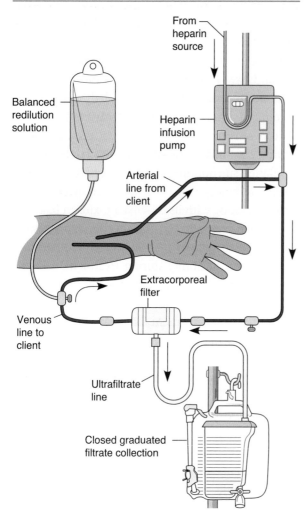

Figure 10.6 Continuous arteriovenous haemofiltration (CAVH).

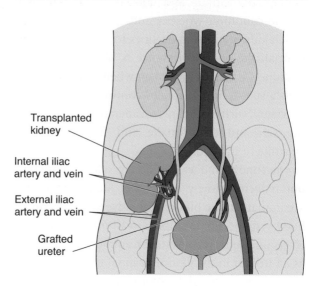

Figure 10.7 Placement of a transplanted kidney.

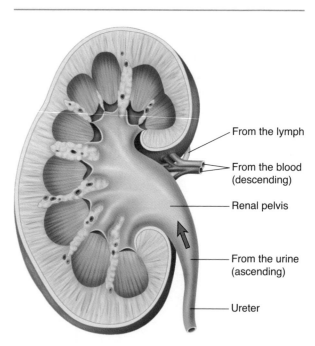

Figure 10.8 Routes of infection for pyelonephritis.

Pyelonephritis

Pyelonephritis is a suppurative urinary tract infection of the kidney and renal pelvis caused by pyogenic (pus-forming) bacteria, including *Escherichia coli*, streptococci and staphylococci. Obstruction of the urinary tract, such as a congenital defect, a kidney stone or an enlarged prostate gland, slows urine flow and increases the risk for infection. The infection may originate in the bladder and ascends up into the kidneys, or it may originate in blood or lymph and descend to the kidneys as is found in tuberculosis. Figure 10.8 shows the possible routes of infection.

In pyelonephritis, abscesses form and rupture, draining pus into the renal pelvis and the urine. Pus in the urine is called **pyuria**, which causes a turbid or cloudy appearance in the urine sample, and may be detected during a **urinalysis procedure**. The abscesses can fuse, filling the entire kidney with pus.

Left untreated, pyelonephritis may lead to renal failure and uraemia. In less severe infections, healing occurs but scar tissue tends to form. Because fibrous scar tissue tends to contract, the kidney shrinks and becomes what is described as a granular contracted kidney.

Symptoms of pyelonephritis include chills, high fever, sudden back pain that spreads over the abdomen, **dysuria** and haematuria. Microscopic examination of the urine reveals numerous pus cells and bacteria. Treatment includes antibiotics such as aminoglycosides or sulfonamides for the infection.

Pyelitis

Pyelitis is an inflammation confined to the renal pelvis, the juncture between the ureter and the kidney. Pyelitis is caused by *E. coli* and other pyogenic bacteria. The bacteria may originate from a urinary bladder infection or the blood. Pyelitis occurs commonly in young children, particularly girls, because the **urethra** in females is much shorter than that of males (approximately 3 cm in length in adult females compared to approximately 25 cm in adult males). Micro-organisms from faecal contamination can enter from the outside and easily travel to the bladder. The infection can then spread up the ureter to the renal pelvis. Dysuria, as well as increased frequency and urgency, are common symptoms of pyelitis. Urinalysis will reveal numerous pus cells.

This disease responds well to treatment with antibiotics, as previously mentioned. Early diagnosis and treatment are important in preventing the spread of the infection into the kidney tissue, which leads to pyelonephritis.

Renal carcinoma

Kidney cancer, also called **hypernephroma**, causes enlargement of the kidney and destroys the organ. Renal carcinoma is a relatively rare type of kidney cancer, comprising only 3% of all adult cancers, but causes 85% of all kidney cancers. Two other types, *transitional cell carcinoma* and *sarcoma*, make up the remaining 15% of kidney cancers. The incidence of kidney cancer in men is twice that for women, and

it normally occurs between ages 50 and 60. Smokers are twice as likely as non-smokers to develop kidney cancer.

The tumour may not manifest itself for several years. Painless haematuria eventually becomes the main sign. When the tumour becomes large, an abdominal mass may be felt. This mass can then be detected on an X-ray as a tumour of the kidney. Metastasis to other organs often occurs before the presence of the kidney tumour is known. The malignancy frequently spreads to the lungs, liver, bones and brain. Besides pain, typical signs include loss of appetite, weight loss, anaemia and an elevated white blood cell count (leucocytosis). Surgical removal (nephrectomy) is the best initial treatment.

A malignant tumour of the kidney pelvis that develops in children, usually diagnosed between ages 2 and 5, is **Wilms' tumour**, an adenosarcoma. A fast-growing tumour, it metastasises through the blood and lymph vessels. Signs and symptoms include haematuria, pain, vomiting and hypertension similar to symptoms of renal carcinoma in an adult. Diagnosis is by **intravenous urography (IVU)** and is confirmed by kidney biopsy. In recent years, without metastasis, surgery and radiation (except stage 1) and chemotherapy treatment that may be intermittent, lasting 6–15 months, offer a good prognosis.

Wilms' tumour, found in 1 in 10 000 individuals, has a genetic connection. It appears that at least three different genes influence the occurrence of this disease. The Wilms' tumour gene 1 (*WT-1*), whose actual function is unknown, seems to play an important role in embryonic development. When this particular gene is missing or mutated, congenital defects appear and this abnormal tissue later becomes the site of cancer.

Kidney stones

Kidney stones, known as **urinary calculi**, predominantly form in the kidney. The prevalence of urinary calculi is approximately 12% for men and 5% for women, and men are almost twice as likely to develop stones with the first episode occurring before the age of 30.

Urinary calculi may be present and cause no symptoms, even when passed through the urinary tract, unless they are larger than 5 mm in diameter, in which case they become lodged in the ureter. The lodged stones cause intense pain that radiates from the kidney to the groin area. In addition to intense pain, other signs and symptoms include haematuria, nausea, vomiting and diarrhoea.

Kidney stones may cause urinary tract infections by blocking urine flow and permitting bacterial growth in the urinary tract. Conversely, a urinary tract infection that blocks urine flow can trigger kidney stone formation because of urine stasis in the renal pelvis. Calculi are formed when certain minerals in the urine form a precipitate; that is, come out of solution and grow in size. Bacteria in urine can serve as sites for calcium deposition. The resulting stones, if small enough, can be passed in the urine, but larger stones may require surgery or other treatment.

Four renal calculi formations are recognised. *Calcium stones* comprise 80% of all kidney stones and consist mainly of calcium salts, calcium oxalate and calcium phosphate. Calcium excess often leads to stone formation. Hyperactive parathyroid glands can cause the excess of circulating calcium, promoting formation of urinary calculi. Therefore, the parathyroids may need to be controlled or surgically removed, especially with rapid recurrence of stones. No evidence suggests that 'hard water' influences kidney stone formation. Men are four to five times more likely than women to form these stones. *Uric acid* stones comprise 10% of all stone formations and occur especially in men subject to gout. Colon surgery increases the risk for uric acid stones. When portions of the colon are removed, the urine becomes more acidic, which enhances the formation of uric acid stones. *Struvite* stones, also called infected stones, comprise nearly 10% of stone formations. Bacterial growth in these kidney stones produces ammonia, making the urine alkaline, which also triggers stone precipitation. When bacteria become encased in minerals, antibiotics are ineffective and the stones tend to enlarge. A stone may become so large that it fills the renal pelvis completely, blocking the flow of urine, and requiring surgical removal. A stone of this type, named for its shape, is the **staghorn calculus** illustrated in Figure 10.9. A kidney containing numerous small calculi is also shown. *Cysteine* stones account for the remaining 1% of renal calculi. These stones are aggregates of the amino acid cysteine, which does not dissolve easily in water. Cysteine stones result from a hereditary disorder in which the kidneys fail to reabsorb cysteine, which builds up in urine, precipitates, and eventually forms stones, more commonly in children.

Stones can also form in the urinary bladder. The presence of bladder stones causes urinary tract infections because they frequently obstruct the flow of urine.

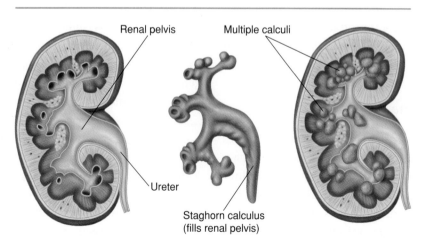

Figure 10.9 Urinary calculi.

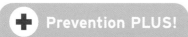
Prevention PLUS!

Kidney stones

To prevent kidney stones or their recurrence, it is recommended that urine output be increased. Drinking greater quantities of fluids, especially water, dilutes the urine and reduces the likelihood of stone formation.

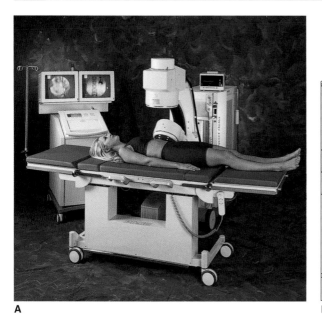
A

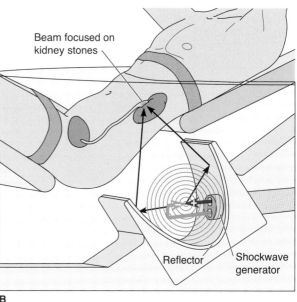
B

Figure 10.10 Extracorporeal shockwave lithotripsy. Acoustic shock waves generated by the shockwave generator travel through soft tissue to shatter the renal stone into fragments, which are then eliminated in the urine. (A) A shockwave generator that does not require water immersion. (B) An illustration of water immersion lithotripsy procedure.

Diagnostic investigations include CT, IVU, renal ultrasound/scan and a KUB that consists of a single X-ray without contrast media to view the abdominopelvic region.

Urinary calculi may be treated with medication that partially dissolves the stone, permitting it to be passed in the urine. **Lithotripsy**, the crushing of kidney stones, is effective for the 20% of kidney stones that do not pass on their own. In lithotripsy, sonic vibrations are applied externally, and focused internally, to crush the stones. If performed while the patient is immersed in a tank of water, the procedure is called **hydrolithotripsy** (Figure 10.10). In this technique, the patient, while partially submerged, is subjected to the sonic waves that shatter the hard stones into sand-sized particles that can be eliminated within the urine flow. Recurrence of stones is not uncommon; after the first stone passes, 14% recur within the first year, about 35% recur within 5 years and up to 52% recur within 10 years. To avoid or reduce recurrence, fluid intake should be increased to keep the urine dilute, and dietary calcium and protein should be reduced.

Hydronephrosis

As a result of urinary calculi, a congenital defect, a tumour, an enlarged prostate gland or other

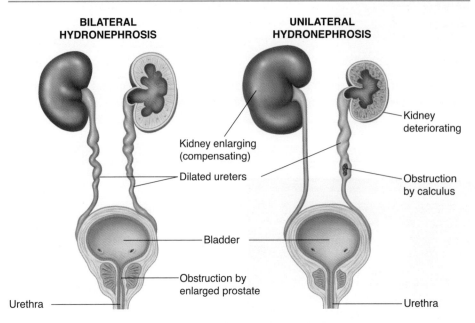

Figure 10.11 Hydronephrosis: bilateral (left); unilateral (right).

obstruction of the renal pelvis, the kidney may become extremely dilated with pockets of urine (fluid). This condition is called **hydronephrosis**. The ureters dilate above the obstruction from the pressure of urine that is unable to pass and are referred to as **hydroureters**. Figure 10.11 shows this dilated condition. A physical cause for hydronephrosis is a **ureterocele**. In this case, the terminal portion of the ureter **prolapses**, or slides into the urinary bladder. When detected, it can be corrected surgically. Haematuria is generally present, and the degree of pain accompanying hydronephrosis depends on the nature of the blockage. If an infection develops because of the stagnation of urine, pyuria and fever occur (Figure 10.12).

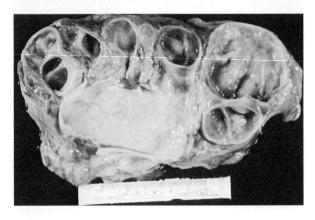

Figure 10.12 Hydronephrosis.
(Courtesy of Dr David R. Duffell)

Polycystic kidney

Solitary renal cysts are relatively common, with sizes varying from a few millimetres to 15 mm (the latter may have little effect on kidney function). However, the polycystic kidney is a congenital defect, an error in development that usually involves both kidneys. An autosomal recessive gene causes polycystic kidney in children, while in adults it is caused by an autosomal dominant gene. Adult polycystic kidney disease affects 1 of every 500–1000 individuals.

The cysts are dilated kidney tubules that do not open into the renal pelvis as they should. Instead, the cysts enlarge, fuse and usually become infected. As the cysts enlarge, they compress the surrounding kidney tissue. The accompanying Side by Side illustrates the polycystic kidney of an adult. By middle age, signs and symptoms appear, including pain, haematuria, polyuria, renal calculi and hypertension. This disease may be diagnosed with a combination of a physical examination, a renal ultrasound or CT, or an IVU (see Diagnostic tests and procedures).

No specific treatment is available. Renal failure eventually occurs, requiring dialysis or kidney transplant.

DISEASES OF THE URINARY BLADDER AND URETHRA

Cystitis

Cystitis is an inflammation of the urinary bladder primarily caused by an infection. It is more common in women than in men because of women's shorter urethra. The chief cause is *E. coli*, which resides in the colon and can reach the urethra and ascend upward into the bladder. Cystitis can also develop following sexual intercourse if bacteria around the vaginal opening spread to the urinary opening. Occasionally, pressure from coughing or exertion squeezes the bladder, which pushes some urine into the urethra and then draws it back to the bladder. This action contaminates the normally sterile fluid within the urinary bladder.

The symptoms of cystitis are increased urinary frequency and urgency, and a burning sensation during urination. Microscopic examination of the urine reveals bacteria, pus, casts and leucocytes. Treatment depends on the type of bacteria and may include a type of penicillin, such as ampicillin or amoxicillin, provided the patient isn't allergic to penicillin.

Urinary incontinence

Very early in life, urinary incontinence (UI) is considered the norm, as it often is in the elderly years. Although adult incontinence is not a disease, it is abnormal and does require attention. Of the total population over 60 years of age, 35% is estimated to be incontinent. This involuntary (or unwanted) release of urine from the urinary bladder is an inconvenience and often an embarrassing problem for those individuals afflicted. Adults may alter their social and physical habits because of this problem.

For the infant, the inability to control micturition occurs because the nerves and muscles have not been coordinated to allow closure of the (voluntary) external urethral valve or sphincter. Automatic reflexive voiding of the urinary bladder occurs because the walls of the bladder expand, and the stretch receptors within the walls signal the internal valve to relax. Otherwise, until the bladder responds to the stretching, the collected urine is retained. A similar mechanism occurs in adults, but conscious

SIDE by SIDE Polycystic kidney

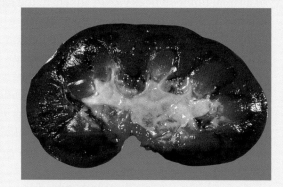

Normal kidney.
(Science Photo Library Ltd/SIU)

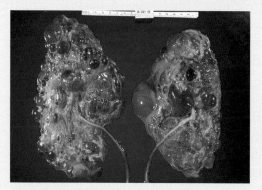

Polycystic kidney.
(Courtesy of the CDC/Dr Edwin P. Ewing Jr, 1972)

efforts allow the voiding signals to be damped down and the external sphincter to remain closed. Urinary retention occurs when the bladder is unable to expel the contained urine fully in a timely fashion owing to weak abdominal muscles or extraneous factors such as anaesthesia (muscles need time to recover). Within the central nervous system, the pons, cerebral cortex and spinal cord coordinate to inhibit micturition, or to allow it to occur. Once the timing is convenient and appropriate, urination proceeds.

A myriad of causes and treatments are found for UI. Obviously, UI is subject to various diseases, like infection or stroke, and heredity. Conditions such as childbirth, pregnancy, hysterectomy and menopause may also be involved. A tumour or enlarged prostate that compresses the urethra, or a prostate surgery, may leave the male incontinent. UI may be inadvertently induced by medications that are used to control hypertension, antihistamines, muscle relaxants and sleeping pills.

Whatever the primary cause, there are three basic forms of adult UI: (1) *overflow incontinence*, in which the bladder overfills and tends to dribble urine out through the urethra; (2) *stress incontinence*, in which the urethral sphincter is weak or damaged and allows leakage upon coughing, sneezing, laughing or increased abdominal pressure; and (3) *urge incontinence*, in which the muscular bladder wall has sudden uncontrolled contractions.

Depending on cause, severity, age and other factors, UI is managed by methods ranging from the very simple to surgical. Wearing incontinence pads should not be considered an adequate intervention for incontinence since many individuals are too embarrassed to seek professional advice. Additional attention to voiding the bladder more often and extending the timing may help, along with exercising the pelvic muscles and the urethral valves. These pelvic manoeuvres are known as **Kegel** exercises and, when performed several times each day, may be sufficient to control some stress-type incontinence.

Collagen injections near the voluntary external sphincter may reduce the urethra passage sufficiently to prevent accidental urine release. Somewhat more invasive surgeries suspend the bladder to a greater degree to allow the bladder neck and urethra to form a better alignment and improve normal functioning. Overflow incontinence may be treated by voiding the bladder more frequently, on demand if possible, or, if needed, by medications like oxybutynin or tolterodine.

When the condition becomes chronic or causes pain or infection, a tubular catheter may be inserted up into the bladder via the urethra to insure voiding the bladder contents. Catheters are small-diameter flexible tubes made of 'plastic' (polyvinyl chloride; PVC) or latex that are primarily inserted through the urethra into the bladder and range from 20 to 44 cm long depending on gender. A balloon device is at the inserted end and is expanded once in place to prevent escape. Externally, a retention bag is attached to the catheter and has a capacity of 0.5–2 l depending on daily and overnight usage. It is important to empty the bag frequently (e.g. every 4 hours) and keep a fresh or cleansed container in place. For more mobility, the external retention bag may be strapped to the thigh, pelvic area or calf position.

The catheter arrangement may be short term (a few days to 2 weeks) or long term depending on the circumstances and agreed management plan. An alternative to urethral catheterisation is a suprapubic catheter, whereby the catheter is surgically introduced through the pelvic wall just superior to the symphysis pubis via an introducer.

Irritation by any tube in the bladder presents the potential for bladder infection (or beyond), bladder calculi and bladder cancer (squamous cell carcinoma of the bladder). Therefore, an external catheter may be used, such as a condom or penile sheath for men or a labial funnel-type device to adhere to the female external genitalia (or **vulva**). Either device is then attached to a tube that drains into a retention bag. Over time the type of catheter arrangement may change depending on situation or preference.

Enuresis, or bedwetting, can occur in children but usually resolves as the child ages. It is more common in boys by a margin of 2 to 3. Usually, it is outgrown within the first 11 years (72%) or by age 15 (99%).

Causes for enuresis include lack of bladder growth or development, heredity (40–70% of cases), heavy sleep and a reduced level of ADH at night. Besides nappies or absorbent pads to prevent bedtime wetting, the youngster may use a nasal spray (e.g. desmopressin acetate) that acts like ADH to prevent bedwetting. Some cases are better served through counselling, urination regimen, reward charts or bladder conditioning to reduce night-time urinating accidents.

Neurogenic bladder

A neurogenic bladder tends to result in urinary incontinence owing to lack of nervous system control. Damage to the nerves supplying the bladder or a breakdown within the central nervous system (CNS) is the root cause of this problem. A common cause is a spinal cord injury from road traffic incident or other trauma. Physical changes such as herniated discs in the lumbar region or tumours compressing on the spinal cord and/or spinal nerves are highly probable causations. Metabolic disorders, especially diabetes mellitus, or cognitive changes such as Alzheimer's disease and other CNS dysfunctions (Parkinson's disease and multiple sclerosis), can also cause bladder impairment.

Symptoms vary with the severity or particular nerve(s) involved and the primary dysfunctional location. The bladder may spasm, fail to empty completely, or lack feeling of fullness or urgency, and thus the signal to evacuate may go undetected. Diagnosis is therefore difficult to ascertain. Beginning with an extensive patient history coupled with a full scale neurological examination and a careful urological evaluation, a probable cause and prognosis may be determined. The goal is to restore bladder function fully, and that may require a major neurological investigation. Urological treatments include indwelling catheters, hygiene training and exercise. Lumbar discs may be repaired and drug treatments for CNS dysfunctions may assist the recovery. However, if nerve damage is severe or permanent, a neurogenic bladder will persist.

Carcinoma of the bladder

Bladder cancer is the seventh most common cancer in the UK, with an estimated 10 000 new cases diagnosed every year. It is more common in men, and the risk of developing bladder cancer increases with age. The leading risk factor is smoking, although exposure to dyes and industrial chemicals have also been linked to development of bladder cancer. There are three types of bladder cancer: transitional cell carcinoma (which is the most common), squamous cell carcinoma and adenocarcinoma.

The tumour grows by sending finger-like projections into the lumen of the bladder. Although these tumours can be seen with a **cystoscope** and removed, 70% recur and 10% of superficial bladder cancers progress to muscle-invasive disease. A more invasive pattern of growth involves infiltration of the bladder wall, which cannot be surgically removed without destroying the bladder.

One treatment involves intravesical chemotherapy using an infusion of BCG solution (Bacillus Calmette Guerin), a weakened tuberculosis bacillus that coats the bladder's internal epithelial surface. This solution causes the inner lining to 'peel off' and be replaced by new surface cells. This treatment lasts from months to years, depending on the status of the patient. If this procedure is not appropriate or is ineffective, then surgical removal of the cancer is required.

If the entire urinary bladder is surgically removed (radical cystectomy), an ileal conduit (Figure 10.13)

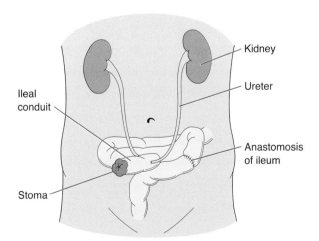

Figure 10.13 Ileal conduit. A segment of ileum is separated from the small intestine and formed into a tubular pouch, with the open end brought to the skin surface to form a stoma. The ureters are connected to the pouch.

is likely to be constructed surgically to store and evacuate urine. See Chapter 4 for more information.

Urethritis

Any part of the urinary tract can become inflamed, and the urethra is no exception. This tubular inflammation is called **urethritis**. In men, the cause may be a gonococcus or other bacteria, viruses or noxious chemicals. A trauma caused by a 'straddle' accident or stressful pressure (e.g. long-distance bicycle riding) may cause irritation and damage to the urethra. Damage to nerves and blood vessels may occur at the same time, and this could cause testicular problems for the male. In women, urethritis frequently accompanies cystitis. An obstruction at the urinary opening may cause the inflammation in women. The symptoms of urethritis include a discharge of pus from the urethra, an itching sensation at the opening of the urethra and a burning sensation during urination. Treatment includes antibiotics such as amoxicillin for bacteria infections.

AGE-RELATED DISEASES

Several changes accompany the aging urinary system. There is less control over urination (the micturition reflex) because the urethral sphincter muscles lose tone, allowing urine to leak. Incontinence tends to be more common with aging, but some suggest that with more conscious effort, training and some medical advice or attention (e.g. minor surgery) numbers of cases might be reduced or prevented by as much as 80%. Brain and spinal cord damage may lead to a weak micturition urination reflex.

Dehydration owing to water loss via the aging kidneys is possible, because the total number of functioning nephrons declines with age, perhaps by as much as 30–40% between ages 25 and 85, and the kidney loses sensitivity to ADH. The reduction of renin and therefore aldosterone activity causes a lack of salt and water retention, allowing more urine to be released by the kidney. Urinary retention occurs because bladders lose muscle tone and are unable to empty completely. Obstruction exacerbates urine retention and is common in men because of prostate enlargement. Urinary retention, in turn, increases the risk for urinary tract infections (UTIs). Cancer increases significantly past age 60 for the kidney, and at age 70 for bladder cancer.

Resources

National Kidney Research Fund: *www.nkrf.org.uk*
MacMillan Cancer Support: *http://www.macmillan.org.uk/Cancerinformation/Cancertypes*
NHS: *www.nhs.uk/conditions*
National Institute of Clinical Excellence (NICE): *http://www.nice.org.uk/*

DISEASES AT A GLANCE Urinary system

DISEASE	AETIOLOGY	SIGNS AND SYMPTOMS	DIAGNOSIS	TREATMENT	PREVENTION	LIFESPAN
Kidney						
Hydronephroma	Idiopathic, radiation	Painless haematuria, later pain, loss of appetite, weight loss, anaemia, elevated white blood count	X-ray	Surgery	Uncertain	Generally increased chance with aging
Wilms' tumour	Idiopathic, genetic (WT-1), chromosome 2	In young children, signs and symptoms similar to hydronephroma in adults	X-ray	Surgery, sometimes radiation	None	At birth and young children
Pyelonephritis	Pyogenic bacteria	Pyuria, chills, high fever, sudden back pain, dysuria, haematuria, eventual renal failure, uraemia	Urinalysis, pus and blood in urine	Antibiotics	Depends on exposure and susceptibility	Especially in younger people, but older people too
Pyelitis	Pyogenic bacteria	Dysuria, frequency, urgency	Urinalysis, numerous pus cells in urine	Antibiotics	Same as above, good hygiene	Usually weaker immunity, age varies
Acute glomerulonephritis	Prior bacterial infection, antigen-antibody complex	Follow strep infection: chills, fever, loss of appetite, weakness, oedema, albuminuria, haematuria, casts	Urinalysis, patient history	Antibiotics, steroids, immune suppression	As above or uncertain	Any age, often younger years
Chronic glomerulonephritis	Hypertension and glomerular destruction	Remission and exacerbation of glomerulonephritis; may end with granular contracted kidneys and uraemia; specific gravity low and fixed in advanced cases	Urinalysis, urine specific gravity low, patient history	Antibiotics, steroids, immune suppression	Prevent negative kidney exposure, or uncertain	Tends to develop with prior infections; middle years +
Acute renal failure	Incompatible blood transfusion, severe dehydration	Sudden oliguria, may become anuria, headache, GI distress, odour of ammonia in breath, muscle weakness	Patient history, blood and urinalysis	Drugs, fluid control, antibiotics, dialysis	Uncertain	Any age
Chronic renal failure	Hypertension, chronic glomerulonephritis, diabetic nephropathy	Slow development, urinary wastes increase in blood, nausea, vomiting, diarrhoea, dim vision, central nervous system affected, convulsions, coma	Patient history, urinalysis, blood analysis	Dialysis, kidney transplant	Implies prior kidney stress	More prevalent in elderly or caused by foreign substances (e.g. poison)

DISEASES AT A GLANCE Urinary system (continued)

DISEASE	AETIOLOGY	SIGNS AND SYMPTOMS	DIAGNOSIS	TREATMENT	PREVENTION	LIFESPAN
Urinary calculi (kidney stones)	Hyperparathyroidism, excess calcium	No symptoms until they block ureter, then intense pain radiating to groin	Patient history, blood and urinalysis, X-ray	Lithotripsy, surgery	Consider family history, prevent dehydration, diet	Usually 30s or 40s for initial onset
Hydronephrosis	Renal obstruction, congenital defect	Pain, haematuria, pyuria and fever if infection present	Urinalysis, IVU cystoscopic examination	Relief of obstruction, surgery	Uncertain, depends on, e.g. obstruction caused by enlarged prostate	Varies; usually teens and beyond
Polycystic kidney	Genetic	Hypertension, eventual renal failure, uraemia	Urinalysis, IVU cystoscopic examination	Kidney transplant	None	Recessive trait – child. Dominant trait – adult
Carcinoma	Idiopathic, radiation, smoking	Early asymptomatic, haematuria may occur, later pelvic pain and frequent urination	Cystoscopy	Surgery	Do not smoke, avoid radiation and other potential carcinogens	Chance increases with age
Urinary bladder						
Cystitis	Usually bacterial infection	Urinary frequency, urgency, burning sensation during urination, blood in urine	Microscopic examination of urine, may be diagnosed by patient's description of typical signs and symptoms	Antibiotics	Uncertain, good hygiene	In women any age; varies for men
Bladder cancer	Idiopathic, smoking, hazardous chemicals	Haematuria, dysuria, fatigue, anorexia	Cystoscope, IVU, X-ray, CT	Fulguration, radiation, surgery	Uncertain; do not smoke, avoid radiation	Middle age and beyond
Urethritis	Microbial agents, viruses, some chemicals	Burning sensation during urination, itching, discharge; in females, accompanies cystitis	Microscopic examination of urine	Antibiotics	Uncertain, good hygiene	Higher incidence among females, any age
Incontinence	Neurological injury, aging	Involuntary loss of urine	Patient history	Exercises for muscles of pelvic floor, antibiotics for infection	Varies; requires treatment	Newborn and elderly

INTERACTIVE EXERCISES

Cases for critical thinking

1. Jane, a nursing student, experienced painful urination and noticed blood in the urine. What can explain her symptoms and haematuria?

2. Britany, a thin 16-year-old, experienced significant weight gain in a 2-week period. Just before the holiday break, she had a bad sore throat, but after a visit to the doctor, those symptoms subsided. Her abdomen was distended and she had oedema of the extremities. She complained of abdominal discomfort and general aches. Urinalysis indicated proteinuria and haematuria. A follow-up blood test found antibodies to streptococcal toxins. What may explain Britany's symptoms?

3. A 52-year-old grandfather's urinalysis revealed blood (haematuria). The X-ray showed a renal mass on the right side. What is the probable cause for the haematuria, and what treatment would be recommended?

Multiple choice

1. Which of the following can cause chronic uraemia?

   a. surgical shock
   b. severe dehydration
   c. complications of pregnancy
   d. diabetes mellitus

2. What is inflammation of the kidney tissue known as?

   a. pyelonephritis
   b. polycystic kidney
   c. hydronephrosis
   d. diabetic nephropathy

3. What is inflammation restricted to the renal pelvis called?

   a. pyelonephritis
   b. glomerulonephritis
   c. pyelitis
   d. congenital cystic kidney

4. Which disease or condition features a breath odour similar to the ammonia-like odour of urine?

   a. glomerulonephritis   b. pyelonephritis
   c. tuberculosis   d. uraemia

5. Which of the following is *true* about urinary tract infections?

   a. are more common in males
   b. usually exhibit dysuria, urgency and frequency
   c. are commonly caused by a virus
   d. do not respond to antibiotics

6. Which form of kidney dialysis permits a patient to retain mobility?

   a. peritoneal dialysis
   b. haemodialysis
   c. haemolysis
   d. ileal shunt

7. The inability to control urination is called

   _____

   a. micturition   b. incontinence
   c. anuria   d. nocturia

8. What dietary restriction helps to prevent uric acid calculi?

   a. protein
   b. dairy products
   c. pasta and citrus
   d. spinach, cabbage and tomatoes

9. What primarily causes the oedema associated with nephritic syndrome?

   a. hypertension
   b. hyperalbuminuria
   c. decreased plasma protein
   d. lower glomerular filtration rate

10. Which of the following includes a reduced sensitivity to ADH, incontinence and increased urination frequency?

    a. overhydration   b. aging
    c. stress   d. excess nitrogen intake

True or false

_____ **1.** A sudden drop in urine volume indicates chronic renal failure.

_____ **2.** Cystitis is often an ascending infection.

_____ **3.** In acute uraemia, fluid intake should be decreased.

_____ **4.** Albuminuria leads to hypoproteinaemia.

_____ **5.** Painful and frequent urination accompanies tuberculosis of the bladder.

_____ **6.** Bacteria are not found in acute glomerulonephritis.

_____ **7.** Pyelonephritis is a suppurative disease.

_____ **8.** The urinary bladder stores urine that may be reused.

_____ **9.** Leucocytes in urine indicate anaemia.

_____ **10.** Calcium (oxalate, phosphate) is the most common form of renal calculus.

Fill-ins

1. _____ is pus in the urine.

2. _____ _____ is a kidney disease resulting from diabetes mellitus.

3. Urinary calculi, or _____ _____, may be present and cause no symptoms until they become lodged in the ureter.

4. _____, the external crushing of kidney stones, is now the preferable procedure to remove kidney stones, replacing the need for surgery.

5. _____ _____ is a congenital anomaly that usually involves both kidneys.

6. Scanty urine or _____ is low urine volume (or formation).

7. Loss of urine at night is called _____.

8. Struvite stones are associated with _____.

9. Adult polycystic kidney is a genetic disease caused specifically by an autosomal _____ gene.

10. An X-ray outline of the urinary system following an injection of solution is the diagnostic technique called _____.

Labelling exercise

Use the blank lines below to label the following image.

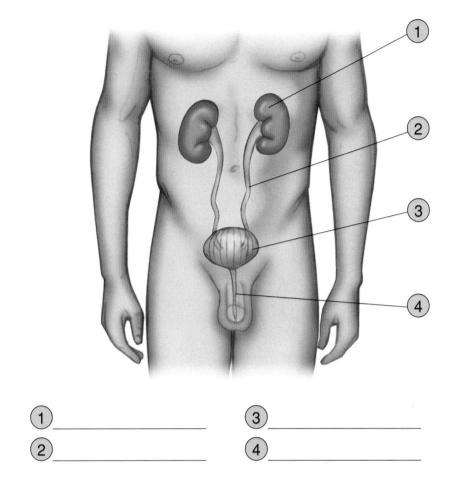

1 _____   3 _____

2 _____   4 _____

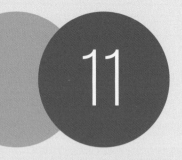

11 DISEASES AND DISORDERS OF THE REPRODUCTIVE SYSTEM

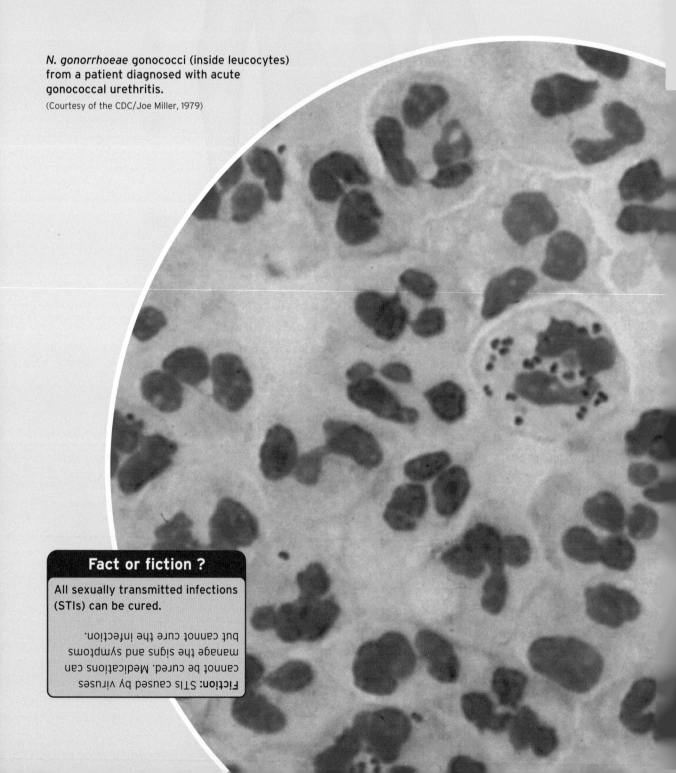

N. gonorrhoeae gonococci (inside leucocytes) from a patient diagnosed with acute gonococcal urethritis.

(Courtesy of the CDC/Joe Miller, 1979)

Fact or fiction ?

All sexually transmitted infections (STIs) can be cured.

Fiction: STIs caused by viruses cannot be cured. Medications can manage the signs and symptoms but cannot cure the infection.

Learning objectives

After studying this chapter, you should be able to:

+ Identify diagnostic procedures used for conditions of the reproductive system
+ Describe the normal structure and function of the reproductive system
+ List signs and symptoms, causes and treatments for diseases and disorders of the reproductive system
+ Describe disorders of pregnancy
+ List signs and symptoms, causes and treatments for sexually transmitted infections
+ List signs and symptoms, causes and treatments for age-related diseases of the reproductive system

Disease chronicle

Tuskegee Institute experiment

In 1932, the US Public Health Service, with the assistance of the Tuskegee Institute, recruited 600 African American men to participate in an experiment involving the effects of untreated syphilis. Of this group, 399 men had been diagnosed with syphilis but were never informed that they had syphilis or that their infection was sexually transmitted. Originally meant to last 6-9 months, the study instead lasted 40 years until the men died. When the story broke in 1972, Congress convened hearings about the Tuskegee study. The hearings resulted in the rewriting of the Department of Health, Education and Welfare's regulations on the use of human subjects in scientific experiments. A $1.8 billion class-action suit was filed on behalf of the Tuskegee participants and their heirs. A settlement for $10 million was made out of court.

ANATOMY OF THE FEMALE REPRODUCTIVE SYSTEM

The female reproductive system consists of the vagina, the uterus, the uterine (Fallopian) tubes and the ovaries. The vagina is a tubular structure extending backward and upward to the cervix, the lowest part of the uterus. It is made up of elastic muscular fibres; its walls are always in apposition and thrown into folds called rugae. The vagina expands during coitus and childbirth. The uterus comprises three layers on its wall: an outer peritoneal covering, the **perimetrium**; a middle layer of smooth muscle, the **myometrium**; and an inner vascular lining, the **endometrium**, which responds to hormonal changes and is the source of the regular menstrual bleed. The expanded, upper portion of the uterus tapers down to form the narrow cervix, giving the organ a pear-shaped appearance. Figures 11.1 and 11.2 show the female reproductive system. The Fallopian tubes extend laterally from each side of the uterus; and the opened, fringe-like projections at the outer ends, the **fimbriae**, receive and propel released ova into the tube.

The ovaries are small, oval-shaped organs, and are anchored by the suspensory ligaments and positioned near the fimbriae. They contain hundreds of thousands of ova, which are present at birth. Surrounding each ovum is a single layer of cells, the **primary follicle**.

The external genitalia (the vulva) include the mons pubis, the labia majora and labia minora, the clitoris and the vaginal opening. The urinary meatus is situated between the clitoris and the vaginal opening. At puberty, the mons pubis, a pad of fat tissue over the symphysis pubis, becomes covered with hair. Extending back from the mons pubis to the anus are two pairs of folds, the labia majora and the labia minora. The clitoris, a tuft of erectile tissue similar to that of the penis, is located at the anterior junction of the minor lips. This structure is removed in **female circumcision** (genital mutilation), practised in some parts of the world. A membranous fold, the

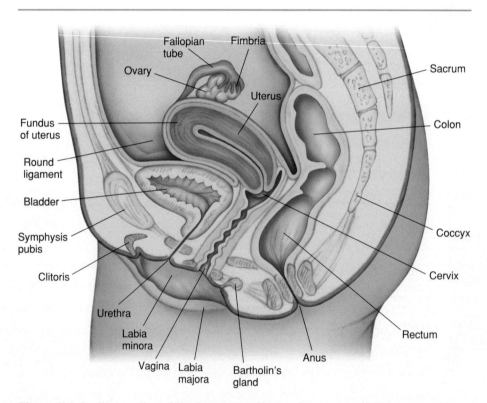

Figure 11.1 Sagittal section of the female pelvis, showing organs of the reproductive system.

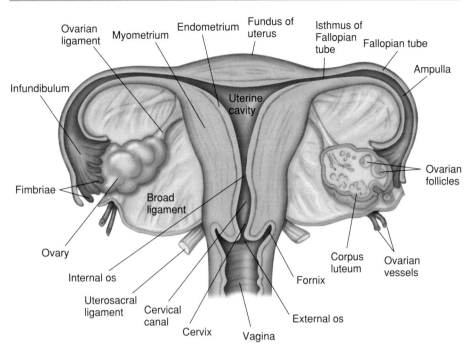

Figure 11.2 The uterus, ovaries and Fallopian tubes.

hymen, partly or completely closes the vaginal opening. Occasionally, this membrane is imperforate or abnormally closed and requires a minor surgical procedure to open it. **Bartholin's glands**, a pair of mucus-secreting glands, are situated at the vaginal entrance; they produce a lubricating secretion during sexual intercourse.

The breasts, accessory organs of reproduction, consist of glandular tissue, supported by connective tissue covered with fatty tissue and skin. The glandular tissue consists of lobes subdivided into lobules with lactiferous ducts which carry milk and converge at the nipple. The nipple is surrounded by a dark pigmented area, the areola, with sparsely distributed elevation, and the Montgomery's glands, which secrete sebum, an oily substance that lubricates the ducts. The breasts overlie the pectoral muscles of the chest.

PHYSIOLOGY OF THE FEMALE REPRODUCTIVE SYSTEM

The female reproductive system is structurally and physically different from that of the male. The gonads (testes in male and ovaries in female) both originate from the **ovotestis** (undifferentiated) before the eighth week of embryonic life. The ovaries have two main functions: the production of the female germ cells, the **ova**, a process called **oogenesis**, and the production of the hormones oestrogen and progesterone.

The cyclical hormonal changes in the life of a woman prepare the uterus monthly for a possible pregnancy. The secretion of the female hormones oestrogen and progesterone is governed by two gonadotrophic hormones – follicle-stimulating hormone (FSH) and luteinising hormone (LH) – of the anterior pituitary gland, which is controlled by the hypothalamus in the brain. Failure of the ovary to secrete sex hormones or to ovulate may result from pituitary disease or disturbances in the central nervous system.

A woman's reproductive life begins with the onset of menstruation, the **menarche**, occurring generally between ages 10 and 15 years. The reproductive years terminate with the cessation of menstrual periods, menopause, which usually begins in the late 40s or early 50s. At the beginning of each monthly cycle, pituitary gonadotrophic hormone stimulates ovarian follicles to develop. The stimulated follicles begin to grow and develop into matured (**Graafian**) follicles, one of which is released at the midpoint of the cycle, through a process called ovulation.

As the follicles grow during the first half of the cycle, the ovary secretes **oestrogen**, which is carried by the blood to the uterus. Oestrogen stimulates the endometrium of the uterus to enter the proliferative phase, in which it thickens and becomes more vascular in preparation for pregnancy.

Once the ovum has been released from the ovary, the empty follicle is converted into the **corpus luteum**, which begins to secrete progesterone. This is the secretory phase of the uterus. Progesterone is pro-gestation as it supports pregnancy by stimulating endometrial growth and promoting the storage of nutrients for nourishing a fertilised ovum.

If fertilisation does not occur, the corpus luteum ceases to secrete hormones approximately 8–12 days after ovulation. At the end of the monthly cycle, the level of oestrogen and progesterone drops, and menstruation, the sloughing of the endometrial lining, occurs. However, if pregnancy occurs, the fertilised ovum (now referred to as the **zygote**) continues its journey to the uterus, during which time it undergoes a mitotic-like cell division called **cleavage**, in which the cell divides while still retaining its outer covering, the **zona pellucida**. It initially divides into two, then four, eight, sixteen and so on; hence it is thought to double at each division, eventually forming a cluster of cells called the **morula**. This cluster of cells is transformed into a **blastocyst**, which comprises an outer layer of cells, the **trophoblast**, and a mass of cells, the **inner cell mass**. The entire structure of the blastocyst resembles an engagement ring with a round ring band and a diamond set on top. It is at this stage, about the sixth day following fertilisation, that the developing pre-embryo arrives and embeds (implants) in the endometrium. The **trophoblast** later develops to form the **placenta** and the **chorion** (one of the embryonic membranes); while the inner cell mass forms the **fetus**, the **amnion** (second membrane) and the umbilical cord. The amniotic

fluid in which the fetus bathes itself is found within the amniotic sac.

The trophoblast invasion of the endometrium during implantation is of significant importance in understanding immunology in pregnancy. The exchange for nutrients, gases and ions between the maternal and fetal circulations takes place at the trophoblast. Human chorionic gonadotrophin (hCG) and other polypeptide hormones are synthesised and secreted directly into the maternal circulation by the trophoblast (Cirrelli *et al.*, 2001). hCG and other enzymes released sustain the corpus luteum which in turn nourishes the developing embryo. Laboratory diagnosis of pregnancy is based on the presence of hCG in the mother's blood or urine.

The corpus luteum enlarges and continues to secrete high levels of progesterone. By weeks 10–12 of pregnancy, the placenta (derived from both maternal and embryonic tissue) gradually assumes the role of the corpus luteum in secreting these hormones.

Near the site of implantation in the uterus, the endometrium greatly thickens, becomes highly vascular and develops large blood sinuses. The chorion develops finger-like projections called villi which dip into the maternal blood sinuses. This interdigitation of embryonic and maternal tissue constitutes the placenta.

The umbilical arteries extend into the chorionic villi, where carbon dioxide and waste are exchanged for oxygen and nutrients. Maternal and fetal bloods do not mix; the exchange of these substances is by diffusion across the blood vessel walls. Oxygen and nutrients return to the fetus through the umbilical vein.

DIAGNOSTIC PROCEDURES

Physical examination of the female reproductive system begins with a pelvic examination that can detect certain cancers in their early stages, infections and other reproductive system disorders. This examination includes inspection of the external genitalia, visual examination of the vagina and cervix through a speculum (an instrument used to spread and hold the vaginal wall in an open position), and palpation of the female internal organs by bimanual examination. During a bimanual examination, the healthcare provider places one hand on the abdomen and inserts fingers of the other hand into the vagina to feel the female organs between the two hands. A bimanual rectal examination allows palpation of the posterior aspect of the uterus and the rectum. During a pelvic examination, a sample for a Papanicolaou (Pap) test may be taken to look for changes in the cells of the cervix. CA125 is a protein tumour marker that is found in greater concentrations in tumour cells than in other body cells and may be used for diagnosis of endometrial and ovarian cancer. In dilatation and curettage (D&C), the cervix is widened (dilatation) and part of the lining of the uterus is removed (curettage). This procedure may be used in the diagnosis of endometrial cancer.

General visualisation of the different parts of the female reproductive system may be done using various techniques; for example, ultrasound or sonography may aid the diagnosis of inflammatory diseases, uterine fibroid tumours, some cancers, **ectopic pregnancy** and menstrual disorders. **Laparoscopy** enables the visualisation of the female reproductive organs; **colposcopy**, the cervix; and **hysteroscopy**, the uterine lining. These techniques may be used to diagnose inflammatory diseases, some cancers, menstrual disorders and endometriosis. **Mammography** is an X-ray examination of breast tissue; if abnormalities or tumours are discovered, a biopsy may be performed.

Sexually transmitted infections are diagnosed by blood or urine cultures, DNA test and antigen or antibody testing. Other laboratory tests include urinalysis and hormone testing.

DISEASES OF THE FEMALE REPRODUCTIVE SYSTEM

Pelvic inflammatory disease

Pelvic inflammatory disease (PID) is an infection or inflammatory condition affecting the upper female genital tract. The pelvic reproductive organs become inflamed because of bacterial, viral, fungal or parasitic invasion. The infection can ascend to the cervix (cervicitis), the endometrium (endometritis), Fallopian tubes (salpingitis) and ovaries (oophoritis). The most common cause of PID is sexually transmitted infections such as gonorrhoea and chlamydia.

Because of vague symptoms, PID goes unrecognised by women and their healthcare providers about two-thirds of the time. Symptoms of PID vary from none to severe; the most common PID symptom is lower abdominal pain. Other signs and symptoms include fever, unusual vaginal discharge that may have a foul odour, painful intercourse, painful urination and irregular menstrual bleeding.

PID is closely linked to non-specific abdominal pain syndrome in fertile women (Gaitan *et al.*, 2002). Untreated bacterial infections may result in scar tissue formation, which in turn blocks or interrupts the normal movement of eggs into the uterus. Total blockage of the Fallopian tubes prevents fertilisation and consequently leads to infertility. Infertility may also result from partial blockage or even slight damage to the Fallopian tubes. About one in eight women with PID become infertile and if a woman has multiple episodes of PID, her chances of becoming infertile increase. In addition, a partially blocked or slightly damaged Fallopian tube may cause a fertilised egg to remain in the tube. If this fertilised egg begins to grow in the tube as if it were in the uterus, this is referred to as an ectopic pregnancy; this may lead to ruptured Fallopian tubes, causing severe pain, internal bleeding and even death. Scarring in the Fallopian tubes and other pelvic structures can also cause chronic pelvic pain that lasts for months or even years. Women with repeated episodes of PID are more likely to suffer infertility, ectopic pregnancy or chronic pelvic pain.

A PID diagnosis is usually based on clinical findings such as lower abdominal pain, in which case a physical examination is performed to determine the nature and location of the pain. Checks for fever, abnormal vaginal or cervical discharge, and evidence of gonorrhoeal or chlamydial infection are essential. Tests to identify the infection-causing organism (e.g. chlamydial or gonorrhoeal infection) or differential diagnosis to distinguish between PID and other problems with similar symptoms may also be performed. A pelvic ultrasound can determine if the Fallopian tubes are enlarged or an abscess is present. In some cases laparoscopy may be necessary to confirm the diagnosis.

Sexually transmitted infections (STIs) are the main preventable cause of PID, hence women should take action to prevent STIs or get early treatment if they are infected. Treatment for PID includes antibiotics; however, antibiotic treatment does not reverse damage to the affected reproductive organs.

Cervical cancer

Cervical cancer is cancer of the cervix that begins in the lining of the cervix, an earlier stage of which is **carcinoma in situ** in which the underlying tissue has not yet been invaded. Some researchers estimate that carcinoma in situ is about four times more common than invasive cervical cancer. Progression from carcinoma in situ to an invasive malignancy

may be slow, followed by ulceration and consequently vaginal discharge and bleeding. The cancer spreads to surrounding organs: the vagina, bladder, rectum and pelvic wall. The accompanying Side by Side shows a normal cervix and a cancerous cervix.

In 2006, 2873 women were diagnosed with cervical cancer in the UK and 941 deaths recorded the following year, 2007. The mortality rate for this condition increases with age, with more over 70+ years compared with only 7% in those under 35 years. This may reduce with increased screening uptake and the use of the HPV vaccine Gardasil (see HPV and genital warts later in this chapter).

The most important risk factor for cervical cancer is infection by the **human papillomavirus (HPV)**. Women who smoke are about twice as likely as nonsmokers to develop cervical cancer, hence its risk can be reduced by avoiding exposure to HPV and smoking. Genital HPV which is sexually transmitted is prevalent in younger women.

Based on scientific evidence and recommendation by the independent Advisory Committee on Cervical

SIDE by SIDE Cervical cancer

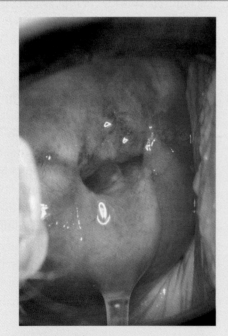

Normal cervix.

(© Isabelle Cartier/Phototake NYC)

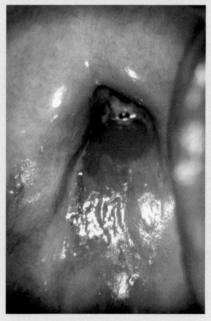

Invasive cervical cancer.

(SIU Bio Med/Custom Medical Stock Photo, Inc.)

Screening (ACCS) and other leading experts and cancer charities, the Department of Health maintains its position on a 25-year age boundary for offering cervical screening. Evidence presented suggests that 2.4% of all cervical cancer cases are in women under 25 years and that lowering the screening age range to 20 years is more harmful than beneficial.

In England, smear tests are offered to women on a 3-yearly basis between ages 25 and 50; thereafter, 5-yearly until age 64. In Scotland and Wales the starting age for screening is 20 years. Cervical cancer can usually be diagnosed early through Pap smear screening.

Diagnosis of cervical cancer may include pelvic examination, Pap smear screening, HPV DNA test and colposcopy. Treatment may include surgery, radiation and chemotherapy.

Endometrial cancer

In the UK, cancer of the endometrium is the most common cancer of the female reproductive organs, the third most prevalent in women in the western world. Women diagnosed with uterine cancer in the UK in 2005 numbered 6891, and in 2007 about 1659 related deaths were recorded. This is compared to a prevalence of approximately 1 in 13 333 women in 2008.

Although the cause of endometrial cancer is not known, most are thought to be hormone-driven. Oestrogen has been highly implicated as a risk factor; however, this has been disputed as it does not seem to account for all associated risk factors (Saidi *et al.*, 2006). A shift in the balance between oestrogen and progesterone toward more oestrogen increases a woman's risk for endometrial cancer. Risk factors for endometrial cancer include total number of menstrual cycles, few pregnancies or infertility, oestrogen therapy, polycystic ovarian syndrome and obesity. The use of oral contraceptives, control of obesity and diabetes, and healthy diet and exercise can reduce the risk of endometrial cancer.

The malignant tumour may grow into the uterine cavity or invade the wall itself, leading to ulcerations, and erosion of blood vessels causes vaginal bleeding. Other signs and symptoms can include vaginal discharge, pelvic pain and weight loss. There are no early detection tests or examinations that can find endometrial cancer in asymptomatic women at average endometrial cancer risk. Diagnosis may include pelvic examination, CA125 blood test, biopsy, hysteroscopy and D&C. Surgery, radiation, chemotherapy and hormone therapy are possible treatments.

Fibroid tumours of the uterus

Benign tumours of the smooth muscle of the uterus, **leiomyomas**, or fibroid tumours, are the most common tumours of the female reproductive system, with between 20% and 40% of women aged 35 and older having fibroid tumours of significant size. Most women with fibroid tumours do not experience any signs and symptoms such as excessive vaginal bleeding, pelvic pressure, abdominal pain, abdominal enlargement and pain during intercourse. Fibroids vary in size from a quarter of an inch to the size of a water melon. The cause of fibroid tumours remains unknown, although their growth is stimulated by oestrogen. Uterine fibroids cannot be prevented and their diagnosis may include pelvic examination, ultrasound, sonography and hysteroscopy. Treatment for fibroid tumours depends on severity of symptoms and childbearing plans. Birth control pills may be used to decrease the bleeding caused by fibroids whereas uterine artery embolisation shrinks the tumours by cutting off their blood supply. Furthermore, focused ultrasound surgery using high-frequency sound waves may be used to destroy fibroids. Endometrial ablation destroys the lining of the uterus and reduces the amount of bleeding during menstruation. Myomectomy is removal of the fibroid or fibroids that are causing symptoms. Hysterectomy may also be necessary; one-third of the 70 000 hysterectomies performed by the NHS in the UK yearly are due to fibroids.

Ovarian cancer

The ovaries are a common site for cancer to develop, and ovarian cancer is the fifth most common cancer occurring in UK females. However, their position deep in the pelvis makes early detection of the tumour difficult. According to Cancer Research UK, about 6600 new cases are identified yearly, a weekly rate of about 125 new cases. It is more common amongst the over-50s, especially those of menopausal age.

Over 204 000 new cases of ovarian cancers are diagnosed worldwide on an annual basis, and 4300 women die in the UK annually because of ovarian cancer.

Extensive metastasis often occurs before there are noticeable symptoms, which include bloating, pelvic or abdominal pain, trouble eating or feeling full quickly, and changes in urinary urgency or frequency. The cause of ovarian cancer is not known, but risk factors include age; obesity; early menstruation; late menopause; not having children or having the first child after age 30; family history of ovarian, breast or colorectal cancer; and a personal history of breast cancer. Oral contraceptives, tubal ligation, hysterectomy, childbearing and breastfeeding may reduce the risk of ovarian cancer.

Currently there is no screening test for ovarian cancer; however, diagnosis may be confirmed by CT or MRI scan or ultrasound. Laparoscopy, biopsy and CA125 blood test may also be performed. Treatment options for ovarian cancer include surgery, radiation and chemotherapy.

Breast cancer

Breast cancer (also discussed in Chapter 4) is the second leading cause of cancer death in women, exceeded only by lung cancer.

Breast cancer is the most common cancer in the UK and affects over 45 500 people annually, with a significant number of these being women; only 300 men are diagnosed per year. It is estimated that, over a lifetime, one in nine women will develop cancer. It is suggested that breast cancer is highest in women who have attained the menopause.

Women living in North America have the world's highest rate of breast cancer; annually approximately 1.3 million women will be diagnosed with breast cancer and 465 000 will die worldwide.

The most common sign of breast cancer is a lump or mass in the breast. Other possible signs and symptoms include swelling of all or part of the breast; skin irritation and dimpling; breast or nipple pain; nipple retraction; redness, scaliness or thickening of the nipple or breast skin; a discharge other than breast milk; and a swelling of a lymph node in the armpit. Breast cancer spreads principally through the lymph system and metastases are frequently found in the lungs, liver, brain and bone. The cause of breast cancer is not known; however, risk factors include gender, age, genetic risk factors, and family or personal history of breast cancer. Approximately 5–10% of breast cancer cases are thought to be hereditary. Women who inherit a *BRCA1* or *BRCA2* mutation have up to an 80% chance of developing breast cancer during their lifetime. A genetic screen for breast cancer is available. Breast cancer risk can be lowered by avoiding alcohol, exercising regularly and maintaining a healthy body weight.

Regular screening and early diagnosis are critical to identify and treat breast cancer. Women are strongly urged to examine their breasts monthly for signs of cancer. Healthcare providers will examine breasts as part of a routine gynaecology examination. Mammography can detect small, early cancers, and the Department of Health recommends that women age 40 and older have a yearly mammogram.

In the UK, the NHS offers a free breast screening programme to all women between ages 50 and 70. By the year 2012 the NHS Breast Screening programme will extend this age range to include 47–73-year-olds. There are over 80 breast screening units located across the UK and this initiative was announced in 2007 as part of the Department of Health's Cancer Reform Strategy.

Ultrasound may be used to target specific areas of concern found on the mammogram. A biopsy of the suspected malignancy confirms the diagnosis or shows the tumour to be benign.

Treatment of breast cancer may include surgery, radiation, chemotherapy, targeted drug therapy and hormone therapy. Lumpectomy removes only the breast lump and a surrounding margin of normal tissue. Partial (segmental) mastectomy or quadrantectomy removes more breast tissue than a lumpectomy. For a quadrantectomy, one-quarter of the breast is removed. For most women with stage I or II breast cancer, breast conservation therapy (lumpectomy/partial mastectomy plus radiation therapy) is as effective as mastectomy. However, breast conservation therapy is not an option for all women with breast cancer. Mastectomy involves removal of all of the breast tissue, sometimes along with other nearby tissues. In a simple or total mastectomy, the surgeon removes the entire breast, including the nipple, but does not remove under-arm lymph nodes or muscle tissue from beneath the breast. Sometimes this is done for both breasts (a double mastectomy), especially when it is done as preventive surgery in women at very high risk for breast cancer. A modified radical mastectomy involves removing the entire breast and some of the axillary lymph nodes. This is the most common surgery for women with breast cancer who are having the whole breast removed. For some women with smaller tumours, one option may be a newer procedure known as a skin-sparing mastectomy, in which most of the skin over the breast (other than the nipple and areola) is left intact. Radical mastectomy is an extensive operation removing the entire breast, axillary lymph nodes and the chest wall muscles under the breast. This surgery was once very common, but because of the disfigurement and side effects it causes and because modified radical mastectomy has been proven to be as effective as radical mastectomy, it is rarely done today.

BENIGN CONDITIONS OF THE BREAST

Benign breast conditions are very common. Unlike breast cancer, these conditions are not life-threatening. Three types of benign breast conditions – **fibroadenomas**, breast cysts and fibrocystic changes – are discussed.

Fibroadenomas

Fibroadenomas are the most common benign tumour of the breast. They are solid and firm and usually painless. Fibroadenomas are most common in young women in their twenties and thirties, but they may occur at any age. The cause is unknown, and there are no known preventative measures. Diagnosis of fibroadenomas may include breast examination, mammogram, ultrasound, fine needle aspiration and biopsy. They often stop growing or even shrink on their own without any treatment, and they may not require removal. Fibroadenoma surgery may involve removing a margin of surrounding breast tissue. However, scarring could occur that distorts the shape and texture of the breast, making future physical examinations and mammography more difficult to interpret.

Breast cysts

Breast cysts are tiny, fluid-filled sacs within the breast tissue. Cysts are oval or round, smooth and firm, and

 Prevention PLUS!

Breast Awareness

The Breast Awareness policy, part of the Department of Health's National Health Services Cancer Reform Strategy (DH 2007), encourages women to be more aware of their bodies, observing what is normal and reporting any deviation in a timely manner. Breast screening is offered to women aged 50 years and above. Awareness of the normal structure of the breast forms the basis of recognising any unusual changes. The Breast awareness programme replaces the routine self examination of the breast abandoned in UK due to lack of scientific evidence of its benefits of early reporting by women and healthcare intervention.

Source: Office for National Statistics (2007) Mortality Statistics, England and Wales, 2007. *www.ons.gov.uk* Accessed 2009.

they move slightly when pressed. Breast cysts are common, especially in women over the age of 35. The cysts may vary in size during the menstrual cycle and may be tender. The cause of breast cysts is not known, and there are no known preventative measures. Diagnosis of breast cysts may include breast examination, mammogram, ultrasound and fine needle aspiration. Cysts may resolve spontaneously or may need to be surgically removed.

Fibrocystic changes

Fibrocystic changes (FCCs) are characterised by breasts that are lumpy. FCCs primarily affect women aged 30–50 years. The cause of FCCs is not known, but oestrogen and progesterone may play a role. FCCs are not preventable. FCCs may be diagnosed by breast examination, mammogram, ultrasound and biopsy. In most women with FCCs there are no symptoms and no treatment is needed. Women with mild discomfort may benefit from wearing a supportive bra or taking over-the-counter pain relievers.

MENSTRUAL DISORDERS

Amenorrhoea is the absence of menstrual periods and is known as primary amenorrhoea if menstruation does not commence by age 16. Primary amenorrhoea affects less than 1% of adolescent girls. The causes include chromosomal abnormalities, problems with the hypothalamus, pituitary disease, lack of reproductive organs or structural abnormality of the vagina. The cessation of menstrual periods for 3–6 months or more once they have begun is termed secondary amenorrhoea. Each year approximately 5% of menstruating women experience 3 months of secondary amenorrhoea. The causes include pregnancy, contraceptives, breastfeeding, stress, medication, chronic illness, hormone imbalance, low body weight, excessive exercise, thyroid disorders, pituitary tumour, uterine scarring and premature menopause. Prevention of amenorrhoea includes maintaining a sensible exercise programme, maintaining a healthy weight, eating a healthy diet,

avoiding excessive alcohol consumption, not smoking and finding healthy outlets for stress. Diagnosis may include pregnancy test, pelvic examination, blood test to check hormone levels and progestin challenge test. Treatment, if any, depends on the cause of amenorrhoea and may include lifestyle changes related to weight, physical activity or stress level; amenorrhoea caused by thyroid or pituitary disorders may be treated with medications.

Dysmenorrhoea is painful or difficult menses and its prevalence is estimated to be between 45% and 95% among reproductive-aged women. Primary dysmenorrhoea does not involve any physical abnormality and usually begins 6 months to a year after the onset of menarche. Secondary dysmenorrhoea involves an underlying physical cause, such as endometriosis or fibroid tumours. Symptoms of dysmenorrhoea include cramping and dull to severe pelvic and lower back pain that may radiate to other areas. Prostaglandins are the cause of primary dysmenorrhoea, whereas the causes of secondary dysmenorrhoea include PID, use of an intrauterine device (IUD), uterine fibroid tumours and endometriosis. Prevention of dysmenorrhoea includes avoiding risk factors for PID, obtaining early diagnosis and treatment of STIs, and not using an IUD. Diagnosis is made based on pelvic examination, ultrasound, laparoscopy and hysteroscopy. Treatment options include antibiotics, oral contraceptive therapy to regulate and decrease menstrual flow, non-steroidal anti-inflammatory medications to reduce pain and surgery to remove fibroid tumours.

Menorrhagia is excessive or prolonged bleeding during menstruation, and is experienced by 35% of women aged between 25 and 44 years (Santer *et al.*, 2005). Clinically, it is defined as total blood loss exceeding 80 ml per cycle or menses lasting longer than 7 days. Menorrhagia is one of the most common gynaecological complaints; gynaecological surveys report that 30% of all premenopausal women perceive their menses to be excessive, and the World Health Organization (WHO) reports that 18 million women aged 30–55 years perceive their menstrual bleeding to be excessive. However, only 10% of these women experience blood loss severe enough to be defined clinically as menorrhagia.

Causes of menorrhagia include hormonal imbalance, fibroid tumours, lack of ovulation, use of an IUD, pregnancy complications, medications (anti-inflammatory and anticoagulants), PID, thyroid disorders, endometriosis and liver or kidney disease. Sometimes the cause of menorrhagia is unknown; however, it may be prevented by avoiding IUD usage, avoiding the risk factors for PID, and through early diagnosis and treatment of STIs. Diagnosis may include pelvic examination, Pap smear test, blood tests, biopsy and ultrasound. Treatment varies according to the cause of the disease and may include iron supplements, non-steroidal anti-inflammatory drugs, oral contraceptives and progesterone. Surgical treatment options include D&C, endometrial ablation or resection, and hysterectomy.

Metrorrhagia is bleeding between menstrual periods or extreme irregularity of the menstrual cycle. This condition may be caused by a hormonal imbalance, endometriosis, infection, miscarriage, ectopic pregnancy, cancer, use of an IUD, thyroid disorders, diabetes and blood clotting disorders. Prevention of metrorrhagia includes early diagnosis, treatment of STIs, and not using an IUD. Diagnosis is based on record of menstrual cycle, pelvic examination, blood tests, hysteroscopy, X-ray, biopsy and ultrasound. The treatment of metrorrhagia depends on the cause of the problem and may include hormone therapy, antibiotics, surgery and other medications.

Premenstrual syndrome and premenstrual dysphoric disorder

Premenstrual syndrome (PMS) is a group of symptoms that start 1–2 weeks before menstruation and cease with the onset of menses. Estimates of the percentage of women affected by PMS vary. According to the Royal College of Obstetricians and Gynaecologists, at least one or two in 20 women experience PMS severe enough to prevent them from carrying out their daily life. This amounts to 5–10% of women and normally improves following menopause. Of menstruating women, 85% have at least one PMS symptom as part of their monthly cycle. Common PMS symptoms include breast swelling and tenderness, acne, bloating and weight gain, headache or joint pain, food cravings, irritability, mood swings, crying spells, fatigue, trouble sleeping, anxiety and depression. The cause of PMS is not known, but hormonal changes trigger the symptoms. Prevention of PMS includes a high intake of calcium and vitamin D. Diagnosis is based on medical history, including symptoms, when symptoms occur, and how much the symptoms interfere with daily life. Although over-the-counter pain relievers may help ease cramps, headaches, backaches and breast tenderness, no single PMS treatment works for everyone. Contraceptives can be used to reduce PMS symptoms. Other measures such as avoiding salt, caffeine and alcohol; exercising; eating healthy foods; getting enough sleep; joining a support group; and managing stress may also help reduce symptoms.

For some women, the symptoms of PMS are severe enough to interfere with their lives and this may be classified as premenstrual dysphoric disorder (PMDD). This affects 3–8% of menstruating women (RCOG, 2007). Evidence shows that the neurotransmitter serotonin plays a role in PMDD, which may present with a number of disabling symptoms. These include feelings of sadness or despair, suicidal thoughts, feelings of tension or anxiety, panic attacks, mood swings, crying, lasting irritability or anger that affects other people, disinterest in daily activities and relationships, trouble thinking or focusing, tiredness or low energy, food cravings or binge eating, having trouble sleeping and feeling out of control. Other physical symptoms may include bloating, breast tenderness, headaches and joint or muscle pain; the patient must have five or more of these symptoms to be diagnosed with PMDD. Prevention of PMDD includes adequate exercise, rest, balanced diet and managing stress. In addition to the PMS treatments listed above, antidepressants that change serotonin levels in the brain have also been shown to help some women with PMDD.

Endometriosis

Endometriosis is a condition in which endometrial tissue from the uterus becomes embedded outside the uterus. During menstruation, the tissue may be pushed through the Fallopian tubes or carried by blood or lymph. The endometrial tissue can embed on the ovaries, the outer surface of the uterus, the bowel or other abdominal organs and appears rarely on other body structures and organs.

The endometrial tissue by nature responds to hormonal changes even when outside the uterus. This tissue goes through proliferative and secretory phases, along with the sloughing with subsequent bleeding. The most common symptom of endometriosis is pelvic pain. Other symptoms can include diarrhoea or constipation, abdominal bloating, menorrhagia, metrorrhagia and fatigue. It is estimated that 30–40% of women with endometriosis are infertile. The aetiology of endometriosis is unknown, and it cannot be prevented. The only certain means of diagnosing endometriosis is by seeing it with laparoscopy. Treatment of endometriosis may include pain relievers, hormone therapy and surgery.

DISORDERS OF PREGNANCY

Ectopic pregnancy

An ectopic pregnancy is a life-threatening gynaecological emergency in which the fertilised ovum implants in a tissue other than the uterus. This condition occurs in 11.1 of 1000 pregnancies in the UK, with about 10 000 cases recorded from 2003 to 2005 (CEMACH, 2007). Overall mortality over this period was 0.35 per 1000 ectopic pregnancies.

The most common site of an ectopic pregnancy is in the Fallopian tubes. In rare cases, ectopic pregnancies can occur in the ovary, cervix and stomach area. An ectopic pregnancy is usually caused by a condition that blocks or slows the movement of a fertilised egg through the Fallopian tube to the uterus. Most cases are a result of scarring caused by a past infection in the Fallopian tubes, surgery of the Fallopian tubes, or a previous ectopic pregnancy. Up to 50% of women who have ectopic pregnancies have PID. Some ectopic pregnancies can be due to birth defects of the Fallopian tubes, endometriosis, complications of a ruptured appendix or scarring

caused by previous pelvic surgery. Symptoms of ectopic pregnancy include lower abdominal or pelvic pain, mild cramping on one side of the pelvis, amenorrhoea, metrorrhagia, breast tenderness, nausea and low back pain. If the area of the abnormal pregnancy ruptures and bleeds, symptoms may get worse and may include severe, sharp and sudden pain in the lower abdominal area; feeling faint or actually fainting; referred pain to the shoulder area; and internal bleeding due to a rupture, which may lead to shock. Shock is the first symptom of nearly 20% of ectopic pregnancies.

Most forms of ectopic pregnancy that occur outside the Fallopian tubes are usually not preventable. Prevention of an ectopic pregnancy in the Fallopian tube includes avoiding risk factors for PID and early diagnosis and treatment of STIs. Diagnosis of ectopic pregnancy is based on symptoms, pelvic examination, ultrasound and measurement of hCG levels. Ectopic pregnancies cannot continue to term, so the pregnancy must be terminated. In cases in which a rupture will occur, the woman may be given a medication called methotrexate that allows the body to reabsorb the pregnancy. In the event of a rupture, laparotomy is performed to stop blood loss and terminate the pregnancy.

Spontaneous abortion or miscarriage

A spontaneous abortion, commonly called a miscarriage, is loss of a fetus before the twentieth week of pregnancy. Most miscarriages result from a genetic abnormality of the fetus. Other possible causes of miscarriage include infection, physical problems in the mother, hormonal factors, immune responses or serious systemic diseases of the mother like diabetes or thyroid disease. It is estimated that up to 50% of all fertilised eggs die and are spontaneously aborted, usually before the woman knows she is pregnant. Among known pregnancies, the rate of miscarriage is approximately 10% and usually occurs between the seventh and twelfth weeks of pregnancy. Possible signs and symptoms of spontaneous abortion include low back pain or abdominal pain that is dull, sharp or cramping; vaginal bleeding; and tissue or clot-like material discharged from the vagina. About 20% of pregnant women have some vaginal bleeding during the first 3 months of pregnancy; approximately half of these women have a miscarriage. Very few miscarriages are preventable. Diagnosis of spontaneous abortion is based on pelvic examination and hCG levels. If all the pregnancy tissue does not naturally exit the body, medication or surgery may be used to help eliminate the remaining tissue.

Pre-eclampsia

Pre-eclampsia is a disease that only occurs during pregnancy. Pre-eclampsia – pregnancy-induced hypertension (PIH) – and toxaemia are essentially interchangeable terms. Pre-eclampsia occurs in 5–10% of all pregnancies. Mild pre-eclampsia is characterised by high blood pressure and the presence of protein in the urine. Severe pre-eclampsia may also include headaches, blurred vision, inability to tolerate bright light, fatigue, nausea, vomiting, urinating small amounts, pain in the upper right abdomen, shortness of breath and the tendency to bruise easily. The cause of pre-eclampsia is not known. Risk factors include family history of pre-eclampsia, being pregnant with twins, young maternal age, never having carried a pregnancy to term, and women who had high blood pressure, diabetes or kidney disease prior to pregnancy. Prevention of pre-eclampsia includes maintaining a healthy weight before pregnancy and taking multivitamins. Diagnosis of pre-eclampsia is based on increased blood pressure and urine protein levels. If close enough to term, the baby will be delivered. However, if a woman has mild pre-eclampsia and is not close enough to term to be delivered, rest, frequent monitoring of blood pressure and urine, reduced salt intake and increased water intake may be recommended. Severe pre-eclampsia may be treated with blood pressure medication.

Gestational diabetes mellitus

Gestational diabetes is diabetes mellitus associated with pregnancy (diabetes mellitus is discussed in detail in Chapter 12). Annually, of about 650 000

women giving birth in England and Wales, 2–5% are diabetic. Of these, 87.5% of pregnancies are complicated by diabetes, all of which are thought to be due to gestational diabetes (NICE, 2008).

Increased metabolic demands during pregnancy require higher insulin levels, but certain normal, maternal, physiological changes during pregnancy can result in insufficient insulin levels, which, if uncorrected, result in diabetes. These changes include increased levels of oestrogen and progesterone, which interfere with insulin action. In addition, the placenta normally inactivates insulin. The normal pregnancy-induced elevation of stress hormones such as cortisol, adrenaline and glucagon raises blood glucose. Insulin requirements continue to rise as pregnancy approaches term. In a normal pregnancy, more insulin is secreted to compensate for these changes, but in some women, insulin levels remain low as blood glucose continues to rise.

Risk factors include a family history of type 2 diabetes, age, gestational diabetes in a previous pregnancy, a previous pregnancy which resulted in a child with a birth weight of 9 pounds or more, diagnosis of prediabetes, impaired glucose tolerance or impaired fasting glucose. Smoking doubles the risk of gestational diabetes. Women at risk for developing gestational diabetes should be screened early and monitored throughout their pregnancy. Signs and symptoms of gestational diabetes are similar to insulin-dependent diabetes mellitus (see Chapter 12) but include maternal hypertension, polyhydramnios (excessive amniotic fluid), excessive weight gain during the last 6 months of pregnancy and a fetus large-for-gestational-age. Prevention of gestational diabetes includes eating a healthy diet, maintaining a healthy weight, not gaining too much weight during pregnancy and engaging in exercise on a regular basis.

The prognosis for gestational diabetes is good if diagnosed and treated early. Diagnosis is made via a glucose tolerance test. Treatment consists of regular blood glucose monitoring, dietary control of blood glucose levels, weight control and, possibly, insulin therapy. Untreated gestational diabetes mellitus entails many risks to mother and fetus. The fetal risks are stillbirth, premature delivery and high or low birth weight. Infants may experience severe hypoglycaemia shortly after birth.

ANATOMY OF THE MALE REPRODUCTIVE SYSTEM

The male reproductive system consists of a pair of testes that produce sperm and hormones; a system of tubules that convey sperm to the outside; and the penis, which transmits the sperm into the female tract. Accessory glands contribute to the formation of semen.

The testes are suspended in the scrotum, a sac-like structure outside the body wall. The testes contain highly coiled tubules called the **seminiferous tubules**, which are the site of sperm development. When the sperm reach a certain maturity, they enter the **epididymis**, a coiled tube that lies along the outer wall of the testis. The epididymis leads into another duct, the **vas deferens**, which passes through the inguinal canal into the abdominal cavity.

Near the base of the urinary bladder, the vas deferens joins a duct of the **seminal vesicle**, an accessory gland, to form the ejaculatory duct. The ejaculatory ducts from each side penetrate the **prostate gland** to enter the urethra. Ducts of the prostate open into the first part of the male urethra. Another pair of glands, the **bulbourethral glands**, secrete into the urethra as it enters the penis. The male reproductive system is illustrated in Figure 11.3.

The penis contains erectile tissue composed of three cylindrical bodies filled with sinuses that become engorged with blood during sexual excitement. The urethra passes through one of these cylindrical bodies as it extends to the outside, and connective tissue supports the erectile structures. The distal, expanded end of the penis is the glans penis. A flap of loosely attached skin covering the glans, the prepuce or foreskin, is sometimes removed shortly after birth, a procedure called circumcision.

PHYSIOLOGY OF THE MALE REPRODUCTIVE SYSTEM

Spermatogenesis, the formation of sperm, begins in the male at puberty and continues through life. The

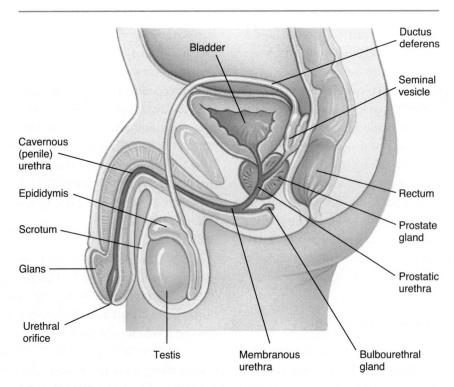

Figure 11.3 The male reproductive system.

development of sperm and the secretion of the male hormone, testosterone, are processes stimulated by gonadotrophic hormones of the anterior pituitary gland. Maturation of sperm continues in the epididymis, where they acquire motility. Sperm are stored in both the epididymis and vas deferens, where they can live for several weeks. Once ejaculated, they live for 24–72 hours in the female reproductive tract.

The accessory glands produce a mucoid secretion, called semen, which nourishes and protects sperm. The seminal vesicles secrete an alkaline fluid that normally constitutes approximately 60% of the volume of semen. The alkaline nature of the seminal fluid helps to neutralise the acidic environment of the male urethra and female reproductive tract. Seminal fluid contains fructose to nourish the sperm and prostaglandins to stimulate uterine contractions and propel the sperm toward the Fallopian tubes. The seminal vesicles release their secretions into the ejaculatory ducts at the same time that the vas deferens empties the sperm. The bulbourethral glands secrete an alkaline fluid into the urethra that neutralises acidic urine in the urethra. At the same time, the bulbourethral glands secrete mucus that lubricates the urethra for easy passage of sperm. The prostate gland surrounds the upper portion of the urethra. The prostate gland secretes a milky fluid that contains citric acid to nourish the sperm and several protein-digesting enzymes such as PSA (prostate-specific antigen). Prostate secretions make up approximately 25% of the volume of semen.

Sexual stimulation of the male transmits impulses into the central nervous system, which initiates the male response. Erection of the penis is the first effect. Nerve impulses cause the dilatation of penile arteries, allowing blood to flow under high pressure into the erectile tissue. The high pressure temporarily impedes the emptying of the penile veins and causes the penis to become hard, elongated and erect.

Intense sexual stimulation causes peristaltic contractions in the walls of the epididymis and vas deferens, propelling sperm into the urethra. Semen typically contains between 50 and 150 million sperm. The seminal vesicles and prostate gland simultaneously release their secretions, which mix with the bulbourethral gland secretions and form the semen. Ejaculation of the semen, the culmination of the sexual act, occurs when contraction of this musculature increases pressure on the erectile tissue and the semen is expressed through the urethral opening.

DIAGNOSTIC PROCEDURES

Physical examination of the male reproductive system includes visual examination of the external genitalia. The testes are palpated to determine the presence of tumours. A digital rectal examination (DRE) allows the physician to palpate the prostate gland. PSA is produced by cells of the prostate gland. The PSA test measures the level of PSA in the blood. Prostate cancer and benign prostatic hyperplasia can increase PSA levels. **Cystoscopy** is used to view the urethra and bladder. If abnormalities or tumours are discovered, a biopsy may be performed.

Sexually transmitted infections are diagnosed by blood or urine cultures, DNA test and antigen or antibody testing. Other laboratory tests that may be performed include urinalysis and hormone testing.

DISEASES OF THE MALE REPRODUCTIVE SYSTEM

Prostatitis

Prostatitis is inflammation or infection of the prostate gland. According to the National Institutes of Health, prostatitis may account for up to 25% of all visits to the GP for complaints involving the genital and urinary systems among young and middle-aged men. Prostatitis has been classified by the National Institutes of Health into four categories: category 1 is acute bacterial prostatitis; category 2 is chronic bacterial prostatitis; category 3 includes the conditions previously known as non-bacterial prostatitis (prostatodynia and chronic pelvic pain syndrome); and category 4 is asymptomatic inflammatory prostatitis. Approximately 5–10% of prostatitis cases are caused by bacterial infection.

The signs and symptoms vary depending on the category of prostatitis. Acute bacterial prostatitis usually comes on suddenly, and signs and symptoms may include fever and chills, flu-like symptoms, pain in the prostate gland, lower back or groin, urinary problems, including increased urinary urgency and frequency, difficulty or pain when urinating, inability to empty the bladder completely, and blood-tinged urine, and painful ejaculation. The signs and symptoms of chronic bacterial prostatitis develop more slowly, usually are not as severe as those of acute prostatitis, and tend to alternate with times when symptoms are worse. Signs and symptoms of chronic bacterial prostatitis include a frequent and urgent need to urinate, pain or burning sensation when urinating, pelvic pain, excessive urination during the night, pain in the lower back and genital area, difficulty starting urination or diminished urine flow, occasional blood in semen or urine, painful ejaculation, slight fever and recurring bladder infections. The signs and symptoms of non-bacterial prostatitis are similar to those of chronic bacterial prostatitis, without fever.

Categories 1 and 2 prostatitis are caused by bacterial infections. The cause of categories 3 and 4 prostatitis is unknown. Prevention includes practising good hygiene, maintaining adequate hydration and seeking early treatment for infections. Diagnosis may include DRE and bacterial cultures of urine or prostate gland fluid. Pain relievers and several weeks of treatment with antibiotics are typically treatment for categories 1 and 2 prostatitis. Treatment for category 3 prostatitis may include alpha blockers to aid in urination, pain relievers and muscle relaxants. Category 4 prostatitis is usually found during examination for another condition and may not require treatment.

Epididymitis

Epididymitis is inflammation of the epididymis. Each year an estimated 1 in 1000 men suffers from epididymitis. Signs and symptoms may include testicular swelling on one or both sides, scrotal pain ranging from mild to severe, tenderness in one or both testicles, tenderness in the groin, painful urination, painful intercourse or ejaculation, fever, penile discharge and blood in the semen. A number of bacterial organisms can cause epididymitis, including gonorrhoea and chlamydia. Other causes of epididymitis may include urinary infections spreading to the epididymis, anatomical abnormalities in the urinary tract or catheter insertion. Prevention of epididymitis includes abstinence, monogamy, use of condoms and dental dams, and early treatment for infections. Diagnosis may include physical examination, DRE, blood and urine tests, bacterial culture, ultrasound and nuclear scan of the testicles. Antibiotics are the treatment for epididymitis.

Orchitis

Orchitis is inflammation of the testes. The most common cause of orchitis is mumps; approximately 30% of male patients will develop orchitis during the course of the illness. Other causes of orchitis include bacterial infections or injury. The signs and symptoms of orchitis usually have an abrupt onset and may include testicular swelling on one or both sides, pain ranging from mild to severe, tenderness in one or both testicles, nausea and vomiting, fever, penile discharge, and prostate enlargement and tenderness. Prevention of orchitis includes vaccination against mumps, abstinence, monogamy, use of condoms and dental dams, and use of a protective cup over the genitals to guard against mechanical injury. Diagnosis may include physical examination, DRE, blood and urine tests, bacterial cultures, ultrasound and nuclear imaging of the testicles. Treatment for viral orchitis is symptomatic and may include pain relievers, non-steroidal anti-inflammatory drugs, bed rest, elevation and application of cold packs to the scrotum. Bacterial orchitis is treated with antibiotics.

Cryptorchidism

Cryptorchidism is not a disease but a failure of the testes to descend from the abdominal cavity, where they develop during fetal life, to the scrotum. Approximately 3% of full-term male newborns have an undescended testicle at birth, and up to 30% of premature male newborns have at least one undescended testicle. Since the testicles typically descend late in fetal development, during the eighth month of gestation, the infant born before this time has a greater chance of having cryptorchidism. In over 50% of boys being seen for cryptorchidism, the testes have descended by the third month, and by the age of 1 year, 80% of all undescended testes have descended into the scrotum. Abnormal testicular development usually causes cryptorchidism. The affected testicles frequently have a short spermatic artery, poor blood supply, or both.

The major sign of cryptorchidism is not being able to feel one or both of the testicles in the scrotum. Cryptorchidism cannot be prevented. Diagnosis of cryptorchidism may involve palpating the scrotum and abdomen to locate the testicles while the patient is in the squatting position or in a warm bath, and testing for testosterone and gonadotrophin in the blood.

Cryptorchidism can cause other complications, including infertility and testicular cancer. It is reported that changes in an undescended testicle occur as early as 6 months of age, with the reported cancer rate in cryptorchidism 22 times higher than in the general population. Treatment may include hormone therapy or surgery.

Testicular cancer

Testicular cancer is cancer in one or both testicles in young men. In about 90% of cases, men have a lump on a testicle that is painless but slightly uncomfortable, or they may notice testicular enlargement or swelling. Men with testicular cancer often report a sensation of heaviness or aching in the lower abdomen or scrotum.

Testicular cancer accounts for approximately 0.7% of all cancers. Approximately 1960 men are diagnosed with the condition each year in the UK. Around 70 people die every year from testicular cancer. Approximately 50 000 men annually will be diagnosed with testicular cancer and 9000 will die worldwide.

The cause of testicular cancer is not known. Risk factors include cryptorchidism (about 10% of

testicular cancer cases occur in men with a history of cryptorchidism), a family history of testicular cancer, age (90% of testicular cancer cases occur in men between the ages of 20 and 54), and race and ethnicity (the risk of testicular cancer among white men is about 5–10 times that of black men and more than twice that of Asian men).

Diagnosis may include physical examination, ultrasound and blood tests. Treatment may include surgery, radiation and chemotherapy.

SEXUALLY TRANSMITTED INFECTIONS

Sexually transmitted infections (STIs), also known as sexually transmitted diseases, are infections spread by sexual contact. Sexual contact includes unprotected oral, anal or vaginal intercourse. STIs are caused by bacteria, viruses and protozoans. The WHO estimates that more than 1 million new cases of sexually transmitted bacterial infections occur worldwide every day. The WHO also estimates that 80–90% of STIs occur in the developing world. Some STIs cause no or relatively minor symptoms, but undetected infections can have serious consequences, including infertility, PID, cervical cancer and adverse pregnancy outcomes.

HIV/AIDS

HIV/AIDS is covered in the discussion of immunity in Chapter 2.

Gonorrhoea

Gonorrhoea is caused by the coccus bacterium *Neisseria gonorrhoea*. Gonorrhoea is transmitted through sexual contact and during childbirth. Gonorrhoea is the second most common STI in the UK, with over 19 000 cases reported in 2006. Young men aged 20–24 and women aged 16–19 years are most affected; the WHO estimates that more than 62 million people worldwide have gonorrhoea.

Although many men with gonorrhoea are asymptomatic, some have some signs or symptoms that appear within 2–5 days after infection; signs and symptoms can take as long as 30 days to appear. Signs and symptoms include a burning sensation when urinating, or a white, yellow or green discharge from the penis, and painful or swollen testicles. Most women who are infected with gonorrhoea are asymptomatic. Even when a woman has symptoms, they can be so non-specific as to be mistaken for a bladder or vaginal infection. The signs and symptoms in women include a painful or burning sensation when urinating, vaginal discharge or vaginal bleeding between periods.

Untreated gonorrhoea can cause serious and permanent health problems in both women and men. In women, gonorrhoea is a common cause of PID. In men, gonorrhoea can cause epididymitis, which can lead to infertility if left untreated. Gonorrhoeal infection in a newborn can cause blindness, joint infection or a life-threatening blood infection. Treatment of gonorrhoea as soon as it is detected in pregnant women will reduce the risk of these complications.

Gonorrhoea can be diagnosed by urine sample, bacterial culture or Gram stain (see Chapter 3). Gonorrhoea is treated with antibiotics. Drug-resistant strains of gonorrhoea are increasing in many areas of the world, and successful treatment of gonorrhoea is becoming more difficult.

Syphilis

Syphilis is caused by the spirochete bacterium *Treponema pallidum*. Syphilis is transmitted through sexual contact, through direct contact with a syphilis **chancre** and during childbirth. In 2006, there were 2766 reported cases in the UK. Syphilis is more common in men than in women, and rates are highest among men who have sex with men. The WHO estimates that worldwide more than 12 million people annually are infected with syphilis.

The time between infection with syphilis and the appearance of symptoms can range from 10 to 90 days. The primary stage begins with the appearance of one or more chancres where *Treponema pallidum* entered the body (Figure 11.4). Chancres are painless lesions that usually last 3–6 weeks and heal without treatment. If no treatment is administered, the infection progresses to the secondary stage. Secondary syphilis is often marked by a skin rash that is characterised by brown sores about the size of a penny. The rash appears anywhere from 3 to 6 weeks after the chancre appears. While the rash may

 Prevention PLUS!

Preventing STIs

- **Reduce your number of sexual partners.**
- **Use condoms.** Protect yourself with a condom *every* time you have vaginal, anal or oral sex. Condoms should be used for any type of sex with every partner. If you're not sure how to use a condom, there are normally instructions on the packet. Alternatively, access the NHS website *www.condomessentialwear.co.uk* or the fpa (Family Planning Clinic) website *www.fpa.org.uk*. For vaginal sex, use a latex male condom or a female polyurethane condom. For anal sex, use a latex male condom. For oral sex, use a dental dam. A dental dam is a rubbery material that can be placed over the anus or the vagina before sexual contact.
- **Know that some methods of birth control, like birth control pills, implants or diaphragms, will not protect you from STIs.** If you use one of these methods, be sure also to use a latex condom or dental dam correctly every time you have sex.
- **Talk with your sex partner(s) about STIs and using condoms.** It's up to you to make sure you are protected. Remember, it's *your* body!
- **Talk frankly with your healthcare provider and your sex partner(s) about any STIs you or your partner have or have had.** Try not to be embarrassed.

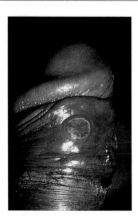

Figure 11.4 Chancre of primary syphilis on the penis.

cover the whole body or appear only in a few areas, the palms of the hands and soles of the feet are almost always involved. Because active bacteria are present in these sores, any physical contact with the broken skin of an infected person may spread the infection at this stage. The rash usually heals within several weeks or months. Other signs and symptoms may also occur, such as mild fever, fatigue, headache, sore throat, as well as patchy hair loss and swollen lymph glands throughout the body. These signs and symptoms may be mild and, like the chancre of primary syphilis, will disappear without treatment. The signs and symptoms of secondary syphilis may come and go over the next 1–2 years.

If untreated, syphilis may lapse into a latent stage during which the disease is no longer contagious and no signs or symptoms are present. Many people who are not treated will suffer no further consequences of the disease. Approximately one-third of those who have secondary syphilis, however, go on to develop the complications of late, or tertiary, syphilis, in which the bacteria damages the heart, eyes, brain, nervous system, bones, joints or almost any other part of the body. This stage can last for years, or even for decades. Late syphilis can result in mental illness, blindness, other neurological problems, heart disease and death.

Syphilis bacteria frequently invade the nervous system during the early stages of infection, and approximately 3–7% of individuals with untreated syphilis develop neurosyphilis (syphilis that has reached the central nervous system). Some patients with neurosyphilis are asymptomatic; others may have headache, stiff neck, fever that results from an inflammation of the lining of the brain and seizures. Patients whose blood vessels are affected may develop symptoms of stroke with resulting numbness, weakness or visual complaints. In some instances, the time from infection to developing neurosyphilis may be up to 20 years.

It is likely that an untreated pregnant woman with active syphilis will pass the infection to her unborn child. About 25% of these pregnancies result in stillbirth or neonatal death. Between 40% and 70% of these pregnancies will yield a syphilis-infected infant. Some infants with congenital syphilis may have signs and symptoms at birth, but most develop symptoms between 2 weeks and 3 months later. These signs and symptoms may include skin sores, rashes, fever, weakened or hoarse crying sounds, swollen liver and spleen, jaundice, anaemia and various deformities.

Prevention of syphilis includes abstinence, monogamy, use of condoms and dental dams, and regular pelvic examinations. Diagnosis of syphilis may include microscopic visualisation of the bacterium from chancre scrapings. Laboratory tests may include antigen or antibody testing. Syphilis is treated with antibiotics; however, development of antibiotic-resistant strains is a serious threat. Treatment will kill the syphilis bacterium and prevent further damage, but it will not repair damage already done.

Chlamydia

Chlamydia is caused by the coccus bacterium *Chlamydia trachomatis*. Between 2007 and 2008, the number of confirmed cases of chlamydia rose from 121 791 to 123 018 in the UK. Young people under 25 are most likely to be infected. Of all new chlamydia diagnoses made in 2008, 65% were in people aged between 16 and 24. The WHO estimates that more than 92 million chlamydial infections occur worldwide each year. Chlamydia is transmitted by sexual contact and during childbirth. It is known as a 'silent' disease because about three-quarters of infected women and about half of infected men are asymptomatic. If signs and symptoms do occur, they usually appear within 1–3 weeks after exposure. Women who have signs and symptoms may have an abnormal vaginal discharge, burning sensation when urinating, lower abdominal pain, low back pain, nausea, fever, pain during intercourse or bleeding between menstrual periods. Men with signs or symptoms may have a penile discharge, burning sensation when urinating, and burning and itching around the urethral orifice.

In women, untreated infection can spread into the uterus or Fallopian tubes and cause pelvic inflammatory disease (PID). This happens in up to 40% of women with untreated chlamydia. Complications among men are rare. Infection sometimes spreads to the epididymis, causing pain, fever and, infrequently, sterility. Rarely, genital chlamydial infection can cause arthritis that can be accompanied by skin lesions and inflammation of the eye and urethra known as Reiter's syndrome. In pregnant women, there is some evidence that untreated chlamydial infections can lead to premature delivery. Babies who are born to infected mothers can develop chlamydial infections in their eyes and respiratory tracts. Chlamydia is a leading cause of early infant pneumonia and conjunctivitis in newborns. Prevention of chlamydia includes abstinence, monogamy, use of condoms and dental dams, and regular pelvic examinations. Diagnosing chlamydia may include bacterial culture and antigen or antibody testing. Antibiotics are used to treat chlamydia.

Trichomoniasis

Trichomoniasis is caused by the protozoan *Trichomonas vaginalis*. Trichomoniasis is transmitted by sexual contact. Most men with trichomoniasis are asymptomatic; however, some men may temporarily have urethritis, epididymitis and prostatitis. Signs and symptoms usually appear in women within 5–28 days of exposure and may include a frothy, yellow–green vaginal discharge with a fishy odour, pain during intercourse and urination, and irritation and itching of the genital area.

Prevention of trichomoniasis includes monogamy and use of condoms. Diagnosis of trichomoniasis may include pelvic examination, microscopic visualisation of the protozoan, protozoal culture, laboratory test and pH test. Treatment of both partners with antiparasitic medication such as metronidazole is effective.

Genital herpes

Genital herpes is caused by the herpes simplex viruses type 1 (HSV-1) and type 2 (HSV-2). HSV-1 can cause genital herpes, but it more commonly causes infections of the mouth and lips, so-called fever blisters. Most genital herpes is caused by HSV-2. Genital HSV-2 infection is more common in women (approximately one out of four women) than in men (almost one out of five). This may be because of male-to-female transmission being more likely than female-to-male transmission.

Most people have no or minimal signs of HSV-1 or HSV-2 infection. Signs of HSV-1 and HSV-2 include one or more blisters on or around the genitals (Figure 11.5). The blisters break, leaving ulcers or tender sores that may take up to 4 weeks to heal. Other signs and symptoms during the first herpes outbreak may include fever, itching, burning or pain in the genital area, vaginal discharge, headache, muscle ache, pain during urination and swollen lymph nodes. The herpes virus becomes latent and can become active from time to time, causing an outbreak of blisters. Over time these recurrences usually decrease in frequency. Active genital herpes has very serious consequences during pregnancy, causing spontaneous abortion or premature delivery and infection of the newborn.

HSV-2 may be diagnosed by physical examination and history, viral culture and antibody testing. Prevention of HSV-1 and HSV-2 includes abstinence, monogamy, use of condoms and dental dams, and regular pelvic examinations. There is no treatment that can cure herpes, but antiviral medications can shorten outbreaks and make them less severe. Taking antiviral medications on a regular basis may stop outbreaks from occurring and may decrease transmission of the virus.

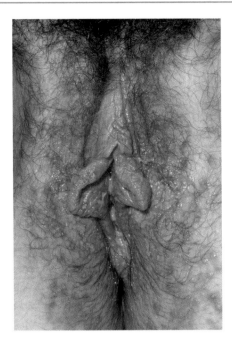

Figure 11.5 Genital herpes blisters as they appear on the labia.
(Mediascan)

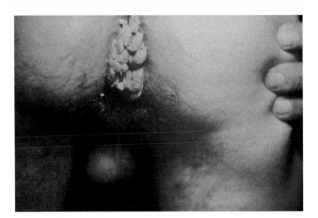

Figure 11.6 Genital warts.
(Courtesy of the CDC/Dr Wiesner, 1972)

Human papillomavirus and genital warts

Human papillomavirus (HPV) is one of the most common causes of STI in the world. At least 50% of sexually active men and women acquire genital HPV infection at some point in their lives. By age 50, at least 80% of women will have acquired genital HPV infection. The WHO estimates the prevalence of genital HPV infection in the world to be 440 million.

More than 100 different types of HPV exist; approximately 30 types are sexually transmitted and are classified as either low risk or high risk. Low-risk types cause genital warts, while the high-risk types may lead to cancer. A person who is infected with HPV but has no signs or symptoms can still spread HPV to a sexual partner. Most people who become infected with HPV will not have any signs or symptoms, and the immune system will clear the infection. Most women are diagnosed with HPV on the basis of abnormal Pap tests or an HPV DNA test.

Genital warts are the most easily recognised sign of genital HPV infection (Figure 11.6). However, many people have a genital HPV infection without genital warts. Genital warts may appear within weeks after sexual contact with an infected partner, or they might not develop for several months. Genital warts are single or multiple growths or bumps that appear in the genital area and are sometimes cauliflower-shaped. Warts can appear on the vulva, in or around the vagina or anus, on the cervix, and on the penis, scrotum, groin or thigh. Genital warts are diagnosed by visual inspection and can be removed by medications, electrocautery (burning), cryosurgery (freezing) and laser surgery.

Prevention of HPV includes use of condoms. There is no cure for HPV or genital warts. In September 2008 a national campaign to vaccinate girls aged 12–13 years against HPV began in the UK.

FEMALE AGE-RELATED DISEASES

In older women, pubic hair thins and greys and the external reproductive genitalia acquire a wrinkled and sagging appearance owing to a decrease in elasticity. Physical changes in the aging female include shrinking of internal reproductive organs, decrease in vaginal secretions and elasticity, and a decrease in breast tissue volume. The pH of vaginal secretions becomes more alkaline, making older women more susceptible to vaginal infections. Increased stimulation and lubrication may be necessary to facilitate sexual intercourse.

Menopause, the cessation of menstrual periods, is not a disease but is a physical change related to ageing. Menopause usually takes place between 45 and 55 years of age. As a woman ages, the ovaries produce less oestrogen and progesterone, causing cessation of ovulation and menstruation. Removal of the ovaries also causes menopause. Common physical signs and symptoms of menopause include hot flushes, night sweats, trouble sleeping, mood swings, trouble focusing, hair loss or thinning, facial hair growth and vaginal dryness. Menopause is diagnosed by signs and symptoms, elevated FSH and low oestrogen. Hormone therapy may help with menopause signs and symptoms; however, each woman and her physician must weigh the benefits and risks of hormone therapy.

Uterine prolapse is the condition of the uterus dropping or protruding downward into the vagina. This condition results from trauma to the fascia, muscle and pelvic ligaments during pregnancy and delivery, or atrophy of the pelvic floor muscles with age. The ligaments and muscles become so overstretched that they can no longer hold the uterus in place, so the uterus falls or sags downward. Symptoms include feelings of heaviness in the pelvic area, incontinence and lower back pain. Diagnosis of uterine prolapse may include pelvic examination and fluoroscopy. Treatment consists of strengthening the pelvic floor muscles (Kegel exercises), inserting a pessary into the vagina to support the uterus, or surgery.

Cystocele is a downward displacement of the urinary bladder into the vagina. This condition results from trauma to the fascia, muscle and pelvic ligaments during pregnancy and delivery, or atrophy of the pelvic floor muscles with age. Symptoms include pelvic pressure, urinary urgency and frequency, and incontinence. Diagnosis is made by pelvic examination. Treatment includes Kegel exercises, inserting a pessary into the vagina, or surgery.

A **rectocele** is the protrusion of the rectum into the posterior aspect of the vagina. This condition results from trauma to the fascia, muscle and pelvic ligaments during pregnancy and delivery, or atrophy of the pelvic floor muscles with age. Symptoms include discomfort, constipation and faecal incontinence. Diagnosis is made by pelvic examination. Treatment includes surgical repair of the posterior wall of the vagina.

MALE AGE-RELATED DISEASES

In older men, pubic hair thins and greys and the external reproductive genitalia acquire a wrinkled and sagging appearance owing to a decrease in elasticity. Testosterone levels decline gradually and the testes decrease in size. Sperm count is slightly reduced and prostate gland secretions are decreased.

A common problem in older males is enlargement of the prostate gland, or **benign prostatic enlargement (BPE)**. BPE affects more than 50% of men over age 60 and as many as 90% of men over age 70. Signs and symptoms of BPE often come on gradually and may include a need to get up during the night and urinate (**nocturia**), need to empty the bladder more frequently during the day, difficulty starting urine flow, dribbling after urination ends, and decrease in size and strength of the urine stream. If the bladder cannot be fully emptied, residual urine provides a medium for bacterial infection, and cystitis can develop. An imbalance of sex hormones frequently causes prostatic enlargement. The level of testosterone generally decreases with age, but oestrogen from the adrenal cortex continues to be secreted, changing the ratio of the two. Diagnosis of BPE may include DRE, urine analysis, PSA blood test (to exclude prostate cancer), ultrasound, and urine flow study, assessment of post-void residual volume, cystoscopy and X-ray.

Treatment options for BPE include watchful waiting, medication to shrink the prostate (5-alpha reductase inhibitors) or to make it easier to pass urine (alpha blockers), and surgery to remove the excess prostatic tissue (for example, transurethral resection of the prostate, or TURP, or variations of this procedure using ethanol, vaporisation or microwaves). BPE can cause urinary tract infections and therefore antibiotics may be required.

Prostate cancer

Prostate cancer is the leading cause of cancer death in British men. Each year approximately 35 000 men will be diagnosed with prostate cancer and 8500 will die. Prostate cancer is also discussed in Chapter 4.

The cause of prostate cancer is not known. Age is the strongest risk factor for prostate cancer; approximately two out of three prostate cancers are found in men over the age of 65. Other risk factors include race (prostate cancer is more common among Afro-Caribbean men than among men of other races and occurs less often in Asian men), and a family history of prostate cancer (having a father or brother with prostate cancer more than doubles a man's risk of developing this disease). The exact role of diet in prostate cancer is not clear, but studies have shown men who eat a lot of red meat or high fat dairy products seem to have a greater risk of developing prostate cancer.

Signs and symptoms include dull pain in the lower pelvic area; urgency of urination; difficulty starting urination; pain during urination; weak urine flow and dribbling; intermittent urine flow; a sensation that the bladder does not empty; frequent urination at night (nocturia); blood in the urine (haematuria); blood in semen (haematospermia); painful ejaculation; general pain in the lower back, hips and upper thighs; loss of appetite and weight; and persistent bone pain. Diagnosis is based on DRE, PSA blood test and biopsy. Because prostate cancer often grows very slowly (the cancer can double in size every 1–3 years), some men (especially those who are older or who have other major health problems) may never need treatment for their cancer. An approach called 'watchful waiting' may be suggested. This approach involves closely watching the cancer (DRE, PSA testing and possible biopsy). Treatment of prostate cancer depends on the stage of the disease, determined by PSA, Gleason score and clinical stage (Table 11.1).

Table 11.1 Assessment of prostate cancer risk.

Risk level	PSA result	Gleason score	Clinical stage
Low	<10 ng/ml	<6	T1-T2a
Intermediate	10-20 ng/ml	7	T2b-T2c
High	>20 ng/ml	8-10	T3-T4

Treatment options include:

- Watchful waiting
- Active surveillance (review every 6 months)
- Prostatectomy (surgical removal of the prostate)
- Brachytherapy (implanting radioactive seeds into the prostate)
- Conformal radiotherapy (external beam radiotherapy to the prostate)
- Cryotherapy (freezing the prostatic tumour)
- High-intensity focused ultrasound (HIFU).

Penile cancer

Penile cancer is an uncommon but devastating tumour for the individual. It is a relatively rare tumour, but has a higher incidence in African, Asian and South American countries. The increase in incidence in these countries is thought to be related to ambient temperature. In the UK, around 400 men are diagnosed with penile cancer each year (Cancer Research UK, 2009). Cancer of the penis has been attributed to chronic irritation of the glans penis caused by smegma, and phimosis which makes washing difficult if the prepuce is not easy to retract.

Treatment for penile cancer depends on the stage of the disease, and includes circumcision (to aid cleaning of the glans penis), chemotherapy and, if the tumour is advanced, partial or total penectomy (amputation of the penis).

Erectile dysfunction

Erectile dysfunction (ED) is defined as the persistent inability to attain and maintain a penile erection adequate for sexual performance. ED commonly has profound negative impact on quality of life in the patient (and his partner), resulting in poor self-image and self-confidence, and depression.

Current epidemiological evidence indicates that 8% of men in their forties report moderate or complete ED and this increases to 40% in men aged 60–69 years.

Historically, causes of ED have been divided into 'organic' and 'psychogenic' factors, although there is growing evidence linking ED and cardiovascular disease. Risk factors for both diseases include obesity, diabetes mellitus, physical inactivity, hypertension, dyslipidaemia and tobacco use. ED is now thought to be a harbinger of cardiovascular disease in younger men (<60 years).

The mean time between onset of ED and cardiac event is approximately 3 years, although if risk factors are modified this becomes longer. Men who initiate physical activity in midlife have a 70% reduced risk for ED relative to those who remain sedentary, and men who engage in regular physical exercise show a significantly lower incidence of ED over an 8-year follow-up period.

First-line pharmacological treatment for ED is with phosphodiesterase type 5 inhibitors (PDE5Is) unless contraindicated. There are currently three types of PDE5I, sildenafil citrate (Viagra), tadalafil (Cialis) and vardenafil (Levitra), that prevent breakdown of nitric oxide, a chemical messenger that promotes relaxation and opening of the blood vessels that supply the corpus cavernosa. Under the influence of nitric oxide, these vessels expand and stay dilated. Increased blood flow makes erectile tissue swell and compresses the veins that carry blood out of the penis, resulting in a full erection. Prior to January 2009 these medicines were only used 'on demand.' Since January 2009 tadalafil once daily has been available in 2.5 mg and 5 mg strengths. These take approximately 5–7 days to reach a steady state in the plasma and are reserved for men with a high demand for sexual activity (>2 per week) who have been successfully treated with a PDE5I already.

Both sildenafil and vardenafil have short half-lives compared with tadalafil. Although the overall efficacy between PDE5Is is similar, for some patients a longer acting PDE5I may reduce performance anxiety (and offer more encounters per tablet), and reduce planning for sexual activity.

Alternative treatments include urethral pellets, intracavernosal injections, vacuum devices, physiotherapy, counselling and penile implant.

Premature ejaculation

Premature ejaculation (PE) is defined as persistent or recurrent ejaculation with minimal stimulation that causes marked interpersonal distress; the estimated prevalence is 22.7%. PE has often been attributed to anxiety where the man ejaculates and experiences orgasm too quickly owing to poor control during sexual activity. Recently there is a growing consensus that there may be a neurobiological cause to PE. Treatment for PE includes careful assessment and examination as prostatitis can also cause the condition. The main treatment options include behavioural therapy (stop/start masturbation exercises, etc.), antidepressants (e.g. selective serotonin reuptake inhibitors) and local anaesthetics (e.g. eutetic mixture of local anaesthetic, EMLA, cream applied to the frenulum).

Delayed ejaculation

Delayed ejaculation can be divided into congenital anorgasmia (without orgasm), which may be related to negative behavioural messages about sexual activity, certain medications (e.g. selective serotonin reuptake inhibitors), excess alcohol consumption and recreational drugs. Treatment for delayed ejaculation includes behavioural therapy/psychotherapy. Alternative strategies include use of vibrotactile stimuli to bombard the pudendal nerve, increasing the amount of stimulation, which may also allow ejaculation.

Retrograde or absent ejaculation

Retrograde ejaculation, where semen is discharged into the bladder, can occur following prostate, bladder or testicular surgery, and is associated with diabetic neuropathy. There is no treatment available for retrograde ejaculation.

Resources

Cancerbackup/Macmillan: *http://www.cancerbackup.org.uk*

Cancer Research UK: *http://www.cancerresearchuk.org*

NHS Choices: *www.nhs.uk/conditions/*

Orchid (Fighting male cancer): *http://www.orchid-cancer.org.uk/*

Sexual Dysfunction Association: *www.sda.uk.net*

Cancer Research, CancerStats, UK Cervical Cancer Mortality Statistics (last updated May 2006): *http://info.cancerresearchuk.org/cancerstats/types/cervix/mortality*

European Society of Human Reproduction and Embryology: *http://healthcarea2z.org*

NHS Direct: *www.nhsdirect.nhs.uk/en.asp*

Clinical Knowledge Summaries: *www.cks.nhs.uk*

Royal College of Obstetrics and Gynaecology: *www.rcog.org.uk/womens-health/clinical-guidance/ management-premenstrual-syndrome-gree-top-48*

National Institute for Clinical Excellence: *www.nice.org.uk*

World Health Organization: *www.who.org*

Cirelli, N., Lebrun, P., Gueuning, C., Delogne-Desnoeck, J., Vanbellinghen, A.M., Graff, G., Meuris, S. (2001) *Physiological concentrations of albumin stimulate chorionic gonadotrophin and placental lactogen release from human term placental explants*. European Society of human reproduction and embryology.

Gaitan, H., Angel, E., Diaz, R., Parada, A., Sanchez, L., Vargas, C. (2002) Accuracy of five different diagnostic techniques in mild-moderate pelvic inflammatory disease. *Infectious diseases in Obstetrics and gynaecology*, 10:171-180.

Saidi, S.A., Holland, C.M., Charnock-Jones, D.S., Smith, S.K. (2006) In vitro and in vivo effects of the PPAR-alpha agonists fenofibrate and retinoic acid in endometrial cancer. Molecular cancer, 5:13. *http://molecular-cancer.com/content5/1/13.*

Santer, M., Warner, P., Wyke, S. (2005) A Scottish postal survey suggested that the prevailing clinical preoccupation with heavy periods does not reflect the epidemiology of reported symptoms and problems. *Journal of Clinical Epidemiology, 58(11):1206-1210.*

Royal College of Obstetrics and Gynaecology (2007) Management of premenstrual syndrome. Royal College of Obstetrics and Gynaecology guideline, December 2007.

CEMACH (2007) Saving Mothers' Lives: Reviewing maternal death to make motherhood safer - 2003-2005. The seventh report of the confidential enquiries into maternal death in the United Kingdom.

NICE (2008) Diabetes in pregnancy. Management of diabetes and its complications from pre-conception to prenatal period. NICE clinical guidelines 63. March 2008. London, National collaborating centre for women's and children's health. *www.nice.org.uk*

Department of Health (2007) NHS Cancer Reform Strategy. Department of Health, London. November, 2007. *www.dh.gov.uk/publications*

Office for National Statistics (2007) Mortality Statistics, England and Wales, 2007. *www.ons.gov.uk* Accessed 2009.

DISEASES AT A GLANCE Reproductive system

DISEASE OR DISORDER	AETIOLOGY	SIGNS AND SYMPTOMS	DIAGNOSIS	TREATMENT	PREVENTION/ LIFESPAN
Pelvic inflammatory disease	Infection	Lower abdominal pain, fever, unusual vaginal discharge that may have a foul odour, painful intercourse, painful urination and irregular menstrual bleeding	Physical examination, positive culture, ultrasound, laparoscopy	Antibiotics	Prevent STIs, early treatment of STIs
Cervical cancer	Human papillomavirus	Vaginal discharge and bleeding	Pelvic examination, Pap smear test, HPV DNA test, colposcopy	Surgery, radiation, chemotherapy	Avoid exposure to HPV, Gardasil
Endometrial cancer	Unknown	Vaginal bleeding, vaginal discharge, pelvic pain, weight loss	Pelvic examination, CA125 blood test, biopsy, hysteroscopy, D&C	Surgery, radiation, chemotherapy and hormone therapy	Use of oral contraceptives, controlling obesity and diabetes, healthy diet, exercise
Fibroid tumours of the uterus	Unknown	Asymptomatic or excessive vaginal bleeding, pelvic pressure, abdominal pain, abdominal enlargement, pain during intercourse	Pelvic examination, ultrasound, sonography, hysteroscopy	Uterine artery embolisation, focused ultrasound surgery, endometrial ablation, birth control pills, myomectomy, hysterectomy	Not preventable
Ovarian cancer	Unknown	Bloating, pelvic or abdominal pain, trouble eating or feeling full quickly, changes in urinary urgency or frequency	CT or MRI scan, ultrasound, laparoscopy, biopsy, CA125 blood test	Surgery, radiation, chemotherapy	Use of oral contraceptives, tubal ligation, hysterectomy, having children, breastfeeding
Breast cancer	Unknown	Lump or mass, swelling of all or part of the breast, skin irritation and dimpling, breast or nipple pain, nipple retraction, redness, scaliness or thickening of the nipple or breast skin, a discharge other than breast milk, swelling of a lymph node in the armpit	Breast exam, mammogram, ultrasound, biopsy	Surgery, radiation, chemotherapy, targeted therapy, hormone therapy	Avoiding alcohol, exercising regularly, maintaining a healthy body weight
Breast cysts	Unknown	Tiny, fluid-filled sacs in breast tissue	Breast examination, mammogram, ultrasound, fine needle aspiration	None, surgery	Not preventable
Fibrocystic changes	Unknown	Lumpy breasts	Breast examination, mammogram, ultrasound, biopsy	None, supportive bra, over-the-counter pain relievers	Not preventable
Fibroadenoma	Unknown	Solid, firm tumour, usually painless	Breast examination, mammogram, ultrasound, fine needle aspiration, biopsy	None, surgery	Not preventable

DISEASES AT A GLANCE Reproductive system (continued)

DISEASE OR DISORDER	AETIOLOGY	SIGNS AND SYMPTOMS	DIAGNOSIS	TREATMENT	PREVENTION/ LIFESPAN
Amenorrhoea	Primary – chromosomal abnormalities, problems with the hypothalamus, pituitary disease, lack of reproductive organs or structural abnormality of the vagina. Secondary – pregnancy, contraceptives, breastfeeding, stress, medication, chronic illness, hormone imbalance, low body weight, excessive exercise, thyroid disorders, pituitary tumour, uterine scarring, premature menopause	No menstrual period	Pregnancy test, pelvic examination, blood test to check hormone levels, progestin challenge test	If needed, lifestyle changes related to weight, physical activity or stress level, amenorrhoea caused by thyroid or pituitary disorders may be treated with medications	Maintaining a sensible exercise programme, maintaining a normal weight, eating a healthy diet, avoiding excessive alcohol consumption, not smoking, finding healthy outlets for stress
Dysmenorrhoea	Primary – prostaglandins. Secondary – PID, use of an IUD, fibroid tumours, endometriosis	Cramping, dull to severe pelvic, lower back pain that may radiate to other areas	Pelvic examination, ultrasound, laparoscopy, hysteroscopy	Antibiotics, oral contraceptive therapy, non-steroidal anti-inflammatory medication, surgery	Not using an IUD, avoid risk factors for PID, early diagnosis and treatment of STIs
Menorrhagia	Hormonal imbalance, fibroid tumours, lack of ovulation, use of an IUD, pregnancy complications, medications (anti-inflammatory and anticoagulants), PID, thyroid disorders, endometriosis, liver or kidney disease, unknown	Excessive or prolonged bleeding during menstruation	Pelvic examination, Pap test, blood tests, biopsy, ultrasound	Iron supplements, non-steroidal anti-inflammatory drugs, oral contraceptives, progesterone, D&C, endometrial ablation or resection, hysterectomy	Not using an IUD, avoid risk factors for PID, early diagnosis and treatment of STIs
Metrorrhagia	Hormonal imbalance, endometriosis, infection, miscarriage, ectopic pregnancy, cancer, IUD use, thyroid disorders, diabetes, blood clotting disorders	Bleeding between menstrual periods, extreme irregularity of menstrual cycle	Record of menstrual cycle, pelvic examination, blood tests, hysteroscopy, X-ray, biopsy, ultrasound	Hormone therapy, antibiotics, surgery, medication	Not using an IUD
Premenstrual syndrome	Unknown but hormonal changes trigger the symptoms	Breast swelling and tenderness, acne, bloating and weight gain, headache or joint pain, food cravings, irritability, mood swings, crying spells, fatigue, trouble sleeping, anxiety, depression	Symptoms, when symptoms occur, and how much the symptoms interfere with the patient's life	Over-the-counter pain relievers, avoiding salt, caffeine and alcohol, exercising, eating healthy foods and getting enough sleep, support groups, stress management, contraceptives	High intake of calcium and vitamin D

DISEASES AT A GLANCE Reproductive system (continued)

DISEASE OR DISORDER	AETIOLOGY	SIGNS AND SYMPTOMS	DIAGNOSIS	TREATMENT	PREVENTION/ LIFESPAN
Premenstrual dysphoric disorder	Unknown but hormonal changes trigger the symptoms	Feelings of sadness or despair, possibly suicidal thoughts, feelings of tension or anxiety, panic attacks, mood swings, crying, lasting irritability or anger that affects other people, disinterest in daily activities and relationships, trouble thinking or focusing, tiredness or low energy, food cravings or binge eating, having trouble sleeping, feeling out of control; physical symptoms, such as bloating, breast tenderness, headaches, joint or muscle pain	Symptoms, when symptoms occur, and how much they interfere with the patient's life	PMS treatments plus antidepressants	Plenty of exercise and rest, eating a well balanced diet, managing stress
Endometriosis	Unknown	Pelvic pain, diarrhoea or constipation, abdominal bloating, menorrhagia, metrorrhagia, fatigue	Laparoscopy	Pain relievers, hormone therapy, surgery	Not preventable
Ectopic pregnancy	PID, surgery of the Fallopian tubes, previous ectopic pregnancy, birth defects of the Fallopian tubes, endometriosis, complications of a ruptured appendix, scarring caused by previous pelvic surgery or unknown	Lower abdominal or pelvic pain, mild cramping on one side of the pelvis, amenorrhoea, metrorrhagia, breast tenderness, nausea, low back pain, severe, sharp and sudden pain in the lower abdominal area, feeling faint or fainting, referred pain to the shoulder area, shock	Signs and symptoms, pelvic examination, ultrasound, measurement of hCG levels	Surgery, medication	In the Fallopian tubes – avoid risk factors for PID, early diagnosis and treatment of STIs. Outside the Fallopian tubes – usually not preventable
Spontaneous abortion or miscarriage	Genetic abnormality of the fetus, infection, physical problems in the mother, hormonal factors, immune responses, diabetes, thyroid disease	Low back pain or abdominal pain that is dull, sharp or cramping, vaginal bleeding, tissue or clot-like material discharged from the vagina	Pelvic examination, hCG levels	Medication, surgery	Not preventable
Pre-eclampsia	Unknown	Mild pre-eclampsia – high blood pressure, and the presence of protein in the urine. Severe pre-eclampsia – also includes headaches, blurred vision, inability to tolerate bright light, fatigue, nausea, vomiting, urinating small amounts, pain in the upper right abdomen, shortness of breath and tendency to bruise easily	Blood pressure, urine protein levels	Delivery of the baby, rest, frequent monitoring of blood pressure and urine, limiting salt, drinking water, blood pressure medication	Healthy weight before pregnancy, taking multivitamins
Gestational diabetes mellitus	Pregnancy	Maternal hypertension, polyhydramnios, excessive weight gain during the last 6 months of pregnancy, a fetus large-for-gestational-age	Glucose tolerance test	Regular blood glucose monitoring, dietary control of blood glucose levels, weight control, insulin injections	Eating a healthy diet, maintaining a healthy weight, not gaining too much weight during pregnancy, regular exercise

DISEASES AT A GLANCE Reproductive system (continued)

DISEASE OR DISORDER	AETIOLOGY	SIGNS AND SYMPTOMS	DIAGNOSIS	TREATMENT	PREVENTION/ LIFESPAN
Prostatitis	Not always known; may be infection	Acute bacterial prostatitis – fever and chills, flu-like symptoms, pain in the prostate gland, lower back or groin, urinary problems, including increased urinary urgency and frequency, difficulty or pain when urinating, inability to empty the bladder completely, blood-tinged urine, painful ejaculation. Chronic bacterial prostatitis – frequent and urgent need to urinate, pain or burning sensation when urinating, pelvic pain, excessive urination during the night, pain in the lower back and genital area, difficulty starting urination or diminished urine flow, occasional blood in semen or urine, painful ejaculation, slight fever, recurring bladder infections. Non-bacterial prostatitis – similar to chronic bacterial without fever	DRE, bacterial cultures	Categories 1 and 2 – pain relievers, antibiotics. Category 3 – alpha blockers, pain relievers, muscle relaxants. Category 4 – may not require treatment	Practise good hygiene, adequate hydration, seek early treatment for infections
Epididymitis	Infection, anatomical abnormalities in the urinary tract, catheter	Testicular swelling on one or both sides, scrotal pain ranging from mild to severe, tenderness in one or both testicles, tenderness in the groin, painful urination, painful intercourse or ejaculation, fever, penile discharge, blood in the semen	Physical examination, DRE, blood and urine tests, bacterial culture, ultrasound, nuclear scan of the testicles	Antibiotics	Abstinence, monogamy, use of condoms and dental dams, early treatment for infections
Orchitis	Infection, injury	Testicular swelling on one or both sides, pain ranging from mild to severe, tenderness in one or both testicles, nausea and vomiting, fever, penile discharge, prostate enlargement and tenderness	Physical examination, DRE, blood and urine tests, bacterial cultures, ultrasound, nuclear imaging of the testicles	Pain relievers, non-steroidal anti-inflammatory drugs, bed rest, elevation and applying cold packs to the scrotum, antibiotics	Vaccinating against mumps, abstinence, monogamy, use of condoms and dental dams, and wearing a protective cup over the genitals to guard against mechanical injury
Cryptorchidism	Abnormal testicular development	Inability to feel one or both testicles	Palpating the scrotum and abdomen, hormone testing	Hormone therapy, surgery	Not preventable
Testicular cancer	Unknown	Lump on a testicle that is often painless but slightly uncomfortable, testicular enlargement or swelling, sensation of heaviness or aching in the lower abdomen or scrotum	Physical examination, ultrasound, blood tests	Surgery, chemotherapy, radiation	Correcting cryptorchidism

DISEASES AT A GLANCE Reproductive system (continued)

DISEASE OR DISORDER	AETIOLOGY	SIGNS AND SYMPTOMS	DIAGNOSIS	TREATMENT	PREVENTION/LIFESPAN
Gonorrhoea	*Neisseria gonorrhoeae*	Men – asymptomatic, burning sensation when urinating, or a white, yellow or green discharge from the penis, painful or swollen testicles. Women – asymptomatic, painful or burning sensation when urinating, increased vaginal discharge or vaginal bleeding between periods	Urine sample, bacterial culture, Gram stain	Antibiotics	Use of condoms/barrier methods of contraception
Syphilis	*Treponema pallidum*	Primary – chancre. Secondary – rash, mild fever, fatigue, headache, sore throat, as well as patchy hair loss, swollen lymph nodes throughout the body, illness, blindness. Neurosyphilis – asymptomatic, others may have headache, stiff neck, fever that results from an inflammation of the lining of the brain, seizures, stroke symptoms. Congenital syphilis – skin sores, rashes, fever, weakened or hoarse crying sounds, swollen liver and spleen, jaundice, anaemia, various deformities	Microscopic visualisation, antigen and antibody testing	Antibiotics	Use of condoms/barrier methods of contraception
Chlamydia	*Chlamydia trachomatis*	May be asymptomatic. Women – abnormal vaginal discharge, burning sensation when urinating, lower abdominal pain, low back pain, nausea, fever, pain during intercourse, bleeding between menstrual periods. Men – penile discharge, burning sensation when urinating, burning and itching around the urethral orifice	Bacterial culture, antigen or antibody testing	Antibiotics	Use of condoms/barrier methods of contraception
Trichomoniasis	*Trichomonas vaginalis*	Men – most are asymptomatic, some have urethritis, epididymitis, prostatitis. Women – frothy, yellow-green vaginal discharge with a fishy odour, pain during intercourse and urination, irritation and itching of the genital area	Pelvic examination, microscopic visualisation, culture, laboratory and pH test	Antiparasitic medication	Use of condoms/barrier methods of contraception
Genital herpes	Herpes simplex type 1 and 2	Blisters	Physical examination and history, culture, antibody testing	Antiviral medication	Use of condoms/barrier methods of contraception
Human papillomavirus and genital warts	Human papillomavirus	Asymptomatic, genital warts	Warts – physical examination. HPV – abnormal Pap tests, HPV DNA test	Warts – medication, electrocautery, cryosurgery, laser surgery	Use of condoms/barrier methods of contraception

DISEASES AT A GLANCE Reproductive system (continued)

DISEASE OR DISORDER	AETIOLOGY	SIGNS AND SYMPTOMS	DIAGNOSIS	TREATMENT	PREVENTION/ LIFESPAN
Menopause	Aging	Hot flushes, night sweats, trouble sleeping, mood swings, trouble focusing, hair loss or thinning, facial hair growth, vaginal dryness	Signs and symptoms, elevated FSH, low oestrogen	Hormone therapy	Occurs with aging
Uterine prolapse	Pregnancy, childbirth, aging	Feelings of heaviness in pelvic area, urinary stress, incontinence, lower back pain	Pelvic examination, fluoroscopy	Kegel exercises, pessary in the vagina, surgery	Occurs with aging
Cystocele	Pregnancy, childbirth, aging	Pelvic pressure, urinary urgency and frequency, incontinence	Pelvic examination	Kegel exercises, pessary in the vagina, surgery	Occurs with aging
Rectocele	Pregnancy, childbirth, aging	Discomfort, constipation, faecal incontinence	Pelvic examination	Surgery	Occurs with aging
Benign prostatic enlargement	Aging, hormone imbalance	Need to get up during the night and urinate, need to empty the bladder often during the day, difficulty starting urine flow, dribbling after urination ends, and decrease in size and strength of the urine stream	DRE, urine analysis, PSA blood test, ultrasound, urine flow study, cystoscopy, X-ray	May not be needed, antibiotics, medications, destroying excess prostate tissue with microwaves or ultrasound, surgery	Occurs with aging
Prostate cancer	Unknown	Dull pain in the lower pelvic area, urgency of urination, difficulty starting urination, pain during urination, week urine flow and dribbling, intermittent urine flow, a sensation that the bladder does not empty, frequent urination at night, blood in the urine, painful ejaculation, general pain in the lower back, hips and upper thighs, loss of appetite and weight, persistent bone pain	DRE, PSA blood test, biopsy	Watchful waiting, surgery, radiation, hormone therapy	Occurs with aging
Erectile dysfunction	Age, psychological, cardiovascular disease, diabetes, obesity, lack of physical activity, surgical complications, urological disorders, medications, premature ejaculation, drug abuse, alcoholism	Inability to achieve and maintain an erection sufficient for sexual intercourse	Medical, sexual and psychosocial history, physical examination, laboratory tests	Medication, lifestyle changes, medication/ counselling	Occurs with aging

INTERACTIVE EXERCISES

Cases for critical thinking

1. A young woman reports severe pelvic pain. Laparoscopic examination found endometrial tissue on the uterine wall and ovaries. Name this disease. What is the cause? What treatments are available?

2. A 16-year-old sexually active woman complains of a green, frothy, fishy-smelling vaginal discharge. What is the possible diagnosis? What test would you perform? What treatment is available?

3. A 63-year-old male says he gets up several times a night to urinate but has difficulty getting urination started. A digital rectal examination reveals an enlarged prostate gland. What are the possible diagnoses? What tests would you perform? What treatment is available?

4. A woman has been infected with genital herpes type 2. Describe how she can reduce the risk of transmission of the infection to her sexual partner.

5. Why do doctors sometimes recommend watchful waiting for prostate cancer?

6. When baby Christopher was born, the paediatrician discovered that his left testicle had not descended into the scrotum. Name this disease. What complications may arise?

Multiple choice

1. Which is the most common tumour among females?
   a. ovarian cysts
   b. breast cancer
   c. uterine fibroids
   d. cervical cancer

2. Syphilis is caused by _____
   a. human papillomavirus
   b. herpes virus
   c. *Trichomonas vaginalis*
   d. *Treponema pallidum*

3. Which statement is *false* about syphilis?
   a. Primary syphilis chancres heal after a few weeks.
   b. A fetus can be infected and born with major physical and mental abnormalities.
   c. Syphilis is only transmitted by sexual contact.
   d. Secondary syphilis is characterised by a non-itching rash.

4. Which of the following can lead to pelvic inflammatory disease?
   a. chlamydia   b. cystitis
   c. prostatitis   d. herpes

5. Excessive or prolonged bleeding during menstruation is known as _____
   a. dysmenorrhoea   b. amenorrhoea
   c. metrorrhagia   d. menorrhagia

6. Protrusion of the rectum into the posterior aspect of the vagina is known as _____
   a. uterine prolapse   b. cystocele
   c. rectocele   d. sepsis

7. Painful or difficult menses is
   _____
   a. amenorrhoea   b. dysmenorrhoea
   c. menorrhoea   d. metrorrhagia

8. Failure of the testes to descend from the abdominal cavity is _____
   a. orchitis   b. prostatitis
   c. cryptorchidism   d. epididymitis

9. Finger-like projections at the outer ends of the Fallopian tubes are known as
   _____
   a. hymen
   b. fimbriae
   c. Graafian follicles
   d. Bartholin's glands

10. Laboratory diagnosis of pregnancy is based on the presence of what hormone?

    a. progesterone
    b. oestrogen
    c. human chorionic gonadotrophic hormone
    d. luteinising hormone

11. Which of the following hormones increases in pregnancy and are hence interpreted as 'supporting pregnancy?'

    a. Oxytocin   b. Progesterone
    c. Prolactin   d. Testosterone

12. Both the male and female gonads originate from _____

    a. Gametes
    b. Ovary
    c. Testis
    d. Ovotestis

13. _____ marks the onset of menstruation.

    a. Menses   b. Menarche
    c. Menopause   d. Menorrhagia

True or false

_____ **1.** Pelvic inflammatory disease can lead to infertility.

_____ **2.** The Pap test detects endometriosis.

_____ **3.** The most important risk factor for cervical cancer is infection by the human papillomavirus.

_____ **4.** Herpes simplex type 2 virus causes syphilis.

_____ **5.** Benign prostatic hyperplasia affects more than 50% of men over age 60.

_____ **6.** Benign breast conditions are common.

_____ **7.** Pre-eclampsia is a disease that occurs during pregnancy.

_____ **8.** The only certain means of diagnosing endometriosis is laparoscopy.

_____ **9.** The most common site for ectopic pregnancy is the ovary.

_____ **10.** The cause of PMS is known.

Fill-ins

1. The site of sperm development is the _____.

2. _____ is inflammation of the testes.

3. The most frequently reported bacterial STI is _____.

4. The _____ surrounds the upper portion of the male urethra.

5. _____ is inflammation of the prostate gland.

6. _____ is an STI caused by a protozoan.

7. The herpes type _____ virus usually causes cold sores; the herpes type _____ virus causes genital herpes.

8. _____ is downward displacement of the urinary bladder into the vagina.

9. _____ is the cessation of menstrual periods.

10. _____ is the inability to achieve and maintain an erection sufficient for sexual intercourse.

Labelling exercise

Use the blank lines below to label the following image.

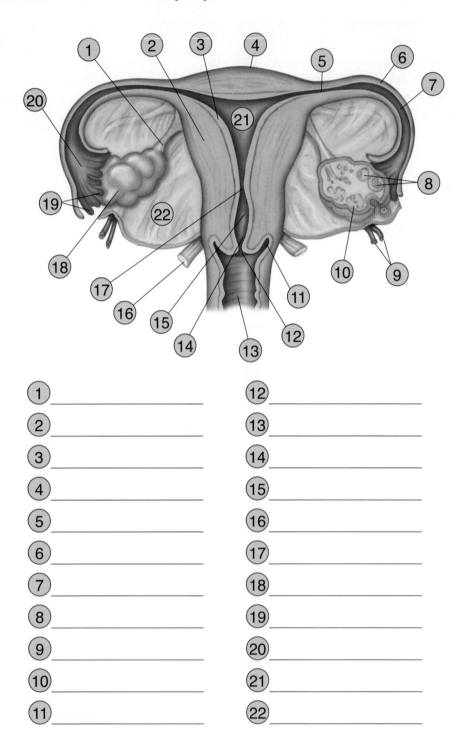

1 _____		12 _____	
2 _____		13 _____	
3 _____		14 _____	
4 _____		15 _____	
5 _____		16 _____	
6 _____		17 _____	
7 _____		18 _____	
8 _____		19 _____	
9 _____		20 _____	
10 _____		21 _____	
11 _____		22 _____	

12 DISEASES OF THE ENDOCRINE SYSTEM

Photomicrograph of a pituitary adenoma.
(© O.J. Staats/Custom Medical Stock Photo)

Fact or fiction ?

The number of patients with type 2 diabetes is expected to increase dramatically and strain the healthcare system worldwide.

Fact: The worldwide prevalence of DM has risen dramatically over the past two decades. The prevalence of type 2 DM is expected to rise more rapidly in the future because of increasing obesity and reduced activity levels. The number of diabetic patients will reach 300 million in 2025. More than 97% of these patients will have type 2 diabetes. The projected increase in the number of diabetic patients will strain the capabilities of healthcare providers worldwide (International Diabetes Federation, 2001).

Learning objectives

After studying this chapter, you should be able to:

✚ Name the major glands of the endocrine system and identify where they are located in the body

✚ Identify the hormones secreted from each endocrine gland and explain their normal functions

✚ Describe the consequences of hyposecretion and hypersecretion of endocrine hormones on various glands and organs

✚ Identify the aetiology, signs and symptoms, diagnostic tests and treatment for type 1 and type 2 diabetes mellitus

✚ Describe the acute and chronic complications of diabetes

✚ Identify age-related changes in endocrine function

Disease chronicle

Diabetes

Ancient Hindu writings record distinctive signs of diabetes thousands of years ago: large volumes of urine, to which ants and flies were attracted; intense thirst; and a wasting of the body. No treatment or cure existed for this mysterious ailment, which killed children and whose complications crippled survivors. It was not until the late nineteenth century, when diabetes was observed in dogs whose pancreas had been removed experimentally, that the disease could be linked to a specific organ. The key functional component of the pancreas was eventually isolated and identified as the protein hormone insulin. Today, instead of treating patients with insulin extracted from dog pancreas, human insulin is synthesised using recombinant DNA technology. Early diagnosis, treatment and effective management have lengthened and greatly improved the lives of diabetics. However, no cure for diabetes exists.

INTRODUCTION

The endocrine system is responsible for the production, storage and secretion of hormones, which are chemical messengers that regulate vital human functions. The major organs of the endocrine system include the pituitary, thyroid, parathyroid glands and the thymus; pancreatic islets; adrenal glands; and gonads (Figure 12.1). Endocrine glands communicate with other organs via complex networks involving the central and peripheral nervous system, hormones, **cytokines** (or regulators of the immune response) and growth factors. Endocrine hormones affect many aspects of body functions, including growth, development, energy metabolism, muscle and fat distribution, sexual development, fluid and electrolyte balance, inflammation and immune responses. Endocrine functions can be affected by anomalies in the primary gland responsible for producing a particular hormone, defects in circulating concentrations of stimulating hormones or releasing hormones, or anomalies in both the primary gland and the target or receiving organ. The result of endocrine abnormalities is either hypofunction or hyperfunction of a gland, hormone or a target organ.

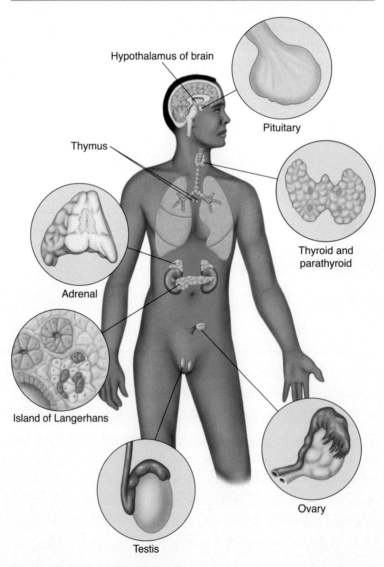

Figure 12.1 The endocrine glands.

Impaired function of an endocrine gland can occur for a variety of reasons. Congenital defects can result in the absence of or impaired development of the endocrine gland or enzymes needed for hormone synthesis can be affected. The gland may be destroyed by **ischaemia** or a disruption in blood flow, infection, inflammation, autoimmune diseases or neoplastic growth. There may be a decline in function with age, or the gland may atrophy as the result of drug therapy or for unknown reasons. Some endocrine-deficient states are associated with receptor defect. Hormone receptors may be absent, receptor binding may be impaired or cellular responsiveness to endocrine hormones may be impaired.

Hormones are released from endocrine glands into the bloodstream, where they affect activity in cells (known as target cells) at distant sites. Some hormones affect the whole body and others act only on target or distant organs. Most hormones are composed of proteins or chains of amino acids; others are steroids or fatty substances derived from cholesterol.

Most glandular activity is controlled by the pituitary, which is sometimes called the master gland. The pituitary itself is controlled by the hypothalamus.

The body is conservative and secretes hormones only as needed. For example, insulin is secreted when the blood sugar level rises. Another hormone, glucagon, works antagonistically to insulin and is released when the blood sugar level falls below normal. Hormones are potent chemicals, so their circulating levels must be carefully controlled. When the level of a hormone is adequate, its further release is stopped. This type of control is called a **negative feedback** mechanism. Its importance becomes clearer as specific diseases of the endocrine system are considered.

Overactivity or underactivity of a gland is the malfunction that most commonly causes endocrine diseases. If a gland secretes an excessive amount of its hormone, it is hyperactive. This condition is sometimes caused by a hypertrophied gland or by a glandular tumour.

A gland that fails to secrete its hormone or secretes an inadequate amount is hypoactive. This condition may be caused by disease or tumour, or it may be caused by trauma, surgery or radiation. A gland that has decreased in size and consequently is secreting inadequately is said to be atrophied. Each endocrine gland is discussed, with an emphasis on normal function and importance. The diseases caused by hypoactivity and hyperactivity of each gland are then explained.

STRUCTURE AND FUNCTION OF THE PITUITARY GLAND

The pituitary gland is a pea-sized organ located at the base of the brain. The gland has an anterior lobe called the **adenohypophysis** and a posterior lobe called the **neurohypophysis**. A stalk called the **infundibulum** connects the pituitary gland to the floor of the hypothalamus. The pituitary gland is regulated by the hypothalamus and feedback control mechanisms in relation to blood concentrations of circulating hormones (Figure 12.2).

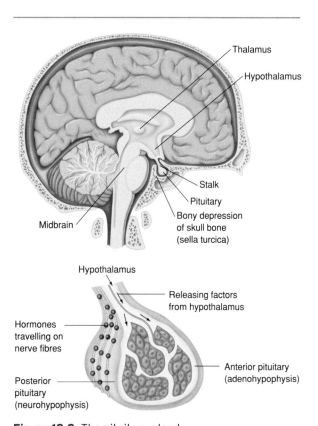

Figure 12.2 The pituitary gland.

HORMONES OF THE ANTERIOR PITUITARY

Growth hormone

Growth hormone (GH; also called somatotropin) affects all parts of the body by promoting growth and development of the tissues. Before puberty, it stimulates the growth of long bones, increasing the child's height. Soft tissues – organs such as the liver, heart and kidneys – also increase in size and develop under the influence of growth hormone. After adolescence, growth hormone is secreted in lesser amounts but continues to function in promoting tissue replacement and repair.

Growth hormone secretion is controlled by complex interactions between the hypothalamus and peripheral organs. Growth hormone releasing hormone (GHRH) is a hypothalamic hormone that stimulates growth hormone synthesis and release. Somatotropin release inhibiting factor (SRIF) is also synthesised in the hypothalamus and inhibits growth hormone secretion. Peripheral hormones that regulate growth hormone include insulin-like growth factors, glucocorticoids and oestrogen. Insulin-like growth factors and glucocorticoids feed back to the hypothalamus to inhibit growth hormone, whereas oestrogen induces growth hormone release.

Thyroid stimulating hormone

The thyroid gland regulates metabolism, the rate at which the body produces and uses energy. The anterior pituitary controls secretion of thyroid hormone by the thyroid gland. The pituitary hormone that stimulates the thyroid gland is thyroid stimulating hormone (TSH; also called thyrotropin). In the absence of TSH, the thyroid gland stops functioning.

Adrenocorticotropic hormone

The anterior pituitary also regulates the adrenal glands. The adrenal glands have an inner region, the

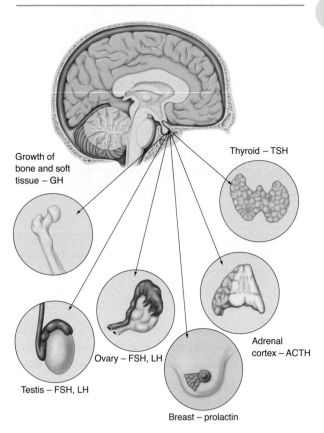

Growth of bone and soft tissue – GH

Thyroid – TSH

Testis – FSH, LH

Ovary – FSH, LH

Breast – prolactin

Adrenal cortex – ACTH

Figure 12.3 Anterior pituitary and its target organs.

The anterior pituitary produces six major hormones: prolactin, growth hormone, adrenocorticotropic hormone (ACTH), luteinising hormone (LH), follicle stimulating hormone (FSH) and thyroid stimulating hormone (TSH). Each of these pituitary hormones elicits a response in target organs (Figure 12.3). The hormones of the posterior pituitary or neurohypophysis are produced in the hypothalamus. The neurohypophysis stores and releases two important hormones: antidiuretic hormone (ADH), also known as vasopressin, and oxytocin. Vasopressin stimulates the elevation of blood pressure by regulating the reabsorption of water in the kidney tubules. The target organ of oxytocin is the smooth muscle of the uterus, where it stimulates uterine contractions, and the mammary glands, where it stimulates milk letdown. Table 12.1 lists the hormones of the pituitary gland, their target organs and the primary effects.

Table 12.1 Hormones of pituitary gland, target organs and primary effects.

Hormone	Target organ	Physiological effects
Anterior lobe		
Follicle stimulating hormone (FSH)	Ovary	In females: stimulates the growth of Graafian follicles of the ovary and secretion of oestradiol
	Testes	In males: stimulates the epithelium of the seminiferous tubules and subsequent spermatogenesis (sperm formation)
Luteinising hormone (LH)	Corpus luteum	In females: triggers ovulation; stimulates production of progesterone by the ovaries
	Interstitial cells of the testes	In males: stimulates production of testosterone
Prolactin	Female mmmary gland	Stimulates milk production after birth
Growth hormone (somatotropin)	All body tissues	Increases the synthesis of protein and promotes the growth of bone and tissues
Adrenocorticotropic hormone (ACTH)	Adrenal cortex, skin, liver and mammary glands	Stimulates the production of corticosteroids; increases metabolism and glycogen storage in the liver
Thyroid stimulating hormone (TSH)	Thyroid gland	Stimulates the production of thyroid hormone
Posterior lobe		
Vasopressin or antidiuretic hormone (ADH)	Smooth muscle of the arterioles and the kidney tubules	Constricts blood vessels, increases blood pressure; stimulates reabsorption of water by the kidney
Oxytocin	Uterus and the mammary glands	Stimulates contraction of the uterus; secretion of milk or 'milk letdown' by the mammary glands

adrenal medulla, and an outer region, the adrenal cortex. The cortex is controlled by the anterior pituitary and the hormone, adrenocorticotropic hormone (ACTH).

Gonadotropins

The anterior pituitary regulates sexual development and function by means of hormones known as the gonadotropins. These are not sex hormones, but they affect the sex organs, the gonads. They are follicle stimulating hormone (FSH), luteinising hormone (LH) and prolactin. These gonadotropins regulate the menstrual cycle and secretion of male and female hormones.

HORMONES OF THE POSTERIOR PITUITARY

Oxytocin

Oxytocin targets the uterus and the mammary glands (breasts). It is a strong stimulant of uterine contractions and is significant only during childbirth and in breastfeeding women.

Antidiuretic hormone (vasopressin)

ADH targets the kidney tubules, which respond by reabsorbing more water from the filtrate and returning it to the circulation. Consequently less urine is produced and blood volume is maintained or increased.

DIAGNOSTIC PROCEDURES FOR ENDOCRINE DISEASES

Indications of pituitary hyperactivity or hypoactivity can be confirmed by serum assays. GH levels can detect hyperpituitarism (gigantism and/or acromegaly) and hypopituitarism (dwarfism). TSH assay is useful in confirming primary hypothyroidism or hyperthyroidism. Activity of the posterior pituitary can be evaluated by the water deprivation and vasopressin test. A urine specimen is taken after controlled water deprivation and a blood sample is drawn. Dilute urine and high osmotic pressure in the blood indicate that water is not being absorbed by the kidney tubules. If vasopressin injection corrects the massive polyuria, diabetes insipidus is confirmed.

Diseases of the thyroid gland are diagnosed on the basis of the levels of the serum thyroid hormones, **tri-iodothyronine (T_3)** and **thyroxine (T_4)** and by the serum level of TSH. An elevated TSH indicates low T_4 function. A low TSH indicates an excess of T_4 caused by a functioning adenoma or carcinoma. A thyroid scan provides visualisation of the thyroid gland after administration of radioactive iodine. It is usually recommended after discovery of a mass, an enlarged gland or an asymmetric goitre. Thyroid ultrasonography evaluates characteristics of thyroid nodules and distinguishes between solid or cystic masses in the gland.

Diagnostic tests for parathyroid gland activity measure parathyroid hormone and calcium levels in the blood and can detect hyperparathyroidism.

Adrenal gland activity can be evaluated by the level of plasma cortisol from the adrenal cortex. Abnormal levels indicate hypersecretion (Cushing's syndrome) or hyposecretion (Addison's disease). Urine tests measure steroid level and detect hyperactivity of the gland.

A fasting blood glucose test helps to detect diabetes mellitus and evaluate the clinical status of diabetic patients. An oral glucose tolerance test challenges the ability of the pancreas to secrete insulin in response to large doses of glucose. A glycated haemoglobin test, also called 'haemoglobin A1c,' is an important blood test that is used to determine how well diabetes is controlled. The test provides an average of blood glucose measurements over a 6–12-week period and is used in conjunction with a patient's home blood glucose monitoring devices.

DISEASES OF THE ANTERIOR PITUITARY

Anterior pituitary insufficiency

Inherited disorders, malignant tumours, inadequate secretion of hormones, inflammation and vascular changes of the pituitary gland can result in hypofunction or insufficiency of the pituitary gland. The manifestations of hypopituitarism depend on which hormones are lost and the extent of the hormone deficiency. Growth hormone deficiency causes growth disorders in children and leads to abnormal body composition in adults. FSH and LH deficiency causes menstrual disorders, infertility and decreased sexual function in women, and loss of secondary sexual characteristics in men. TSH deficiency causes growth retardation in children and features of hypothyroidism in both adults and children. ACTH deficiency leads to decreased production of adrenal cortical hormones.

Pituitary dwarfism

Pituitary dwarfism results from a growth hormone deficiency. Growth retardation may become evident in infancy and persists throughout childhood. The child's growth curve, which is usually plotted on a standardised growth chart, may range from flat, indicating no growth, to shallow, indicating minimal growth. Normal puberty may or may not occur, depending on the degree to which the pituitary gland can produce sufficient hormone levels other than growth hormone. Some cases are due to a tumour known as a craniopharyngioma. This is a rare tumour with an overall incidence of about 0.5–2 per 100 000 per year in the UK. A rare form of this disease may be caused by an inherited autosomal recessive gene. Similar to pituitary insufficiency, pituitary dwarfism may also be associated with deficiencies in all pituitary hormones.

Symptoms of this disorder include slowed growth before the age of 5 years, absent or delayed sexual development, and short stature and height for age. Confirmation of the diagnosis is made by evaluation of blood pituitary hormone levels. Hand X-rays help determine bone age and cranial X-rays are useful for identifying any abnormalities of the skull that may contribute to this condition. MRI scans provide detailed images of the pituitary and the hypothalamus.

Replacement therapy with injections of growth hormone is currently used to treat children with pituitary dwarfism who have isolated growth hormone deficiency. In cases of pituitary insufficiency, other associated hormone deficits should be corrected, especially glucocorticoids, thyroid hormone and sex steroids. Treatment regimens that mimic physiological hormone production allow for maintenance of satisfactory growth and metabolic homeostasis.

Adult growth hormone deficiency

Adult growth hormone deficiency (AGHD) is a rare condition that is usually caused by damage to the pituitary gland or the hypothalamus. Adults at risk for AGHD are those with a history of pituitary surgery, a previous tumour of the pituitary or hypothalamus, history of radiation to the head and previously documented growth hormone deficiency in childhood.

Clinical features of AGHD include changes to body composition such as increased body fat, reduced exercise capacity, impaired heart function, reduced muscle mass, abnormal lipid profile and atherosclerosis. Patients usually experience decreased energy and drive and a decreased ability to concentrate.

Radiographic imaging studies are used to diagnose masses or structural damage to the pituitary gland. Blood serum hormone concentrations of growth hormones are suppressed, and concomitant gonadotropin, thyroid hormone and ACTH deficits may be evident.

Replacement of growth hormone in AGHD is associated with body composition changes such as increased muscle mass and lower body fat. Women generally require higher doses of synthetic growth hormone than men.

Hyperpituitarism

Gigantism Gigantism is a rare condition of growth hormone excess that occurs during childhood. Prior to closure of the epiphyseal growth plate, excess growth hormone stimulates excessive linear growth. The most common cause of this disorder is a benign tumour of the pituitary gland.

The appearance of gigantism is usually dramatic, as all growth parameters are affected and accelerated linear growth occurs. Facial features may thicken, and the hands and feet may be disproportionately large.

Treatment of gigantism depends on the aetiology of growth hormone excess. In cases of well defined tumours, surgical resection may be curative. Radiation therapy may be used in conjunction with surgery or in cases where surgery is not possible. Medications that reduce growth hormone secretion are also used for cases where surgery is not possible.

Acromegaly Acromegaly is a condition that results from excess growth hormone secretion after growth plate fusion has occurred. Worldwide, acromegaly occurs at a rate of 2.4–4 cases per million. The mean age at the time of diagnosis is between 40 and 45 years.

The most common cause of acromegaly is a pituitary tumour. Other aetiologies are excess release of growth hormone releasing hormone caused by hypothalamic tumours, or excess growth hormone releasing hormone secretion by non-endocrine malignant tumours.

Acromegaly has an insidious onset, and symptoms are usually present for a number of years before a diagnosis is made. The disease is characterised by weight gain, growth of the soft tissues, and enlargement of the small bones of the hands, feet, face and skull. Prominent facial features include development of a bulbous nose, a protruding jaw and slanted forehead, and changes in bite with difficulty chewing. Bony changes to the spine lead to **kyphosis**, or hunchback. Bone overgrowth eventually results in degenerative arthritis to the hips, knees and spine.

The metabolic effects of acromegaly are numerous and life-threatening. Excess growth hormone stimulates release of free fatty acid from fat tissue. Glucose intolerance and diabetes mellitus ensues, with changes in carbohydrate metabolism.

The treatment for acromegaly focuses on correcting metabolic abnormalities, improving adverse clinical features and correcting the underlying cause. Surgical resection of tumours of the pituitary or hypothalamus is the treatment of choice. Medications that decrease growth hormone secretion may be administered prior to surgery or in cases where surgery is not possible to shrink the tumour. Radiation is also used to shrink the tumour and is used when medication therapy fails and in cases where surgery is not an option.

HYPOFUNCTION OF THE POSTERIOR PITUITARY

Diabetes insipidus

Decreased secretion or action of ADH results in the syndrome of diabetes insipidus. The leading symptom of diabetes insipidus is the production of abnormally large amounts of urine, or **polyuria**. The polyuria produces symptoms of urinary frequency, disturbed sleep owing to bed-wetting, and daytime fatigue. Excessive urination is accompanied by extreme thirst and a corresponding increase in fluid intake, or **polydipsia**.

The most common cause of diabetes insipidus is destruction of the neurohypophysis for unknown reasons. Diabetes insipidus can also occur when ADH levels are normal. This condition, nephrogenic diabetes insipidus, involves a defect in the kidney tubule that interferes with the reabsorption of water. The kidney fails to concentrate urine in response to the instructions of ADH. Figure 12.4 illustrates the normal action of ADH; Figure 12.5 illustrates the effects of ADH deficiency.

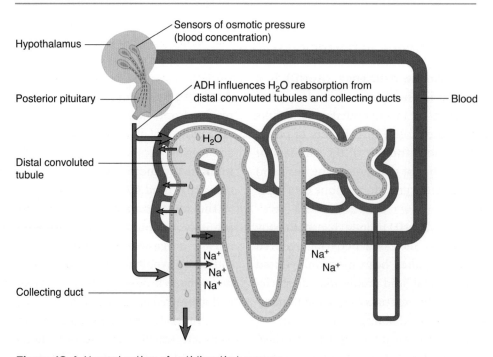

Figure 12.4 Normal action of antidiuretic hormone.

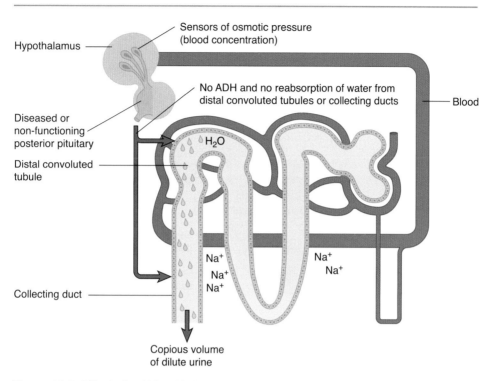

Figure 12.5 Effect of antidiuretic hormone deficiency.

The diagnosis of diabetes insipidus is based on the patient's history, physical examination and results of urine tests. An MRI of the pituitary gland or the hypothalamus assists in identifying the aetiological basis of the diabetes insipidus.

Treatment of diabetes insipidus is aimed at removing the primary cause and treating the symptoms to prevent dehydration. Cranial diabetes insipidus may be controlled with desmopressin (a form of vasopressin) which is administered as either a nasal spray or tablets. Vasopressin is ineffective for nephrogenic diabetes insipidus. Treatment of nephrogenic diabetes insipidus requires compensatory fluid intake with effort to correct the underlying aetiology.

STRUCTURE AND FUNCTION OF THE THYROID GLAND

The activity of the thyroid gland affects the whole body. It regulates the metabolic rate, the rate at which calories are used. The thyroid gland, through its hormone **thyroxine**, governs cellular oxygen consumption and thus energy and heat production. The more oxygen that is used, the more calories are metabolised ('burned up'). Thyroxine ensures that enough body heat is produced to maintain normal temperature even in a cold environment.

Structure of the thyroid gland

The thyroid gland is located in the neck region, with one lobe on either side of the trachea. A connecting strip, or isthmus, anterior to the trachea connects the two lobes. The thyroid gland lies just below the Adam's apple, the protrusion formed by part of the larynx (Figure 12.6). Internally, the thyroid gland consists of follicles, or microscopic sacs. Within these protein-containing follicles, the thyroid hormones thyroxine (also known as T_4) and tri-iodothyronine (also known as T_3) are stored. Thin-walled capillaries run between the follicles in a position ideal for receiving the thyroid hormones.

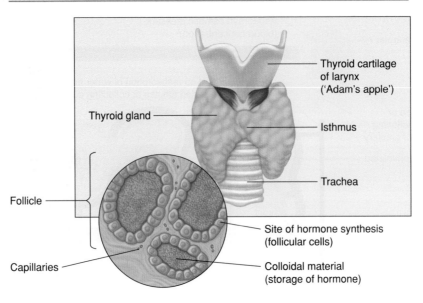

Thyroid cartilage of larynx ('Adam's apple')

Thyroid gland

Isthmus

Trachea

Follicle

Site of hormone synthesis (follicular cells)

Capillaries

Colloidal material (storage of hormone)

Figure 12.6 The thyroid gland.

Function of the thyroid gland

The thyroid gland synthesises, stores and releases thyroid hormones, which contain iodine. Most of the iodide ions of the body are taken into the thyroid gland by a mechanism called the iodide trap. Iodine combines with an amino acid and the thyroid hormones are formed.

The hormones are stored in the thyroid gland until needed and then released into the blood. Tests to determine the activity of the thyroid gland are based on tri-iodothyronine (T_3) and thyroxine (T_4) levels in the plasma.

Effects of thyroid hormones

Although there is more than one thyroid hormone, for clarity the thyroid hormones are referred to here as thyroxine, or T_4, the hormone that is secreted in the largest quantity. Thyroxine stimulates cellular metabolism by increasing the rate of oxygen use with subsequent energy and heat production.

Secretion of thyroxine leads to a compensatory increase in cardiac output. Faster cellular metabolism increases the cell's demand for oxygen, so more oxygen must be circulated to the cells. Nutrients are converted to energy in the presence of oxygen,

and the waste products of metabolism, including carbon dioxide, are formed. These must be carried away from the cells. The circulatory system can meet these needs by increasing blood flow to the cells. Increased blood flow is obtained by greater cardiac output, or more heart activity.

As cellular metabolism increases, respiration increases. The greater need for oxygen and a corresponding accumulation of carbon dioxide stimulate the respiratory centre of the brain. Stimulation of the respiratory centre results in a faster rate and greater depth of breathing.

Thyroxine increases body temperature. Heat is produced through cellular metabolism, and thyroxine stimulates this process. In a cold environment, thyroxine secretion increases to ensure adequate body heat. If excessive body heat is produced, it is dissipated in two ways. Blood vessels of the skin dilate, increasing blood flow at the body surface and giving the body a flushed appearance. As the blood flows through the skin's blood vessels, excess heat escapes. The body is also cooled by the perspiration mechanism. Body temperature is controlled by the hypothalamus in the brain.

Thyroxine also has a stimulatory effect on the gastrointestinal system. It increases the secretion of digestive juices and the movement of food through

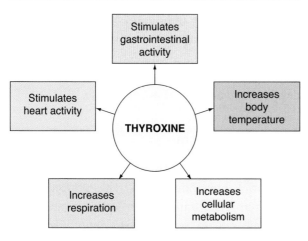

Figure 12.7 Effects of thyroxine.

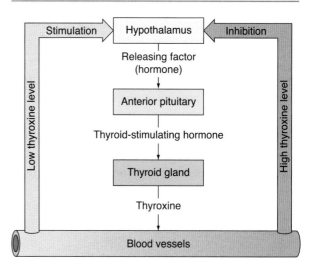

Figure 12.8 Control of thyroxine secretion through negative feedback.

the digestive tract. Absorption of carbohydrates from the intestine is also increased under the influence of thyroxine, assuring adequate fuel for cellular metabolism. The effects of thyroxine are illustrated in Figure 12.7. Many symptoms of thyroid diseases can be related to the effects of inadequate or excessive thyroxine secretion.

Control of circulating thyroxine level

The anterior pituitary gland stimulates the thyroid by releasing TSH. The thyroid, in turn, releases thyroxine, which circulates in the blood to all cells and tissues. When the level of circulating thyroxine is high, the anterior pituitary is inhibited and stops releasing TSH. This is an example of a negative feedback mechanism. An adequate level of thyroxine prevents further synthesis of the hormone. When the level of thyroxine falls, the anterior pituitary is no longer inhibited and once again sends out TSH. This feedback mechanism is shown in Figure 12.8.

At times, this control mechanism fails, constituting one basis for a thyroid disease. The thyroid gland also functions abnormally if the body's iodine supply is inadequate, if the gland is overstimulated or understimulated by the anterior pituitary, or if the thyroid gland itself becomes diseased. Some of these conditions are discussed in the following section.

DISEASES OF THE THYROID GLAND

Hypothyroidism

Hypothyroid, or thyroid hormone deficiency, may affect almost all body functions. The severity of hypothyroidism ranges from mild and unrecognised symptoms to striking symptoms such as mental status changes, extreme and prolonged fatigue, weight gain, swelling or complaints of cold in the hands and feet, menstrual irregularities, muscle aches and hair thinning.

The aetiology of hypothyroid disease may be a primary disease in the thyroid gland or a lack of pituitary TSH. Primary hypothyroidism is the most common form of this condition and is generally caused by autoimmune disease, use of radioactive iodine, destruction or removal of the thyroid gland, dietary iodide deficiency, overtreatment with thyroid medications and medical treatment for bipolar disorder with the drug lithium. Secondary hypothyroidism is caused by inadequate secretion of TSH caused by a disease of the pituitary gland.

Hypothyroid disease occurs more frequently in women. The average annual rate of autoimmune hypothyroidism is up to 4 per 1000 women, and

1 per 1000 men. The average age at onset of hypothyroid is around 60 years, and the prevalence continues to increase with age.

The most severe form of hypothyroidism is myxoedema coma. **Myxoedema** is a medical emergency with a high mortality rate. It is caused by hypothyroidism, but is usually precipitated by an acute illness or trauma. Physical signs may include severe hypotension, unresponsiveness, **bradycardia** (slow heart rate), shallow and slow breathing, convulsions, extremely low body temperature and decreased oxygen delivery to vital organs such as the brain.

Thyroid hormone replacement therapy is often required for the duration of the patient's life. Regular blood tests to measure circulating levels of thyroxine are required to regulate the dose of thyroid replacement medication. Treatment of myxoedema requires hospitalisation and intensive administration of intravenous fluids, intravenous administration of thyroid hormone, warming, mechanical ventilation and cardiac support.

Congenital hypothyroidism

Hypothyroid of the newborn, also known as cretinism, is most often the result of **hypoplasia** (underdevelopment), **aplasia** (absence), and failure of the thyroid gland to migrate to its normal anatomical position. Maternal factors such as excessive iodine intake and ingestion of antithyroid medications during pregnancy can cause hypothyroidism in both the mother and the fetus.

Most newborns with congenital hypothyroidism generally appear normal at birth and gain weight normally for the first 3–4 months of life. Symptoms that follow include physical and mental sluggishness, constipation, poor muscle tone, umbilical hernia and a protruding abdomen, hypothermia, bradycardia and growth retardation. Physical growth retardation includes short stature, preservation of infantile facial features and delayed dental eruption. Severe impairment of intellectual development with retardation of brain development is a severe consequence of untreated congenital hypothyroidism.

Congenital hypothyroidism is diagnosed by neonatal screening techniques, usually within the first few days of birth. Adequate treatment with thyroid hormone supplementation started as soon as possible improves the prognosis of intellectual development and function later in life.

Hyperthyroidism

Hyperthyroidism is a hypermetabolic condition of thyroid hormone excess. The symptoms of hyperthyroidism range from mild increases in metabolic rate to severe hyperactivity. The term **thyrotoxicosis** refers to the clinical manifestations and aetiologies associated with excess systemic thyroid hormone.

Graves' disease is the most common aetiology of thyrotoxicosis. It is an autoimmune disease that is more common in women than in men. The onset of Graves' disease is between the ages of 20 and 40 years, and it is often associated with other autoimmune diseases, such as diabetes mellitus. Thyrotoxicosis is also caused by high levels of hormones secreted during pregnancy, pituitary tumours with excess secretion of TSH and ingestion of excessive amounts of thyroid hormone medication.

Symptoms of thyrotoxicosis include nervousness, restlessness, heat intolerance, increased sweating, fatigue, weakness, muscle cramps and weight loss. Women frequently report menstrual irregularities. Cardiac manifestations of thyrotoxicosis include a rapid pounding heartbeat, cardiac arrhythmias and heart failure, especially in older individuals with longstanding mild hyperthyroidism.

Treatment of hyperthyroid disease depends on the severity, aetiology and presence of complications. The goal of treatment is to bring the metabolic rate to within a normal range with minimal complications. Medications, radioactive iodine and surgery are used to treat hyperthyroidism. Drugs that inhibit the formation of thyroid hormone are administered until thyroid function returns to normal. If thyroid levels cannot be maintained, radiation or surgery may be performed. Medications that control heart rate and blood pressure are administered to prevent complications of thyrotoxicosis.

Thyroiditis

Thyroiditis, or swelling of the thyroid gland, is associated with viral or bacterial infections, auto-immune disease and aging. **Subacute thyroiditis** affects younger women and is usually associated with a viral infection. **Hashimoto's thyroiditis** is an autoimmune disease characterised by infiltration of leucocytes and progressive destruction of the thyroid gland.

Subacute thyroiditis commonly occurs in younger women and may or may not be associated with hyperthyroidism. Symptoms of pain, swelling and thyroid tenderness last weeks or months and then disappear. Symptomatic management includes the use of anti-inflammatory and pain medications, observation and treatment for severe symptoms of hyperthyroid.

Hashimoto's thyroiditis, or an enlargement of the thyroid gland – known as a goitre, most often occurs in women around 40–50 years of age (Figure 12.9). The goitre is painless, although local symptoms may develop owing to compression of the oesophagus, trachea, neck veins or laryngeal nerves. The goitre disrupts the function of the thyroid gland. Treatment of Hashimoto's thyroiditis is directed toward relief of compression symptoms by surgical removal of the goitre. Thyroid hormone supplementation is used if hypothyroid develops.

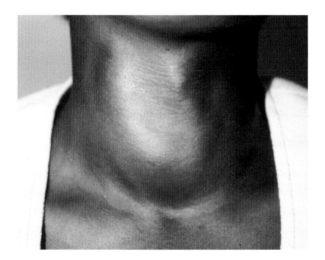

Figure 12.9 Thyroid goitre.
(Science Photo Library Ltd/Dr Ken Greer/Visuals Unlimited)

STRUCTURE AND FUNCTION OF THE PARATHYROIDS

Structure of the parathyroids

The parathyroids are four tiny glands located on the posterior side of the thyroid gland. Before the function of the parathyroid glands was understood, they were sometimes removed with a thyroidectomy. The hormone secreted by the parathyroids is **parathormone**, also called parathyroid hormone (Figure 12.10).

Function of the parathyroids

The parathyroid glands are extremely important in regulating the level of circulating calcium and phosphate. Ninety-nine per cent of the body's calcium is in bone, but the remaining 1% has many important functions. Calcium is essential to the blood-clotting mechanism. It increases the tone of heart muscle and plays a significant role in muscle contraction and the transmission of nerve impulses.

There is a constant exchange of calcium and phosphate between bone and the blood. Two kinds of cells are at work within bone: **osteoblasts**, which form bone tissue, and **osteoclasts**, which resorb salts out of bone, dissolving them. These salts are then released into the blood. The balance between

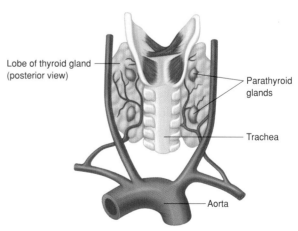

Figure 12.10 Parathyroid glands.

these two processes, osteoblastic and osteoclastic, is governed by the parathyroid hormone.

When the blood calcium level falls, parathormone is secreted. The hormone acts at three distinct sites to raise the blood level of calcium to normal. Parathormone increases the amount of calcium that is absorbed out of the digestive tract by interaction with ingested vitamin D. It prevents a loss of calcium through the kidneys and releases calcium from bones by stimulating osteoclastic activity. When the proper level of circulating calcium is restored, parathormone is no longer released. An excess or a deficiency of calcium can have disastrous results. These conditions are usually the result of hyperactivity or hypoactivity of the parathyroid glands.

DISEASES OF THE PARATHYROID GLAND

Hyperparathyroidism

Hyperparathyroidism, or excessive secretion of parathyroid hormone, is often caused by benign parathyroid tumours. The size of the tumour often correlates with the amount of parathyroid hormone secreted into the blood. Hyperparathyroidism occurs most frequently in persons over the age of 50 years and is more common in women than in men.

Excessive parathormone raises the level of circulating calcium above normal, a condition called **hypercalcaemia**. Much of the calcium comes from bone resorption mediated by parathormone. As the calcium level rises, the phosphate level falls.

With the loss of calcium, the bones are weakened. They tend to bend, become deformed and fracture spontaneously. Giant cell tumours and cysts of the bone sometimes develop. Excessive calcium causes formation of kidney stones because calcium forms insoluble compounds. Calcium deposited within the walls of the blood vessels makes them hard. Calcium may also be found in the stomach and lungs.

Hyperparathyroidism, with its concurrent excess of calcium, causes generalised symptoms. There may be pain in the bones that is sometimes confused with arthritis. The nervous system is depressed and muscles lose their tone and weaken. Heart muscle

---

Box 12.1

Complications of hyperparathyroidism: hypercalcaemia

- Kidney stone formation
- Calcification of blood vessel walls
- Calcification of organ walls
- Spontaneous fractures

---

is affected and the pulse slows. Symptoms include gastrointestinal disturbances, abdominal pain, vomiting and constipation. These symptoms result from deposits of calcium in the mucosa of the gastrointestinal tract. Deposits of calcium sometimes form in the eye, causing irritation and excessive tearing. Hyperparathyroidism usually results from a tumour. If the tumour is removed, parathormone secretion returns to normal, and the level of circulating calcium is again properly controlled. See Box 12.1 for complications of hyperparathyroidism.

The most common laboratory findings in patients with hyperparathyroidism are elevated levels of blood serum calcium and excessive loss of phosphate in the urine. Imaging studies are used to locate the parathyroid tumour(s) and to guide surgical resection.

Medical treatment of hyperparathyroidism is aimed at lowering serum calcium level. This is accomplished through medication and intravenous hydration therapy. Medications called biphosphanates are potent inhibitors of bone resorption and can temporarily treat the hypercalcaemia. Surgical resection is recommended for patients with severe chronic and recurrent symptoms.

Hypoparathyroidism

Hypoparathyroidism is mostly a transient condition that commonly occurs in patients following surgical resection of the thyroid gland. Parathyroid deficiency can also be the result of damage from heavy metals such as copper or iron, or it can result from immune disorders and infections.

The principal manifestation of hypoparathyroidism is **tetany**, a sustained muscular contraction. In hypoparathyroidism, the muscles of the hands

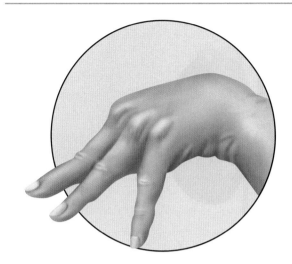

Figure 12.11 Tetany of the hand in hypoparathyroidism.

and feet contract in a characteristic fashion. The typical tetanic contraction of the hand is seen in Figure 12.11. Symptoms of chronic disease include lethargy, personality changes, anxiety, blurred vision and trembling of the limbs.

Common laboratory findings include low serum calcium, high serum phosphate levels and low urine calcium. Imaging studies may show excessive calcification of bone and increased bone mineral density.

Acute hypoparathyroid tetany is a medical emergency that occurs after surgery and requires immediate treatment. Emergency replacement of calcium, magnesium and vitamin D is used to maintain blood calcium in the appropriate range.

STRUCTURE AND FUNCTION OF THE ADRENAL GLANDS

The adrenal glands are located on top of each kidney. Each of the glands consists of two distinct parts: an outer region (the adrenal cortex) and an inner region (the adrenal medulla). The cortex and medulla secrete different hormones. The adrenal cortex is stimulated by ACTH from the anterior pituitary gland. The adrenal glands are shown in Figure 12.12.

The adrenal cortex secretes many steroid hormones, which can be classified into three groups. One group, the **mineralocorticoids**, regulates salt

balance. The principal hormone of this group is aldosterone. **Aldosterone** causes sodium retention and potassium secretion by the kidneys. Another group, the **glucocorticoids**, helps regulate carbohydrate, lipid and protein metabolism. The principal hormone of this group is **cortisol** or **hydrocortisone**. The third group of hormones is sex hormones: **androgens**, the male hormones, and **oestrogens**, the female hormones.

The adrenal medulla secretes adrenaline (epinephrine) and noradrenaline (norepinephrine). These hormones are secreted in stress situations when additional energy and strength are needed. Adrenaline causes vasodilatation and increases heart rate, blood pressure and respiration. Noradrenaline brings about general vasoconstriction. Together, adrenaline and noradrenaline help shunt blood to vital organs when required.

Hyperactivity of the adrenal cortex is usually caused by hyperplasia (enlargement of the glands) or a tumour. Hyperactivity may also result from overstimulation by the anterior pituitary gland.

Hypoactivity of the adrenal cortex sometimes results from a destructive disease such as tuberculosis. Some steroid hormones can cause the adrenal glands to atrophy by interfering with the normal control mechanism for corticosteroid release.

DISEASES OF THE ADRENAL CORTEX

Hypoadrenalism

Primary adrenal insufficiency, or **Addison's disease**, was first described in 1855 when Thomas Addison described symptoms associated with destruction of the adrenal glands. Addison's disease can result from any disease process that damages the entire adrenal cortex; however, approximately 75–80% of all cases are caused by an autoimmune process. Other common causes of adrenal insufficiency include infectious diseases such as tuberculosis, fungal disease, opportunistic infections associated with AIDS, certain cancers and haemorrhage of the adrenal gland secondary to anticoagulation medication.

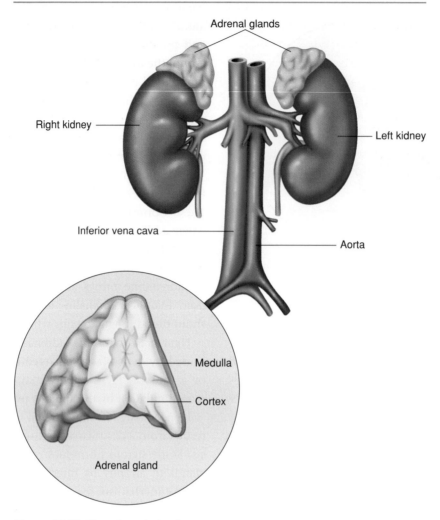

Figure 12.12 The adrenal glands.

The prevalence of Addison's disease is low, occurring in approximately 8 in every million people in the UK. It is more common in females, with a female to male ratio of 2:1, and is usually diagnosed in people aged between 20 and 50 years of age.

The lack of cortisol, aldosterone and adrenal androgens contribute to the symptoms of Addison's disease. Weight loss, fatigue and anorexia occur with a deficiency in cortisol. The most distinctive sign is hyperpigmentation found in non-sun-exposed areas of the body such as the gums and in the creases of the palms of the hands. Gastrointestinal symptoms include anorexia or loss of appetite, abdominal discomfort, vomiting and diarrhoea. Fluid loss from these symptoms may contribute to low blood pressure or hypotension. Hypotension is often associated with dizziness, lack of blood sodium and **syncope**, or fainting.

Diagnostic tests for Addison's disease include a 24-hour urine test for cortisol or blood tests for serum cortisol level. An ACTH stimulation test measures adrenal gland response to an intravenous dose of ACTH. An abnormal response to ACTH stimulation establishes adrenal insufficiency.

Addison's disease can result in a life-threatening condition known as acute adrenal insufficiency. It may occur in patients with chronic adrenal insufficiency in the setting of another acute illness such as infections, trauma or severe physical stress such as surgery. Symptoms develop rapidly and include nausea, vomiting, abdominal pain and severe hypotension. Death can result from shock and cardiovascular collapse. Immediate rehydration with salt solution along with intravenous glucocorticoid replacement is essential to prevent death.

The treatment of chronic adrenal insufficiency includes lifelong replacement of both glucocorticoids and mineralocorticoids. During stress, patients may require additional medication as they are not able to increase endogenous cortisol production.

Hyperadrenalism

Hyperadrenalism, or Cushing's syndrome, refers to the manifestations of excessive corticosteroids. The prevalence of Cushing's syndrome is approximately 0.7–2.4 per million population per year in the UK. The aetiology of Cushing's syndrome is most often benign pituitary adenomas causing hypersecretion of ACTH with excess stimulation of the adrenal glands. Other causes include non-pituitary neoplasms, such as small cell lung carcinoma that produce excessive amounts of ACTH and adrenal tumours that cause excessive secretion of cortisol.

Excess cortisol secretion results in a number of metabolic abnormalities, including hyperglycaemia, hyperlipidaemia, fluid retention, weight gain, weakness, fatigue and hypertension. Clinical signs of cortisol excess include central obesity, 'moon face', fat accumulation behind the shoulders (also known as a buffalo hump), impaired wound healing, loss of elastic tissues, thinning of the skin and emotional distress, including depression and psychosis (Figure 12.13). Untreated Cushing's syndrome can produce serious morbidity and even death. The patient may suffer from complications of hypertension or diabetes or from susceptibility to infections.

Laboratory tests for Cushing's syndrome include blood tests for diabetes, electrolyte abnormalities and signs of infection. Urine tests provide evidence for diabetes and excess cortisol. Radiographic tests, including MRI and CT scans, provide evidence for pituitary tumours or other tumours in the chest or abdomen that may be the source of excess ACTH.

The goal of treatment for Cushing's syndrome is to correct hypersecretion of adrenal hormones. Removal of pituitary tumours is accomplished

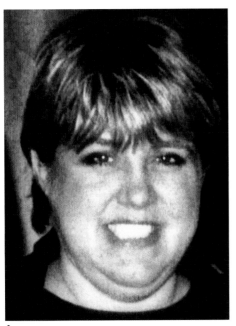
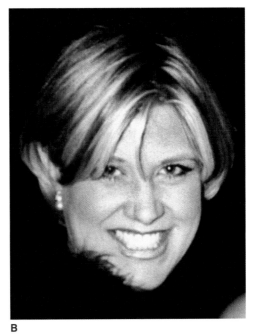

A   B

Figure 12.13 A patient with Cushing's syndrome (A) before and (B) after receiving treatment.
(Sharmyn McGraw)

through microsurgery or radiation therapy. Medications are administered to treat symptoms of diabetes, hypertension, hyperlipidaemia, psychosis and depression. Medications that block the synthesis of corticosteroids are useful in patients for whom surgery is not appropriate.

DISEASES OF THE ADRENAL MEDULLA

Phaeochromocytoma

Phaeochromocytoma is a rare adrenaline and noradrenaline-producing tumour that occurs equally in men and women in the fourth and fifth decades of life. Most phaeochromocytomas (85–90%) are located in the adrenal medulla.

Excess release of adrenaline and noradrenaline is responsible for the signs and symptoms of this disease. The most common clinical sign is hypertension. Headache, excessive sweating and palpitations are also common symptoms. Some patients may also suffer from anxiety, constipation, low energy level and exhaustion.

Phaeochromocytomas are diagnosed by biochemical evidence in both blood and urine of overproduction of adrenaline and noradrenaline. Imaging studies such as CT or MRI scan are essential for detection and localisation of this tumour.

Surgery provides an effective cure by removing the tumour. Medication therapy is used to stabilise blood pressure and to treat associated symptoms. Often various combinations of medications are necessary to stabilise the patient's blood pressure.

ENDOCRINE FUNCTION OF THE PANCREAS

The pancreas is a long organ that lies across the middle of the abdominal cavity, below the stomach. It is divided into a head, body and tail, with the head nearest to the duodenum and the opening of the pancreatic duct (see page 199 in Chapter 9). The pancreas carries out two types of functions: exocrine and endocrine. Most of the pancreas is devoted to exocrine secretion of digestive enzymes; the cells providing the endocrine function of the pancreas make up a smaller part. The endocrine functions of the pancreas consist of synthesis, storage and release of two main hormones, insulin and glucagon.

Insulin is secreted by certain cells of the pancreas called **beta cells**, located in patches of tissue named the islets of Langerhans or pancreatic islets. **Glucagon** is secreted by the **alpha cells** of the islets. Insulin and glucagon work antagonistically to each other. Insulin lowers the level of blood glucose, and glucagon elevates it. The combined effect of these hormones maintains the normal level of blood glucose.

Insulin is secreted when the blood glucose level rises. Insulin facilitates the entry of glucose into the cells, where it is primarily stored as glycogen and metabolised for energy. Glucose enters primarily skeletal muscle cells and fat cells.

As glucose enters cells and is converted to glycogen by the liver, the level of blood glucose falls. The normal level of glucose in the blood is about 4–8 mmol/l.

When the level of blood glucose falls below normal, glucagon is released. Glucagon circulates to the liver and stimulates the release of glucose from its stored form, glycogen. This raises the level of blood glucose to normal. The control of glucose is illustrated in Figure 12.14.

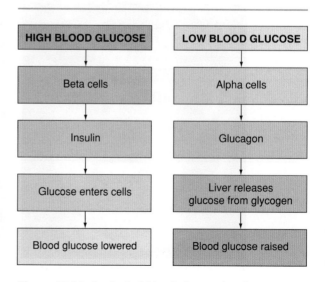

Figure 12.14 Control of blood glucose level.

HYPOSECRETION OF THE PANCREAS

Diabetes mellitus (hyperglycaemia)

Diabetes mellitus (DM) is an endocrine disease of impaired glucose regulation and hyperglycaemia caused by complex interactions of genetics, environmental factors and lifestyle choices. Depending on the underlying aetiology of DM, factors contributing to hyperglycaemia may include an absolute insulin deficiency, reduction in insulin secretion, decreased glucose utilisation and increased glucose production.

DM is classified on the basis of the underlying pathology that leads to hyperglycaemia. The two broad categories of DM are designated as type 1 and type 2. **Type 1 diabetes** is characterised by an absolute insulin deficiency and often results from autoimmune destruction of the insulin-producing beta cells of the pancreas. **Type 2 diabetes** often develops later in life and is associated with variable degrees of insulin resistance, impaired insulin secretion and increased glucose production; this condition is associated with obesity. Diabetes may develop during pregnancy, a condition called **gestational diabetes**. Resistance to the effects of insulin is related to the metabolic changes of pregnancy associated with increased requirements for insulin.

Over 1 767 000 people in the UK have DM. Type 1 diabetes accounts for approximately 5–10% of cases; type 2 diabetes accounts for 90–95% of diabetic cases. Gestational diabetes occurs in approximately 4% of pregnancies annually. Most women revert to normal glucose tolerance following pregnancy but continue to have a considerable risk for developing diabetes later in life.

Type 1 diabetes Type 1 diabetes mellitus (T1DM) is characterised by total or near total absence of insulin production. This type of diabetes often appears between the ages of 10–14 years. Patients with T1DM require continuous insulin supplementation and glucose monitoring to sustain life.

T1DM occurs when an autoimmune process develops in individuals who are genetically susceptible and exposed to some unknown environmental trigger. In T1DM, the immune system attacks and destroys beta cells. This destruction typically occurs over several months, although it may be more rapid or last for years. Once 80% or more of beta cell function is destroyed, patients no longer have sufficient insulin capacity to control blood glucose, so they develop the hyperglycaemia of diabetes. Eventually, patients lose the ability to produce insulin and depend on insulin injections to survive. Because type 1 diabetics cannot produce insulin, they are susceptible to severe metabolic derangements such as **diabetic ketoacidosis (DKA)**.

Symptoms of T1DM include **polyuria**, or excessive urination, **polydipsia**, or excessive thirst, and **polyphagia**, or excessive hunger and weight loss. Because of water's movement by concentration gradients, water is lost through the kidneys as glucose concentrations rise. To compensate for fluid loss, patients develop extreme thirst. Although blood glucose levels are high, the body's tissues are unable to take up the glucose and use it effectively as an energy source owing to the lack of insulin. Patients develop extreme hunger in the presence of hyperglycaemia, leading to excessive eating with a paradoxical weight loss. Patients experience rapid weight loss despite increased food intake.

As T1DM progresses without treatment, alternative metabolic pathways are stimulated, causing depletion of protein and fat stores. Metabolism of fat produces molecules called **ketones**. During starvation, ketones serve as an alternative energy source; however, in T1DM these molecules accumulate to dangerous levels owing to excessive fat metabolism. DKA results when ketone build-up is associated with blood glucose levels greater than 15 mmol/l. DKA can lead to coma and death if not treated immediately as a medical emergency. See the discussion of DKA in the section 'Complications of diabetes mellitus.'

Type 2 diabetes Unlike T1DM, type 2 diabetes (T2DM) is not associated with destruction of pancreatic beta cells. T2DM results from defects in insulin secretion by the pancreas and insulin utilisation in target tissues. Insulin resistance occurs when the tissues' normal response to insulin is impaired. This insulin resistance leads to increased insulin secretion by the beta cells, with eventual insulin decline or insulin deficiency relative to blood glucose levels.

Insulin resistance can be induced by hormones such as cortisol, growth hormone and adrenaline, or target tissue defects. Insulin receptor defects include disruption of glucose transport by free fatty acid accumulation common in obesity. Glucotoxicity, or high levels of blood glucose, results in structural and functional damage to the beta cells, reducing the ability of the beta cells to secrete sufficient insulin in response to glucose.

Type 2 diabetics retain some insulin-producing capacity. The primary defects leading to T2DM are insulin resistance in liver, muscle and fat cells; reduced insulin secretion by the pancreas; and increased glucose production by the liver. Obesity contributes to insulin resistance, and weight reduction may help improve insulin resistance and lower blood glucose in obese patients. As T2DM progresses, insulin levels eventually decrease owing to the inability of the pancreas to continue producing large amounts of insulin.

Risk factors for the development of T2DM include a family history of diabetes, older age, obesity, history of gestational diabetes, sedentary lifestyle, and history of high blood pressure and high cholesterol, or hyperlipidaemia.

Treatment of T2DM includes diet and weight management and oral medications, and insulin for patients who cannot control their diabetes with diet and oral medications. Oral medications increase insulin release from the beta cells, improve insulin utilisation and decrease insulin resistance. Patients often require more than one oral medication to control their diabetes, and some progress to lifelong insulin injections.

Complications of diabetes mellitus

Acute complications of diabetes are related to excessive hyperglycaemia and include DKA and hyperosmolar hyperglycaemic state (HHS). DKA occurs in patients with T1DM, whereas HHS is a rare complication of T2DM.

DKA can be the initial presenting problem in a newly diagnosed patient with T1DM. More commonly, DKA is caused by acute illnesses such as the flu or common cold or physical and emotional stress. During stress, the production of stress hormones such as adrenaline and noradrenaline inhibits insulin action and stimulates glucose production. Without adequate amounts of insulin, the body continues to break down all forms of stored energy to glucose. Eventually the liver uses fatty acids to produce ketone bodies. As ketone bodies accumulate, the blood becomes acidic. Symptoms of DKA include nausea, vomiting, polyuria, polydipsia, dehydration, mental status changes and rapid breathing. DKA treatment includes continuous intravenous infusions of fluids, electrolytes and insulin until the ketosis is reversed and the acidity is corrected.

HHS typically occurs in older, debilitated type 2 diabetic patients. Similar to DKA, HHS is associated with acute stress from infections, medical illnesses or surgery. Because T2DM patients have some insulin function, ketone body formation is prevented; however, patients often present with pronounced hyperglycaemia. Treatment of HHS is aimed at rehydration and correction of hyperglycaemia and electrolyte disturbances. Aggressive intravenous fluid and electrolyte replacement is necessary as patients can lose up to 10 litres of fluid within a short period of time. Administration of intravenous insulin is essential to improve glucose utilisation and correct the hyperglycaemia.

Chronic complications of diabetes are caused by chronic pathological insults to the microvasculature, or small blood vessels, and to the macrovasculature, or large vessels. Microvascular disease occurs primarily in the eyes, kidneys and nerves. Hyperglycaemia damages the endothelial cell lining of blood vessels, resulting in progressive narrowing and occlusion of large and small vessels. Cells die when vessel occlusion cuts off blood supply. Macrovascular damage leads to cardiovascular disease, the leading cause of death in patients with diabetes.

Microvascular disease of diabetes includes retinopathy, nephropathy and neuropathy. Diabetic retinopathy is the leading cause of blindness among adults aged 20–74 years. Diabetic nephropathy occurs in approximately 20–30% of patients with diabetes and is the leading cause of end-stage kidney disease. About 60–70% of patients with diabetes have nerve damage or neuropathy. Typical symptoms of neuropathy include numbness or tingling in the hands and feet and/or severe, burning muscle aches. The loss of sensation in the feet and poor circulation can lead to severe infections requiring amputations. More than 50% of non-traumatic limb amputations in the UK occur annually in people with diabetes.

Macrovascular disease includes the development of coronary vascular disease, peripheral vascular disease and stroke. Death rates due to heart disease are two to four times higher for adults with diabetes compared to persons without diabetes; stroke is two to four times more likely. Approximately 75–80% of patients with diabetes die because of the complications of cardiovascular disease. Treatment of the underlying factors that lead to cardiovascular disease is essential for the long-term health of patients with diabetes. Research has shown that reducing blood glucose as measured by blood levels of haemoglobin A1C, blood pressure and cholesterol levels reduces morbidity and mortality from cardiovascular disease in patients with diabetes.

See Table 12.2 for warning signs of type 1 and type 2 diabetes.

Tests for diabetes mellitus

A simple urine test can show the presence or absence of glucose or ketones in the urine. Urine

Table 12.2 Warning signs of diabetes.

Type 1 or insulin-dependent diabetes mellitus	Type 2 or non-insulin-dependent diabetes mellitus
Frequent urination	Any of the type 1 symptoms
Excessive thirst	Frequent infections
Extreme hunger	Recurring skin, gum or bladder infections
Weight loss	Blurred vision
Fatigue	Cuts and bruises that heal slowly
Irritability	Numbness or tingling sensations in the hands or feet

Source: American Diabetes Association website: *www.diabetes.org/risk-test.jsp* (accessed 25 August 2008).

tests are helpful for initial screening and for those who are prone to ketoacidosis. Fasting blood glucose levels, glucose tolerance testing and glycosylated haemoglobin testing are used to monitor and diagnose diabetes. For the fasting blood glucose level test, a sample of blood is taken after the person has fasted for 8 hours. The glucose tolerance test challenges the body's ability to secrete and use insulin. The test is performed after a 10-hour fast. The patient drinks a standard glucose solution, and blood and urine samples are taken and analysed for the next 3 hours. No glucose should appear in the urine, and the blood glucose levels should not exceed 9.5 mmol/l of blood if insulin is being produced and utilised. Glycosylated haemoglobin determination is a simple blood test that is used to monitor long-term control of diabetes. It generally indicates the average blood glucose levels over the

 Prevention PLUS!

Obese children and type 2 diabetes

A report on diabetes in the UK estimated that the number of children with type 2 diabetes could be as high as 1400. This estimate was based on a survey of the number of overweight and obese schoolchildren in the UK.

These children have an increased risk of developing heart disease and cancer in the future. It is therefore vital that children are provided with appropriate activities and healthy food to prevent them becoming overweight in the first place.

Source: *http://www.diabetes.org.uk/Guide-to-diabetes/Introduction-to-diabetes/What_is_diabetes/Type_2_diabetes_in_children/* (accessed 14 December 2009).

past 90 days. Normal values should be below 6%, and levels for diabetics should be less than 7%.

Education of the diabetic patient

The diabetic who understands the disease knows the importance of weight control, diet, exercise and either insulin or oral agents in leading a normal life.

ABNORMALITIES IN SECRETION OF SEX HORMONES

The gonads (ovaries and testes) are endocrine glands as well as the source of the ova and sperm. They secrete the hormones oestrogen and testosterone directly into the blood.

Hypergonadism (hypersecretion)

Abnormally increased functional activity of the gonads before puberty produces precocious sexual development in both sexes. In a male child, excessive production of testosterone may be caused by a tumour in the testes. This causes rapid growth of musculature and bones but premature uniting of the epiphyses and shaft of long bones. Normal height, therefore, is not attained. Hypersecretion of ovarian hormones in the female is rare because negative feedback stimulation of gonadotrophic hormones stops ovarian hormone secretion.

Hypogonadism in the male

Several factors can cause hypogonadism, or decreased functional activity of the gonads. A person may be born without functional testes, the testes may fail to descend and thus may atrophy, or the testes may be lost through castration. Testes fail to develop because of lack of gonadotrophic hormone.

Loss of the male gonads before puberty causes the condition of eunuchism, in which sexual characteristics do not develop. Development of male traits depends on testosterone secreted by the testes. Castration after puberty causes some regression of secondary sexual characteristics, but masculinity is retained. Hormonal therapy, the administration of testosterone, can be effective.

Hypogonadism in the female

Hyposecretion of hormones by the ovaries may be caused by poorly formed or missing ovaries. When ovaries are absent or fail to develop, female eunuchism results. Secondary sexual characteristics do not develop. A characteristic of this condition is excessive growth of long bones because the epiphyses do not seal with the shaft of the bone, as normally occurs at adolescence.

AGE-RELATED DISEASES

Some changes in endocrine function occur normally with aging. Of these, none are significant causes of disease. However, some changes make the aging person more susceptible to disease.

Growth hormone level decreases with age. This is manifested in men after age 30 as a decrease in lean body mass and decreases in thickness and strength of bone matrix. As the body fat level increases, the growth hormone level decreases further. Increased body fat is correlated with greater risk of diabetes, heart disease and cancer. Decreased bone density makes bones more susceptible to fracture.

A slight decrease in T_3:T_4 ratio is seen with age, resulting in decreased metabolic rate. The incidence of autoimmune disease of the thyroid among females increases with age.

Although aldosterone levels remain relatively steady, an age-related decline in the kidneys' sensitivity to aldosterone occurs, accompanied by a diminishing capacity of the kidneys to secrete renin when needed. The body is less able to deal with the stress of changes in blood pressure, dehydration and disease in general. There is an increased incidence of abnormalities in blood pressure, sodium and potassium levels, acid–base balances and osmotic pressure.

The pancreas retains the ability to secrete insulin at normal levels with age, but tissue responsiveness to insulin decreases. Insulin resistance leads to a greater incidence of T2DM. It is estimated that T2DM occurs in 10% of those over age 56, 20% of those between 45 and 76, and 40% of people over age 85. Although T1DM is somewhat less common than T2DM and its occurrence is unrelated to aging, it remains among the ten leading causes of death among people over age 65.

Androgen and oestrogen levels drop with age, although this is considered a normal process of aging.

Resources

http://www.diabetes.org.uk/Guide-to-diabetes/Introduction-to-diabetes/What_is_diabetes/Type_2_diabetes_in_children/

DISEASES AT A GLANCE Endocrine system

DISEASE	AETIOLOGY	SIGNS AND SYMPTOMS	DIAGNOSIS	TREATMENT	PREVENTION	LIFESPAN
Pituitary dwarfism	GH hyposecretion beginning in childhood due to pituitary damage or ischaemia	Normal mental development, slow growth, sexual development lacking	Serum assay for GH	Hormone replacement therapy	Unknown	Diagnosed in childhood and persists through life
Adult growth hormone deficiency	Damage to the pituitary or hypothalamus	Increased body fat, reduced exercise capacity, impaired heart function, reduced muscle mass and abnormal lipid profile	X-ray, serum assay for GH	Hormone replacement therapy	Unknown	Occurs in adults
Gigantism	GH hypersecretion beginning in childhood due to adenoma of anterior pituitary	Bone length increases rapidly, delayed sexual development	Serum assay for GH	None	Unknown	Diagnosed in childhood, persists for life
Acromegaly	GH hypersecretion beginning in adulthood due to adenoma of anterior pituitary	Enlargement of feet, hands, face as bones grow in diameter; soft tissue growth; nose, lips, lower jaw protrude; tongue and skin thicken	Serum assay for GH	None	Unknown	Occurs in adults
Diabetes insipidus	Central: hyposecretion of ADH by hypothalamic nuclei owing to vascular lesion, neoplasm, trauma to base of skull, or inherited abnormality on chromosome 20. Nephrogenic: kidney insensitive to ADH due to X-linked gene or due to polycystic disease or pyelonephritis	Polyuria, polydipsia	Urinalysis in water deprivation vasopressin test	Administer ADH	Unknown	Can occur at any age
Hyperprolactinaemia	Pregnancy, stress, infections, liver disease	Hypogonadism and reduced fertility	Serum assay for prolactin	Treatment of the underlying cause	Unknown	More common in women of childbearing years
Hypothyroidism	Primary disease of the thyroid gland, autoimmune disease, radioactive iodine, dietary iodine deficiency, lithium	Hypotension, weakness, fatigue, weight gain, complaints of cold in hands and feet	Serum assay for thyroxine and TSH	Thyroid hormone replacement	Prevention of iodine deficiency by consumption of iodised table salt	Can occur at any age
Congenital hypothyroidism	Excessive maternal iodine intake during pregnancy	Physical and mental sluggishness, poor muscle tone, umbilical hernia, protruding abdomen, bradycardia and growth retardation	Serum assay for thyroxine and TSH	Thyroid hormone replacement	Unknown	Diagnosed in infancy

DISEASES AT A GLANCE Endocrine system (continued)

DISEASE	AETIOLOGY	SIGNS AND SYMPTOMS	DIAGNOSIS	TREATMENT	PREVENTION	LIFESPAN
Thyrotoxicosis	Autoimmune, pituitary tumours, pregnancy	Nervousness, restlessness, heat intolerance, increased sweating, fatigue, weakness, muscle cramps and weight loss	Serum assay for thyroxine and TSH	Radioactive iodine, surgery to remove tumours, radiation	Unknown	Usually diagnosed in adulthood, though can occur at any age
Thyroiditis	Autoimmune, or viral infection	Pain, swelling, thyroid tenderness, goitre	Swelling and pain in neck region of thyroid gland	Anti-inflammatory medications, pain medications	Unknown	Can occur at any age
Addison's disease	Damage to the adrenal cortex, infections, opportunistic infections associated with AIDS, cancer, haemorrhage of the adrenal gland	Weight loss, fatigue, anorexia, abdominal discomfort, vomiting, diarrhoea	24-hour urine assay for cortisol	Replacement of glucocorticoids and mineralocorticoids	Unknown	Can occur at any age, though more common in adults
Cushing's syndrome	Benign pituitary adenomas	Hyperglycaemia, hyperlipidaemia, fluid retention, weight gain, weakness, fatigue, hypertension	Serum assay for diabetes, electrolyte disturbance, X-rays to diagnose tumour	Surgery, radiation, medications to treat hypertension, diabetes and hyperlipidaemia	Unknown	Occurs in adults
Phaeochromocytoma	Tumour	Hypertension	X-ray, CT scan, MRI	Antihypertensive medication	Unknown	Occurs mostly in adults
Hyperparathyroidism	Neoplasm	Weak bones deform and fracture easily, kidney stones, pain in bones, depressed nervous system, weak muscles, slow heart rate, abdominal pain, vomiting, constipation	High serum calcium, patient history, kidney stones	Surgical removal of tumour, medication to lower calcium	Unknown	Can occur at any age, though mostly diagnosed in adults
Hypoparathyroidism	Complication of thyroidectomy; also rare X-linked syndrome	Overexcited muscular and nervous system, characteristic tetany in hands, laryngeal spasm	Low serum calcium, patient history	Administer vitamin D and calcium	Unknown	Can occur at any age, though mostly diagnosed in adults
Type 1 diabetes mellitus	Autoimmune destruction of the beta cells of the pancreas	Polyuria, polydipsia, polyphagia, weight loss	Serum assay for glucose, haemoglobin A1C	Insulin	Unknown	Can occur at any age, though mostly diagnosed prior to the age of 20 years
Type 2 diabetes mellitus	Obesity, hypertension, hyperlipidaemia	Polyuria, polydipsia	Serum assay for glucose, haemoglobin A1C	Weight loss, exercise, oral antidiabetic medication, insulin	Control of weight, healthy eating, exercise	Diagnosed in adulthood
Hypergonadism	Hypersecretion of sex hormones caused by tumours	Precocious sexual development	Serum sex hormones	Administration of sex hormones	Unknown	Can occur at any age
Hypogonadism	Hyposecretion of sex hormones caused by undeveloped gonads	Lack of sexual development, eunuchism	Serum sex hormones	Administration of sex hormones	Unknown	Can occur at any age

INTERACTIVE EXERCISES

Cases for critical thinking

1. A mother brings her 5-year-old son to the paediatrician with complaints that her son has been wetting the bed consistently. The child has a good appetite, drinks a lot of water and has a high metabolism, according to the mother. On examination, the doctor notes that the child has lost 3 kilograms since his last examination 6 months ago. What diseases should be ruled out?

2. A 59-year-old woman reports to the GP's office with a chief complaint of terrible headaches, especially between her eyes. Her blood pressure, blood sugar and cholesterol level are high. The doctor also notes a terrible bruise on her leg that was there since her last examination 2 months ago. What diseases should be ruled out?

3. A 45-year-old man reports to accident and emergency with severe dehydration. He has a yellowish appearance and can hardly stand without assistance. His blood level of potassium is extremely high and his legs feel tingly. His heartbeat is very rapid, and his breathing is shallow. What diseases might this man have?

Multiple choice

1. Acromegaly results from hyperactivity of the
   _____
   a. thyroid   b. parathyroid
   c. anterior pituitary   d. posterior pituitary

2. Which hormone increases the blood calcium level?
   a. glucagon   b. parathormone
   c. androgen   d. insulin

3. Hypoglycaemia is a sign in _____
   a. Cushing's disease   b. Addison's disease
   c. diabetes   d. Graves' disease

4. The trunk is obese in _____
   a. Graves' disease   b. Cushing's disease
   c. Addison's disease   d. Conn's disease

5. A deficiency of ADH is the cause of
   _____
   a. IDDM   b. NIDDM
   c. diabetes insipidus   d. ketoacidosis

6. Which of these is associated with hypersecretion of thyroxine?
   a. Graves' disease   b. gigantism
   c. cretinism   d. myxoedema

7. Which gland secretes adrenaline and noradrenaline?
   a. pancreas   b. parathyroid
   c. testes   d. adrenal

8. A deficiency in corticosteroids is associated with
   _____
   a. Addison's disease   b. Conn's disease
   c. diabetes insipidus   d. Phaeochromocytoma

9. An absolute insulin deficiency is characteristic of
   _____
   a. type 1 diabetes   b. gestational diabetes
   c. type 2 diabetes   d. all of the above

10. Iodine is required for the body to make
    _____
    a. bone   b. insulin
    c. thyroxine   d. glucose

True or false

_____ **1.** Kidney stones are likely to form in hypoparathyroidism.

_____ **2.** Hypercalcaemia causes tetany.

_____ **3.** Glucagon prevents hyperglycaemia.

_____ **4.** Steroids that suppress the inflammatory response, as in arthritis, are produced by the thyroid.

_____ **5.** Hypertension accompanies Addison's disease.

_____ **6.** Myxoedema results from thyrotoxicosis.

_____ **7.** A person with Graves' disease is very sensitive to cold.

_____ **8.** Dehydration can develop in diabetes mellitus.

_____ **9.** Cushing's syndrome results from an excess of glucocorticoids.

_____ **10.** Glucagon elevates blood glucose level.

Fill-ins

1. Overproduction of growth hormone before puberty is called _____.

2. An overproduction of growth hormone after puberty is called _____.

3. The posterior pituitary secretes _____ and _____.

4. Microvascular disease is a chronic complication of _____.

5. A tumour of the adrenal medulla, or _____, causes overproduction of adrenaline and noradrenaline.

6. Insulin is secreted by cells of the pancreas called _____ _____.

7. Elevated blood levels of calcium are associated with excess _____ hormone.

8. Tropic hormones are secreted by the _____ _____.

9. Dwarfism is associated with hyposecretion of _____ _____.

10. Sexual characteristics do not develop in the rare condition called _____ _____.

Labeling exercise

Use the blank lines below to label the following image.

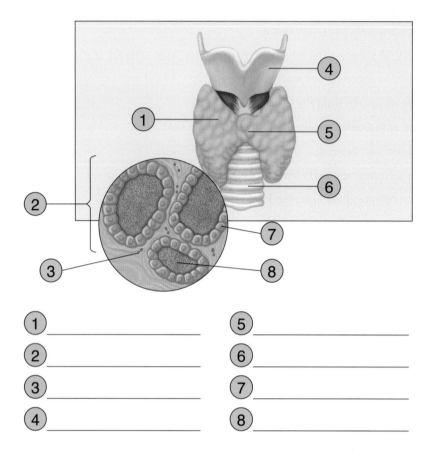

1 _____

2 _____

3 _____

4 _____

5 _____

6 _____

7 _____

8 _____

DISEASES OF THE NERVOUS SYSTEM AND THE SPECIAL SENSES

Photomicrograph of a neurofibrillary tangle.

(© O.J. Staats/Custom Medical Stock Photo)

Fact or fiction ?

Benign brain tumours are not very serious and therefore are not cause for concern.

Fiction: Benign tumours tend to grow and crowd out precious cranial space and, thus, apply pressure or restrict blood flow to particular brain regions. If these benign growths are inoperable or uncontrolled, they will kill the victim. Malignant brain tumours may be lethal, but they may also be surgically removed or reduced with medication or radiation. All brain tumours require attention and may be lethal if left untreated. Treatment with surgery, medication or radiation is most successful for slowly growing, encapsulated tumours.

Learning objectives

After studying this chapter, you should be able to:

✚ Recognise the basic structure and functions of the nervous system and major sensory elements

✚ Describe the aetiology, signs and symptoms, diagnostic tests and treatment of different types of headache

✚ Describe the aetiology, signs and symptoms, diagnostic tests and treatment of infectious diseases of the nervous system

✚ Describe degenerative diseases of the central nervous system, including multiple sclerosis, Parkinson's disease and amyotrophic lateral sclerosis

✚ Discuss inherited and congenital diseases of the nervous system

✚ Describe the effects of trauma on the brain and sensory organs

✚ Discuss the aetiology, signs and symptoms, diagnostic tests and treatment of seizure disorders

✚ Discuss the aetiology, signs and symptoms, diagnostic tests and treatment of CVA (stroke) or related cerebrovascular disorders

✚ Discuss the definitions, the purpose and the physiology of pain

  ✚ Describe the aetiology, signs and symptoms, diagnostic tests and treatment of selected eye and ear diseases

Disease chronicle

Death to a killer

Not so long ago, your great-grandparent or grandparent may have suffered from this tragic disease or feared it within his or her community. Your parents' generation began to break free from the grip of this disease, and for today's generation this disease has been nearly eradicated. What is this devastating killer disease? Poliomyelitis. Poliomyelitis thrived around the world until the 1950s, especially impacting on the post-war 'baby boom' generation. By 1955, Dr Jonas Salk and Dr Albert Sabin had formulated vaccines that put this disease on the shelf. How was that incredible feat accomplished?

Dr Jonas Salk's vaccine consisted of inactivated poliovirus injected intramuscularly, which stimulated production of antibodies against the polio virus. With the institution of large scale immunisation programmes, cases of polio dropped immediately. Dr Albert Sabin developed an oral vaccine more convenient to administer, particularly to large groups, and it is extremely effective. The Sabin vaccine is taken orally and stimulates the production of antibodies within the digestive system, where the viruses reside. Unlike the Salk vaccine, the Sabin vaccine destroys the viruses in the digestive system, thus preventing transmission and eliminating carriers. Many researchers believe, however, that the Salk vaccine is the better choice because it employs killed virus and ensures that the vaccine itself will not transmit polio, especially secondarily to compromised patients such as those with HIV.

The World Health Organization projects that in the near future polio will be eradicated worldwide. Between 1988 and 1998, polio declined 85% worldwide, and today, polio has been eliminated from much of the world. In 2003, only 700 cases of polio were found in the world, and three-quarters of these cases were in Nigeria, India and Pakistan, where undervaccination has enabled numerous outbreaks to occur. Clearly, it remains important to continue immunisation, both locally and globally, to end this devastating disease.

STRUCTURAL ORGANISATION OF THE NERVOUS SYSTEM

The nervous system monitors the external and internal environment of the body and, along with the endocrine system, controls many of the body's functions, like breathing rate and alertness.

The basic organisation of the nervous system includes two major divisions: the central nervous system (CNS) and the peripheral nervous system (PNS). The CNS is composed of the brain and spinal cord. It integrates information and controls the PNS. The PNS comprises all those nerves outside the CNS, beginning with the 12 pairs of cranial nerves and 31 pairs of spinal nerves. The nerves carry information to and from the CNS. Nerves consist of motor nerves, which carry information to muscles and glands, and sensory nerves, which carry sensory information from sense receptors to the CNS.

Certain organs are highly specialised for gathering sensory input; these are called organs of the special senses and include the eyes, ears and nose. Diseases of the eye and ear will be discussed in this chapter; diseases of the nose were described in Chapter 8.

The basic unit of the nervous system is the **neuron**, or nerve cell. The neuron consists of a cell body with attached filamentous extensions called dendrites that carry information toward the cell body, and a filamentous axon that carries information away from the cell body. A neuron is shown in Figure 13.1. Receptors attached to sensory neurons are capable of detecting environmental changes and transmitting messages to the brain or spinal cord (e.g. touch or pain). Motor neurons convey messages from the CNS out to muscles, causing contraction, or to glands, triggering secretion. The axons of sensory and motor neurons are insulated by a lipoprotein covering called **myelin** that forms a sheath, which insulates and protects the neuron. Deterioration of this sheath decreases the impulse velocity and impairs function. When the myelin degeneration becomes profuse it characteristically causes a misfiring, or incomplete impulses as in multiple sclerosis.

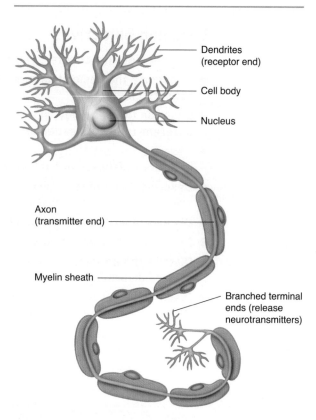

Figure 13.1 Typical neuron.

The brain

Three membranous coverings, called the **meninges**, protect the delicate nerve tissue of both the brain and spinal cord. The innermost covering is the pia mater, the middle layer is the arachnoid, and the toughest outermost covering is the dura mater. Meningitis is a potentially life-threatening disease caused by an inflammation of these coverings.

The brain has three major anatomical areas: the cerebrum, cerebellum and brainstem. The largest portion of the brain is the cerebrum, comprised of two cerebral hemispheres. The cerebral surface is highly convoluted with many elevations (gyri) and depressions (sulci). The outer surface of the brain, the cortex, consists of grey matter, where nerve cell bodies are concentrated. The inner area consists mostly of white matter, the nerve fibre tracts. Deep within the interior of the white matter are clusters of nerve cell bodies known as **basal ganglia**, also called basal nuclei, which help control position and subconscious movements. It is the basal ganglia (also grey matter) that are defective in Parkinson's disease, because they fail to produce sufficient quantities of the neurotransmitter dopamine.

Within the brain are four cavities called ventricles, where **cerebrospinal fluid** (CSF) is formed. These ventricles all interconnect and are continuous with the central canal of the spinal cord. CSF is derived from plasma and flows out of the ventricles through small openings to circulate over the brain and spinal cord, forming a watery, protective cushion. CSF is reabsorbed into the venous sinuses of the dura mater, and new fluid is formed. Obstruction of CSF circulation results in hydrocephalus, a condition commonly called 'water on the brain' in the newborn.

The cerebellum controls voluntary movements, such as riding a bicycle. The brainstem is called the 'vitals centre' because it regulates heart and breathing rates. These three major brain areas will be examined as part of the CNS along with the spinal cord.

The spinal cord

The spinal cord is housed within the vertebral column and is continuous with the brainstem (Figure 13.2). Numerous tracts of nerve fibres within the spinal cord ascend to and descend from the brain, carrying messages to and from muscles, organs and glands.

The autonomic nervous system

One division of the PNS is the autonomic nervous system (ANS). This system controls internal functioning of the body. The ANS houses the sympathetic and the parasympathetic nervous systems, which often work antagonistically to each other. The **hypothalamus**, located within the brain, controls certain activities of the ANS and is known as the centre for homeostasis. Homeostasis is the foundation of all fundamental principles in the study of physiology. The ANS controls arterial blood pressure, heart rate, gastrointestinal functions, sweating, temperature regulation and many other involuntary

actions. Whereas some peripheral nerves affect skeletal or voluntary muscle, the ANS acts on smooth or involuntary muscle and cardiac muscle. Diseases of the digestive system such as stress ulcers, regional enteritis and ulcerative colitis (Chapter 9) are influenced by the ANS. As mentioned earlier, the overall function of the nervous system is to monitor and regulate the various body systems. This monitoring allows the body to adjust to the surrounding environment both internally and externally, and much of this is done by the ANS.

The sensory nervous system

Sensations detected by receptors and carried by sensory neurons from specialised organs such as the eye and ear, as well as in skin, muscles, tendons and internal organs, are transmitted to the CNS. The spinal cord receives simple sensations and directs simple reflex responses, as when one touches a hot stove and quickly withdraws the hand. Complex sensory information must travel to specialised parts of the brain. Impulses reaching the brainstem and cerebellum bring about many unconscious automatic actions, but sensory information involving thought processes must reach the highest area of the brain, the cerebral cortex.

The cerebral cortex has specialised areas to receive sensory information from all parts of the body, such as the feet, the hands and the abdomen. Visual impulses are transmitted to the posterior part of the brain, whereas olfactory and auditory impulses are received in the lateral parts. Association areas of the brain interpret deeper meaning of the sensations, and many of the sensory messages are integrated and stored as memory. Creative thought becomes possible through use of sensory input.

The motor nervous system

Just as the cerebral cortex has areas specialised for the reception of sensory information, it also has areas that govern motor activity. The primary motor cortex is the frontal lobe that controls discrete movements of skeletal muscles. Because the nerve fibres cross over in the medulla or spinal cord,

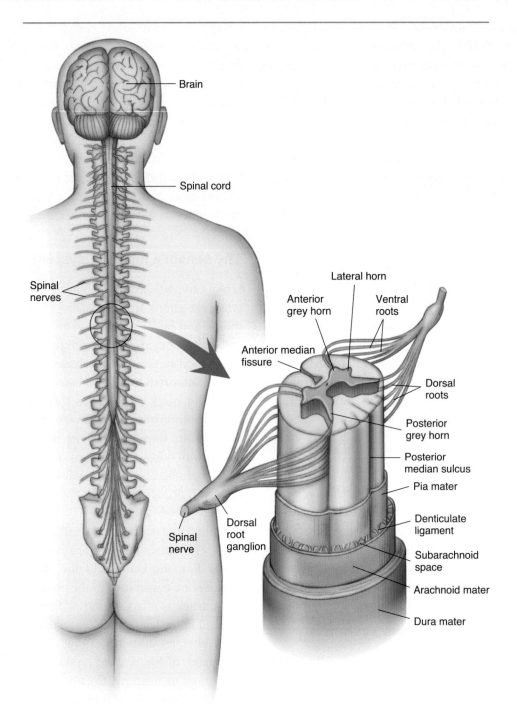

Figure 13.2 The brain, spinal cord and spinal nerves. An expanded view of the spinal cord is shown.

stimulation on one side of the cerebral cortex affects particular muscles on the opposite side of the body.

Anterior to the primary motor cortex is the premotor cortex, which controls coordinated movements of muscles. This process is accomplished by stimulating groups of muscles that work together. The speech area is located here and is usually on the left side, especially in right-handed people. Specialised areas of the brain are shown in Figure 13.3.

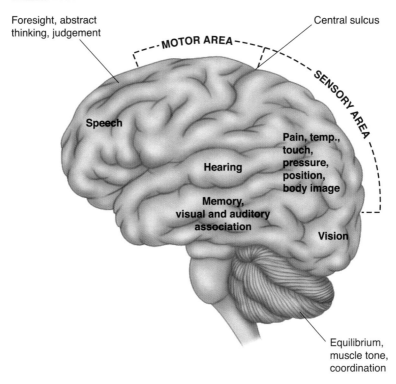

Foresight, abstract thinking, judgement

Central sulcus

MOTOR AREA

SENSORY AREA

Speech

Pain, temp., touch, pressure, position, body image

Hearing

Memory, visual and auditory association

Vision

Equilibrium, muscle tone, coordination

Figure 13.3 Specialised areas of the brain.

DIAGNOSTIC PROCEDURES FOR THE NERVOUS SYSTEM

Neurological laboratory tests include CSF examination obtained by a lumbar puncture, as previously described. Angiography allows visualisation of the cerebral circulation through the injection of radio-opaque material. Computerised tomography (CT) scans are particularly valuable for diagnosing pathological conditions such as tumours, haemorrhages, haematomas and hydrocephalus. **Electromyelography (EMG)** is a radiographic process by which the spinal cord and spinal subarachnoid space are viewed and photographed after injection of contrast medium into the lumbar subarachnoid space. Myelography is used to identify spinal lesions caused by trauma or disease, such as amyotrophic lateral sclerosis (ALS). **Electroencephalography (EEG)** records the electrical activity of the brain (brain waves). It is used to diagnose lesions or tumours, and seizures, in impaired consciousness. Magnetic resonance imaging (MRI) uses magnetic fields in conjunction with a computer to view and record tissue characteristics at different planes. MRI is excellent for visualising brain soft tissue, spinal cord, white matter diseases, tumours and haemorrhages. Where a disease is idiopathic or without cure, the diagnosis is directed at relief of symptoms, as in Parkinson's disease.

For the eye, ophthalmoscopy is used for routine eye examinations. This may determine cataracts when viewing through the slit-lighted feature of the scope. Tonometry procedures are used for glaucoma determination. Audio examinations with tuning fork and electronic audio signals help discover tone quality and hearing loss.

DISEASES OF THE NERVOUS SYSTEM

Common headache

Moderate to severe head pain characterises the common headache. Tension or inflammation of muscles in the head, eyes, neck and shoulders may cause the common headache. Other causes include dilatation or constriction of cerebral blood vessels, allergies, chemical fumes, extreme temperatures and constipation. Simple unintended actions like coughing and laughter may trigger a headache, as may an intracranial mass of tumour or lesion. Nausea, vomiting and sensitivity to noise and light may accompany the common headache and more severe cases.

Common household treatments are rest and NSAIDs (non-steroidal anti-inflammatory drugs) such as aspirin or ibuprofen. Resting in a dark, quiet room and applying a cold compress may be beneficial for many sufferers, especially if time and space are available. Two of the more intense and episodic forms of headache are the cluster headache and the migraine.

Cluster headache

Cluster headache affects 1–4 per 1000 individuals, and men, especially middle-aged men, are five times more likely to be affected than women. The cluster headache occurs suddenly, producing severe, sharp and stabbing pain particularly near one eye or temporal area. The headaches are caused by blood vessel abnormalities and may occur two to three times per day for weeks, or may occur intermittently over a span of 1–3 months, subside, and recur months or years later. The pain may develop at any time but usually occurs at night and tends to last from 30 minutes to several hours. The pain is so severe that many individuals cannot lie down or be idle and may pace about. In contrast with migraine, however, light intensity, sounds or strange odours do not elicit nausea or vomiting.

Often there is no family history of cluster headache, although this condition tends to run in families. As of this writing, genetic factors have not been determined. Alcohol and nicotine tend to trigger these painful headaches, along with stress, ingestion of specific foods and glare. Treatment requires medications like subcutaneous or intranasal sumatriptan (Imigran); inhalation of 100% oxygen and ergotamine works well, as well as biofeedback and reduction of stress. Ergotamine tartrate is used as a prophylactic agent given in various modes of delivery.

Migraine headache

Migraine headaches are more common in women than in men and usually begin in the teen years or early twenties. The symptoms are throbbing (moderate) pain on one or both sides of the head plus sensitivity to light and noise or certain odours. Because migraines tend to cause nausea and vomiting, they are referred to as a 'sick headache'. Sometimes an aura or premonition precedes the migraine onset. Additional symptoms include numbness, dizziness and visual blurring. The headaches last from a few hours to a few days and may recur once a month or once every few years. A history of the symptoms helps diagnose migraine. Daily or weekly patient logs of activities, especially timing of migraine onset and subsequent events, helps reduce episodes and the need for medication.

Specific causes have not been identified, although there may be a natural abatement in some women when they discontinue birth control pills or attain menopause. The concentration of the neurotransmitter serotonin appears to have a role in the pathogenesis of migraines, and nitric oxide (NO), a vasodilator, may be implicated as well. When NO or serotonin are blocked, migraine pain subsides.

One of the most recently discovered causes related to migraine headache is a developmental or congenital defect in the heart that occurs as much as 25% of the time in those affected. The normal connection between the two atria in a fetal heart, the foramen ovale, happens to remain open (at least partially) instead of slapping shut at the time of birth. This fetal remnant is called a patent foramen ovale (PFO). Surgeons found that when this defect was closed in their adult patients, migraine episodes resolved. Clinical trials are currently scheduled to evaluate this new development.

Heredity is now known to be a primary factor in the case of migraine. It has been documented that a gene on chromosome 1 contributes to sensitivity of sound; on chromosome 5 a gene is recognised as one that allows pulsating headaches and sensitivity to light; and a gene on chromosome 8 is related to vomiting and nausea.

Bed rest and sleep in a dark, quiet room seems to benefit most migraine sufferers. Drug treatment is aimed at prevention and relief of symptoms. NSAIDs may not provide adequate relief, but prescription drugs like opioids and codeine are often effective. Imigran, mentioned previously, helps relieve pain and reduce nausea and sensitivities to light and sound. Cardiac medications like beta blockers (Atenolol) or calcium channel blockers (Diltiazem) help, but the exact mechanism is not fully understood, and tricyclic antidepressants have shown positive results as well.

INFECTIOUS DISEASES OF THE NERVOUS SYSTEM

Certain pathogenic micro-organisms are neurotropic in that the virus or bacterium has an affinity for nervous tissue. Pathogens obtain access to the nervous system by many routes, including wounds or trauma, and systemic infections entering from the thinner paranasal sinuses or mastoid regions.

Meningitis

Meningitis is an acute inflammation of the first two meninges that cover the brain and spinal cord: the pia mater and the arachnoid mater. A contagious disease, it usually affects children and young adults and may have serious complications if not diagnosed and treated early.

There are many forms of meningitis, and some are more contagious than others. The most common bacterial causes are *Haemophilus influenzae*, *Neisseria meningitidis* (also called meningococcus), and *Streptococcus pneumoniae*. However, other bacteria, as well as viruses, cause meningitis. **Enteroviruses** account for most of the cases when the virus is identified; in aseptic meningitis no bacterium is found and thus it is usually considered a viral condition. The infecting organisms can reach the meninges from the middle ear, upper respiratory tract or frontal sinuses; they can also be carried in the blood from the lungs or other infected sites. Healthy children may be carriers of the bacteria and

spread the organisms by sneezing or coughing. Viral or aseptic meningitis is considered the cause in 30% of the cases involving non-immunised individuals, primarily caused by contracted mumps, and it affects males two to five times more frequently than females. This form is normally a mild case of meningitis that may not require specific treatment. Other cases may be caused by the waning poliomyelitis virus and occasionally by herpes simplex, and non-infectious cases may result from lymphoma, brain cancer or leukaemia.

In the UK, the number of bacterial cases of meningitis is about 2300 per year, while viral cases are more common but less severe. Causative agent, the geographical region and accessibility to medical coverage influence prevalence; in addition, some agents become resistant to penicillin (*S. pneumoniae*) and others have been reduced because of the vaccine (Hib) for *Haemophilus influenzae* type B.

The symptoms of meningitis are high fever, chills and a severe headache caused by increased intracranial pressure. A key symptom is a stiff neck that holds the head rigidly. Movement of neck muscles stretches the meninges and increases head pain. Nausea, vomiting and a rash may also be symptomatic. The high fever often causes delirium and convulsions in children, and they may lapse into a coma.

Diagnosis of meningitis is made by performing a **lumbar puncture** (Figure 13.4), in which a hollow needle is inserted into the spinal canal between vertebrae in the lumbar region. This procedure is possible because the spinal cord terminates as a solid structure at or near the first lumbar vertebra, although a sac containing CSF extends down to the sacrum. In addition, a lumbar puncture may reveal the relative pressure of CSF. The infected fluid contains an elevated protein level, numerous polymorphs/leucocytes and infecting agents. When the level of glucose in the CSF is below normal, bacteria may have used the sugar for their own growth and metabolism.

The prognosis depends on the cause of meningitis and a prompt diagnosis and treatment. Treatment with antibiotics like rifampicin, cefotaxime or ceftriaxone is very effective if the meningitis is bacterial.

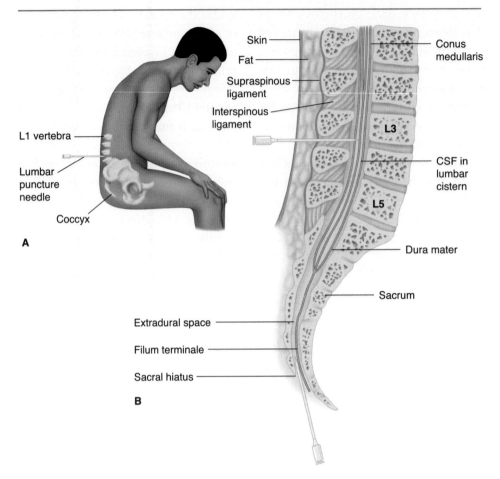

Figure 13.4 (A) Lumbar puncture, also known as spinal tap. (B) Section of the vertebral column showing the spinal cord and membranes. A lumbar puncture needle is shown at L3–4 and in the sacral hiatus.

If not treated, about 15% of those affected suffer permanent brain damage that manifests by sight or hearing loss, paralysis, mental retardation or death. Another complication is blockage of the fourth ventricle by a pyogenic (bacteria) infection, which results in the accumulation of CSF in the brain, a form of **hydrocephalus**. Preventive measures include vaccines like Hib or meningococcal group C conjugate vaccine.

Encephalitis

Encephalitis, an inflammation of the brain and meninges, is caused by several types of viruses. Some of these viruses may be harboured by wild birds and transmitted to humans by mosquitoes, commonly called arboviruses (carried by arthropods, including insects). These cases are mostly seasonal and are represented by regional variations.

Symptoms of encephalitis range from mild to severe, such as headache, sudden fever, stiff neck and drowsiness, to more severe cases that include cerebral dysfunction, disordered thought patterns and seizures in 5% of the cases. Most cases resolve themselves within 1–2 weeks with no specific treatment required except for mild, flu-like symptoms. In serious cases involving extensive brain damage, convalescence is slow and requires prolonged physical rehabilitation. Some nerve damage may cause paralysis, as occurs in 10% of these cases. Personality changes or other emotional disturbances may occur that require therapy.

Diagnosis of encephalitis is made by lumbar puncture. Brain imaging CT or MRI may be used to check for brain swelling. Treatment is essentially aimed at controlling high fever and intracranial pressure, maintaining fluid and electrolyte balance, and carefully monitoring respiratory and kidney function. In individuals generally in good health except for the virus, the prognosis is positive with supportive treatment.

There are many forms of the disease, and they may occur in epidemics. Lethargic encephalitis, or 'sleeping sickness,' is one type of encephalitis characterised by persistent drowsiness and delirium that sometimes results in coma. Secondary encephalitis may develop from viral childhood diseases such as chickenpox, measles and mumps, or herpes. In the case of herpes simplex encephalitis (HSE), type 1 is most common, but type 2 may cause infection in newborns or immunocompromised people like those with HIV or who have received an organ transplant. In the latter case, the patient may be treated with aciclovir or valaciclovir medications.

Prevention depends on control of mosquitoes and deterring contact through use of repellents, clothing and timing of outdoor activities. Other sources may be unavoidable, but early treatment is crucial to reduce neurological severity and deficits or death.

Poliomyelitis

Poliomyelitis, commonly called polio, is an infectious disease of the brain and spinal cord caused by an enterovirus. Motor neurons of the medulla oblongata and pons, which houses the respiratory centre, and the spinal cord are primarily affected. As a result, muscle tissue is not stimulated; it weakens and finally atrophies. If the respiratory muscles are depressed, then an artificial means of respiration is required.

Symptoms of poliomyelitis are stiff neck, fever, headache, sore throat and gastrointestinal disturbances. When diagnosed and treated early, severe damage to the nervous system and paralysis can be prevented. Those who survive paralytic polio may be left with a limp or need a walking aid such as crutches or a wheelchair. Excessive fatigue, muscular

weakness, pain and other difficulties such as muscle atrophy and scoliosis may occur 20–30 years after the onset of the disease. The recurrence of these symptoms is known as post-polio syndrome (PPS). Age seems to be an integral factor, although the exact cause of PPS remains unknown. Additional rest seems to offer some necessary relief from PPS symptoms.

In the 1940s and early 1950s, polio was a highly prevalent disease around the world that crippled or killed thousands, primarily children. This devastating disease has nearly been eradicated worldwide through the development of the Salk and Sabin vaccines (see the Disease chronicle at the start of this chapter).

Rabies

Rabies is an infectious disease of the brain and spinal cord caused by a virus that is transmitted by secretions (saliva, urine) of an infected animal. Rabies is very rare in the UK because of animal and human vaccines in addition to animal control efforts. Rabies can be lethal, and is primarily a disease of warm-blooded animals such as dogs, cats, raccoons, skunks, wolves, foxes and bats, but it can be transmitted to humans through bites or scratches from a rabid animal that licks its fur or feet. The virus may be airborne as a mist from urine in caves and in faecal matter, allowing for transfer to fur, feet or saliva.

The virus passes from the wound site along peripheral nerves to the spinal cord and brain, where it causes acute encephalomyelitis. The incubation period is long, 1 month to perhaps a year, depending on the distance of the wound from the brain or degree of breached surface. Bites on the face, neck and hands are the most serious. The mode of tetanus and rabies transmission to the CNS is illustrated in Figure 13.5.

Symptoms of rabies include fever, pain, mental derangement, rage, convulsions and paralysis. Rabies affects the areas of the brain that control the muscles in the throat required for swallowing and also the muscles used for breathing. As a result, spasms occur within the throat and voice box, causing a painful paralysis. Because of the inability to swallow or clear

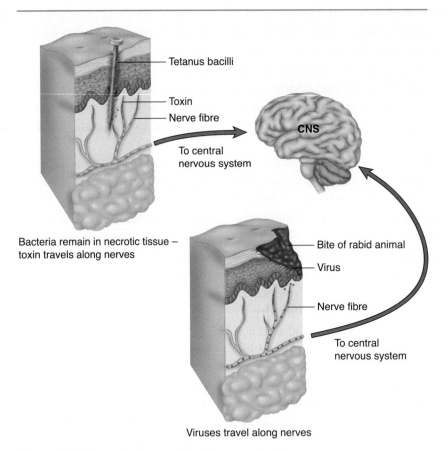

Figure 13.5 Nerve involvement in tetanus and rabies.

the throat effectively, the infected animal or human produces a profuse, sticky saliva and thus tends to 'foam' at the mouth. Hydrophobia is an aversion to water often linked to rabies. The disease is fatal in humans once it reaches the CNS and the symptoms described have developed.

In the case of an animal bite, it is extremely important to know if the animal is rabid, and a detailed investigation of the animal must be made as soon as possible. If rabies is suspected, immunisation and globulin injections are started on the infected person. The victim receives repeated injections of an altered virus to stimulate antibody production and an immune serum to provide a substantial passive immunity. The severity of rabies explains the critical need for the vaccination of dogs and cats against the disease.

Prevention of rabies is achieved by taking a series of three vaccinations over 28 days. The vaccine is required for field workers and medical associates who work with animals and tissues that may carry the rabies virus.

Shingles (herpes zoster)

Shingles is an acute inflammation of sensory neurons caused by the latency effect of the chickenpox virus, herpes zoster. It may even be caused by shingles exposure itself without a reactivation of the chickenpox virus, but that scenario is less common. Shingles is manifested by pain and a rash characterised by small water blisters surrounded by a red area. The lesions follow a sensory nerve, forming a streak toward the midline of the torso, generally across the shoulder, chest or trunk area. The rash is usually confined to one side of the body and does not cross the midline. Blisters fade and the lesions dry up and become encrusted. The encrusted areas cause severe itching and pain and may result in scarring; this after-effect is called **post-herpetic neuralgia** and is caused by the release of substance P (pain agent). The optic nerve can be affected, causing severe conjunctivitis. If not properly treated, ulcerations can form on the cornea, especially from zoster keratitis, and cause scarring or blindness.

Shingles can develop from exposure to a person with shingles in the infectious stage. It may also develop from exposure to chickenpox, which has an incubation period of about 2 weeks. It sometimes accompanies other diseases, such as pneumonia or tuberculosis. Shingles may also result from trauma or reaction to certain drug injections.

Treatment of shingles is directed toward relieving the pain and itchiness. Dry ice pads and lotions such as calamine may provide relief. Glucocorticoids may also be prescribed to suppress the inflammatory reaction, and antiviral agents like aciclovir (Zovirax) are used. Two-thirds of cases of shingles occur in those over the age of 50, and one half are in those aged 85 or more. Repeat occurrences are mostly found in immunocompromised patients.

Prevention includes immunisation against chickenpox.

Reye's syndrome

Reye's syndrome is a potentially devastating neurological illness that sometimes develops in children after a viral infection. Viruses associated with Reye's syndrome include Epstein–Barr, influenza B and varicella, the group which causes chickenpox. Use of aspirin during these infections is associated with Reye's syndrome. The actual cause of the disease is unknown.

Manifestations of Reye's syndrome include persistent vomiting, often a rash and lethargy about 1 week after a viral infection. Neurological dysfunction can progress from confusion to seizures to coma. The encephalopathy includes cerebral swelling with elevated intracranial pressure.

Management is geared toward lowering intracranial pressure and monitoring of vital signs, blood gases and blood pH. The outcome is very satisfactory when diagnosed and treated early, with a recovery rate of 85–90%.

Tetanus

Tetanus is an acute infectious disease, commonly called 'lockjaw', characterised by rigid, contracted muscles that are unable to relax. Tetanus is caused by the tetanus toxin, which is produced by a rod-like tetanus bacillus that lives in the intestines of animals and human beings. The organisms are excreted in the faecal material and persist as spores indefinitely in the soil. The bacilli are prevalent in rural areas and in garden soil fertiliser containing manure, especially from horse farms or race tracks. In developing countries neonatal tetanus kills about 250 000 per year and is called 'the silent death' because the infants die before the birth is recorded.

A laceration, puncture or animal bite introduces the bacterium deep into the tissues, where it flourishes in the absence of oxygen. Thus, deep wounds with ragged, lacerated tissue contaminated with faecal material (manure or contaminated soils) are the most dangerous type.

Tetanus has an incubation period ranging from 1 week to a few weeks. The toxin travels slowly, so the distance from the wound to the spinal cord is significant. The tetanus toxin (see Figure 13.5) anchors to motor nerve cells and stimulates them, which in turn stimulate muscles. Muscles become rigid, and painful spasms and convulsions develop. The jaw muscles are often the first to be affected (hence the name *lockjaw*, also called **trismus**). Because these muscles cannot relax, the mouth clamps tightly closed. The neck is stiff, and swallowing becomes difficult. If the muscles of respiration are affected, asphyxiation occurs. Death can result from even a minor wound if the condition is not treated.

Treatment includes a thorough cleansing of the wound and removal of dead tissue and any foreign substance. Immediate immunisation to inactivate the toxin before it reaches the spinal cord is crucial. The type of immunisation administered depends on the patient's history. If the patient has had no previous immunisation, tetanus antitoxin is given.

If 5 years have elapsed since the previous tetanus injection, the person receives a booster injection of **tetanus toxoid** to increase the antitoxin level.

Additional treatment includes the administration of antibiotics such as metronidazole or benzylpenicillin to prevent secondary infections. Sedatives may be used to decrease the frequency of convulsions. Oxygen under high pressure is also used because the bacillus is anaerobic; that is, it thrives in the absence of oxygen.

Tetanus may be prevented by adequate immunisation. Tetanus toxoid, which stimulates antibody formation, should be given to infants and small children at prescribed times. This inoculation may be done in combination with the diphtheria toxoid and pertussis vaccine (the latter prevents whooping cough).

Abscesses of the brain

Pyogenic organisms such as streptococci, staphylococci, amoebae and *E. coli* can travel to the brain from other infected areas and cause a brain abscess. Infections of the middle ear, skull bones or sinuses, including the mastoid, as well as pneumonia and endocarditis, are potential sources for brain abscess. Figure 13.6 shows abscesses of the brain.

The symptoms of brain abscess may be misleading, because the symptoms may include fever and headache, which can suggest a tumour. Analysis of

 Prevention PLUS!

Reye's syndrome

Reye's syndrome (RS) appeared in the 1950s and virtually disappeared by the 1980s. It has been suggested that the disappearance of RS is related to the recognition of metabolic inborn errors that parallel RS in various clinical manners. RS may be misdiagnosed because of mitochondrial dysfunction that allows various metabolites (e.g. liver enzymes and ammonia) that cause RS-type symptoms and conditions to increase. However, prescribing paracetamol instead of aspirin will prevent this syndrome.

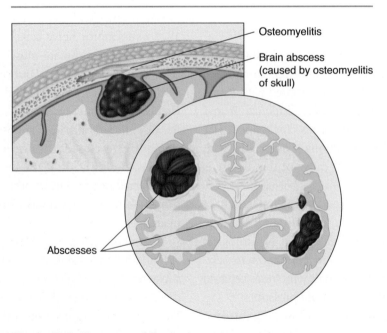

Figure 13.6 Abscesses of the brain.

CSF shows increased pressure and the presence of neutrophils and lymphocytes, indicating infection.

Once the diagnosis of a brain abscess has been made, the abscess must be opened surgically and drained, and the patient must be treated with penicillin-like antibiotics. Brain abscesses are not as common today in the developed world because most infections are held in check by antibiotics. Prevention may be unavoidable owing to accidental trauma situations, but monitoring current infectious situations helps prevent the spread of any disease.

DEGENERATIVE NEURAL DISEASES

Some diseases of the nervous system involve the degeneration of nerves and brain tissue. Abnormalities in muscle and sensory function often result from degeneration of nervous tissue. For example, note that Alzheimer's disease is also discussed in Chapter 14, although it, too, can be considered a type of neurodegenerative disease. Therefore, the description of Alzheimer's in this section focuses on the degenerative aspects of nervous tissue.

Alzheimer's disease

The most common cause of **dementia** (a syndrome of brain abnormalities) in the elderly is Alzheimer's disease (AD), a progressive degenerative brain disease. The incidence of AD rises with age, and the prevalence doubles about every 5 years. Those aged 60–64 have a prevalence of at least 1%, while that number rises to 30–40% for those individuals older than age 85.

The root cause of Alzheimer's disease is genetic, although most cases seem to appear in a random or sporadic manner. Familial cases, or those linked within families, account for about 5–10% of the cases. Chromosomes 1, 10, 12, 14, 19 and 21 have shown genes which affect protein production for specific enzymes or structural components within nerve cells. In the neuron, a support scaffolding of microtubules helps the cell maintain its integrity and to be functionally sound. The directional protein making these microtubules may be corrupted by a malformed compound known as the tau protein. This corruption causes a malformation of microtubules that normally form the linear feature of a neuron and results in a contracted mass known as neurofibrillary tangles. These tangles are not unique to Alzheimer's disease but do indicate a significant breakdown of functioning. These elements are apparent upon autopsy inspection, which is required to confirm a diagnosis of Alzheimer's disease.

Although autopsy is the confirming manner for this devastating disease, a combination of clinical assessment, modern imaging methods and family history can accurately diagnose AD in 80–90% of cases. Within 5–10 years of onset, the person tends to become disabled, immobile and muted; the person usually dies of pneumonia.

Multiple sclerosis

Multiple sclerosis (MS) is a chronic, progressive, degenerative disorder of the CNS. It usually affects young adults between the ages of 20 and 40. The frequency of occurrence is rare, at about 0.1%, and MS currently afflicts about 1 million worldwide.

At first, the disease manifests itself by muscle impairment, beginning with a loss of balance and coordination. Tingling and numbness ensue and are accompanied by a shaking tremor and muscular weakness. Walking is reduced to a shuffle or a cane is used, and occasionally a wheelchair or a more permanent assistance is required. Speech becomes difficult, and urinary bladder dysfunction often develops.

Vision may suddenly become impaired, and double vision frequently occurs. Lesions on the optic nerve can lead to blindness. The individual acquires **nystagmus**, an involuntary, rapid movement of the eyeball. Emotional changes are common owing to less independence and functional control. Signs and symptoms of MS vacillate between periods of remission and exacerbation and proceed at different rates as the disease progresses.

The disease is difficult to diagnose in the early stages, as many disorders of the nervous system have similar symptoms. Diagnosis is based on the specific tissue changes that accompany MS.

The degeneration of nervous tissue in MS involves the breaking up or erosion of the neuronal (myelin) sheath because of chronic inflammation. The nerve tracts do not degenerate in a regular pattern or to the same degree. Therefore, patchy areas of demyelination appear and become sclerotic. A myelin sheath protects the neuron and acts as an insulator to ensure the direction and velocity of the nerve impulse transmission. Any degradation of myelin impairs nerve conduction. MRI demonstrates plaques of demyelinated nerve fibres.

The disease takes one of three potential directions once established: relapsing–remitting involves about 85% of those affected, where flare-up episodes of worsening conditions are followed by partial or complete recovery periods; primary progressive is exhibited by a slow, gradual deterioration at variable rates of speed with minor plateaus of improvement, and involves about 10% of patients; secondary progressive, or progressive–relapsing, involves about 5% of patients and is characterised by steadily progressing deterioration and acute relapses with or without recovery.

The cause of MS is still uncertain, and although it is considered an autoimmune disease, it has been attributed to various viruses or immunological reactions to a virus, bacteria or trauma and heredity. To date, there is no specific treatment for MS that works effectively for long periods. Physical therapy enables the person to use the muscles that are controllable. Muscle relaxants help reduce spasticity, and steroids are often helpful. Some success has been found with beta interferon, and exercising in a pool of cold water seems to be beneficial for some individuals. Psychological counselling is advantageous in dealing with the emotional changes brought about by the disease.

Amyotrophic lateral sclerosis

Amyotrophic lateral sclerosis (ALS), also known as Lou Gehrig's disease, is a chronic, terminal neurological disease noted by a progressive loss of motor neurons and supportive astrocytes. ALS occurs late in life, most commonly in those in their 50s and 60s, and is slightly more common in men than in women. The prevalence of ALS is 2–3 per 100 000 people.

ALS is characterised by disturbances in motility and atrophy of muscles of the hands, forearms and legs because of degeneration of neurons in the ventral horn of the spinal cord. Also affected are certain cranial nerves, particularly the trigeminal (V), facial nerves (VII) and hypoglossal (XI), which impair muscles of the mouth and throat. Swallowing and tongue movements are affected, and speech becomes difficult or impossible.

The cause of ALS is not known. It is diagnosed by an electromyogram (EMG), which shows a reduction in the number of motor units active with muscle contraction. Motor units are motor neurons and their connection to a host of muscle fibres. Also observed are **fasciculations**, the spontaneous, uncontrolled discharges of motor neurons seen as irregular twitching.

ALS requires early education of the patient and the patient's family so that a proper management system may be provided to anticipate and prevent certain hazards. Specifically, the prevention of upper airway obstruction and pathological aspiration – drawing of vomitus or mucus into the respiratory tract – is the main focus. Aspiration can occur from weakened respiratory musculature and ineffective cough. Death usually occurs within 3–5 years after onset of symptoms and generally results from pulmonary failure. However, as the renowned British scientist Stephen Hawking attests, survivorship of ALS does vary.

Prevention of ALS is uncertain because 90% of the cases are indeterminate as to origin, while 10% have an autosomal dominant gene on chromosome 21.

Parkinson's disease

Parkinson's disease (PD) is a degenerative disease that affects muscle control and coordination. PD normally strikes at midlife, about age 45. Approximately 0.2% of the UK population are affected with PD, with 10 000 people diagnosed every year. More men than women are affected, and as the cause of Parkinson's disease is still unknown, environmental factors, particularly undetected viruses, are suspected.

A very small percentage of PD cases are hereditary as either autosomal dominant or recessive genes. The resultant cause is related to a loss of cells and the neurotransmitter dopamine in the substantia nigra of the basal nucleus within the core of the brain. Dopamine suppresses undesired movements that skeletal muscles may be instructed to do but are normally held in check or dormant. Therefore, when dopamine is not present, the unrestrained signals call for an uncoordinated 'shaky' tremor.

Symptoms are progressive and include tremor, rigid muscles and loss of normal reflexes. The tremors are called 'tremors at rest', meaning they occur while the patient is inactive and subside when the muscles are put into motion. A mask-like facial expression is noticed along with faltering gait and mental depression in approximately 10–15% of patients.

In the earlier stages, physical therapy and exercise help maintain flexibility, motility and mental well-being. Relaxation is particularly important for PD patients because stressful situations worsen the condition. Figure 13.7 summarises possible effects of PD.

Treatment includes the administration of levadopamine (L-dopa), a form of dopamine that passes the blood–brain barrier and is similar to the natural form. The drug does not stop the degeneration, but it restores dopamine levels in the brain and reduces symptom severity. Other similar drugs like pergolide and co-careldopa (Sinemet) may be used, as well as anticholinergic medications like orphenadrine for treatment.

In later stages, physical therapy, including heat and massage, helps reduce muscle cramps and relieve tension headaches caused by the rigidity of neck muscles. Psychological support is needed while learning to cope with the disability. In terminal stages, an increased risk for suicide has been noted.

Deep brain stimulation with electrodes implanted into the thalamus has become an additional tool for controlling tremors. The patient may turn on/off the implanted pulse generator by passing a magnet over

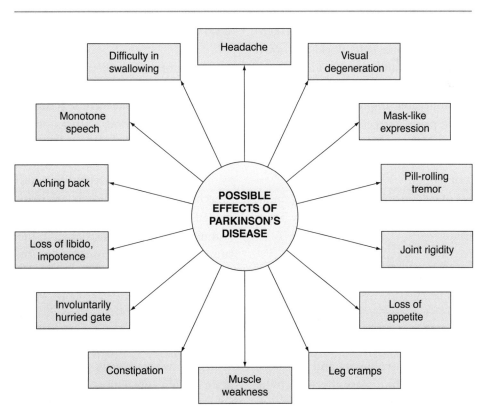

Figure 13.7 Summary of Parkinson's disease effects.

it. The small, pacemaker-like device is implanted under the collar bone. Normally, a constant trickle of charge is sent to the thalamus to interrupt tremor-causing signals, similar to surgical techniques that destroy part of the thalamus to limit involuntary movements.

Another future treatment being suggested is a sort of 'brain transplant', in which dopamine-producing neural tissue from a mouse or pig is implanted in the brain to replenish the missing dopamine. Most PD patients are unaware of the initial agent(s) that bring about this disorder, and prevention is not an option in hereditary cases. Pesticides are suspected causative agents.

Essential tremor

This disorder is often confused with Parkinson's disease even though it usually becomes symptomatic in adolescence. Like PD, essential tremor progresses with the passage of time; at rest the problem abates. Moving or shaking of the head and hands and a halting or quivering voice are characteristic of this condition. There is a familial pattern, but the genetics are not clear. Drugs like beta blockers, known for heart regulation, tranquillisers like Valium and botox injections help approximately 40% of the patients, and a noticeable improvement occurs in about 60% of the patients receiving brain implant devices. Still, some of those afflicted choose to leave the disease untreated until it interferes with the basic routines of living.

Prevention is uncertain and there may be familial links, but these associations are not clearly identified at this time.

Huntington's disease (Huntington's chorea)

Huntington's chorea is a progressive degenerative disease of the brain that results in the loss of muscle control. *Chorea* refers to involuntary and ceaseless, rapid, jerky movements. The disease affects both the mind and body. Physical disabilities include speech loss and a difficulty in swallowing, coupled with involuntary jerking, twisting motions and muscle

spasms. Personality changes include carelessness, poor judgement and impaired memory, ultimately deteriorating to total mental incompetence.

World prevalence is about 5 per 100 000 people. Huntington's disease is an inherited disease, but symptoms may not appear until middle age (ages 30–50). If either parent has the disease, the children have a 50% chance of inheriting it because it is an autosomal dominant trait (see Chapter 5 for a discussion of genetic transmission). The responsible gene has been identified on chromosome 4. The abnormality causes the neurotransmitter dopamine to be produced in excess, and insufficiencies of acetylcholine underlie the dementia and abnormal muscle activity. To reduce dopamine action, the drug tetrabenazine can be used. Given its genetic component, prevention is not an option. There is no cure for Huntington's chorea. When desired, carriers can be identified with gene testing. Following onset, death normally occurs 15–20 years afterward, with a progressive deterioration.

CONVULSIONS

A convulsion is a sudden, intense series of uncontrollable muscular contractions and relaxations. Causes of convulsions include accumulation of waste products in the blood, such as occurs in uraemia, toxaemia of pregnancy, drug poisoning or withdrawal from alcohol. Infectious diseases of the brain, such as meningitis and encephalitis, and high fevers, especially in young children, are frequently accompanied by convulsions. The basis for convulsions is abnormal electrical discharges in the brain, which stimulates muscles to contract abnormally.

Epilepsy

Epilepsy is a group of uncontrolled cerebral discharges that recurs at random intervals. The seizures associated with **epilepsy** are a form of convulsion. Brain impulses are temporarily disturbed, with resultant involuntary convulsive movements. Epilepsy can be acquired as a result of injury to the brain, including birth trauma, a penetrating wound or depressed skull fracture. A tumour can irritate the brain, causing abnormal electrical discharges to be released. Alcoholism can also lead to the development of epilepsy. Most cases of epilepsy are idiopathic, but a predisposition to epilepsy may be inherited.

Epilepsy is one of the more common, yet controllable, neurological disorders, with European studies showing that 40–70 adults per 100 000 have a first unprovoked seizure. Childhood prevalence is rather higher, especially under 10 years old, and involves proportionally more boys than girls.

Epilepsy may manifest itself mildly, particularly in children. Loss of consciousness may last only a few seconds, during which time the child appears in a state of shock or absent-mindedness (amnesia). Some muscular twitching may be noticed around the eyes and mouth, and the child's head may sway rhythmically, but the child may not fall to the floor. This form of epileptic seizure is known as absence (or petit mal) and usually disappears by the late teens or early twenties.

Major seizures, called tonic clonic or grand mal, involve a sudden loss of consciousness during which the person falls to the floor. *Tonic* refers to the increased muscle tone or contraction phase, while *clonic* involves alternating contracting and relaxing muscle activities. Absence and tonic forms are considered generalised convulsions and range from mild to severe, with violent shaking and thrashing movements lasting about 1 minute. Hypersalivation causes a foaming at the mouth. The individual tends to lose control of the urinary bladder and sometimes bowels. Sometimes there are repeated seizures, without a recovery period, that may last 30 minutes. This condition is known as status epilepticus.

Individuals sometimes have a warning of an approaching seizure that gives them time to lie down or reach for support. This warning, known as an **aura**, may come as a ringing sound in the ears, a tingling sensation in the fingers, spots before the eyes or various odours. The signs described are characteristic of the absence or clonic form of seizure. After a seizure, the person is fatigued, groggy and unaware of what happened. Seizures last for varying lengths of time and appear with varying frequencies.

Epileptic seizures may take different forms. The International Classification of Epileptic Seizures, adopted by the World Health Organization, classifies seizures into four categories:

1. Partial seizures begin locally and may or may not involve a larger area of brain tissue.
2. Generalised seizures are bilaterally symmetrical and without local onset.
3. Unilateral seizures generally involve only one side of the brain.
4. Unclassified epileptic seizures are less defined in origin and degree.

Diagnosis of epilepsy can be made on the results of an electroencephalogram (EEG), a recording of brain waves. X-ray films are also used to identify any brain lesions. Family histories of epilepsy are very important in diagnosing the condition. The diagnosis of epilepsy and the seizure type has become more accurate with new techniques for imaging the brain. CT scans, using X-rays, and MRI, using magnetic fields, visualise brain anatomy.

Medication is very effective in controlling epilepsy, particularly anticonvulsant drugs, such as carbamazepine. Alcohol must be avoided with anticonvulsant medication. Molecular neurobiology research is providing new information on how nerve cells control electrical activity, thus making development of more effective antiepileptic drugs possible. It is now known which drugs are best for treating the various kinds of seizures. Assistance or treatment during a seizure is directed toward preventing self-injury. Finally, epilepsy does not appear to interfere with mental prowess or creative talents for those afflicted. A consistent medication regimen usually prevents epileptic episodes.

DEVELOPMENTAL ERRORS OR MALFORMATIONS

Spina bifida

Spina bifida, a neural tube defect (NTD), is a developmental error in which one or more vertebrae fail to fuse, leaving an opening or weakness in the vertebral column. The consequences of spina bifida depend on the extent of the opening and the degree to which the vertebral column, usually in the lumbar area, is exposed and the involvement of the spinal cord. One form of spina bifida, spina bifida occulta (hidden), may not be apparent at birth. In this mildest case, a slight dimpling of the skin and tuft of hair over the vertebral defect indicates the site of the lesion.

Lesions of spina bifida occulta show internal weakness or backbone breaks that can be readily seen on X-ray films. Other malformations, such as hydrocephalus, cleft palate, cleft lip, club foot and **strabismus** (crossed eyes), tend to accompany this developmental error and may occur simultaneously or separately. Any single malformation may point to spina bifida and trigger closer observations of the individual even without noticeable disability. Muscular abnormalities, such as incorrect posture, inability to walk or lack of urinary bladder and bowel control appear later.

A second form of spina bifida noticeable at birth is a **meningocele**. In this condition, meninges protrude through the opening in the vertebra as a

sac filled with CSF. The spinal cord is not directly involved in this case.

Meningomyelocele is a serious anomaly in which the nerve elements protrude into the sac and are trapped, thus preventing proper placement and development. The child with this defect may be paralysed, fail to develop, lack sensation and experience mental retardation. The consequences of the defect depend on the region and size of the spinal cord affected. Surgical corrections of the various forms of spina bifida have been very effective. Some procedures are intrauterine, to repair the defect of the fetus, and these new operations look promising. Physical rehabilitation may allow for a more normal lifestyle, depending on severity.

The most severe form of spina bifida is **myelo-cele**, in which the neural tube itself fails to close and the nerve tissue is totally exposed and disorganised. This condition is usually fatal. The various forms of spina bifida are shown in Figure 13.8.

Hereditary and environmental influences or idiopathic instances are possible causes of spina bifida. Worldwide, the occurrence rate of spina bifida is about 1 per 1000 births, but is higher in

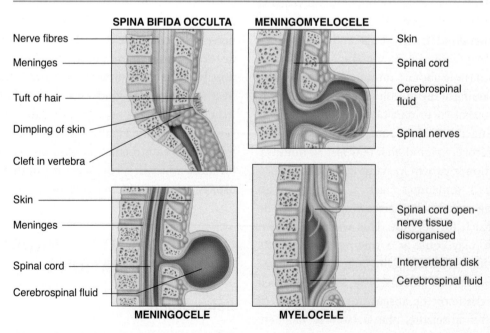

Figure 13.8 Forms of spina bifida.

the UK, at about 2–3 per 1000 births. However, since the introduction of folate into the neonatal care regimen, the number of cases has been cut significantly. Spina bifida and other NTD cases may be detected by ultrasound and elevated blood levels of alpha fetoprotein.

Hydrocephalus

Hydrocephalus is a consequence of excess CSF trapped within the brain. The formation, circulation and absorption of CSF were described earlier in this chapter. In hydrocephalus, this fluid and pressure increases abnormally, causing the ventricles to enlarge and press the brain against the skull, which forces it to enlarge greatly, especially in the case of newborns.

An obstruction in the normal flow of CSF is the usual cause of hydrocephalus. A congenital defect causes stenosis (narrowing) of an opening from the ventricles, or an acquired lesion can block the CSF flow. Meningitis, a tumour or birth trauma may result in acquired hydrocephalus. The error may also be a failure to absorb the fluid into the circulatory system.

There are two types of hydrocephalus: *communicating* and *non-communicating*. In the communicating type, the excess CSF enters the subarachnoid space. In non-communicating hydrocephalus, the increased pressure of the CSF is confined within the ventricles and is not evident in a lumbar puncture (LP).

The head of a child born with hydrocephalus may appear normal at birth, but it will enlarge rapidly in the early months of life as the fluid accumulates.

The brain is compressed, the cranial bones are thin, and the sutures of the skull tend to separate under the pressure. A hydrocephalic infant exhibits a prominent forehead, bulging eyes and a facial expression of fright or pain. The scalp is stretched and the veins of the head are prominent. The weight of the excessive fluid in the head makes it impossible for the baby to lift its head. Infant growth is stunted, as is mental development.

There have been cases of self-arrested hydrocephalus in which expansion of the head stops. A balance is reached between production and absorption of the CSF fluid. The cranial sutures knit together and the skull bones thicken. The extent of brain damage before the expansion stops determines the degree of mental retardation.

The number of cases involved is difficult to attain because of causes, ages and matters of degree, especially when tabulated in combination with other diseases. For example, an obvious case at birth is noted, but trauma or a tumour or encephalitis cases may not be accounted for and may simply be considered cerebral oedema. The incidence of hydrocephalus in the UK is approximately 6.46 per 10 000 per year. Success in relieving the excessive CSF can be achieved by placing a shunt between the blocked cerebral ventricles and the jugular vein (Figure 13.9), to the heart or placed into the peritoneal cavity. This connection facilitates the reduction in cranial pressure and allows the fluid to enter the general circulation. Prevention is difficult owing to the uncertainty of events that gradually lead to this crucial disorder.

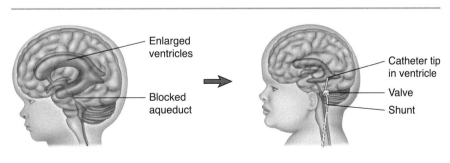

Figure 13.9 Hydrocephalus.

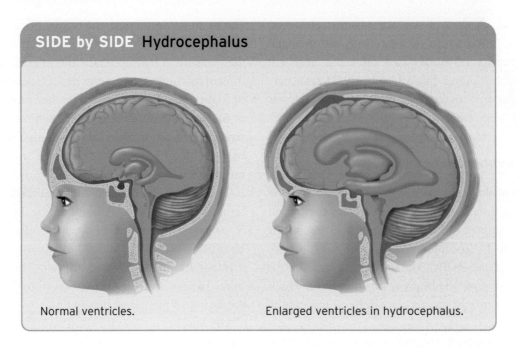

SIDE by SIDE Hydrocephalus

Normal ventricles.

Enlarged ventricles in hydrocephalus.

BRAIN INJURY

Cerebral palsy

Cerebral palsy is not a disease but a functional disorder of the brain manifested by motor impairment that may induce varying degrees of mental retardation; it usually becomes apparent before age 3. The assault causing brain damage may be due to injury at or near the time of birth, a maternal infection such as rubella (German measles) or infection of the brain even after birth. Reduced levels of oxygen, primarily caused by reduced blood flow or incompatible blood type or Rhesus (Rh) factor, may cause brain injury. For example, a pinched umbilical cord against the birth canal may shut off blood and starve the fetus of necessary oxygen. With incompatibilities, a Rh⁻ mother may produce antibodies against the blood of a Rh⁺ fetus. The result is excessive destruction of fetal blood cells that causes hyperbilirubinaemia; bilirubin is toxic to the brain and causes damage. Often, cerebral palsy is idiopathic. Cerebral palsy affects 2–4 per 1000 infants in industrialised countries and is 10 times more often found in premature and low birthweight babies.

There are four recognised forms of cerebral palsy: spastic, choreoathetoid, atactic and mixed. However, it is not easy to diagnose a specific type before the infant is at least 18 months old because the signs may be subtle and attributed to immature development. The largest percentage of cerebral palsy type (70%) is the spastic version in which muscles are tense and reflexes are exaggerated. In the athetoid form, constant, purposeless movements are uncontrollable. A continuous tremor or shaking of the hands and feet is common. Cerebral palsy sufferers with the atactic form have poor balance and are prone to fall. Poor muscular coordination and a staggering gait are characteristic of this form of the disorder.

Depending on the area of the brain affected, there may be seizures along with visual or auditory impairment. If the muscles controlling the tongue are affected, speech defects result. Intelligence may be normal, but often there is reduced mental capacity.

Treatment depends on the nature and the severity of the brain injury. Anticonvulsant drugs reduce seizures, and casts or braces may aid walking. In addition, muscle relaxants can relieve spasms along with traction or surgery, which is necessary in some cases. Muscle training is the most important therapy, and the earlier it is started, the more effective it is. Prevention may depend on circumstances such as sterile environment and strict monitoring of fetal status at the time of birth.

STROKE OR CEREBROVASCULAR ACCIDENT

The main cause of cerebral haemorrhage is hypertension. Prolonged hypertension tends to result from atherosclerosis, which leads to arteriosclerosis, explained in Chapter 6. The combination of high blood pressure and hard, brittle blood vessels is a predisposing condition for cerebral haemorrhage. **Aneurysms**, weakened areas in vascular walls, are also susceptible to rupture (Figure 13.10). Surrounding the pituitary gland is the circle of Willis, a major crossroads of cerebral vascularity, vulnerable to weakness, especially aneurysms. If the rupture or leakage occurs here, the collection of blood within the cranial cavity increases and the intracranial pressure increases proportionally to dangerous levels. When this pressure increase is controlled or alleviated early, brain damage and death is unlikely. The pressure relief may come in the form of medication or emergency surgical procedure. Any subsequent haemorrhage into the brain tissue damages the neurons, causing a sudden loss of consciousness. Death can follow, or, if the bleeding stops, varying degrees of brain damage can result. When detected, swift surgical repairs of aneurysms save lives.

Cerebrovascular accident (CVA) is the second leading cause of death in the UK, the first being heart attacks. Prevention includes not smoking, maintaining proper diet and exercise and monitoring blood pressure; some people take an aspirin each day if they are not taking blood thinners like coumarins. CVAs are basically of two varieties; those due to a haemorrhage or to a blood clot. Most CVAs result from the blood clot or occlusion and will be addressed in the next section.

Thrombosis and embolism

Blood clots that block the cerebral arteries cause infarction of brain tissue. **Thromboses** are blood clots that develop on walls of atherosclerotic vessels, particularly in the carotid arteries. These clots take time to form, and some warning may precede the occlusion of the vessel. The person may experience blindness in one eye, difficulty in speaking or a generalised state of confusion. When the cerebral blood vessel is completely blocked, the individual may lose consciousness.

An **embolism** is a travelling clot that may suddenly occlude a blood vessel and cause ischaemia. The embolism is most frequently a clot from the heart, aorta or carotid artery, but it can travel from another part of the body, such as the deep veins of the leg. Consciousness may be lost suddenly. When this event occurs, a thrombolytic drug (alteplase), called a 'clot buster', may be used to dissolve clots and restore blood flow in occluded vessels. However,

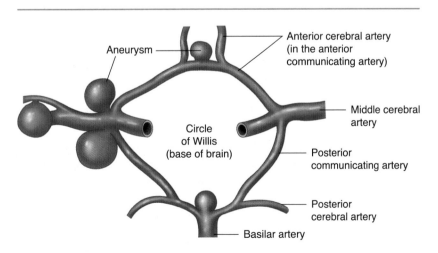

Figure 13.10 Aneurysms.

if this is given in haemorrhagic cases of CVAs, intracranial bleeding and increasing pressure continue and the individual could die. Crucial decisions must be made in acute cases, and because most CVAs are of the ischaemic form, alteplase is a reliable and available agent for the physician.

The site and extent of the brain damage, regardless of its cause, determines the outcome for the patient. Gradually consciousness is regained, but immediately after the **stroke**, speech is often impaired. Loss of speech, or **aphasia**, is normally temporary but may require therapy to assist in a full recovery.

Damage to the motor nerves at the point passing down the spinal cord causes weakness (**paresis**) or paralysis on the side of the body opposite the brain lesion owing to the crossover of nerve tracts in the brainstem. Paralysis on one side of the body is referred to as **hemiplegia**.

Various procedures make it possible to determine the site of blockage in a cerebral blood vessel. Angiography, a process in which radio-opaque material is injected into cerebral arteries, allows X-rays to locate the lesion.

A blockage in a carotid artery can be treated surgically. **Endarterectomy**, the more common procedure, removes the thickened area of the inner vascular lining. Carotid bypass surgery removes the blocked vascular segment, and a graft is inserted to allow blood flow to the brain. Other vascular replacement may be performed in other areas, such as the aorta, to reduce the risk of haemorrhage.

Transient ischaemic attack

Transient ischaemic attacks (TIAs) are caused by brief but critical periods of reduced blood flow in a cerebral artery. TIAs may be thought of as 'mini' strokes resulting from blood clots occluding vessels or vessel spasms that interrupt blood flow and thus impair neurological functioning. The individual may lose feeling in the face or extremity or have tingling sensations for a brief time. Factors influencing the constrictions are similar to CVA, and with prior TIAs there is a tenfold chance of a stroke. Reduced flow may be caused by an atherosclerotic narrowing

of the blood vessel or to small emboli that temporarily lodge in the vessel. The attacks may last less than a minute or two or up to several hours, with the average attack lasting 15 minutes. Manifestations are often abrupt and can include visual disturbances, transient hemiparesis (muscular weakness on one side) or sensory loss on one side. Lips and tongue may become numb, causing slurred speech. Multiple TIAs often precede a complete stroke and may serve as warning of a cerebral vascular disturbance. Further diagnostic testing, such as a cerebral angiogram or CT scan, may be indicated. Prevention of a TIA is uncertain, but their occurrence may alert the person to see a doctor and prevent further damage caused by a full-scale stroke by taking 'blood thinning' medications.

TRAUMATIC DISORDERS

Concussion of the brain

A **concussion** is a transient shaking of the brain resulting from a violent blow to the head or a fall. The person typically loses consciousness and cannot remember the events of the occurrence. Although the brain may not actually be damaged, the whole body is affected; the pulse rate is weak, and when consciousness is regained, the person may experience nausea and dizziness. A severe headache may follow, and the person should be watched closely, since a coma may ensue, and that could be life-threatening.

In the UK, about 8 per 100 000 people every year suffer severe traumatic brain injuries (TBIs), another 18 per 100 000 suffer moderate TBIs, and 250–300 per 100 000 suffer mild TBIs. About 6–10 per 100 000 TBI victims die per year in the UK, and TBI is a leading cause of death for those under the age of 45. There are many causes of TBI, from falling and vehicle accidents to sports injuries.

A person suffering from a concussion should be kept quiet, and drugs that stimulate or depress the nervous system, such as painkillers, are contraindicated. The condition usually corrects itself with time and rest. Prevention is difficult because of the unpredictability of some situations, but vehicular accident-related concussions are down owing to the use of seatbelts and child car seats.

Contusion

In a **contusion**, there is a bruising to brain tissue even though the skin at the site of the trauma may not be broken, as it is in a skull fracture. The brain injury may be on the side of the impact or on the opposite side, where the brain is forced against the skull. Blood from broken blood vessels may accumulate in the brain, causing swelling and pain. The blood clots and necrotic tissue form and could block the flow of CSF, causing a form of hydrocephalus.

Efforts must be made to reduce intracranial pressure, and surgery may be necessary to alleviate pressure and to remove blood clots. Simple pain reduction measures, such as ice packs, may help until professional help arrives. Along with observation, rest will be necessary for full recovery, although some pain medications may be prescribed if needed.

Skull fractures

The most serious complication of a skull fracture is damage to the brain. A fracture at the base of the skull is likely to affect vital centres in the brainstem. The pressure that increases because of accumulation of CSF or blood must be reduced by emergency medical intervention. Another danger of skull fractures is that bacteria may be able to access the brain directly.

Haemorrhages

Haemorrhages can occur in the meninges, causing blood to accumulate between the brain and the skull. A severe injury to the temple can cause an artery just inside the skull to rupture. The blood then flows between the dura mater and the skull; this is known as an **extradural** or **epidural** haemorrhage (Figure 13.11). The increased pressure of the blood causes the patient to lose consciousness. Surgery is required immediately to seal off the

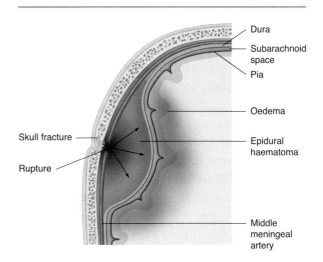

Figure 13.11 Extradural haematoma.

bleeding vessel and remove the blood. No blood would be found in a lumbar puncture because the blood accumulation is outside the dura mater.

A haemorrhage under the dura mater is a **subdural** haemorrhage or haematoma (Figure 13.12), and is caused by a rupture of a cranial vein, or the large venous sinuses of the brain, rather than an artery. This breach may occur from a severe blow to

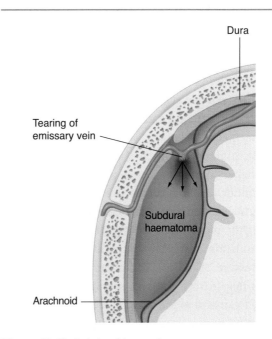

Figure 13.12 Subdural haematoma.

the front or back of the head. The blood clots and CSF accumulates in a cyst-like formation. Intracranial pressure increases, but the cerebral symptoms may not develop for a time. Subdural haemorrhages are sometimes chronic occurrences in cases of alcoholic abuse (owing to falling accidents) and in battered or violently abused individuals.

The surface membrane of the brain may be torn by a skull fracture, causing a **subarachnoid** haemorrhage. Blood flows into the subarachnoid space, where CSF circulates. Blood is found in the CSF with a lumbar puncture. Rupture of an aneurysm can also cause a subarachnoid haemorrhage.

Many haemorrhages are accidental and unpredictable. Therefore, prevention is not easy to project, but prior symptoms may be used as indicators to reduce occurrences.

BRAIN TUMOURS

Tumours of the brain may be malignant or benign. Because benign tumours may grow and compress vital nerve centres, they are considered serious growths. Benign tumours are usually encapsulated, and they can be completely removed surgically. Malignant tumours have extensive roots and are extremely difficult or impossible to remove in their entirety. Most malignant tumours of the brain are metastatic from other organs, especially the lung and breast. Primary malignant tumours of the brain are called **gliomas**, tumours of the glial cells that support nerve tissue rather than growths of the neurons themselves.

Brain tumours manifest themselves in different ways depending on the site and growth rate of the tumour. **Astrocytomas** are basically benign, slow-growing tumours. **Glioblastomas multiforme** are highly malignant, rapidly growing tumours. Brain function is affected by the increased intracranial pressure. Mannitol, corticosteroids and cranial shunts help relieve the pressure symptoms. Blood supply to an area of the brain may be reduced by an infiltrating tumour or by oedema, and this causes dysfunctional activity as well as causing the tissue to become necrotic.

Symptoms of brain tumours typically include a severe headache because of the increased pressure of the tumour. Personality changes, loss of memory or development of poor judgement may give further evidence of a brain tumour. Visual disturbances, double vision or partial blindness often occur, and the ability to speak may be impaired. An upright person may be unsteady while standing or become drowsy. Seizures often develop and may progress into a coma.

Diagnostic measures include MRI and CT scans plus a full array of skull X-rays. Treatment depends on growth type and location. When possible, surgery (see Chapter 4) is followed by radiation and/or chemotherapy. Radiosurgery uses a gamma knife, and the radiation is beamed through designated holes in a helmet that directs the radiation specifically to the target. A limitation of gamma knife surgery is that a special nuclear facility is required for this procedure.

CRANIAL NERVE DISEASE

Trigeminal neuralgia

Any one of the twelve pairs of cranial nerves may be subject to impairment. Individual cranial nerves may be affected by degeneration or unknown causes and is thus involved with various ailments. The fifth (V) cranial nerve, or trigeminal nerve, may become inflamed, causing severe intermittent pain, usually on one side of the face. This condition, known as trigeminal neuralgia or *tic douloureux*, affects 10 people per 100 000 in the UK (Figure 13.13). The cause of *tic douloureux* is often idiopathic but may be caused by stress, tumours compressing the nerve or, in young individuals, may be an indication of multiple sclerosis barring other neurological signs. Those affected are usually age 40 or older and complain of severe pain, especially around the oral cavity (the tongue, lips and gums). This recurring pain may or may not respond readily to pain medication. Anticonvulsive agents like phenytoin or carbamazepine are generally prescribed. In very severe and resistant cases, surgery may be considered.

Sensory distribution

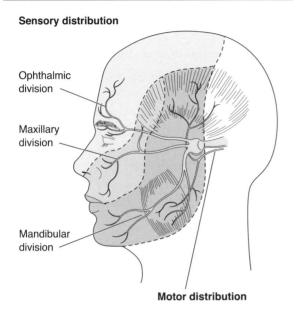

Figure 13.13 Sensory and motor distribution of the trigeminal nerve. There are three sensory divisions: ophthalmic, maxillary and mandibular.

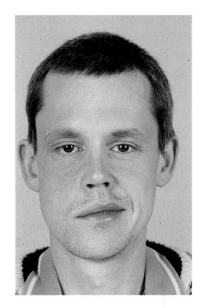

Figure 13.14 Bell's palsy, showing typical drooping of one side of the face.
(NIH/Phototake NYC)

Ablation or microvascular decompression of the nerve as it exits the skull will reduce the pain, as will using glycerol, radiofrequency or even radiation to damage the sensory root elements and give pain relief in a procedure called **rhizotomy**.

Bell's palsy

Bell's palsy involves the inflammation of the seventh (VII) cranial nerve, or facial nerve. The aetiology is usually unknown, but viruses, autoimmunity and vascular ischaemia are probable factors. This nerve may also be traumatised, compressed or invaded by pathogens. Because the seventh cranial nerve innervates facial muscles and salivary glands, attacks cause sagging of the facial muscles on one side of the face and a watery eye. The person may drool and have slurred speech (Figure 13.14). In these cases, massage or heat treatment may help. Recovery may take weeks. The occurrence of Bell's palsy is about 25 per 100 000 in the UK.

Some corticoid medications such as prednisone or antiviral agents (aciclovir) are given if herpes simplex 1 (HSV1) is suspected. Therefore, relief of symptoms may not always be quick or simple. Bell's palsy is rare in children. Usually it strikes between ages 25 and 50. If the situation fails to be resolved, a facial contracture develops. The prognosis is generally good, although complete healing may take many months to a year.

PAIN

Pain and pain perception are integral parts of nervous system function. In this section, we will discuss the following:

- Definition of pain
- The function or purpose of pain
- Types and characteristics of pain
- The physiology of pain
- Pain assessment
- Pain management
- Other methods of pain control

Pain means different things to different individuals. Pain includes a major degree of perception and is therefore subjective. This symptom requires a level of threshold and therefore acts as a gauge of tolerance, plus learned behaviours, that rely on past experience and culture. Threshold accounts for the initial level of pain that an individual acknowledges, while tolerance suggests the point at which the same individual requires treatment in dealing with the pain. Thus, pain may be thought of as an individualistic occurrence.

In neurophysiology, pain is described as a result of some form of tissue damage. However, this simple definition does not account for emotional pain or pain resulting from some functional disorders. When physical breakdowns or lesions are apparent, it is easier to ascertain an accompanying pain criterion. Functional disparities are not always found or determined through superficial observation (e.g. a microscope), but many forms of psychogenic pain are well recognised and treated.

Regardless of definition, perception or understanding, pain is a sensation of hurt or a strong discomfort, typically from some form of noxious stimulus. Therefore, pain is caused by injury or disease and is transmitted throughout the body to associated cortical areas in the brain for interpretation and prospective recourse.

Pain does have a purpose and function. Its primary purpose is to warn the person of an abnormal state, like inflammation, infection, body trauma or injury. Second, it is a signal not to pursue any activity that causes additional pain and thus may cause any more damage. This pause will assist the healing process by allowing the body to rest and conserve resources for recovery and homeostasis. Pain is considered the most common cause that forces individuals to the doctor's surgery.

There is a rare alternative to pain sensation, known as 'congenital insensitivity to pain', found in individuals who are born without a sense of pain. In these cases, the nervous system is not equipped to instruct the person about injurious conditions or accidents and may allow continual walking on broken limbs or permit advanced infections to go untreated. There is a natural reluctance to pain, but without it life may be less safe.

Categories and characteristics of pain

Various categories of pain usually refer to origination or duration. The pain origin includes areas such as cutaneous (skin), somatic (body), visceral (organ), neuropathic or referred (redirected site). Somatic pain involves blood vessels, nerves, muscles and joints (e.g. sprained ankle), while cutaneous pain may emanate from a pinprick or sunburn. Visceral pain may be diffuse or poorly localised. In the case of appendicitis, pain is referred to the surface of the right lower quadrant of the abdomen, even though the problem is internal (see Table 13.1).

Neuropathic pain may not be caused by a commonly held noxious agent but tends to be delayed and induce a generalised burning sensation and occasionally stabbing pain, as found in the legs of some diabetics.

Pain duration is acute (immediate) or chronic. Acute pain has a relatively short time of activity (e.g. within 6 months), whereas chronic pain exceeds the 6-month time frame and may last for years. Severity and specific descriptions, like pounding, throbbing, and sharp or dull, help to qualify the situation as well.

Pain importance may be ascribed to the fact that pain receptors (**nociceptors**) are the most abundant sensory receptor in the skin; there are as many as 1300 per square inch. Compared to touch or thermal receptors, pain reception is scattered around to ensure basic protection and homeostatic balance. Nociceptors consist of free nerve ending elements

Table 13.1 Body regional pain.

Body region	Pain manifestations
Cranial	Headache – common, migraine Oral – toothache Facial – Bell's palsy
Cervical – neck	Whiplash – may become chronic pain
Torso	Chest – heart pain, lung Abdominal – gastric (e.g. ulcer) Appendix, gallbladder – stones Lumbar – lower back, pinched nerve Pelvic – ovary, urinary bladder
Extremities – limbs	Muscle and joint pain (e.g. arthritis)

(not encapsulated) attached to a sensory neuron. Pain receptors are found in the viscera, or internal organs, as well, as noted by gas pains or gastric burning sensations, and in the muscles and joints.

The physiology of pain and the pain theory concept

The most commonly supported theory by which pain is exhibited is called the gate control theory. The physiological process begins with an afferent nociceptor that responds to the stimulus of pain. This information then travels along a neuronal fibre as an impulse. There are differences in the size or diameter of the neuronal fibres. They can be insulated with myelin or unmyelinated and this causes a variance in the conduction velocity of their impulse. The largest diameter fibre type is the A-beta form, which responds to light touch in the skin and therefore normally does not cause a pain response. The small diameter myelinated A-delta and unmyelinated C fibres are found in nerves of the skin and deeper somatic (body) and visceral structures. These fibres are missing in individuals with congenital insensitivity to pain. Some designated areas, like the cornea, have only A-delta and C fibre neurons because they respond maximally only to intense and painful stimuli. For the most part, afferent nociceptors respond to heat and intense mechanical stimuli (e.g. pinching and noxious or irritating chemicals). When these fibres are blocked from responding, then no pain sensation is expressed.

The gate control theory holds that pain impulses are transmitted from specialised nociceptors within the skin, muscle or joints to the spinal cord. These impulses are carried by large A and small C fibres to a specialised area within the superior horn of the spinal cord known as the substantia gelatinosa. This area acts as a gate that regulates transmission for impulses to the CNS. Stimulation of the larger fibres (A) causes cells within the substantia gelatinosa to 'close the gate' and therefore diminish pain perception. The smaller fibre elements (C) do the reverse and thus enhance pain perception. Depending on the degree of opening and closing, the CNS regulates

pain output. Similarly, the thalamus, functioning as a relay station, tends to delegate or transmit some pain activity and alternately inhibit other pain transmission. The quick-acting myelinated large nerve fibres (A) tend to carry impulses for well localised, sharp pain, while the unmyelinated C fibres carry sensations more slowly, as in a diffuse burning or aching feeling (Figure 13.15). Note that amplified or continual outside impulses interfere with pain input, as when we bang our head against a wall or pound our fist; the force of the activity delays or diverts the pain sensation.

Another concept, known as the nociceptor pain process, extends the gate control theory. It consists of four primary features: transduction, transmission, perception of pain and modulation; these will be discussed here. These features parallel physiological nerve conduction operations.

In transduction, the nociceptors distinguish among the various stimuli as to noxious or harmful versus innocuous inputs. Transduction also converts the noxious stimuli into sensory nerve ending impulses to the spinal cord and describes how pain is perceived by the body. Transmission is the movement of the transduced stimuli into impulses that ascend up the spinal cord to the brainstem and thalamus. From here the dispatched impulse proceeds to the proper cortical lobe or area (e.g. parietal lobe) for pain interpretation. Some impulses may be challenged or blocked from relay as well. Perception of pain means the sensation has become a conscious feeling. The overall perception and response process is not well understood, especially among different individuals. Again the reminder here is that pain is an individual-type sensation. Modulation is the manipulation that the brain imposes on signals to modify or inhibit pain impulses. In this case, the brain naturally releases compounds that produce relief (analgesia) called **endorphins** and **enkephalins**. These compounds are often referred to in the case of marathon runners who feel a sense of euphoria miles into a race. Both of the prevailing concepts of pain attempt to incorporate basic neurological processes or principles with a means to envision a mechanism for interpretation and control.

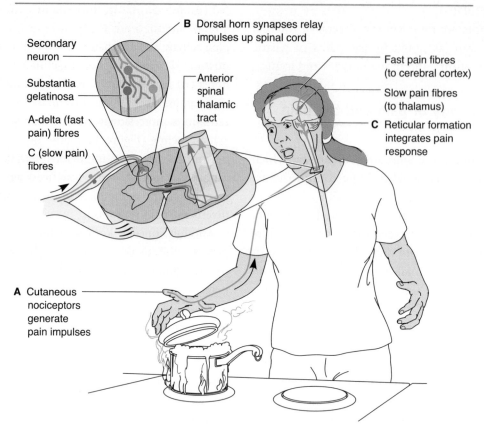

Figure 13.15 (A) Cutaneous nociceptors generate pain impulses that travel via A-delta and C fibres to the spinal cord's dorsal horn. (B) Secondary neurons in the dorsal horn pass impulses across the spinal cord to the anterior spinothalamic tract. (C) Slow pain impulses ascend to the thalamus, while fast pain impulses ascend to the cerebral cortex. The reticular formation in the brainstem integrates the emotional, cognitive and autonomic responses to pain.

Pain assessment and management

The most reliable indicator of the presence and degree of pain is reported by the person experiencing it. Pain must also be assessed. During the assessment process, there are a variety of considerations: language barriers, children and developmental stage, and those with hearing limitations or who are intubated. A variety of tools are used to assess pain. These tools include simple pictorial or numeric scales or mnemonics that can help convey vital information from the patient to the healthcare assistant or clinician (Figure 13.16). Culture, age and past experience with pain can also influence assessment findings.

Chronic pain causes fatigue and interferes with the routines of working, eating, sleeping and concentrating. In the case of cancer, chronic pain may become the central concern. The cancer may become secondary to pain for some stricken individuals, because it may be exacerbated by treatment and fear. Cancer-related pain can be acute or chronic, but accurate assessment of pain is essential as it influences treatment. Counselling and group therapy may help relieve some anxiety and uncertainty, especially in cases of little or no family support.

Pain management depends on a number of variables, but the focus is to control pain without serious side effects. Over-the-counter and prescription

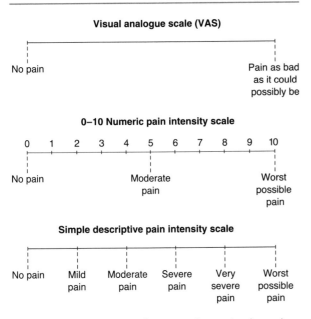

Figure 13.16 Examples of commonly used pain scales.

medications such as opiates are often needed to treat acute or chronic pain. See Table 13.2 for a summary of alternative treatments.

The body has its own endogenous opioid agents, called endorphins or enkephalins, to counteract pain-causing symptoms such as induced by substance P, an agent that is thought to be released from a pain source. However, it is the medication that tends to act on a specific target. Aspirin is a widely used drug; others include NSAIDs, like paracetamol, ibuprofen or naproxen, all of which work to reduce or stop pain primarily in the PNS. Opiates or narcotic-type drugs work best in the CNS by blocking or interfering with pain receptors or pathways (e.g. oxycodone or pethidine). Chronic pain requires stronger remedies like morphine.

Table 13.2 Alternative pain therapies.

Therapy	Methodology/purpose
Acupuncture	Ancient Eastern method may stimulate release of endorphins
Aromatherapy	Oils and scents along with bath or massage
Biofeedback therapy	Electrothermal devices plus training for pain (e.g. migraine)
Heat and cold packs	Pain relief in traumas such as sprains and burns
Humour	Acts as a distraction and comfort, at least temporarily
Hypnosis	Extends pain relief or blocks pain perception
Imagery	Induces relaxation; may induce endorphins and reduce stress
Massage	Promotes muscle relaxation and blood flow for comfort
Music and art	Provide soothing atmosphere in clinics and help to calm patient fears
Relaxation techniques	Reduce muscle tension and increase pain threshold; reflexology is an example
Transcendental meditation (TM)	Solitary introspection for calming relaxation
Transcutaneous electrical nerve stimulation (TENS)	Electrical stimulation through skin patches to interfere with pain release and timing activities
Yoga	Body manipulation, mind relaxation and mind control technique

DISEASES OF THE SPECIAL SENSES: EYE AND EAR

Special senses include the nose for olfaction or sense of smell; the tongue for gustatory or taste sensations; the eyes for vision; and the ears for acoustics or hearing. Diseases related to the nose and nasal cavity were discussed in Chapter 8; diseases of the eye and ear are covered in the sections that follow.

The eye

Our discussion starts with protective coverings of the eye, called eyelids and associate glands, and continues to the eye surface or conjunctiva, the clear area known as the cornea, the photoreceptors and the retina, and the optic nerve (Figure 13.17). The ear disorders will also be covered from the external to the internal components.

Eyelids and associate glands One of the most noticeable lesions found on the eyelid is the common **stye** or **hordeolum**. This reddish tender lump is caused by a local staphylococcus abscess on the upper or lower lid. Smaller styes tend to be external to the lid surface and on the margin, while internal styes tend to jut toward the eye surface. Sometimes they resolve themselves, but when the lesion is large enough to cause irritation or a reduced field of vision, treatment is required. A warm compress or application of an antibiotic ointment usually resolves the situation. Because of oversight or lack of attention, these common bumps tend to recur, especially in youngsters.

Similar to the stye is a hardened internal lesion called a **chalazion**. This inflammation impacts a deeper oil gland (**meibomian**) and feels tender and irritated. The oil secreted by the meibomian gland is necessary to prevent the watery tear fluid from evaporating. When the oil is absent, a dry eye develops, which causes pain and potential for a coarse sclera and corneal surface or superficial cracks. As in cases of exophthalmia, found in Graves' disease (Chapter 12), eye drops help relieve the dryness. When given extended, albeit untreated, time, the condition may resolve itself, but hot compresses normally help, with a gentle massage, repeated twice daily for best results. If the condition does not improve, vision may be impaired and a corticosteroid injection may be needed or the cyst may need to be lanced to let it drain. Once resolved, the problem seems to subside and, with increased awareness, the occurrence is reduced.

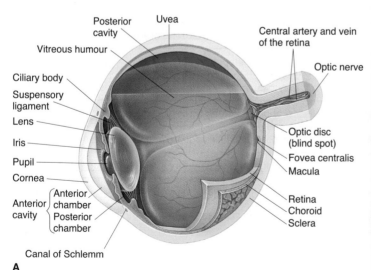
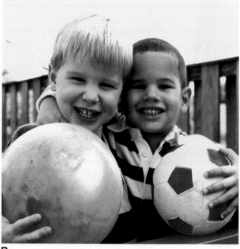

Figure 13.17 (A) Human eye anatomy and (B) normal vision image.
(National Eye Institute)

Blepharitis is a common chronic inflammation, with or without ulcers, often involving both eyelid margins and perhaps becoming bilateral (occurring in both eyes). This bacterially initiated problem resembles seborrhoea of the scalp and eyebrows or perhaps acne rosacea (see Chapter 16). Itching and burning sensations are caused by oozing pus, and a thick crust develops, especially after sleep. The potential for ulceration of the cornea is serious, and treatment is warranted. Antibiotic ointment such as polymyxin B may be used for known microbe types and, if other skin conditions are factors, they should be addressed as well. Preventive measures include good hygiene, with consistency, and proper training to keep hands away from nose, mouth and especially eyes.

Dacryocystitis is an infection and obstruction of the nasolacrimal apparatus for tear production and drainage. Common skin flora like *Staphylococcus aureus* or the beta version of streptococcus and yeast infection (e.g. *Candida albicans*) are all potential sources. Symptoms include swelling, tenderness and pain. If chronic, tearing and pus discharge are cause for surgical relief, and antibiotics may continue, although they may have been unable to dry up the ducting network initially. Spontaneous healing can occur in some patients.

Prevention of common infectious conditions is achieved through hygiene and retraining of old habits, like unnecessary finger and hand contact with the eye. If known allergies are recognised, they must be avoided or eliminated if possible.

Conjunctivitis Conjunctivitis is an inflammation of the conjunctiva, the superficial covering of the visible sclera (white of the eye) and the inner linings of the eyelids. Red, swollen eyes with discharge and some discomfort are the usual symptoms. About 30% of all eye complaints are conjunctivitis, commonly called 'pink eye', yet many cases go unreported, and children are the primary source group.

Various fumes, such as from peeled onions or bathroom cleansers, may initiate an inflammatory or allergic response. However, viruses and various bacteria, including the normal bacterial flora such as *Staphylococcus aureus*, or fungi commonly cause

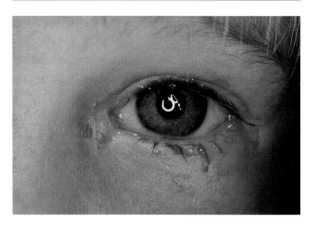

Figure 13.18 Conjunctivitis.
(© Dorling Kindersley)

conjunctivitis. Unfortunately, these viral and bacterial infections are quite contagious, and therefore patients, usually children, are instructed to stay home from school or social activities. Reinfections may occur owing to lack of hygiene and to rubbing or touching the eye unnecessarily. Often the inflammation subsides on its own accord, but it may progress into *inclusion conjunctivitis*, which is caused by particular bacteria (e.g. *Chlamydia trachomatis*) and is longer lasting. For diagnosis and determination of infective agents, ocular swabs are taken to culture and suggest favourable antidotes. Topical antibiotics or eye drops, such as chloramphenicol (even in viral cases, to prevent secondary infection) or antihistamines and cold compresses help control the 'pink eye' (see Figure 13.18).

Chronic conjunctivitis, or **trachoma**, results when the infecting agent invades the conjunctiva. These cases tend to be highly contagious and, when severe, may disrupt the corneal surface and impair vision. The infective agent in this case is *Chlamydia trachomatis*, mentioned previously, the same organism responsible for the STI chlamydia (see Chapter 11). Infected mothers pass on this infection to the newborn. Tetracycline is usually administered to resolve trachoma.

Prevention of conjunctivitis is best achieved by reducing hand to eye contact, disposing of contaminated materials such as contact lenses and beauty products (e.g. mascara), and avoiding known allergic agents or persons with conjunctivitis.

Glaucoma Glaucoma is an insidious, painless disease that typically results from pressure building up in the anterior chamber of the eye or the space in front of the lens. This condition is known as chronic glaucoma and will be discussed here; however, another condition is acute glaucoma, which is accompanied by intense pain and blurriness. In acute cases intraocular pressure must be relieved immediately to reduce pain and to save vision.

The aqueous humour made by the ciliary body apparatus is produced at a fairly constant rate and normally drains away. But in glaucoma, fluid accumulates and increases the pressure within the eye. Pressure exceeding twice the normal intraocular pressure (8–21 mmHg) causes the retina to start losing its ability to distinguish images clearly. This progression of events continues until a partial to total blindness develops. Peripheral vision is severely reduced if the condition is untreated; then it is lost and 'tunnel vision' ensues as the photoreceptors on the retina are destroyed and continue to deteriorate visual quality (eyesight) (Figure 13.19).

A glaucoma gene, *GLCA1*, on chromosome 1 may account for some of the 172 000 new referrals each year, of which about a third become confirmed cases in the UK. Worldwide, glaucoma affects about 66.8 million individuals. Most congenital glaucoma is hereditary, while secondary glaucoma is caused by systemic diseases, such as infections, or drugs like corticosteroids. This disease increases in prevalence over the age of 40. In South East Asia glaucoma is quite common, considering a host of tropical infections and lack of treatment. Individuals with a family history or with diabetes should have frequent eye checkups.

The ophthalmoscope is the primary portable tool used by the ophthalmologist to view the interior of the eyeball for general inspection. However, to diagnose glaucoma, a non-contact ('air-puff') **tonometer** helps to screen for the disease by bouncing a puff of air off the cornea that flattens it slightly and allows a quick register of intraocular pressure. After first using numbing droplets on the eye, a more accurate measurement is done with **applanation tonometry**, which allows the instrument to touch the cornea lightly. The pressure required to indent the corneal surface is measured, and using a slit lamp (magnifying) device allows the ophthalmologist to explore the whole interior of the eye with bright light and obtain a three-dimensional view. In this case, the lighted interior tends to show a cupping of the optic disc, where the optic nerve enters the back of the eye.

Drugs such as timolol reduce fluid production, and pilocarpine promotes aqueous humour flow. Surgery involves piercing the anterior chamber with a laser, which promotes draining and reduction in pressure and improves vision. Prevention is basically genetically determined but includes a healthy diet with adequate intake of vitamin A, and good vision care (e.g. reducing infections via limited hand–eye contact, and wearing eye protection such as sunglasses).

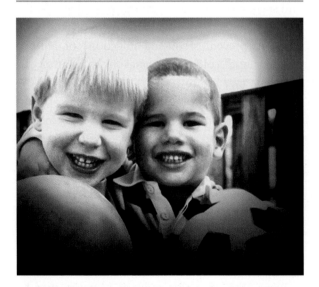

Figure 13.19 Glaucoma visual image reveals tunnel vision.

(National Eye Institute)

Uveitis The uvea is the second layer of the eye known as the vascular or pigmented layer and includes the ciliary body and the coloured part of the eye known as the iris. Inflammation of the uvea may be caused by infectious agents, especially in reduced immune conditions, but uveitis itself has an immunological or neoplastic basis.

Symptoms include pain, redness, photophobia and blurred vision. If the inflammatory attack is in front of the lens (anterior) or behind it (posterior), different approaches are taken to ensure the best outcome. Anterior inflammation accounts for about 90% of the cases and usually lends itself to topical corticosteroids. Posterior uveitis requires systemic (internal) medications or intravitreal (in uvea) corticosteroid therapy, and, if bacterial agents are present, then appropriate antibiotics are used. This primarily immune disorder is related to or accompanies many other conditions or diseases, from psoriasis to Crohn's disease. Prevalence is estimated at 38 per 100 000 in the western world, with approximately 9100 new cases per year in England and Wales.

Light and refractory distortions

Astigmatism Light enters the clear curved cornea. If the cornea is pitted from prior ulceration or is asymmetrical or has thick and thin sections, it transmits light to the lens and retina in irregular wavelengths. Similarly, if the lens is warped or irregular, the transmitted light is uneven. Both scenarios give a blurry or unclear image when the light (image) strikes the retinal surface. This refractory condition is called **astigmatism**. It may be associated with any other eye condition, like myopia, and may affect one eye or both. The objects viewed might be recognisable, but there is always some degree of distortion to the overall image. Corrective lenses, including contact lenses, help but may not fully repair the condition, especially if the irregularities are with the internal lens. Cornea adjustments may be made surgically, or the lens can be replaced. Most individuals tend to ignore the minor deficiency and adjust to it.

Myopia and hyperopia (nearsightedness and farsightedness) The more common types of eye problems involve distance. An acuity test done by the famous Snellen chart (E letters) allows determination of a 20/20 (normal) or a range from 20/200 to 20/10 reading for different distance levels. Nearsightedness, or myopia, and farsightedness, or hyperopia, as well as astigmatism, described earlier, are outlined in Figure 13.20.

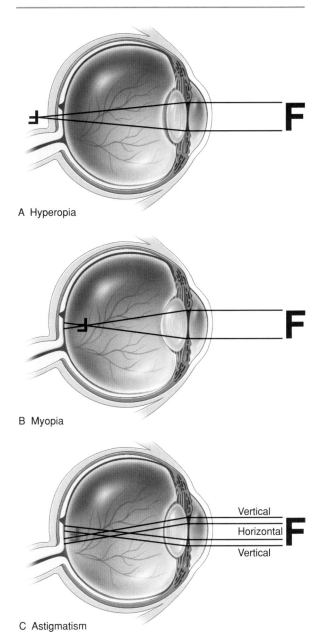

A Hyperopia

B Myopia

C Astigmatism

Figure 13.20 In hyperopia light rays focus behind the retina, making it difficult to focus on objects at close range. In myopia light rays focus in front of the retina, making it difficult to focus on objects that are far away. In astigmatism light rays do not uniformly focus on the eye owing to abnormal curvature of cornea or lens.

Compared to normal vision, myopia or nearsightedness is noticed when close objects are clear and sharp while more distance objects are blurred. The eyeball is longer than normal, so the image falls short (thus the term short/nearsightedness) and does not reach the retina sufficiently, leaving a blurry image. It may be that the lens is too thick and thus the image would fall in front of the retina. To correct myopia, a concave lens is required to stretch incoming light rays to reach the retina and give a clear picture. Approximately 5 million people in the UK have myopia.

In the case of hyperopia (hypermetropia), objects at a distance are clear, but those images close up are blurry. About twice as many people have hyper-metropia as have myopia in the UK. The eyeball appears too short, or the lens may be too thin. A convex lens is required to bend the light waves more quickly or shorter to strike the retina in a clearly focused fashion. Contact lenses work well, and laser treatments may shave layers off the cornea or lens to improve sight. LASIK surgery, a type of cornea surgery, holds great promise for long-term relief. LASIK surgery eliminates or reduces use of eyeglasses or contact lenses for most normal activities requiring near- or far-sighted vision. For some tasks, reading glasses may still be required. With either case, astigmatism may be an additional part of the visual correction, and that would require a special lens or glasses to offer a sharper image at the retinal surface. The astigmatism may be in one or both eyes and be of varying degree.

Presbyopia Presbyopia is an age-related and refractive disorder. At about age 45, the crystalline lens of the eye loses its flexibility and causes a reduc-tion in the ability to focus images on the retina. This may happen rather suddenly, but the lens has been growing from birth and continues to grow throughout life, so by the time of death the lens has increased in weight by about four times. This change is a normal modification to the eye caused by aging, and individuals notice the problem when they hold pictures and written material at arm's length to obtain a better view. Optometrists can fit corrective lens like bifocals or trifocals or contact lenses for better vision. Because things continue to change, so must the corrective lenses.

Cataracts Cataracts are the result of a clouding of the lens. There are three types of cataracts that correspond to the three layers of the lens. The outer layer is a clear membrane or capsule, the middle zone is composed of soft clear material called the cortex, and the core is the least flexible site called the nucleus. The cause of cataracts is not known, but they have been attributed to a congenital defect, eye trauma, the effects of toxins and aging. The main symptom is fading and distortion of vision. Additional lighting is useful early on, especially for printed material, and this helps clue the person as to an impending visual impairment.

By age 65, some degree of cataracts and thus impaired vision has occurred in a large portion of the population, increasing in numbers further after age 75. Usually by the eighth decade, cataracts have become more evident or ripe. A routine (general) eye examination, using ophthalmoscopy, normally detects early stages of cataracts. This detection allows planning for treatment if needed or preven-tative measures to reduce the progression of cataract development, such as avoiding bright light and wearing sunglasses. A new measuring device called an **aberrometer** allows a better record of the status of the eye and assists the preparation of LASIK surgery to match or exceed what glasses or contact lenses do for sight. The patient looks at a pattern of faint red lights, and the machine makes detailed optical measurements as it inspects the interior of the eyeball. This procedure is simple and painless. In the past, treatment was usually non-specific or withheld, and with time the lens was surgically replaced. Outpatient surgery for lens replacement, including lenses for 20/20 vision or bifocals, has become a routine procedure, and vision is restored to normal in patients 95% of the time. Prevention is almost impossible for an age-related condition or in the face of a concurrent disease (e.g. diabetes or syphilis). However, avoiding harmful drugs or chemicals and direct sunlight can postpone this common disorder (see Figure 13.21).

Retinal image defects
Macular degeneration Macular degeneration is the reduction or loss of acute vision. Macular degen-eration develops in 10% of the elderly and affects both eyes, affecting only central vision and leaving

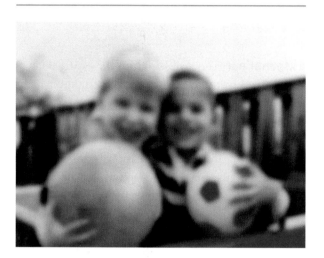

Figure 13.21 Cataracts show the whole image as blurry.
(National Eye Institute)

peripheral vision intact. There are two forms of macular degeneration: the atrophic (dry) version, comprising 70+% of the cases, and the exudative (wet, haemorrhagic) type, a more destructive version (see Figure 13.22).

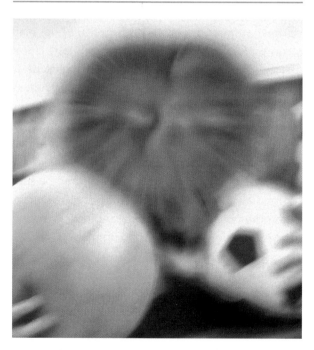

Figure 13.22 Age-related macular degeneration demonstrating loss of central vision.
(National Eye Institute)

Causes for this degeneration are not well understood, but it is known that obstructed blood flow, followed by revascularisation (as occurs in atherosclerosis), compromises the area of the retina responsible for acute vision. Other contributing factors are injury, inflammation, infection and heredity.

Diagnosis is by direct eye examination with ophthalmoscope and fluorescein angiography, which reveal leaking vessels in the subretinal area. There is no cure for the atrophic case, but 5–10% reduction in the exudative condition can be accomplished by using an argon laser to cause photocoagulation.

Diabetic retinopathy About 40% of diabetes type 1 patients will be diagnosed with diabetic retinopathy within 3 years of diagnosis. Depending on the intensity of the diabetes and patient's age, it may be a mild abnormality or a major factor causing loss of eyesight. It is the leading cause of new blindness in adults aged 20–65. In type 2 diabetes, about 20% of cases have diabetic retinopathy at the time of diagnosis. Screening involves dilated pupils and ophthalmoscopy, which may become routine annual events with eye checkups. Special attention must be given to those pregnant or attempting to become pregnant. This monitoring is performed primarily through diabetes control measures, such as blood glucose levels and kidney functioning plus blood pressure measurements. In exudative cases, leakage can be abated by using an argon laser to cause photocoagulation. Prevention is unlikely considering the universal effect over the body that diabetes mellitus presents.

Retinitis pigmentosa Retinitis pigmentosa is a genetic disease either as a recessive or dominant trait on the X chromosome. Other forms may exist, but it is a rare, progressive retinal degeneration that eventually causes blindness. The symptoms of weakened sight start in childhood and slowly encroach peripherally and cause tunnel vision, somewhat like glaucoma. A special electroretinogram that measures the retina and its response to light determines the disease and its status. No particular treatment is known, although some success has been noted with fetal retinal tissue transplant. Retinal detachment is possible here as well, and that causes more complications for treatment.

The optic nerve may be a part of the visual disturbance pattern, and that may be caused by physical strain, such as trauma or pressure (stretching) in the event of exophthalmos, as found in hyperthyroidism. With various toxins (especially heavy metals), low oxygen levels and drugs (including Viagra), the optic nerve is sensitive to many factors injurious to eyesight. Blindness normally develops when light is blocked to the retina as in cataracts and when there is increased intraocular pressure as in glaucoma, optic nerve damage or image failure recognition by the occipital cortex. Regardless of cause, the best way to prevent visual impairment is to practise good hygiene (e.g. avoid unnecessary hand–eye contact), observe safety precautions and seek medical help with any noticeable eye problem.

The ear

Hearing loss is a major problem for those with normal acoustic function, and there are three categories of hearing loss: conductive, mainly a blockage or physical problem; sensory loss owing to inner ear elements being lost or compromised; and neural hearing loss from damage to the auditory nerve (VIII). Age can be a major factor in hearing disabilities, along with the environmental workplace and modern instrumentation, including mobile phones and personal audio devices that put a significant stress on hearing abilities. Almost 9 million people in the UK are deaf or have some hearing loss; that is, about one in seven of the population, particularly the elderly.

Conductive hearing loss is commonly caused by excess ear wax build-up (cerumen impaction), a tumour, or pus build-up in the auditory canal or middle ear from infection (external otitis, otitis media). The middle ear bony ossicles may stiffen as in arthritis, called **otosclerosis**, and a perforated ear drum is a frequent occurrence. All of these situations reduce hearing abilities and require different modes or procedures to correct them. External and middle ear infection are common events, especially

in children, and these dysfunctional disorders are now addressed.

External ear The visible part of the external ear is known as the **auricle** or **pinna** and it enhances hearing perception by a small amount (2–4%). It assists hearing by collecting sound waves and funnelling them down the auditory canal and is subject to skin cancer, primarily from sun exposure, and trauma from accidents or athletic activities, e.g. rugby. Skin cancer is treated mainly by surgery. Trauma cases may require surgery as well and to prevent disfigurement (such as a 'cauliflower' appearance). Cosmetically, auricle design or size may be an issue, especially for children when the auricles are extra large or protrude and appear asymmetrical. Infections can occur when pierced ear ring sites are not properly cleaned, and some metals cause allergic reactions. Protecting the ear from severe environmental extremes and using ear plugs for noise reduction are effective preventive measures for reducing hearing loss (see Figure 13.23).

Cerumen impaction Wax is necessary for the soft texture and flexibility of the ear drum. However, cerumen impaction or excess wax build-up may recur, especially in youngsters or the elderly. Upon first appearance of wax building, better hygiene is required. The build-up is usually alleviated by heated water, oil treatment, hydrogen peroxide (3%) or alcohol drops as simple remedies. However, on occasion a suction action or mechanical removal is necessary. It is imperative to have an intact ear drum when performing any treatment, and be sure to dry the ear area completely following treatment. Prevention is possible through routinely checking the ear canal for signs of wax accumulation.

External otitis External otitis, or 'swimmer's ear', is an infection caused by bacteria and fungi. Symptoms and signs include pain, pruritis, fever and (temporarily) hearing loss.

The pathogens responsible for external otitis are found in contaminated swimming pools or beaches. Drying the external ear opening after bathing or swimming and cleaning ear phones,

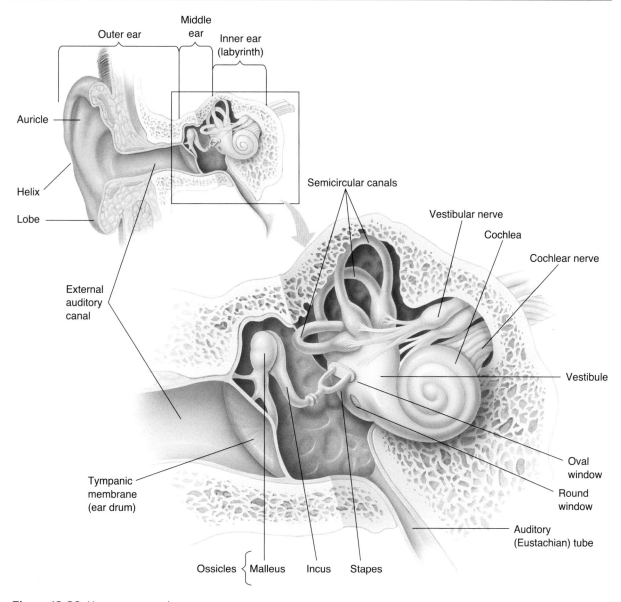

Figure 13.23 Human ear anatomy.

ear plugs and ear muffs can prevent it. Treatment with antibiotics is effective for bacterial infections, but some fungus infections may be more stubborn to control.

Otitis media Acute otitis media is a middle ear infection that affects primarily infants and children because of weak immune systems and perhaps the lack of breastfeeding. Symptoms include pain and oedema, with pus and, left unchecked, the condition may cause perforation of the tympanic membrane (ear drum). Otitis media often follows pneumonia or an upper respiratory tract infection (URTI), such as laryngitis. Most often, bacteria are the cause. Children are more susceptible than adults to middle ear infections because their nearly horizontal auditory tubes prevent adequate drainage. Diagnosis is primarily performed by observation of pus in the ear canal and complaint of earache. Pain can be controlled with analgesics, and swelling is reduced by use of decongestants. To relieve pressure and allow pus to drain, small ear tubes like tiny cylinders are placed through the ear drum (tympanic membrane) to allow air into the middle ear. They are called tympanostomy tubes or myringotomy tubes, or grommets. In recurrent cases, scarring of the ear drum, auditory ossicles and inner ear components can occur. There is potential for invasion of the nearby mastoid area, a honeycombed sinus area, and this penetration results in **mastoiditis**. With mastoiditis comes a fever and the possibility of brain infection or abscess formation because of the relatively thin membrane between the sinus area and the brain vault. In developing countries with inadequate access to healthcare and antibiotics, chronic otitis media and its complications is very common among both adults and children. Penicillin-type antibiotics help, but in some resistant cases, such as those caused by *Pseudomonas aeruginosa*, stronger agents are required.

For chronic otitis media there may be relief. A clinical test study published in 2005, using a device called the EarPopper, had an efficacy (effectiveness) rate of about 85% for those tested. This tool sends a gentle stream of air into the nasal cavity and, as the individual swallows, it forces the Eustachian tube (or auditory tube) open and equalises the pressure within the middle ear. If fluid is present, it may take two treatments per day for a few weeks, but the benefit is that ear surgery is not required. This device is safe, basically pain-free, and can be used by anyone, including children.

Inner ear The inner ear consists of the semicircular canals (which register changes in equilibrium) and the snail-like device called the cochlea. The semicircular canals give a sense of balance and of being upright. In addition, at the base where the three semicircular canals meet and form a connection with the cochlea, stiff ciliated (brush-like) elements attached to neurons line a common chamber. In this same chamber of fluid are grains called **otoliths** that tumble or float down like an hourglass and thereby stimulate the sensory elements to signal the brain about body positioning or orientation (e.g. turned head). Along with the cerebellum and visual cues, the body maintains a normal standing or sitting posture or comprehends body location.

Some infections may interfere with the functioning of semicircular canals. In the case of fever or various drug interactions and electrolyte imbalances, the viscosity of the internal fluid may be altered. Vertigo or dizziness may cause nausea, headache or accidental stumbling or falling. Acute cases of imbalance that may become episodic or longer term vertigo need to be addressed.

The cochlea houses coiled tubes filled with fluid that rushes over miniature hair cells collectively called the **organ of Corti** which triggers signals to the auditory nerve. When the organ of Corti is damaged or lost, the hearing loss is permanent. Loud noises or sounds from heavy equipment, airplanes and loud music or ototoxic drugs like some chemotherapy drugs, and various infective agents leave a scar on the hearing apparatus.

As with sight and age, hearing too has its limitations; this is called **presbycusis**. This condition is the most common cause of sensorineural hearing loss in adults. The actual cause is not known, but the condition tends to run in families and progresses with age. Constant exposure to loud noises gives ample reason to wear devices (ear plugs) to protect the natural hearing mechanism. About 25% of those aged 65–75 have measurable hearing loss, in part due to age, and about half of those over age 75 have presbycusis. Hearing aids help restore some sound, but clarity is somewhat sacrificed.

Neural loss involving the eighth cranial nerve (vestibulocochlear) or auditory nerve has many possibilities. If the nerve is damaged by trauma, high fever, toxins or other agents, the loss may be permanent.

Deafness can have a genetic component, e.g. when a baby is born deaf, and cochlear implants can be used to overcome deafness. Inheritance of deafness may be either dominant or recessive, and over 100 genes have been identified as instrumental in this deficiency. The *connexin-26* mutation has been suggested as a prevalent form of recessive hearing loss. Mitochondrial (cell organelle) disorders and hearing loss also play a significant role in the complex mechanism of auditory challenge. Whatever the circumstance, it is critical to save and protect all areas of the auditory pathway for the melodies of sound; cochlear implants are a viable alternative when hearing is lost.

Ménière's disease The occurrence of **Ménière's disease** is about 1 per 1000 and it usually occurs in the mid to late forties. Primarily considered idiopathic, some cases may be initiated by trauma, tumour or autoimmune diseases that impact the cochlear apparatus whereby fluid and delicate sensory hairs are altered or degenerated. Ménière's disease is characterised by intermittent hearing loss, tinnitus (see below) and episodes of vertigo or dizziness. Therapy is focused on vertigo. Diuretics and restricted salt intake control fluid levels and short-term glucocorticoids reduce inflammatory activity. Surgery may be a later option, but some loss of hearing may occur. Many individuals live with this disease if dizzy spells are reasonably under control.

Tinnitus Tinnitus is defined as the perception of ringing, buzzing or roaring sounds from an environment void of sound. The cause or pathophysiology of tinnitus is not well known, perhaps because there are many causes and tinnitus may be just one indication among many of other disease attributes. At least 1% of the UK population have tinnitus, and some have it severely enough that it interferes with daily life. This development may involve either conductive or sensorineural hearing loss. A full examination of the ear, nose and throat is required to discern problems such as infection, trauma or growths, plus family history and any drug regimen. Diagnosis is similar to other ear investigation and begins with the **Weber and Rinne tuning fork** test. Not only are the frequencies or pitch of the sound noted, but more so, whether the limitation is conductive or sensorineural. The stem of the vibrating fork is placed on the skull near the mastoid process (just behind and under the ear), or maybe the teeth, to tell if a sound is louder or softer compared to the sound in air. If the sound is louder in air versus the contacted bone, then it appears to be a sensorineural insufficiency, and if louder by bone contact, it appears to be a conduction defect.

Tinnitus is known to be affected by, or is part of, a hearing loss problem because of excessive loud noise exposure, poor reaction to some medications or various other health concerns. Treatment by the **otolaryngologist** includes hearing aids to overpower the background sounds, sound-masking devices to cancel or reduce the ringing noises, amplifier devices on phones, or electronic equipment to pick up better quality sound, plus medications and relaxing techniques. People with tinnitus should avoid loud sounds and be patient; some may find that lipoflavanoid supplementation is helpful. Lipoflavanoid is a dietary supplement used since the 1960s to specifically improve the microcirculation within the inner ear. Therefore, the flexibility of the sensory hair cells responsible for sound transmission to the brain is maintained and the fluid within the cochlear canals flows easier. Lipoflavanoid improves inner ear health and reduces the intensity of ear ringing found in tinnitus as well as symptoms found in Ménière's syndrome.

All senses make for a more enjoyable life. Any reduced stress promotes better homeostasis, and that means a healthier and better existence. The olfactory sensation, mentioned in Chapter 8, may add pleasure or displeasure to the environment and is necessary for detecting methane gas or rotten odours from spoiled food sources; thus a sense of smell could help prevent illness or save a life. Similarly, the sense of taste (gustatory) is necessary to detect rotten, toxic or pleasurable attributes of our living arena. Taste and smell often diminish with age, disease and drugs like chemotherapy treatments. Zinc supplements seem to offer some relief in the case of reduced gustatory abilities and allow for a more pleasant taste of life.

AGE-RELATED DISEASES

Neurological disease affects individuals at all stages of life. Glaucoma and cataracts are age-related visual problems, as is presbyopia, a lens condition that occurs usually in the mid 40s. In presbyopia, the lens becomes less resilient and remains relatively flat, leaving distance vision intact but impairing near vision. Corrective lenses are very common after age 43–45. Macular degeneration typically comes along with age, as do cataracts and difficulty hearing (called presbycusis). Tinnitus, an ear ringing sensation, normally develops in later years owing to environmental or unknown factors. Cranial nerve dysfunction usually occurs in young and middle-aged adults. Alzheimer's disease (see Chapter 14) is a prominent concern for the elderly. The incidence of dementia and Parkinson's disease increases with age. In trisomy 21 (Down's syndrome), patients who live past age 45 tend to develop dementia.

Finally, with age, the 3-pound brain reduces in weight and size, with concurrent loss of neurons and synapses. Thus, it is understandable that functional losses in hearing, sight and coordination will be experienced in the elderly. Reaction times are reduced, and so is agility, which increases risks for injury.

Resource

National Institutes of Allergy and Infectious Diseases: *www.nei.nih.gov*

DISEASES AT A GLANCE Nervous system and special senses

DISEASE	AETIOLOGY	SIGNS AND SYMPTOMS	DIAGNOSIS	TREATMENT	PREVENTION	LIFESPAN
Glioma, glioblastoma	Idiopathic	Severe headache, personality changes, loss of speech, unsteady movement, seizures, coma	CT scan, MRI	Surgery, chemotherapy, radiation	Uncertain	Any age, usually adult
Meningitis	Bacterial, viral	High fever, chills, severe headache, stiff neck, nausea, vomiting, rash, delirium, convulsions, coma	Lumbar puncture	Antibiotics if bacterial infection	Be aware, avoid contact	Can occur at any age
Encephalitis	Viral	Mild to severe headache, fever, cerebral dysfunction, disordered thought, seizures, persistent drowsiness, delirium, coma	Lumbar puncture	Control fever, control fluid and electrolyte balance, monitor respiratory and kidney function	Depends on circumstance	Can occur at any age
Poliomyelitis	Viral	Stiff neck, fever, headache, sore throat, GI disturbances, paralysis may develop	Physical examination	Supportive; preventive vaccination	Vaccine	Usually younger to early adult
Tetanus	*Clostridium tetani*	Rigidity of muscles, painful spasms and convulsions, stiff neck, difficulty swallowing, clenched jaws	Physical examination, patient history	Antitoxin, symptom relief, preventive vaccination	Vaccine	Can occur at any age
Rabies	Viral	Fever, pain, mental derangement, rage, convulsions, paralysis, profuse sticky saliva, throat muscle spasm produces hydrophobia	Physical examination, history of animal bite	Vaccination before disease develops; fatal once CNS involved	Vaccine, be alert	Can occur at any age
Shingles	Varicella, herpes zoster	Painful rash of small water blisters with red rim, lesions follow a sensory nerve, confined to one side of body, severe itching, scarring	Physical examination	Alleviation of symptoms and pain relief, steroids	Avoid contact, vaccine	Usually 50+
Reye's syndrome	Idiopathic or viral; Epstein-Barr, influenza B, varicella	Persistent vomiting, rash, lethargy about 1 week after a viral infection, may progress to coma; linked with use of aspirin in children under 16 years of age	Patient history, liver enlargement, hypoglycaemia, ammonia in blood	Supportive; close monitoring necessary	Avoid aspirin in children, seek care	Infants, young children
Abscess	Pyogenic bacteria	Fever, headache	Lumbar puncture	Surgical draining of abscess, antibiotics	Quick treatment	Can occur at any age
Multiple sclerosis (MS)	Idiopathic, suspect viral or autoimmune	Muscle impairment, double vision, nystagmus, loss of balance, poor coordination, tingling and numbing sensation, shaking tremor, muscular weakness, emotional changes, remission and exacerbation	Physical examination, patient history, MRI	None effective; physical therapy and muscle relaxants, steroids, counselling	Basically autoimmune and polygenetic	Midlife
Amyotrophic lateral sclerosis (ALS), or Lou Gehrig's disease	Idiopathic	Disturbed motility; fasciculations; atrophy of muscles in hands, forearms and legs; impaired speech and swallowing; death from pulmonary failure in 3-4 years	Electromyelography (EMG)	Supportive	Uncertain	Midlife

DISEASES AT A GLANCE Nervous system and special senses (continued)

DISEASE	AETIOLOGY	SIGNS AND SYMPTOMS	DIAGNOSIS	TREATMENT	PREVENTION	LIFESPAN
Huntington's disease (Huntington's chorea)	Genetic	Involuntary, rapid, jerky movements; speech loss; difficulty swallowing; personality changes; carelessness; poor judgement; impaired memory; mental incompetence	Patient history (inherited disease) and physical examination	No cure; genetic counselling for family	Totally genetic	Age 35+
Convulsion: epilepsy	Trauma, chemical, idiopathic, genetic	Involuntary contractions or series of contractions; a seizure is a sign of illness, not a disease. Petit mal: brief loss of consciousness, 'absence seizure'. Grand mal: often preceded by aura (various sensations), total loss of consciousness, generalised convulsions, hypersalivation; incontinence may occur	Observation of seizure, electroencephalogram (EEG), X-ray, family history, CT scan, MRI	Removal of cause once detected; anticonvulsive drugs	Avoid cranial trauma; use helmet or headgear	Can occur at any age
Spina bifida	Congenital, lack of folate	Opening in vertebral canal. Spina bifida occulta – hidden; meningocele – meninges protrude; meningomyelocele – nerve elements protrude; myelocele – nerve tissue disorganised	Physical examination, CT scan, MRI, EEG	Surgical, physical therapy	Variable, folate supplements	Middle-aged mother
Hydrocephalus	Congenital, idiopathic	Enlarged head develops	Physical examination, CT scan, MRI, lumbar puncture	Implant shunt to drain CSF	Variable to pathogen exposure	Can occur at any age, but more prevalent among newborns
Cerebral palsy	Birth trauma, rubella infection	Seizures, visual or auditory impairment, speech defects. Spastic – muscles tense, reflexes exaggerated. Athetoid – uncontrollable, persistent movements, tremor. Atactic – poor balance, poor muscular coordination, staggering gait	Physical examination	Muscle relaxants, anticonvulsive drugs, casts, braces, traction, surgery, physical therapy	Variable, birth caution	Can occur at any age
Transient ischaemic attacks (TIA), 'mini strokes'	Ischaemia, aneurysm, hypertension	Visual disturbances, transient muscle weakness on one side, sensory loss on one side, slurred speech; attacks last minutes to hours, average 15 minutes	Cerebral angiogram, CT scan	Depends on cause; surgical treatment of blocked vessels	Blood pressure monitoring, uncertain	Usually middle age
Cerebrovascular accident (CVA) stroke, brain attack	Trauma	Severe, sudden headache; muscular weakness or paralysis; disturbance of speech; loss of consciousness	Angiography, CT scan, MRI	Clot-dissolving drugs, surgery, endarterectomy	Uncertain, family history, keep low blood pressure levels	Usually mid life+
Alzheimer's disease	Idiopathic, but genetically connected	Memory loss, moody, indigent	Behavioural, clinical screening	Care facilities, medications	None with long survival	Onset middle age, progressive with time

DISEASES AT A GLANCE Nervous system and special senses (continued)

DISEASE	AETIOLOGY	SIGNS AND SYMPTOMS	DIAGNOSIS	TREATMENT	PREVENTION	LIFESPAN
Special senses: eye						
Conjunctivitis	Viral, bacterial	Inflamed eye surface, oozing	Eye inspection, environment, eye fluids	None or ointment or eye drops	Contagious, avoid contact	Usually young child, but not determined by age
Glaucoma	Poor aqueous fluid drainage	Elevate intraocular pressure, dim vison	Ophthalmoscope and slit-scope	Eye drops	None, 10% genetic	Middle age+
Uveitis	Infectious agents	Eye discharge, pain, low vision	Eye examination	Corticoids	Basically autoimmune	Variable
Astigmatism	Irregular cornea or lens	Blurry vision	Chart examination, eye inspection	Corrective lenses	None	Variable
Cataracts	Cloudy lens	Blurred, dim vision	Ophthalmoscope	Some laser, lens replacement	None, avoid sunlight, STIs	Usually elderly
Macular degeneration	Idiopathic	Central vision lost	Ophthalmoscope	Non-specific	None	Older persons
Diabetic retinopathy	Diabetes	Blurred, cloudy vision to blinded	Ophthalmoscope and fluorescein angiography	Some laser, control diabetes and blood pressure	Perhaps control diabetes	More likely with aging
Retinitis pigmentosa	X chromosome	Weakened sight gradual blindness	Electroretinogram	Non-specific	None	From birth
Special senses: ear						
External otitis	Infection	Discharge, pus	Ear inspection	Antibiotic, cleanse area	Depends, use good hygiene, keep ear canal dry	Can occur at any age
Otitis media	Infection	Internal fluid pressure, fever	Ear inspection	Drain tube, antibiotics	Depends, use good hygiene	Children+
Presbycusis	Increased age	Hard of hearing	Audio testing	Hearing aids	None	Worse with age
Ménière's disease	Idiopathic, trauma, autoimmune?	Vertigo, disorientated, tinnitus	Hearing test and examination	Glucocorticoids, low salt diet	Uncertain	Age 40+
Tinnitus	Idiopathic, may be blood pressure-related, loud sounds	Ringing, roaring internal sounds without real sounds externally	Hearing test	Sound aids, low sound makers for interference	Depends	Usually middle aged, but expected in younger people following loud music performances

INTERACTIVE EXERCISES

Cases for critical thinking

1. John has had a severe headache for the past 12 hours, a fever of 102°F, plus a stiff neck. Following a lumbar puncture, *Streptococcus pneumoniae* was found in culture along with low sugar levels and higher protein values. What disease best explains these findings? What is the prognosis and treatment?

2. At age 78, Karen started rubbing her eyes and constantly cleaning her (old) glasses for a better view. The right eye particularly was not very good, and she hoped the problem, which she first noticed months ago, would finally go away. The vision in the right eye was foggy, dim and not focused. There was essentially no pain. What do the symptoms suggest? What are the prognosis and treatments for this woman?

3. Trevor complained of an earache, and after a recent bout with a bad cold, he was rather irritable. The ear was 'beet red' and felt warm. He could hardly hear on that side, but he knew there was nothing intentionally or accidentally poked into the ear. What disease best explains these symptoms? Give some recommendations for treatment.

Multiple choice

1. What is the infective agent for rabies?
   a. bacterium   b. virus
   c. fungus   d. tick

2. Which of the following may cause epilepsy?
   a. a birth trauma
   b. injury to the brain
   c. a penetrating wound
   d. all of these

3. What functions are controlled by the brainstem?
   a. sensory function   b. muscle action
   c. memory   d. heart rate and breathing

4. What is called an acute inflammation of the first two meninges of the brain and spinal cord, the pia mater and the arachnoid?
   a. thrombophlebitis   b. meningitis
   c. prostatitis   d. encephalitis

5. Which of the following is true of polio?
   a. it is caused by a virus
   b. it affects sensory neurons
   c. it is found in most people by age 80
   d. it was wiped out in 1976

6. Which of the following applies to MS?
   a. it occurs only in males
   b. it occurs primarily in east European cultures
   c. it results from a damaged myelin sheath
   d. it strikes adults age 20 or beyond

7. Within 3-4 hours, what clot buster may be used to treat the most common form of CVA?
   a. aspirin   b. TPA
   c. ATP   d. haemolase

8. What disease has a seizure symptom known as petit mal?
   a. polio   b. MS
   c. epilepsy   d. encephalitis

9. What is the lesion in Parkinson's disease?
   a. no dopamine   b. no myelin
   c. autoimmunity   d. cerebral blood clot

10. Paul, in Year 7, woke one morning to discover a blood-shot right eye and a yellowish mass near the medial corner of his eye. What is the correct diagnosis?
    a. common cold   b. trachoma
    c. conjunctivitis d. osteitis

True or false

_____ 1.   Rabies is a viral infection.

_____ 2.   The Sabin vaccine works in the digestive tract.

_____ 3.   Oxygen under high pressure is effective in treating rabies.

_____ 4.   Blood is not normally found in cerebrospinal fluid.

_____ 5.   Dopamine deficiency causes epilepsy.

_____ 6.   Transient ischaemic attacks are characterised by loss of consciousness.

_____ 7.   An aura is a flashback of previous contusion events.

_____ 8.   Viral meningitis requires quarantine isolation procedures.

_____ 9.   Excess Dilantin may cause Parkinson's disease.

_____ 10. Conjunctivitis is usually a viral attack in adults.

Fill-ins

1.   _____, commonly called lockjaw, is an infection of nerve tissue caused by the tetanus bacillus that lives in the intestines of animals and human beings.

2.   Amyotrophic lateral sclerosis is diagnosed by _____.

3.   _____ _____ is a chronic, progressive disease of the central nervous system with myelin destruction.

4.   _____ _____, also known as shaking palsy, is a disease of brain degeneration that appears gradually and progresses slowly.

5.   The common drug given to victims of Parkinson's disease is _____.

6.   _____ headaches are severe, are unilateral, involve the periorbital and orbital area, and typically occur in men.

7.   _Tic douloureux_, or _____ _____, causes severe pain elicited from cranial nerve V.

8.   _____ _____ is a unilateral dysfunction of muscles in the face that leaves the person with slurred speech and a watery eye.

9.   _____ is called Lou Gehrig's disease.

10. _____ is the worst form of spina bifida.

Labelling exercise

What processes does each labelled part of the diagram control?

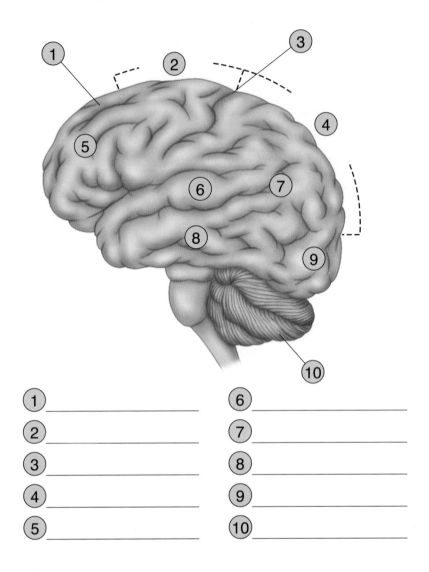

1 _____   6 _____

2 _____   7 _____

3 _____   8 _____

4 _____   9 _____

5 _____   10 _____

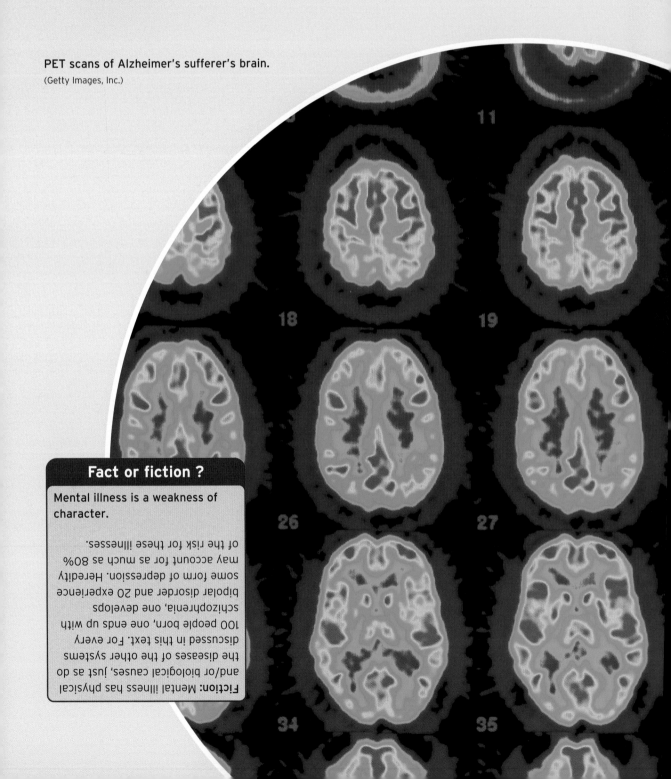

14 MENTAL ILLNESS AND COGNITIVE DISORDERS

PET scans of Alzheimer's sufferer's brain.
(Getty Images, Inc.)

Fact or fiction ?

Mental illness is a weakness of character.

Fiction: Mental illness has physical and/or biological causes, just as do the diseases of the other systems discussed in this text. For every 100 people born, one ends up with schizophrenia, one develops bipolar disorder and 20 experience some form of depression. Heredity may account for as much as 80% of the risk for these illnesses.

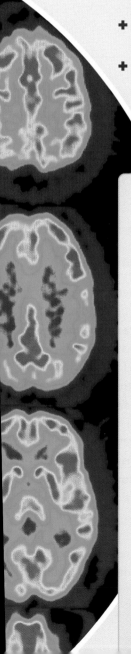

Learning objectives

After studying this chapter, you should be able to:

✚ Describe the warning signs of mental illness

✚ Identify signs, symptoms, aetiology and treatment of the following:
  - developmental disorders
  - disruptive behaviour disorders
  - mood disorders
  - substance use disorders
  - schizophrenia
  - anxiety disorders
  - eating disorders
  - personality disorders

✚ Recognise environmental, genetic and biological factors associated with mental illness

✚ Describe diagnostic approaches for mental illness

  ✚ Identify the warning signs of suicide

Disease chronicle

Post-traumatic stress disorder and modern psychiatry

The human brain has evolved to cope with intermittent ordinary stressors, such as hunger, pain and isolation, but the brain is not well adapted to handle stressors that are outside the realm of normal human experience. Certainly such extreme stressors occurred occasionally in the human evolutionary past; however, the modern world presents humans with abundant opportunities to experience extreme stress; for example, the sort of stress associated with post-traumatic stress disorder. These experiences include war, rape or sexual abuse, being hit or harmed by someone in your family, violent crime, airplane or car crashes, hurricane, tornado or fire, any event in which you thought you might be killed or witnessing any of these events. Today we know that post-traumatic stress disorder is a real disorder with severe consequences; to appreciate the significance of this, remember that until recently this disorder and many mental illnesses were misunderstood. Prior to the twentieth century, mental illnesses were primarily attributed to human fault and hostility, magic or divine forces. The mentally ill were treated by confinement in prisons and asylums. Reforms in the treatment of the mentally ill started after the French Revolution with Franz Mesmer, an Austrian physician, who established rapport with patients. Emil Kraepelin began the modern classification of psychiatry in the nineteenth century. Modern psychiatry, founded in the twentieth century by Sigmund Freud, is credited with a comprehensive approach to understanding development, emotion, behaviour and psychiatric illness. Psychological theory, treatment options and scientific advancements continue to evolve, contributing to further understanding of the biological, chemical, environmental, social and behavioural mechanisms of mental illness.

MENTAL ILLNESS

Mental illness refers to a group of psychiatric disorders characterised by severe disturbances in thought, mood and behaviour. **Psychiatry** is the medical specialty that diagnoses and prescribes medical treatment for mental illness, whereas **psychology** is the discipline that studies normal and abnormal behaviour and applies counselling methods to treat mental illness.

Mental illness affects one of every four people in the UK, and is associated with social stigma, disability and death. Many people suffering from mental illness may not look as though they are ill, while others may appear detached and withdrawn from society. Warning signs of mental illness are listed in Box 14.1.

Over 200 psychiatric diagnoses for adults and children are categorised in the *Diagnostic and Statistical Manual of Mental Disorders*, or DSM. The DSM-IV is the most recent edition and is used internationally to classify, assess and guide treatment for mental illness. Because it is difficult to provide a single definition that accounts for all mental illness, disorders are categorised in the DSM-IV according to groups of symptoms or diagnostic criteria. Psychiatric disorders are assigned a diagnosis in one of five axes, and each axis is a grouping of

---

Box 14.1

Warning signs of mental illness

- Aggression
- Changes in eating or sleeping habits
- Confusion
- Decline in school or work performance
- Depression
- Euphoria alternating with depression
- Excessive fear
- Frequent complaints of physical illnesses
- Hearing voices
- Substance abuse
- Thoughts of suicide
- Withdrawal from family and friends

Source: *Diagnostic and Statistical Manual Text Revision IV*. American Psychiatric Association, 2000.

Box 14.2

The five-axis system of psychiatric diagnoses

Axis I – Primary diagnosis (clinical disorders and other conditions that may be a focus of clinical attention)

Axis II – Primary diagnosis (personality disorders, mental retardation, learning disabilities)

Axis III – General medical conditions

Axis IV – Psychosocial and environmental problems

Axis V – Global assessment of functioning

Primary psychiatric diagnosis is indicated on axis I or II.

Source: *Diagnostic and Statistical Manual Text Revision IV*. American Psychiatric Association, 2000.

---

developmental, medical, psychosocial and overall adaptive disorders (Box 14.2). All DSM-IV diagnoses require evidence that the symptoms impair academic achievement, occupational performance and social relationships.

CAUSES OF MENTAL ILLNESS

Biological basis for mental illness

Current biological theories of mental illness implicate anatomical differences, genes and chemical messengers or **neurotransmitters** in mental illness. Anatomical differences such as brain size and altered neural connections develop from physical insults to the brain, degenerative processes and genes. Genes within the brain's DNA are inherited from both parents and contain all the necessary information to build the structures that mediate the specialised function of neurotransmitters.

Neurotransmitters are produced, stored and released from **neurons**, or nerve cells, within the central and peripheral nervous systems. Voluntary and involuntary physical and psychological processes, such as heart rate and blood pressure, behaviour, emotions, mood, sleep and sex drive, are regulated

Table 14.1 Neurotransmitters, regulatory actions and associated psychiatric disorders.

Neurotransmitter	Regulatory action	Mental illness
Dopamine	Mood, behaviour, thought process, muscle movement, physical activity, heart rate, blood pressure, feeding, appetite, satiety	Schizophrenia, depression, ADHD, bipolar disorder, eating disorder, autism, Tourette syndrome
Noradrenaline	Mood, anxiety, vigilance, arousal, heart rate, blood pressure	Depression, anxiety disorders, ADHD, bipolar disorder
Serotonin	Pain perception, feeding, sleep-wake cycle, motor activity, mood, sexual behaviour, temperature regulation	Depression, aggression, suicidal, bipolar disorder, eating disorders
Acetylcholine	Learning, memory, muscle tone	Alzheimer's disease, Parkinson's disease, Huntington's chorea, Tourette syndrome
Gamma aminobutyric acid (GABA)	Interacts with a wide range of neurotransmitters to enhance inhibition	Anxiety disorders, alcoholism, Tourette syndrome, sleep disorders, epilepsy

Source: Kaplan, G.B. and Hammer R.P. (2002). *Brain Circuitry and Signaling in Psychiatry: Basic Science and Clinical Applications.* American Psychiatric Association.

by intricate neurotransmitter activity. Inadequate regulation of neurotransmitters and excess neurotransmitter activity in distinct areas of the brain are associated with mental illness. The regulatory action of neurotransmitters and their associated mental illnesses are listed in Table 14.1.

Environment and mental illness

Environmental causes of mental illness have informed the diagnosis and treatment of mental illness for many years. Family interactions, age, gender, race, culture and socioeconomic status alter biological and psychological vulnerability for mental illness and define learned behaviours, attitudes and perception of health and illness.

Age and gender are determining factors for some mental health problems and illnesses. Mood disorders such as depression, anxiety disorders and eating disorders occur more frequently in women, whereas disorders with outwardly directed behaviours such as antisocial personality disorder and associated substance abuse are more common in males. Attention deficit hyperactivity disorder (ADHD) is a developmental behavioural disorder that appears more commonly in boys before the age of 7 years. Degenerative disorders involving memory and dementia, such as Alzheimer's disease

and Huntington's chorea, occur most commonly among older adults.

Mental illness affects all cultures, races and socioeconomic classes. Access to medical care and acceptance of psychiatric illness is also influenced by race, cultural beliefs and socioeconomic status. The highest rates of mental illness are found among the lowest socioeconomic classes, which are associated with adverse living conditions, increased social stress and limited access to medical and psychiatric care.

Mental illness in children and adolescents

Mental illness in childhood can have far-reaching academic, social, developmental and physical consequences. Common complications of childhood-onset mental illness include learning delays and poor performance in school, low self-esteem, impaired relationships with family and friends, and social rejection and withdrawal.

Although many psychiatric disorders begin in childhood, they may not be diagnosed until adulthood. In the UK, about 10% of children and adolescents have a mental disorder.

Some disorders have slightly adapted criteria for children. Unlike adults, children often do not verbalise their feelings and may present with behavioural problems such as boredom, irritability, and conduct problems. The outcome of childhood mental illness depends on the ability of the family to cope and seek treatment, the severity of the illness, and the ability of the child to compensate for and adapt to mental health deficits.

DIAGNOSTIC TESTS FOR MENTAL ILLNESS

Comprehensive evaluations, including a medical history and physical examination, psychosocial history, mental health examination and family history, are essential for diagnosis of mental illness. A thorough medical history and physical examination should identify physical illnesses and metabolic and hormonal stresses that mimic symptoms of mental illness. A patient history obtained from family and friends with major timelines of life events can help form a diagnosis. Observation of the patient alone or within a family environment is used to assess emotional responses, physical appearance and reactions, speech and language abilities, clinical estimate of intelligence and level of judgement and insight. A number of standardised questionnaires and rating scales supplement the clinical evaluation by providing a systematic review and standard score to describe behaviours and emotions.

DISORDERS OF INFANCY, CHILDHOOD OR ADOLESCENCE

Disruptive behaviour disorders

Disruptive behaviour disorders, including **conduct disorder** and **oppositional defiant disorder**, are characterised by wilful disobedience. Conduct disorders affect males more often than females and commonly overlap with other psychiatric disorders. A single cause cannot be identified; however, many of these children come from unstable or dysfunctional families and are exposed to domestic violence, poverty and shifting parental figures. The risk for disruptive behaviour disorders increases with inconsistent parenting and punitive disciplinary techniques, parental alcohol and drug abuse, and parental antisocial personality disorder. Harsh parental discipline with physical punishment appears to lead to aggressive behaviour; however, genetic heritability of antisocial and aggressive behaviours has been identified.

Signs include defiance of authority, fighting, school failure and destruction of property. During adolescence, fire setting, theft, sexual promiscuity and criminal behaviours may develop. Treatment involves individual and family counselling as well as medication if appropriate.

Attention deficit hyperactivity disorder

Attention deficit hyperactivity disorder (ADHD) is characterised by prominent symptoms of inattention and/or hyperactivity and impulsivity. ADHD affects males more often than females and persists into adolescence and adulthood. The cause is unknown, but family and twin studies provide evidence of genetic susceptibility, and molecular DNA studies implicate the role of genes in ADHD. Imaging techniques show anatomical and metabolic differences in the brains of ADHD subjects compared to non-ADHD subjects.

DSM-IV defines three subtypes of ADHD: predominantly inattentive, predominantly hyperactive-impulsive, and combined inattentive, hyperactive and impulsive. Children with the inattentive subtype tend to be described as 'spacey' and socially withdrawn, and they have fewer conduct and behavioural problems than the hyperactive-impulsive subtype. The term ADD (attention deficit disorder) was once used to describe children with these symptoms, but ADD is no longer a DSM diagnosis. Even so, at times ADD is still used informally today to describe children with the predominantly inattentive subtype of ADHD. Hyperactive ADHD children tend to run around excessively, fidget and have difficulty playing or engaging in quiet activities. Impulsivity in ADHD is characterised by the inability to wait turns, blurting out answers and interrupting others.

Table 14.2 Clinical specialists in treatment and diagnosis of ADHD.

Clinical specialty	Can diagnose	Can prescribe medication if needed	Provides counselling or training
Psychiatrists	Yes	Yes	Yes
Psychologists	Yes	No	Yes
Paediatricians or family physicians	Yes	Yes	No
Neurologists	Yes	Yes	No

Source: National Institutes of Mental Health: *www.nimh.org*.

Contrary to common belief, ADHD is not limited to childhood. ADHD has a chronic lifelong course and, if untreated, results in school and work failure, substance use disorders, legal difficulties, car accidents and fatalities and sexual indiscretions. ADHD commonly occurs with depressive disorders, anxiety disorders, conduct disorder, oppositional defiant disorder and learning disorders. Like many psychiatric disorders, ADHD often requires multimodal treatment that may include medication, cognitive behavioural therapy, counselling and collaboration among a variety of clinical professionals (Table 14.2). The majority of children with ADHD are effectively treated with stimulant medications. Stimulant medications are the oldest and most established pharmacological agents in children with ADHD (Table 14.3). Behaviour therapy can improve academic achievement and reduce targeted conduct problems, especially in children with a co-occurring conduct disorder.

DEVELOPMENTAL DISORDERS

Mental retardation

Mental retardation is defined by the presence of low intelligence accompanied by deficits in social and language skills and adaptive functioning. The most common biological cause of mental retardation is fragile X syndrome, an inherited defect of the X chromosome that affects 1 in 2000 males and 1 in 4000 females in all races and ethnic groups. However, in some cases the exact cause cannot be

Table 14.3 Medications used in treatment of ADHD.

Trade name	Generic name	Approved age
Strattera	atomoxetine	6 and older
Concerta XL (long-acting)	methylphenidate	6 and older
Dexedrine	amphetamine	3 and older
Ritalin	methylphenidate	6 and older
Equasym XL	methylphenidate	6 and older
Medikinet XL	methylphenidate	6 and older

The medication Strattera, or atomoxetine, works on the neurotransmitter noradrenaline; whereas the stimulants primarily work on dopamine. Both of these neurotransmitters are believed to play a role in ADHD. More studies will need to be done to contrast Strattera with the medications already available but the evidence to date indicates that over 70% of children with ADHD given Strattera manifest significant improvement in their symptoms.

Sources: National Institutes of Mental Health: *www.nimh.org*; Food and Drug Administration: *www.fda.gov*.

identified. Treatment focuses on occupational therapy to maximise the development of cognitive and behavioural skills.

Autistic disorder

Autistic disorders (autism) include deficits in reciprocal language and social interactions and are characterised by repetitive stereotyped behaviours. Autism affects nearly one child in 100 in the UK, although this is subject to debate. Autism often goes unrecognised during infancy and first becomes apparent after 3 years of age. The cause of autism is unknown. Central nervous system changes have been postulated, and a number of genes are now associated with the disorder.

The concordance rate for autism in twins is about 90%, and the rate of autism is higher in families with a history of language-related disorders.

The most notable deficits in autism are severe deficits in reciprocal social interactions. These include minimal eye contact with caregivers, delayed language development and disinterest in social interactions with peers, usually first observed during the toddler years. When speech does develop, it is usually illogical and echo-like, as words that are heard are repeated. Repetitive and stereotypic behaviours include odd posturing, hand-flapping, self-injurious behaviour, abnormal patterns of eating and drinking and unpredictable mood changes.

Widely accepted as effective when begun early, applied behaviour analysis (ABA) has been shown to improve behaviour and communication skills. ABA utilises intensive and frequent one-on-one interaction with a therapist. No medications are approved for treatment of children with autism. Medications for behaviour and mood have been used and these include antidepressants, anxiolytics and antipsychotics. As with other childhood illnesses, parental guidance and assurance is critical to obtain appropriate medical and psychosocial support. Informed parents contribute to the child's learning of self-care and adaptive skills and to positive long-term outcomes.

Tic disorders

A **tic** is a sudden, rapid, involuntary stereotyped movement or vocalisation that may be temporarily suppressed by conscious efforts. Tics are exacerbated by stress, anxiety, boredom or fatigue, and typically decrease in severity when the child is concentrating on an enjoyable task. Tics occur more commonly in boys than girls and are presumed to result from a neurotransmitter imbalance. Tourette syndrome is a common tic disorder characterised by patterns of motor and vocal tics which affects 1–3% of children and adolescents in the UK.

Complications of tic disorders include embarrassment and impaired self-esteem that results from being teased and rejected by peers and adults. Severe symptoms may interfere with forming intimate friendships. The unemployment rate in adults with tics has been reported to be as high as 50%.

Transient tics usually do not require treatment. Complicated tic disorders require carefully titrated medication therapy. No medication eliminates tics, but some can modulate tic severity. The dopamine blockers risperidone and haloperidol can reduce the severity of tics.

Dementia

Dementia is a degenerative syndrome characterised by deficits in memory, language and mood. The most common form of dementia is **Alzheimer's disease**, which develops gradually and occurs most commonly after the age of 60 years. **Vascular dementia** has a more abrupt onset and is caused by physical insults from high blood pressure, diabetes and strokes. Poor nutrition, head injuries, and chronic alcohol intake may result in alcohol-related dementia. Parkinson's disease is a degenerative neurological movement disorder characterised by dementia in late stages of the disease (see Chapter 13).

Alzheimer's disease In 1906 Dr Alois Alzheimer first recorded certain abnormalities in the brain of a woman who died from dementia. Alzheimer's disease is a degenerative and progressive form of dementia that seriously disrupts daily living activities, behaviour and mood.

The two most significant risk factors for Alzheimer's disease are advanced age and family history. Each year 163 000 new cases of dementia occur in England and Wales. The prevalence of Alzheimer's disease increases with age, with the risk increasing over the age of 60, but Alzheimer's disease is not a normal part of aging. Alzheimer's affects about 5% of men and women aged 65–74 and about 50% of those over the age of 80. Causes remain unknown, but certain mutations in chromosomes and inheritance of two high risk genes are associated with a greater risk for developing Alzheimer's disease.

Alzheimer's disease can only be diagnosed definitively by autopsy. However, it is important to recognise the disease early, and so a tentative diagnosis is made using a number of different sources of information. The patient, caregivers and family members should be interviewed to determine the patient's history, information about the person's general health, past medical problems and ability to carry out daily activities. Standard psychological tests are given to assess memory, problem-solving, attention, counting and language. Finally, brain scans (positron emission tomography, or PET scans) can evaluate brain function.

The earliest manifestation of Alzheimer's disease is loss of short-term memory. Psychosis, aggression and profound personality changes are associated with advanced disease. With severe disease, judgement is lost, personal care is neglected and physical illnesses may ultimately lead to death.

Physical findings in Alzheimer's disease include degeneration of neurons and plaque formation on and around neurons. Plaques or deposits of proteins build up around neurons and interrupt communication between neurons by neurotransmitters. Abnormal collections of proteins form **neurofibrillary tangles** that are detected by brain scans. **Acetylcholine** is the neurotransmitter that is most affected by Alzheimer's disease. Decreases in acetylcholine are correlated with memory loss. Alterations in noradrenaline, GABA and serotonin have been documented and may play a role in mood, behaviour and aggression.

Medications can slow the progression of early and middle stages of Alzheimer's disease, but they do not cure the disease or stop its progression. These medications include Aricept and Exelon. Associated symptoms of depression, aggression and anxiety may be treated with antidepressants and anxiolytics. Social support is needed to improve the quality of life and maximise personal care. Vitamin E may prevent the progression of Alzheimer's disease by decreasing oxygen free radicals that accelerate cell death. In spite of treatment, the disease remains progressive, often ending in death 8–10 years after onset of symptoms.

SUBSTANCE ABUSE DISORDERS

Substance abuse disorders include drug and alcohol abuse and addiction. Drug and alcohol abuse and addiction have many adverse medical, emotional and economic outcomes. Commonly abused substances include alcohol, cocaine, amphetamines, LSD, prescription drugs like benzodiazepines and

Table 14.4 Commonly abused drugs.

Stimulants	Street names
Cocaine	Coke, snow, crack, crank
Amphetamines	
Amphetamine sulphate	Bennies, grennies, cartwheels
Methamphetamine	Speed, meth, crystal
Dextramphetamine sulphate	Hearts, oranges, dexies
Hallucinogens	
LSD (lysergic acid diethylamide)	Angel dust, rocket fuel, elephant tranquilliser, peace pill
Depressants	
Alcohol	Beer, wine, distilled drinks like whisky, gin, vodka
Benzodiazepines	Dolls, yellow jackets
Barbiturates	Barbs, downers, reds
Opiates	Heroin: junk, horse, H, smack; Morphine: M, morph
Cannabinoids	
Marijuana	Pot, grass, weed, reefer, joint, THC

painkillers, barbiturates, opiates like codeine and morphine and marijuana (Table 14.4). Substance abuse and addiction occur at all ages, affect all socioeconomic groups and worldwide are among the most common causes of disability and death.

Symptoms of drug and alcohol dependence include compulsive use, physical and psychological cravings and dependence, tolerance and withdrawal. The addict cannot function without the use of drugs and/or alcohol, and daily activities centre on obtaining the substance. The key sign of substance abuse is persistent use that is physically damaging and continues in spite of adverse medical, social, economic and legal consequences.

Some signs and symptoms are specific to the type of substance abused and include behavioural and physical changes. Long-term alcohol abuse and addiction are characterised by denial and attempts to hide the addiction and temporarily lead a functional life. A patient history reveals a pattern of alcohol use to maintain normal functioning and the inability to refrain from drinking or becoming intoxicated. The physical effects of long-term alcohol abuse include malnutrition, cirrhosis, neuropathy, brain damage and cardiomyopathy. See Chapter 9 for more on the physical effects of alcohol addiction.

Behavioural and physical changes accompanying addiction and abuse involving other substances also depend on the type of substance abused, and this lies beyond the scope of this text.

Causes and risk factors that lead to substance abuse include stressful events, untreated mental illness, genetic predisposition and, in children and adolescents, peer pressure, poor self-esteem, depression and even boredom. Legitimate medicinal use of drugs rarely leads to abuse or addiction. Underlying addiction and abuse are seeming alterations in the dopamine reward centres of the brain where alcohol or drugs simulate pleasure and reward in susceptible individuals. Family and twin studies have implicated genes in addiction.

Treatment of alcohol and substance abuse

Treatment of alcohol abuse and addiction must include total abstinence from drinking. Supportive individual and group therapy and counselling, including Alcoholics Anonymous (AA), is effective for some alcoholics. Medical treatments such as acamprosate (Campral EC) reduce craving for alcohol and are effective at reducing relapses when used in combination with supportive therapy. Treatment of other types of substance abuse and addiction depends on the type of substance but must also include a treatment plan that leads to complete abstinence.

SCHIZOPHRENIA

Schizophrenia is a complex mental illness that affects about 1% of the UK population. The onset of **schizophrenia** is often first noted in late teenage years or early adulthood. Signs and symptoms of schizophrenia include hallucinations, delusions,

disordered thinking, movement disorders, flat affect, social withdrawal and cognitive deficits. These symptoms fall into three categories: positive, negative and cognitive, and include fairly complex and pervasive disturbances in behaviour and thinking (Box 14.3). The suicide rate among schizophrenics is 10%, and the average life expectancy is lower than that of the general population.

Schizophrenia diagnosis is based on a detailed history and family interviews. Medical causes such as tumours or endocrine disorders may be ruled out. The pattern of characteristic signs and symptoms is key to diagnosis. The characteristic signs of schizophrenia are a gradual withdrawal from people, activities and social contacts, with increasing concern for abstract and sometimes eccentric ideas. Some patients experience only a single episode and remain symptom-free for most of their lives. The course of the illness can fluctuate over many years and can become worse if episodes recur. Depression, anxiety, suspiciousness, difficulty in concentrating and restlessness are among the early symptoms of schizophrenia, and they intensify or diminish as the illness progresses.

Disturbances in perception, or **hallucinations**, and false beliefs, or **delusions**, are reflected in behaviour and thoughts that are vague and detached from reality. Schizophrenics may experience auditory or visual hallucinations in which they may hear or see things that are not present. Delusions are commonly **persecutory** (belief that they are being watched, followed or plotted against), **grandiose** (belief that they have special powers, influence or wealth), or **somatic** (physical belief that something is rotting inside their bodies).

Affect, or 'feeling tone', refers to the outward expression of emotion. The schizophrenic affect may be extremely unstable, with rapid shifts from sadness to happiness for no obvious reason, or it may be flattened, with no signs of emotion in tone of voice or facial expression. Patients may state that they no longer respond to life with normal intensity or that they are 'losing their feelings'.

Motor disturbances in schizophrenia may be **catatonic** or rigid, or disorganised or agitated. Catatonic

Box 14.3

Signs and symptoms of schizophrenia

Positive symptoms

Positive symptoms are easy-to-spot behaviours not seen in healthy people. They include hallucinations, delusions, thought disorder and disorders of movement. Positive symptoms can come and go. Sometimes they are severe and at other times hardly noticeable, depending on whether the individual is receiving treatment. Examples include the following.

- Hallucinations
- Delusions
- Thought disorders
- Disorders of movement.

Negative symptoms

The term negative symptoms refers to reductions in normal emotional and behavioural states, and usually involve a loss of contact with reality.

- Flat affect (immobile facial expression, monotonous voice)
- Lack of pleasure in everyday life
- Diminished ability to initiate and sustain planned activity
- Speaking infrequently, even when forced to interact
- Neglect of basic hygiene
- Help needed with everyday activities.

Cognitive symptoms

Cognitive symptoms are subtle and are often detected only when neuropsychological tests are performed.

- Poor 'executive functioning' (the ability to absorb and interpret information and make decisions based on that information)
- Inability to sustain attention
- Problems with 'working memory' (the ability to keep recently learned information in mind and use it right away).

Source: *Diagnostic and Statistical Manual Text Revision IV*. American Psychiatric Association, 2000, and the National Institute of Mental Health: *www.nimh.gov*

---

features may range from a total reduction in movement, or 'zombie-like state', to a wild, aggressive and agitated state. Disorganised conduct is usually **blunted** or dull, bearing no relationship to social signals. The causes of schizophrenia are complex and include genetics and environment. While schizophrenia occurs in 1% of the population, it occurs in 10% of those who have a first-degree relative with schizophrenia and occurs at a high rate among identical twins. In spite of these observations of genetic risk for developing schizophrenia, no genes have been definitively linked to schizophrenia, but many are under investigation. Environmental risks include exposure to viruses or malnutrition in the womb, problems during birth and psychosocial factors, like stressful environmental conditions. Levels of the neurotransmitters dopamine and glutamate, and changes in brain metabolism and structure point to the biological basis for schizophrenia.

Treatment includes antipsychotic medications such as risperidone and olanzapine. Treatment must include illness management therapy, psychosocial therapy and cognitive behavioural therapy, and must often include family therapy.

MOOD DISORDERS

Mood disorders are characterised by marked periods of sadness and euphoria. While it is normal for people to experience ups and downs, those who have **major depression** or **bipolar disorder** experience debilitating symptoms that result in vocational failure, social withdrawal and dysfunctional relationships.

Major depression

Complaints of sadness and hopelessness are commonly expressed by depressed individuals. Major depression occurs at any age and, if untreated, may result in suicide. Between 8% and 12% of people in the UK suffer from depression. Women are diagnosed with major depression about twice as often as men. Depression in the elderly is often masked by concurrent physical illness and is attributed to normal aging processes. Poor performance in school, irritability, loss of appetite, social withdrawal and pretending to be sick are signs of depression in children.

A major depressive disorder consists of at least one episode of serious mood depression accompanied by a number of changes in behaviour. Complaints frequently include a loss of interest and pleasure, and withdrawal from activities. Feelings of guilt, worthlessness, anxiety and shame are reported because individuals with major depression view their illness as a moral deficiency. Physical symptoms that suggest emotional distress include unexplained weight loss or weight gain, disturbed sleep, decreased energy, poor eye contact, monosyllabic speech and indifference to pleasure or joy.

Subcategories of depression include **seasonal affective disorder**, **postpartum depression**, **dysthymia** and **premenstrual dysphoric disorder**. Seasonal affective disorder is believed to be caused by decreased sunlight exposure during the winter months. Postpartum depression usually occurs 2 weeks to 6 months following the birth of a child. Persistent care of the newborn, sleep deprivation, social stresses and hormonal changes all play a role in the development of postpartum depression.

Chronic depression or dysthymia is diagnosed when symptoms persist for more than 2 years. Cyclic depressive symptoms prior to menstruation may occur regularly for some women.

Heredity is currently the most important predisposing factor for major depression. The risk for major depression is higher in families with a history of mood disorders. Depression in a parent contributes to depression in genetically vulnerable children. While stressful life events trigger sadness, despair and grief, stressful factors alone do not cause major depression (Box 14.4).

The most prominent theory for depression focuses on regulatory disturbances in neurotransmitters. The neurotransmitters serotonin, noradrenaline and dopamine are widely distributed in the central nervous system and are implicated in regulation of mood, arousal, movement and sleep. Medications that increase serotonin, noradrenaline and dopamine effectively reduce symptoms of depression.

Major depression may occur with a number of physical and psychological disorders. Physical disorders such as thyroid disease or Cushing's disease

---

Box 14.4

Symptoms of major depression

- Prolonged sadness or unexplained crying spells
- Significant changes in appetite and sleep patterns
- Irritability, anger, worry, agitation, anxiety
- Pessimism, indifference
- Loss of energy, persistent lethargy
- Unexplained aches and pains
- Feelings of guilt, worthlessness and/or hopelessness
- Inability to concentrate
- Indecisiveness
- Inability to take pleasure in former interests
- Social withdrawal
- Excessive consumption of alcohol or use of chemical substances
- Recurring thoughts of death or suicide

Source: Diagnostic and Statistical Manual Text Revision IV. American Psychiatric Association, 2000.

induce depression by altering hormone levels. Chronic heart disease and cancer can produce depressive symptoms from associated disability, fatigue and physical pain. Direct physical causes of depression include HIV infections and seizure disorders that damage the brain and central nervous system. Psychological disorders such as anxiety disorders, eating disorders and developmental disorders are often referred to as **comorbid disorders** because they commonly occur with major depression.

Various prescription medications and substance abuses induce depression by altering brain function and regulation of hormones and neurotransmitters. Heart medications, for example, alter neuronal responses to noradrenaline, leading to fatigue and depressive symptoms. Corticosteroid medications induce behavioural changes, psychosis and major depression, especially in susceptible individuals. Alcoholic beverages as well as many commonly abused substances depress the central nervous system.

A trial of antidepressant medication that restores regulation of noradrenaline, dopamine and/or serotonin is indicated for most cases of major depression. These drugs elevate the levels of these neurotransmitters; the drugs are commonly called selective serotonin reuptake inhibitors (SSRIs), noradrenaline reuptake inhibitors (NRIs), serotonin and noradrenaline reuptake inhibitors (SNRIs), monoamine oxidase inhibitors (MAOI) and tricyclics. Optimal reduction of symptoms is usually noticed 14–21 days after starting medication. Psychosocial treatment is often required to improve social functioning and to change depressive thought processes. Depression that is resistant to drug treatment may respond to electroconvulsive therapy, in which electrodes apply current to the brain. Severe depression may be accompanied by psychosis, which requires the use of antipsychotic medications.

Bipolar disorder

Bipolar disorder, or manic depressive illness, is a mood disorder that causes unusual shifts from depression to **mania**, or an overly elevated,

Box 14.5

Symptoms of mania

- Increased physical and mental activity and energy
- Heightened mood, exaggerated optimism and self-confidence
- Excessive irritability, aggressive behaviour
- Decreased need for sleep without experiencing fatigue
- Grandiose delusions, inflated sense of self-importance
- Racing speech, racing thoughts, flight of ideas
- Impulsiveness, poor judgement, distractibility
- Reckless behaviour such as spending sprees, rash business decisions, erratic driving and sexual indiscretions
- In the most severe cases, delusions and hallucinations

Source: Diagnostic and Statistical Manual Text Revision IV. American Psychiatric Association, 2000.

energetic, irritable mood. Periods of highs and lows are called *episodes* of mania and depression. Bipolar disorder affects about 1% of the population. Bipolar disorder typically develops in late adolescence or early adulthood. However, some people have their first symptoms during childhood, and some develop them late in life. Bipolar disorder is often not recognised as an illness, and people may suffer for years without a diagnosis or proper treatment (Box 14.5).

Mania can vary from extreme elation, hyperactivity and irritability to extreme aggression, with little need for sleep, and risky behaviours that are later regretted. An overly enthusiastic mood at times may attract others; however, mood shifts with delusions may lead to alienation of friends and family and to irresponsible behaviours such as spending one's life savings or engaging in sexual indiscretions.

A distinct period of an abnormally elevated mood that is not induced by the physiological effects of a drug substance followed by a distinct period of depression is central to diagnosis of a bipolar disorder. Different categories of bipolar disorder are determined by patterns of symptoms or severity of highs and lows. Bipolar I disorder is associated with periods of intense mania and depression that last for several weeks. Bipolar II disorder is associated with less severe episodes of mania, but depression may continue for several weeks. A chronic fluctuating mood, with mild symptoms of both depression and mania, or cyclothymic disorder, is often undiagnosed and may eventually result in a more severe form of bipolar disorder.

The causes of bipolar disorder are unclear, though genetic, biochemical and environmental causes have been identified. Like other mental illnesses, several genes acting together may ultimately identify patients who will develop bipolar disorder. Bipolar disorder runs in families, and stressful experiences may trigger some symptoms. Changes in neurotransmitter regulation that lead to bipolar disorder may be affected by the presence of another illness, stress, substance abuse, changes in diet and exercise and hormonal changes.

Medical treatment of bipolar disorder is complex. Patients often require prolonged treatment with medications called mood stabilisers, such as lithium or certain antiepileptic medications, antidepressants, sedative medications or 'sleep aids', and major tranquillisers or antipsychotic medications. Family and individual patient counselling improves social functioning by providing psychological support and treatment that stabilises extreme characteristics of mania or depression.

ANXIETY DISORDERS

Anxiety disorders include a number of disorders in which the primary feature is abnormal or inappropriate anxiety that interferes with daily school, work, recreational and family activities. Anxiety is a normal phenomenon in which our mind and body reacts to flee from danger, also known as 'fight or flight'. Heart rate, respiratory rate, blood pressure and muscle tension increases at the onset of a stressful event. Symptoms of anxiety become a problem when they occur without any recognisable cause or when the cause does not require an intense response.

Anxiety disorders affect adults and children and may persist for many years without proper treatment. As with many other mental illnesses, family and friends often label those that suffer anxiety disorders as weak and unable to 'snap out of their condition'. Some people's lives become so restricted that they avoid normal, everyday activities such as grocery shopping or driving. In some cases, they become housebound.

The genetic basis for anxiety disorders originates from family studies. Anxiety disorders are common among relatives of affected individuals. The risk for phobias is greater in relatives of individuals with both depression and panic disorder. In cases of post-traumatic stress disorder (PTSD), genetic factors may explain why only certain individuals exposed to trauma develop PTSD.

Head injuries, an overactive thyroid gland, cardiovascular disease, respiratory disease, altered regulation of neurotransmitters and certain medications may cause anxiety disorders. Individuals with anxiety disorders are more sensitive to medications that increase heart rate, blood pressure and fear behaviour. Abnormal neurotransmission of the neurotransmitter serotonin is recognised as a cause of obsessive compulsive disorder (OCD) by a reduction of symptoms with medications that increase serotonin.

Types of anxiety disorders

Physical symptoms and behaviours vary slightly with each subtype of anxiety disorder. Panic disorder, generalised anxiety disorder, phobic disorders, social phobia, OCD and PTSD share the common theme of excessive, irrational fear.

Panic disorder A panic attack involves a sudden onset of fear and terror accompanied by physical symptoms in vital organs such as the heart and lungs. Shortness of breath, chest pains and palpitations peak within 10 minutes and usually resolve within 30–60 minutes. Because of the unpredictability of a panic attack, people who have them develop anticipatory anxiety, or a persistent pattern of worry regarding when and where the attack will take place. Physical complaints often lead patients to seek emergency medical care.

Generalised anxiety disorder Severe persistent worries that are out of proportion to the circumstance describe a typical day for sufferers of generalised anxiety disorders. Common worries related to work, money, health and safety are difficult to control. Additional complaints of restlessness, fatigue, muscle tension, impaired concentration and disturbed sleep may often be misdiagnosed as depression.

Phobic disorders An irrational fear of something, or a specific phobia, that poses little or no danger is the most common type of anxiety disorder. Some phobias, such as a fear of the dark, of strangers or of large animals, begin in childhood and disappear with age. Hyperventilation, or rapid breathing, may accompany a fear of heights, flying, closed spaces, insects and rodents. Although adults with phobias realise that these fears are irrational, they often find that facing the feared object or situation brings on a panic or severe anxiety attack.

Social phobia Social phobia involves excessive worry and self-consciousness in everyday social situations. Intense fears of being humiliated in social situations interfere with ordinary activities. Physical symptoms that accompany social anxiety include blushing, profuse sweating, nausea and difficulty talking.

Obsessive compulsive disorder Anxious, irrational thoughts and images, also known as obsessions, lead to the need to perform rituals to prevent or get rid of the obsessive stimulus. Rituals are patterns of irrational behaviours, or compulsions, that provide temporary relief from the anxiety. Obsessions centred on cleanliness and fear of germs, for example, may lead to compulsive hand washing. Other rituals may include the need to repeat certain words and phrases to ward off danger, or repetitive counting of objects. Patients with OCD are aware that their compulsion and corresponding ritual is irrational but cannot stop it. OCD affects both men and women, and symptoms may ease over time with appropriate treatment.

Post-traumatic stress disorder Exposure to an overwhelming traumatic incident such as the events of 11 September 2001, or encounters of trauma such as rape, violence, child abuse or war, may lead to symptoms and diagnosis of PTSD. Victims of trauma develop persistent frightening thoughts and memories months or years after the event. The traumatic event is repeatedly experienced as nightmares and flashbacks or numbing recollections of the event throughout the day. The individual avoids reminders of the event, startles or feels frightened easily and may feel detached and numb. PTSD sufferers may lose interest in things they used to enjoy, avoid affection and become irritable or aggressive. Individuals with PTSD often feel guilty about surviving the event or about behaving destructively, as in the case of veterans of war.

Imaging techniques have focused on the role of brain structures that mediate communication and process information to memory. The **amygdala** is an almond-shaped structure located deep within the brain, and it may play a role in fear and phobias. The **hippocampus** is a structure of the brain that processes and stores information to memory. The hippocampus appears smaller in those with PTSD, which may explain the memory deficits and flashbacks in these individuals.

Treatment of anxiety disorders

Anxiety, as a learned response to a stimulus and corresponding biochemical changes in brain chemistry, responds to treatment with medications and psychotherapy. Medications that increase serotonin are effective in the treatment of OCD, though psychotherapy is often required to gain understanding of underlying emotional conflict. Antianxiety medications that increase the effect of the neurotransmitter gamma aminobutyric acid (GABA) have a calming effect and work quickly. The use of antianxiety medications is limited, however, by their potential for addiction.

EATING DISORDERS

Eating disorders involve serious disturbances in eating behaviour. Fashion trends, ad campaigns, social attitudes and athletics promote leaner body weight and a preoccupation with body shape and weight. Extreme attitudes surrounding weight and food, combined with psychological and medical complications, define the disabilities that meet the criteria for eating disorders.

Symptoms of eating disorders

Anorexia nervosa and **bulimia nervosa** occur primarily in young women who develop a paralysing fear of becoming fat. In anorexia nervosa, fear of obesity causes excessive restriction of food, resulting in emaciation. Bulimia involves massive binge eating followed by purging or excessive dieting and exercise to prevent weight gain.

Anorexia nervosa *Anorexia* means 'lack of appetite'. Ironically, individuals with anorexia nervosa are hungry and yet are preoccupied with dieting and limiting food intake to the point of starvation. There is an intense fear of gaining weight or becoming fat even though anorectics become dangerously thin. The process of eating becomes an obsession, with rituals centred on meal plans, calorie counts, compulsive exercise and self-induced vomiting despite little food intake.

The typical anorectic is an adolescent female who has lost 15% of her body weight, fears obesity, stops menstruating and otherwise looks healthy. Other notable signs include low blood pressure, decreased heart rate and **oedema**, or swelling of tissues. Metabolic changes, including dehydration and depletion of electrolytes (sodium, potassium and chloride), can result in abnormal heart rhythm, heart failure, sudden cardiac arrest and death.

The individual denies that anything is wrong and typically does not seek medical care until prompted into treatment by friends and family. Depression is common as anorectics withdraw from social affairs involving food and festivities.

Bulimia nervosa Similar to anorexia nervosa, bulimics are excessively concerned with body weight and physical shape. Unlike anorectics, bulimics **binge** by eating an excessive amount of food within a restricted period of time, followed by compensatory **purging** behaviour such as self-induced vomiting or misuse of laxatives or diuretics. Rigorous dieting and exercise may also follow binges to prevent weight gain. There is a feeling of loss of control during the binging episode, followed by intense distress and guilt. Body weight may be normal, which makes it easy for bulimics to hide their illness.

The medical consequences of bulimia nervosa can be devastating. Stomach acid and digestive enzymes from vomiting erode tooth enamel and cause injury and inflammation to the oesophagus and salivary glands. Severe dental caries and gum disease eventually require removal of teeth. Vomiting, laxative and diuretic abuse lowers blood potassium levels, causing muscle cramping and abnormal heart rhythms. In cases of severe potassium loss, death may result from cardiac arrest. Prolonged and excessive laxative abuse may severely damage the bowel. If the bowel ceases its function, surgery is required to form a **colostomy**, an opening from the bowel to the abdominal wall to allow removal of the faeces into a bag attached to the outer abdominal wall.

Bulimics are aware of their behaviour and feel intense guilt and shame. Bulimics are generally outgoing, impulsive and prone to depression and alcohol or drug abuse. Unlike anorectics, bulimics are more likely to talk about their illness and desperately seek help from physicians and friends.

Patterns of psychological and interpersonal issues most consistently provide insight into the causes of eating disorders. Low self-esteem and persistent feelings of inadequacy shape attitudes of perfectionism for the anorectic and severe self-criticism for the bulimic. Troubled family relationships, difficulty expressing feelings and emotions, and a history of physical or sexual abuse are reported more often in bulimics than anorectics. Social attitudes that value thinness and limit beauty to specific body weight and shape influence body image and contribute to extreme dieting and exercise for both anorectics and bulimics.

The biological basis for eating behaviour involves a complex network of brain structures and neurotransmitters. The hypothalamus regulates hunger, monitors fullness of the stomach and determines how much food is eaten. The limbic system influences emotions and selection of foods to appease the appetite. The prefrontal region of the brain controls decisions about when, where and how to eat. Future studies on the biology of appetite control and behaviour may lead to development of new medications to treat eating disorders.

Successful treatment of and recovery from eating disorders requires the realisation that starvation, binging and purging is destructive. Medical treatment to restore nutrition and replace fluids and electrolytes is crucial to prevent death from organ failure. Medication to relieve depression and anxiety may improve mood and thought processes. Group, family, individual and nutritional counselling provides support to break down delusions that shape eating behaviour and distortions in body image.

PERSONALITY DISORDERS

Persistent, inflexible patterns of behaviour that affect interpersonal relationships describe **personality disorders**. Personality disorders appear in adolescence or early adulthood and remain stable throughout an individual's lifetime. DSM-IV describes three major categories of personality disorders based on 'clusters' of symptoms.

Personality disorders occur along with medical and psychiatric illnesses. Relations with family, friends and caregivers are often strained by inflexible and maladaptive personality characteristics. People with severe personality disorders are more vulnerable to psychiatric breakdowns and are at risk for alcoholism, substance abuse, reckless sexual behaviour, eating disorders and violence.

Symptoms of personality disorders

Cluster A: paranoid and schizoid
Paranoid personality The paranoid personality type is indifferent, suspicious and hostile. His or her relationships are shallow because of a tendency to respond to positive acts or kindness with distrust. The paranoid personality type interprets positive statements such as 'You look like a million bucks' to mean 'My friend is after my money.'

Schizoid personality People with a schizoid personality appear cold and isolated. Often called introverted, schizoid personality types appear self-absorbed and withdrawn. They often deal with their fears through superstitions, magical thinking and unusual beliefs.

Cluster B: antisocial, borderline, histrionic and narcissistic
Antisocial personality Callous disregard for others and manipulation of people for personal gratification characterise antisocial personality types. Antisocial personality may start as a conduct problem in childhood, manifested as disrespect for authority and for personal and public property. Adolescents and adults with antisocial personalities are at risk for alcoholism, drug abuse, sexual improprieties and violence.

Borderline personality Borderline personality disorders often occur in women who were deprived of adequate care during childhood. Their moods are unstable and characterised by crisis and anger alternating with depression. Threats of real or imagined abandonment elicit impulsive behaviours such as promiscuity and substance abuse. The individual with a borderline personality disorder is vulnerable to brief psychotic episodes, substance abuse and eating disorders.

Histrionic personality The histrionic personality is characterised by theatrical and exaggerated emotional behaviour. Friendships are initially formed because others are attracted to the histrionic personality's energetic and entertaining behaviour. Hysteria and flamboyant behaviours often result in negative responses and feelings of rejection.

Narcissistic personality The narcissistic personality type has an exaggerated self-image and a tendency to think little of others. Narcissists expect others to admire their grandiosity and feel they are entitled to have their needs attended to. When rejected by others through criticism or defeat, the narcissist becomes enraged or severely depressed.

Cluster C: avoidant, dependent and obsessive compulsive

Avoidant personality Avoidant personality types appear shy and timid, as if they have a social phobia. They fear relationships, although they have a strong desire to feel accepted. They are hypersensitive to criticism and rejection and are susceptible to depression, anxiety and anger for failing to develop social relationships.

Dependent personality Dependent personality types have an extremely poor self-image. They appoint others to make significant decisions out of fear of expressing themselves or offending others. Extended illness may bring out a dependent personality in adults.

Obsessive compulsive personality The obsessive compulsive personality types are dependable, meticulous, orderly and intolerant of mistakes. They are often high achievers, attending to details while failing to complete the task at hand. Individuals with an obsessive compulsive personality avoid new situations and relationships because these new elements cannot be methodically controlled.

Treatment of personality disorders

Most people with personality disorders do not see a need for treatment. Often, secondary medical and psychiatric illnesses force persons with personality disorders to seek treatment. Rigid thoughts and behaviour often complicate compliance with treatment and are frustrating for healthcare providers.

Individual, family and group therapy is required to point out consequences of behaviour. Antianxiety, antidepressant and antipsychotic medications may be required to treat accompanying symptoms of anxiety, depression and psychosis.

SUICIDE

Suicide is almost always associated with mental illness. People consider suicide when they feel hopeless and are unable to see alternative solutions to confusion, mental and physical anguish and chaos in their life. Risks for suicide include substance abuse, previous suicide attempts, a family history of suicide, a history of sexual abuse and impulsive or aggressive character. More than four times as many men as women die by suicide; however, women attempt suicide more often. Suicidal behaviour occurs most often when people experience major losses and stressful events such as divorce, loss of a job, incarceration and chronic illness.

Unlike physical illnesses, mental illness has no visible wounds and so is associated with social stigma, isolation and personal faults. Those with mental illness contemplating suicide may talk about their distress at the risk of being judged, ignored and isolated. Warning signs of suicide include withdrawal, talk of death, giving away cherished possessions and a sudden shift in mood. A severely depressed person may unexpectedly appear better, or a schizophrenic may progressively develop delusions about death prior to a suicide attempt. A suicide attempt or completed suicide is devastating to families, friends and caregivers, who commonly experience remorse and guilt for failing to avert the suicide attempt or death.

AGE-RELATED DISORDERS

Mental illness can occur at any age. Some disorders occur first in childhood and adolescence, such as ADHD, conduct disorder and oppositional defiant disorder. Others are developmental disorders usually first recognised in childhood but which continue throughout life; these disorders include mental retardation, autistic disorders and tic disorders. Some are strongly associated with adolescence, including bulimia nervosa and anorexia nervosa. Other disorders clearly associated with advanced age include dementia and Alzheimer's disease. Many other disorders can first occur at any time during adulthood from young adult through to advanced age. These include depression, anxiety, schizophrenia and substance abuse disorders.

Resources

Food and Drug Administration: *www.fda.gov*

National Alliance for the Mentally Ill: *www.nami.org*

National Institutes of Mental Health: *www.nimh.org*

World Health Organization: *www.who.org*

 Prevention PLUS!

Suicide warning signs

Mentally ill people may have self-destructive thoughts and may exhibit suicidal behaviours. Patients with depressive symptoms in particular are more likely to have suicidal thoughts. Thus it is important for healthcare workers and families of the patient to watch for suicide warning signs. The following are signs of suicidal behaviour and require immediate attention:

- Withdrawal and isolation
- Saying goodbye to close friends and family
- Indirectly expressed suicide messages or wishes
- Depression
- Giving away or discarding personal possessions
- Explicit suicide messages

Source: National Institutes of Mental Health: *www.nimh.org*

DISEASES AT A GLANCE Mental illness and cognitive disorders*

DISORDER	AETIOLOGY	SIGNS AND SYMPTOMS	DIAGNOSIS	TREATMENT	LIFESPAN
Disruptive behaviour disorders	Genetics, biology, environment	Wilful disobedience, defiance of authority, aggression	Psychosocial and medical evaluation, psychometric testing; diagnosed in childhood	Cognitive behavioural psychotherapy, pharmacotherapy: stimulants, atypical antipsychotic medications	Onset in early childhood
Attention deficit hyperactivity disorder	Genetics, biology, environment	Hyperactivity, impulsivity, inattention	Psychosocial and medical evaluation, psychometric testing; diagnosed prior to the age of 7, with approximately 50% persistence into adulthood	Cognitive behavioural psychotherapy, pharmacotherapy: stimulants	Onset in early childhood; more prevalent in boys
Mental retardation	Genetics, biology, environment	Social language deficits, below average intelligence	Psychosocial and medical evaluation, psychometric testing; diagnosed usually before 3 years of age	Behavioural therapy, occupational therapy, social support services	Usually first recognised in childhood
Autistic disorder	Genetics, biology, environment	Reciprocal language deficits, repetitive stereotypical behaviours	Psychosocial and medical evaluation, psychometric testing; diagnosed usually around 3 years of age	Behavioural therapy, occupational therapy, social support services; pharmacotherapy or other supportive care to manage aggression or self-injurious behaviour	Usually first recognised by age 3
Tic disorder	Genetics, biology, environment	Rapid involuntary repetitive movement or vocalisation	Psychosocial and medical evaluation, psychometric testing; diagnosed usually before adulthood	Behavioural therapy; pharmacotherapy: certain antidepressants or atypical antipsychotic medications	Can develop at any age; usually first recognised in childhood and adolescence
Dementia	Genetics, biology, environment, toxins	Language, memory and mood deficits	Psychosocial and medical evaluation; diagnosed most commonly after age 60	Behavioural, cognitive, family psychotherapy; social supportive care services; pharmacotherapy: memory enhancers	Onset in older adults
Substance abuse disorders	Genetics, environment	Compulsive use, physical and psychological cravings, tolerance and withdrawal	Diagnosis may follow social, medical or legal consequences imposing psychosocial evaluation	Behavioural therapy, 12-step programmes supporting abstinence (such as Alcoholics Anonymous or Narcotics Anonymous); sometimes pharmacotherapy	
Schizophrenia	Genetics, biology, environment	Loss of contact with reality, severe disturbance in social functioning, bizarre thoughts, withdrawal from social interactions, hallucinations, delusions	Psychosocial and medical evaluation, psychometric testing, unpredictable behaviour	Pharmacotherapy: antipsychotic medications, behavioural therapy, occupational therapy, social support services	Usually first recognised in late adolescence and early adulthood

*Prevention of a disorder and its complications depends on screening and intervention, especially in at-risk persons.

DISEASES AT A GLANCE Mental illness and cognitive disorders (continued)

DISORDER	AETIOLOGY	SIGNS AND SYMPTOMS	DIAGNOSIS	TREATMENT	LIFESPAN
Major depression	Genetics, biology, environment	Prolonged sadness, significant changes in sleep and appetite, irritability, feelings of guilt and anxiety	Psychosocial and medical evaluation, psychometric testing	Cognitive behavioural therapy, psychotherapy, social supportive care; pharmacotherapy: antidepressants, tranquillisers, sleep medications	Usually first recognised in late adolescence and early adulthood
Bipolar disorder	Genetics, biology, environment	Mania (episodic elation, inflated sense of self) alternating with depression	Psychosocial and medical evaluation, psychometric testing	Cognitive behavioural therapy, psychotherapy, social supportive care; pharmacotherapy: mood stabillisers, atypical antipsychotic medications, sleep medication	First seen in young adults
Anxiety disorder	Genetics, biology, environment	Inappropriate fear response with avoidance of daily work, family, life, school and recreational activities	Psychosocial and medical evaluation, psychometric testing	Cognitive behavioural therapy; pharmacotherapy: antianxiety medications and certain antidepressants	Usually first recognised in late adolescence and early adulthood
Eating disorders	Genetics, social trends, attitudes, stresses	Anorexia: persistent dieting, starvation, excessive exercise, body weight 15% less than ideal body weight Bulimia: binge followed by purging behaviour, overuse of laxatives, excessive dieting, body weight normal or thin	Psychosocial and medical evaluation, psychometric testing	Psychosocial therapy, pharmacotherapy	Most prevalent in late childhood and adolescence, young adulthood; mostly in girls and women
Personality disorders	Environment	Inflexible patterns of behaviour with strained relationships; may occur with substance use disorders, reckless sexual behavior, eating disorders and violence	Psychosocial and medical evaluation, psychometric testing	Cognitive behavioural therapy, social support, social services; pharmacotherapy for coexisting depression, anxiety, agitation, aggression, delusions or psychosis	Onset in early adulthood; more prevalent in females

INTERACTIVE EXERCISES

Cases for critical thinking

1. Bill is a 17-year-old male with above average intelligence. As an infant, he was colicky and difficult to put to sleep. He learned to walk at 12 months of age. At home, Bill seemed to run on a motor: he scurried around the house, frequently bumping into furniture. Bill had a hearing test at school at 5 years of age because teachers felt that he may have been hard of hearing, but the test was normal. His marks were average during the primary and secondary school years. When he went to college Bill's marks dropped dramatically. He frequently appeared distracted, irritable and angry. He preferred to eat lunch alone and spent much time in his room. His parents feared that he was abusing drugs because he had a history of a 'poor choice of friends'. His college counsellor recommended a psychiatric evaluation for Bill. His parents were offended at this recommendation.

   a. What are the advantages and disadvantages of a full mental health evaluation?
   b. What potential disorders do you suspect Bill is experiencing?
   c. What are the potential causes of his disorders?

2. Anne-Marie is a 10-year-old girl with a history of 'poor' school marks and fighting in class. She has a brother with ADHD. Her parents divorced when she was 5 years old, and she has been raised with a nanny because her mother travels frequently with her job. Anne-Marie is very athletic – she is a member of the travelling netball team and a competitive ballet dancer. She has voiced frustration over her marks, as she feels that although she works hard, she cannot 'get the marks'. She fears disappointing her mother by stopping dance and netball and she feels like a failure. Although Anne-Marie is a very talented dancer, she trembles and feels her heart pound prior to competition. Her appetite has been poor, and she has been observed picking at her food.

Anne-Marie's mother is concerned and has made an appointment with a doctor.

   a. Does Anne-Marie have warning signs of a potential mental illness? What symptoms and behaviours point to a potential problem?
   b. Would you recommend an evaluation for Anne-Marie?
   c. What type of treatments are available for Anne-Marie?

3. David is a 46-year-old man who recently moved his family across the country. His mother recently died of complications from Alzheimer's disease, and he is executor of her estate. David moved his family because of a great job opportunity. Although he loves his job, he regrets moving his family from the town they lived in for 20 years. He has been spending much of his free time alone in his office and has been ignoring his wife and children. David's father was an alcoholic, and his wife fears that his recent stress may drive him to drink. He has lost interest in sex and recently declined an invitation to a golf outing that he had enjoyed in the past. David has been talking to himself a lot and claims that at times he has seen his mother in his sleep. He awoke abruptly one night from sleep and has been complaining of having nightmares. David sometimes appears frozen and indifferent to conversations and behaves as though something is bothering him. His wife feels that David is mourning the loss of his mother, since his mother was never the person he always longed for. His mother had been abusive to David, who was conceived out of wedlock. His mother made sure that he had 'proper' upbringing with strict discipline and often punished David rather harshly if he failed to follow directions.

   a. What signs of mental illness does David have?
   b. What condition do you think David has?
   c. What recommendations would you give to David's wife?

Multiple choice

1. Reforms in the treatment of the mentally ill started after the French Revolution with an Austrian physician named _____
   a. Sigmund Freud   b. Franz Mesmer
   c. Emil Kraepelin   d. Sybil Dorsett

2. Psychiatric diagnoses are categorised in a book named the _____
   a. PDR   b. AMA
   c. DSM   d. Axis

3. Which of the following neurotransmitters is implicated in schizophrenia, depression and ADHD?
   a. adrenaline
   b. serotonin
   c. gamma amino butyric acid (GABA)
   d. dopamine

4. Which of the following regarding ADHD is false?
   a. ADHD is limited to children
   b. ADHD is a neurobiological disorder
   c. ADHD is more common in males than in females
   d. There are three subtypes of ADHD

5. Medications that replace _____ are effective in improving memory in persons with Alzheimer's disease.
   a. dopamine   b. serotonin
   c. acetylcholine   d. GABA

6. A false belief that one is being watched or punished is also known as a _____ delusion.
   a. persecutory   b. somatic
   c. grandiose   d. affective

7. Binge eating followed by purging behaviour such as self-induced vomiting most commonly occurs in _____
   a. anorexia nervosa
   b. bulimia nervosa
   c. binge eating disorder
   d. all of the above

8. Periods of intense mania and depression that last for several weeks are also known as _____
   a. cyclothymic disorder   b. bipolar I
   c. bipolar II   d. all of the above

9. Adults with bipolar illness may be treated with all of the following types of medications except _____
   a. sedatives
   b. antidepressant medications
   c. stimulant medications
   d. antipsychotic medications

10. Anxious, irrational thoughts and images are also called _____
    a. compulsions   b. delusions
    c. hallucinations   d. obsessions

True or false

_____ **1.** Bipolar disorder is a behavioural disorder with extreme highs and lows.

_____ **2.** ADHD is an emotional disorder associated with depression, anxiety and hyperactivity.

_____ **3.** Persons of different age groups are at risk for different types of mental illness.

_____ **4.** Childhood conduct disorder is also known as childhood antisocial personality.

_____ **5.** People with high blood pressure and diabetes have a higher risk for dementia.

_____ **6.** Substance abuse is a conscious choice to use drugs or alcohol.

_____ **7.** Hallucinations and delusions are symptoms of post-traumatic stress disorder.

_____ **8.** Children are at risk for major depression.

_____ **9.** Individuals with a schizoid personality disorder are distant, introverted and tend to hallucinate.

_____ **10.** Primary psychiatric diagnoses are indicated in all the five axes of diagnosis according to the DSM.

Fill-ins

1. _____ is the medical specialty that diagnoses and prescribes medical treatment for mental illness.

2. Chemical messengers, or _____, are implicated in mental illness.

3. Mood, thought processes, appetite, movement, heart rate and blood pressure are regulated by the neurotransmitter _____.

4. Below average intelligence accompanied by deficits in language and adaptive functioning is diagnostic for _____.

5. Rapid stereotyped movements that may be suppressed by conscious effort are known as _____.

6. Alzheimer's disease is mostly caused by impaired regulation of _____ neurotransmitters.

7. Core symptoms of drug and alcohol abuse include _____, _____, _____ and _____.

8. An individual's emotional state in mental illness is referred to as _____.

9. _____ is caused by decreased sunlight exposure during the winter months.

10. Decreased need for sleep, with excessive irritability and grandiosity, is symptomatic for _____.

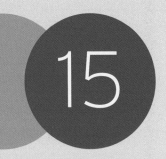

15 DISEASES OF THE MUSCULOSKELETAL SYSTEM

Duchenne's muscular dystrophy. Cross-section of gastrocnemius muscle shows extensive replacement of muscle fibres by adipose cells.

(Courtesy of the CDC/Dr Edwin P. Ewing Jr, 1972)

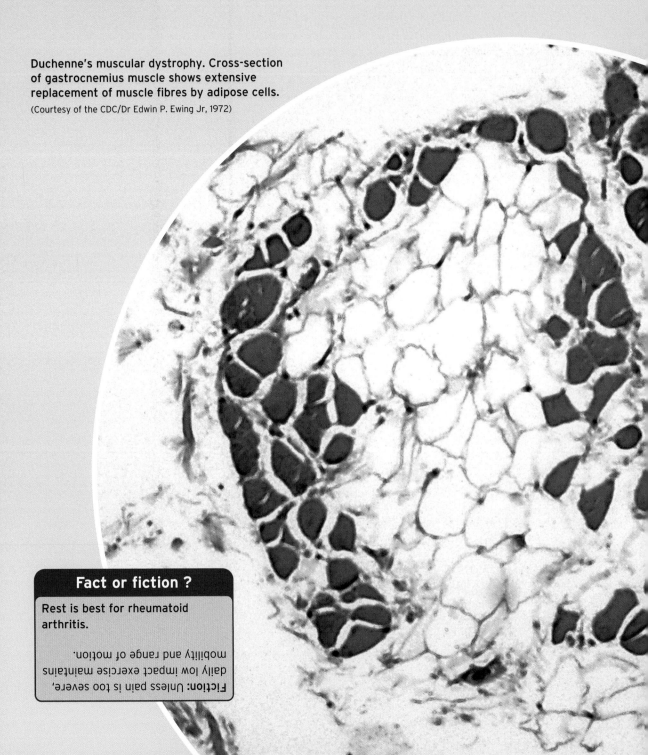

Fact or fiction ?

Rest is best for rheumatoid arthritis.

Fiction: Unless pain is too severe, daily low impact exercise maintains mobility and range of motion.

Learning objectives

After studying this chapter, you should be able to:

+ Understand the normal structure and function of bones, joints and muscle
+ Describe the aetiology, signs and symptoms, diagnostic tests and treatment of infectious diseases of bone
+ Explain how vitamin and mineral deficiencies can lead to bone disease
+ Describe the aetiology, signs and symptoms, diagnostic tests and treatment of bone cancer
+ Describe the aetiology, signs and symptoms, diagnostic tests and treatment of the common types of arthritis, gout and bursitis
+ Identify the aetiology, signs and symptoms, diagnostic tests and treatment of dislocations, sprains, strains and carpal tunnel syndrome
+ Describe the aetiology, signs and symptoms, diagnostic tests and treatment of muscular dystrophy and myasthenia gravis
+ Understand age-related changes and diseases of the musculoskeletal system

Disease chronicle

Arthritis

Arthritis in its various forms has a long history. Prehistoric human and dinosaur remains both display evidence of joint disease. As often happens when a nasty and frequent problem has no cure, multiple folk remedies were suggested: in Norfolk, a stone with a hole in it placed under the bed was deemed to do the trick. Other ideas included drinking cider turning to vinegar. More modern remedies, however, can appear equally unscientific: over a dozen herbal remedies and nutritional supplements carry claims that they help relieve arthritis, and many people wear copper bracelets in the hope of controlling the grinding pains of joint disease. Our understanding and treatment of arthritis has progressed significantly, but a cure is still a long way off. Thus unscrupulous individuals and companies continue to espouse expensive treatments that have little evidence of success, and prey upon vulnerable people.

INTERACTION OF BONES, JOINTS AND MUSCLES

Bones, joints and muscles work together. The bones of the skeleton provide the body with a sturdy framework. Bones are held together by a variety of joints, some of which permit movement at parts of the skeletal framework. Because skeletal muscle is attached via tendons to bones, when muscle contracts, or shortens, it moves the skeleton. Thus, the muscles that span a joint bring about action at that joint. Groups of muscles may have opposite or antagonistic actions on a joint. For example, one group of muscles extends (straightens) the knee, while another group flexes (bends) the knee. Still other muscles stabilise joints, preventing undesired movements. In this chapter, the principal diseases and disorders of bone, joints and muscles – the musculoskeletal system – are explained although the diseases described are diseases of *voluntary* muscle. Because muscle action requires nerve stimulation, some nervous system diseases are manifested in muscles. These diseases are discussed with the nervous system in Chapter 13. This chapter discusses a few muscle diseases that are not directly caused by nervous system disease. Smooth muscle, or involuntary muscle, is a different type of muscle found in the walls of the internal organs and the walls of blood vessels. Cardiac muscle is an involuntary striated muscle and is present only in the heart (see Chapter 6). This chapter does not address cardiac or smooth muscle disease.

STRUCTURE AND FUNCTION OF BONES, JOINTS AND MUSCLES

Bone may appear inert, but changes constantly occur within it. Bone development, growth and homeostasis rely on interplay among its constituent minerals, proteins and living cells. **Calcium** and **phosphate**, bone's primary minerals, are embedded in **collagen**, bone's main protein. The minerals confer hardness and rigidity to bone, while the collagen imparts flexibility. Mature bone cells, **osteocytes**, along with bone-forming cells, **osteoblasts**, and bone reabsorbing cells, **osteoclasts**, reside within this bony matrix. The cells receive nutrients by an organised system of blood vessels that run throughout the bone.

Bones can be either long, flat, or irregularly shaped. Most are covered with a layer of a type of bone tissue called **compact bone**. The cells, minerals, proteins and blood vessels of compact bone are arranged in a regular, organised fashion. Another type of bone tissue, **spongy bone**, contains many spaces filled with bone marrow.

Bone marrow may be red or white. In babies, most bone marrow is red, but in adults red bone marrow is confined to the ends of long bones and is the site of formation of all blood cells. Yellow bone marrow consists primarily of fat and is found in the **medullary cavity** of the long bones of the arms and legs.

The increase in length of the long bones of a growing child occurs at the **epiphyses**, or growth plate, an area of cartilage near each end of the bone (Figure 15.1). At this site, new bone is formed, pushing the ends apart from each other until full growth is achieved, at which time the cartilage turns into bone, a process called **ossification**, and no further increase can occur. Damage to the growth plate before maturity tends to prevent the bone from reaching its mature length.

The **periosteum** is a highly vascular layer of fibrous connective tissue that covers the surface of bones. It contains cells that are capable of forming new bone tissue following injury, and serves as a site of attachment for tendons or muscles.

Joints are the articulating sites between bones. Various degrees of movement, called *range of motion*, are possible in different kinds of joints. The amount and type of movement at a joint is defined by the shapes of bones and the type of connective tissue holding the bones together at the joint. The shoulder (joint between humerus and scapula) is the most freely movable joint, but it is also the one most easily dislocated.

Articulating bones are held together by **ligaments**. Dense strands of collagen impart great strength to ligaments. A joint capsule consisting of ligaments and connective tissue surrounds the bone ends.

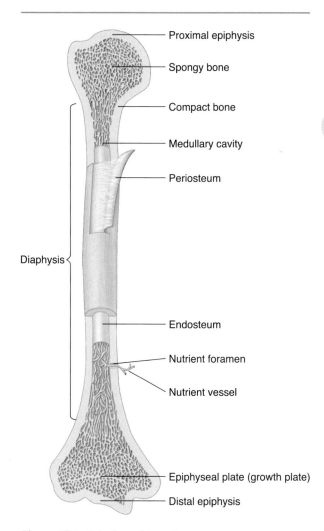

Proximal epiphysis

Spongy bone

Compact bone

Medullary cavity

Periosteum

Diaphysis

Endosteum

Nutrient foramen

Nutrient vessel

Epiphyseal plate (growth plate)

Distal epiphysis

Figure 15.1 Cut view of long bone.

tissue. When stimulated by nerves at the myoneural junction, muscle fibres contract, and because muscles are attached to bones, the shortening of the muscles moves the bones.

DIAGNOSTIC TESTS FOR MUSCULOSKELETAL DISEASES

X-rays can reveal fractures, joint dislocations, bone deformities and calcification, measure bone density and detect signs of other bone damage. MRI (magnetic resonance imaging) uses strong magnetic fields to visualise details of joint anatomy and can show trauma and arthritis damage. CT (computed tomography) scans show details of soft tissues like tendons and ligaments as well as muscle. Arthroscopy involves passing an endoscope into the joint – such as the knee, a particularly complex joint – to visualise the inside of the cavity. Joint fluid can be aspirated for microscopic and chemical analysis. Myelography detects abnormalities of the spinal cord by visualising the distribution of a radio-opaque contrast medium injected into the subarachnoid space. Myelography can detect tumours and herniated discs. Electromyography measures electrical activity of muscles and reveals some abnormalities of muscle function. Biopsy can show muscle tissue abnormalities.

DISEASES OF BONE

Bone can be affected by disease in various ways. Infectious agents can enter bone through a compound fracture, transmission in the blood or extension from an adjacent infection. Mineral and vitamin deficiencies prevent proper formation or maintenance of bone structure. Bones **atrophy** with disuse and fracture, or spontaneously in certain diseases. Tumours can also develop in bone.

Infectious diseases of bone

Osteomyelitis is an inflammation of the bone, particularly of the bone marrow in the medullary

The inner surface of the capsule is lined with a **synovial membrane** that secretes **synovial fluid**, which lubricates the joints. Pockets of this fluid, the **bursae**, are situated near some joints, such as the shoulder and knee, where they reduce friction during movement. The articulating surfaces of the bone ends are covered with a layer of cartilage, which also reduces friction. A typical joint is illustrated in Figure 15.2.

Skeletal muscle (which can also be termed striated or **voluntary muscle**) tissue is found in muscles that are firmly attached to bones by **tendons**. Some voluntary muscles (the facial muscles, for example) are attached to soft tissue. Muscles consist of bundles of muscle fibres held together by connective

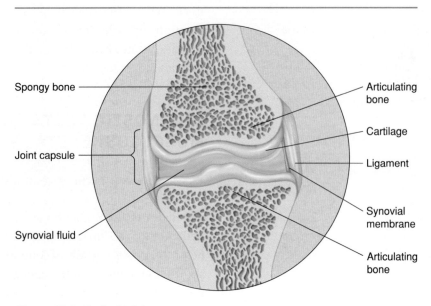

Spongy bone

Joint capsule

Synovial fluid

Articulating bone

Cartilage

Ligament

Synovial membrane

Articulating bone

Figure 15.2 Typical joint.

cavity and the spaces of spongy bone. Osteomyelitis affects 1 in 5000 people, principally children and adolescents, whose bones are still growing. In children, the long bones – the femur, the tibia and the humerus – are most frequently affected near their ends at the growth plate. In adults, osteomyelitis usually affects the pelvis and vertebrae following trauma and surgery. The main risk factor for developing osteomyelitis is a recent bacterial infection that may have escaped treatment, permitting the bacteria to become bloodborne.

Osteomyelitis is caused by bacteria, usually *Staphylococcus aureus* and occasionally *Streptococcus pyogenes*, *Pneumococcus* or *Escherichia coli*. The bacteria are carried by blood to the bone from some other site in the body, such as infection adjacent to the bone. Hence, the chief risk factor for osteomyelitis includes infections, including open wounds of a compound fracture.

In osteomyelitis, the infection develops into an abscess in the bone, which compresses small blood vessels, reduces circulation and causes bone necrosis. Infections may spread under the periosteum, lifting sections of it from bone surface, further reducing circulation to bone. In an attempt to heal, bone may be deposited around this area of necrosis.

Local symptoms of bone infection include pain, redness and heat. Systemic symptoms of chills, fever and leukocytosis, tachycardia, nausea and anorexia also occur. Diagnosis begins with history and physical examination and can be confirmed with white blood cell count, an elevated erythrocyte sedimentation rate, blood culture of causative micro-organism and magnetic resonance imaging or bone scans. An X-ray will not reveal early infections.

Early antibiotic therapy is an effective treatment and has reduced the incidence of advanced serious cases. Surgery may be required to remove necrotic bone tissue (Figure 15.3).

Tuberculosis of bone is rare and is associated with untreated pulmonary tuberculosis. This infection occurs when bacteria spread to the bones from other tissues, principally the lungs. Commonly affected areas are the ends of long bones and knees. Usually seen in children, Pott's disease is tuberculosis of the vertebrae, leading to deformity and paralysis. As in the lungs, tuberculosis of bone leads to the formation of hollow cavities within the bone and tissue destruction (see Chapter 8). The infection can be treated with antibiotics, although strains of *Mycobacterium tuberculosis* have developed multiple drug resistance. Surgery may be able to correct bone deformities.

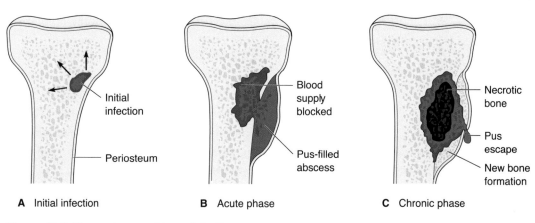

Figure 15.3 Three phases of bone infection.

Bone disease and vitamin and mineral deficiencies

Vitamins and minerals are essential to bone health. Calcium and phosphorus are required in appropriate quantities for proper bone formation and maintenance. However, dietary calcium cannot be absorbed from the digestive tract without vitamin D. Thus, mineral or vitamin D deficiencies may result in soft, malformed or fragile bones.

Rickets is a disease of infancy or early childhood in which the bones do not properly ossify, or harden. Rickets was considered an obsolete disease, but appears to be increasing again. In one year, a programme in Birmingham identified 24 children with rickets severe enough to warrant further treatment. A child with rickets develops bones that are soft and tend to bend. Over time, the weightbearing bones of the body become deformed: the legs become bent ('bow-legged' or 'knock-kneed') and the vertebral column becomes misaligned. The sternum projects forward, and bony nodules form on the ends of ribs and at wrists, ankles and knees. The skull is large and square. The pelvic opening in a girl may narrow, leading to problems with childbirth later. Other signs and symptoms of rickets include flaccid muscles, delayed teething and a characteristic potbelly. Each of these symptoms can be explained by calcium deficiency.

Rickets occurs where there is a lack of calcium or vitamin D (or sunlight, see below) in the diet, or in

malabsorption syndromes. It can also, rarely, be the result of an inherited metabolic problem, or a complication of kidney disease. It can be prevented with vitamin D-fortified milk and exposure to sunlight. Sunlight converts a substance (dehydrocholesterol) in the skin to vitamin D in the body. This need for sunlight explains the higher incidence of rickets in large, smoky cities where buildings are close together and shut out the sun, and in people who, for cultural reasons, do not expose their skin to daylight. Furthermore, people with dark skin require more sunlight to manufacture the required amounts of vitamin D. Ironically, concerns about the risk of sunlight causing skin cancer may be leading to problems related to lack of vitamin D, including rickets, osteomalacia and certain cancers. Children with rickets respond well to sunlight exposure and treatment with vitamin D concentrate.

Osteomalacia is the same softening or decalcification of bones, but in adults. Similar to rickets, its prevalence may be underestimated. It is most common in Asia among women who have had multiple births, eat a cereal-based diet and have little exposure to sunlight. Symptoms include muscle weakness, weight loss and bone pain. Bones of the vertebral column, legs and pelvis become susceptible to bending and fracturing with mild stress.

Osteoporosis is a disease characterised by porous bone that is abnormally fragile and susceptible to fracture. Of those affected by osteoporosis, 80% are women. While some bone loss is expected with

Box 15.1

Risk factors for osteoporosis

- Low bone mass
- Low calcium intake
- Female
- Vitamin D deficiency
- Small frame
- Sedentary lifestyle
- Family history
- Cigarette smoking
- Postmenopausal
- Excessive alcohol use
- Hysterectomy
- Caucasian or Asian
- Amenorrhoea

aging, the cause of the accelerated bone loss observed in osteoporosis is unknown. However, risk factors for osteoporosis have been identified, and these include being female, advanced age and having a small frame (Box 15.1).

Unfortunately, osteoporosis can quietly become advanced because no symptoms accompany bone loss until bones weaken enough to fracture. Weightbearing bones of the vertebrae and pelvis are especially susceptible and accumulated compression fractures in these bones cause a decrease in height and bending of the spine (Figure 15.4). Compressed vertebrae press on spinal nerves, causing great pain. Fractures are also common in the hips and wrists.

Osteoporosis is diagnosed using patient history and bone density tests. No cure exists, so prevention is strongly recommended. A lifelong diet rich in calcium and vitamin D along with weightbearing exercise stimulates the development of dense and strong bone and slows progression of the disease. Smoking should be avoided, and alcohol and

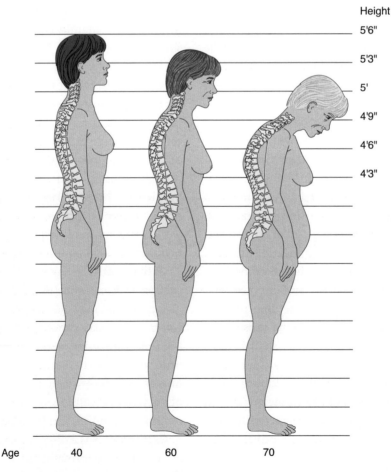

Figure 15.4 Spinal changes caused by osteoporosis.

SIDE by SIDE Osteoporosis

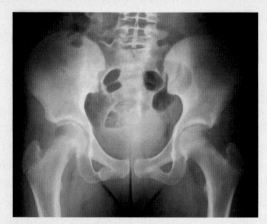

X-ray of pelvis in 18-year-old female showing normal bone density.
(Science Photo Library Ltd)

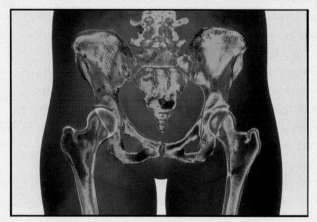

X-ray of female pelvis with osteoporosis. Note greatly decreased bone density, especially visible in hip bones.
(Chris Bjornberg)

caffeine consumption should be minimised. Treatment requires medication. Various drugs facilitate calcium uptake in bone and include oestrogens, calcitonin, parathyroid hormone as well as oestrogen receptor modulators and bisphosphonates.

Other bone deformities

Paget's disease, or **osteitis deformans**, is a condition in which the normal cycle of bone formation and reabsorption is disrupted, particularly in the skull, vertebrae and pelvis. Paget's disease is rare worldwide, but, for unknown reasons, is more common amongst white people of British descent. It is an age-related condition. In the UK it affects 1–2% of white adults over 55 years of age, rising to 5–8% of white people over 80 years of age, although most of these are asymptomatic. The cause of Paget's disease is unknown, but approximately 20–30% of cases are genetically based.

The disease begins with bone softening, which is followed by bone overgrowth. The new bone tissue is abnormal and tends to fracture easily. The excessive bony growth causes the skull to enlarge, which often affects cranial nerves; thus, vision and hearing

are affected. Abnormal bone development causes curvatures in the spinal column and deformities in legs. Another complication of this disease is **osteogenic sarcoma**; see the following discussion.

Paget's disease is diagnosed by examination, X-rays, bone scan and bone biopsy. Treatment requires calcitonin and etidronate, which reduce bone reabsorption, and mithramycin, which decreases calcium. Sufferers may also require analgesia. Surgery may be appropriate to correct deformities.

Scoliosis is an abnormal lateral curvature of the spine that occurs to varying degrees of severity and is usually first identified during childhood. Scoliosis may be caused by abnormal development that results in fusion of the vertebrae. Scoliosis may also have a neuromuscular origin. Weak or asymmetric muscle development can pull the spine laterally. This can result from diseases such as polio, muscular dystrophy, spina bifida or cerebral palsy. Scoliosis may be idiopathic. Symptoms may include low back pain and fatigue. Diagnosis is based on history, physical examination and X-rays. Mild curvatures of less than 20° are common in adolescents and may not require treatment. More severe curvatures of 30° in growing adolescents must be treated with braces to prevent further curving of the verte-brae. Curves of 40° require surgery to correct the misalignment. The outcomes are promising follow-ing treatment although neuromuscular scoliosis may be more difficult to treat because it is usually accompanied and caused by another disease.

Kyphosis, an exaggerated posterior curve of the thoracic spine, sometimes called hunchback, occurs most commonly in adults and becomes more noticeable in the elderly (Figure 15.5). It is most often caused by collapse of vertebrae affected by osteoporosis and by degenerative changes associ-ated with arthritis of the vertebrae. Symptoms include mild back pain, back fatigue, perhaps tenderness and, in severe cases, difficulty breathing because of compression of the thoracic cage. It can be diagnosed with physical examination and X-rays. Treatment options are few and provide no cures. Treatment of the underlying osteoporosis can slow progression of kyphosis. Treatment of underlying arthritis can relieve pain and immobility but only to a limited degree.

These two conditions can occur together, when it is termed **kyphoscoliosis**.

Lordosis is an inward curvature of the lumbar vertebrae. Some degree of curvature is normal and most cases of lordosis are benign. Any unusual pain or curvature should be investigated.

Bone cancer

Malignant bone tumours Bone cancer is rare, comprising 1% of malignancies. Most bone cancer is secondary and results from metastasis from a tumour located elsewhere in the body. Primary malignancy of bone occurs most often in males, especially children and adolescents. One type of bone cancer, **osteogenic sarcoma**, arises in the bony tissue itself and frequently affects the ends of long bones, frequently at the knee, where enlargement of the bone is observed. The cause of osteogenic sarcoma is unknown. Signs and symptoms include dull localised bone pain that intensifies at night. Masses may be noted and fractures accompany

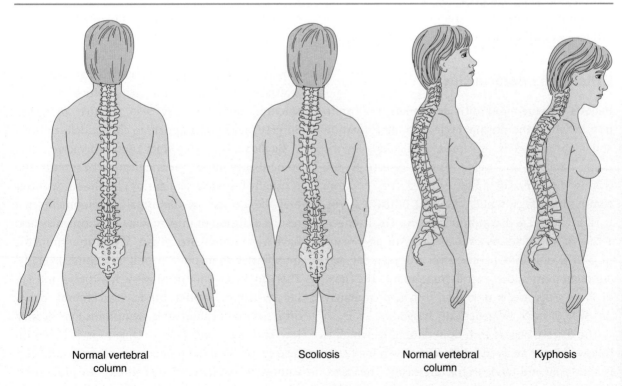

Normal vertebral column   Scoliosis   Normal vertebral column   Kyphosis

Figure 15.5 The two most common deformities of the spinal column are scoliosis and kyphosis.

sarcomas. Bone cancer is diagnosed with biopsy. X-rays and CT scans are used to locate and measure tumours. Treatment may involve chemotherapy to reduce tumour size followed by surgical removal. See Chapter 4 for a discussion of cancer.

Bone trauma: fractures

Several diseases and disorders discussed in this chapter may result in bone loss or other damage that can result in fracture. Trauma, however, is also a common cause of bone fractures: a loss of continuity in the structure of the bone. Excessive force, twisting or compression can lead to bone fractures. The chief signs and symptoms of a fracture include the following.

- Visibly out-of-place or mis-shapen limb or joint
- Swelling, bruising or bleeding

- Intense pain
- Numbness and tingling
- Broken skin with bone protruding
- Limited mobility or inability to move a limb.

These signs and symptoms require diagnosis and medical attention to promote healing and to prevent infections. A variety of fractures can occur (Figure 15.6). Most fractures require immobilisation with a splint or cast, while others, like open fractures, require surgery, pins and plates to promote healing.

DISEASES OF THE JOINTS

Joints permit movement of the skeleton; thus diseases of the joints cause pain and limit mobility. Joints that bear weight – the lower vertebrae, hips and knees – receive a great deal of stress and are

FRACTURE TYPE	DESCRIPTION	COMMENTS	FRACTURE TYPE	DESCRIPTION	COMMENTS
Closed 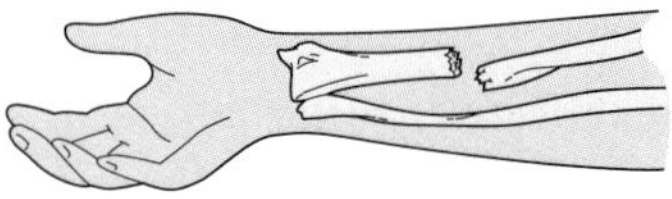	Bone breaks cleanly but does not penetrate skin	Also called a simple fracture	Depressed	Broken bone is pressed inward	Common in skull fractures
Open 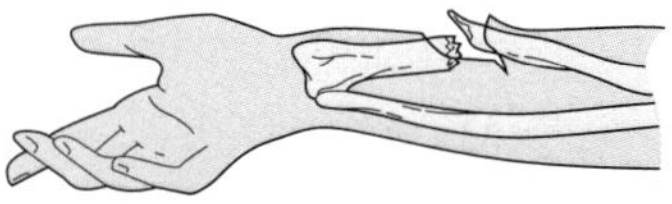	Broken ends of bone protrude through soft tissues and skin	Serious; may result in osteomyelitis. Also called a compound fracture	Spiral	Jagged break owing to twisting force applied to bone	Common fracture owing to sports injuries
Comminuted 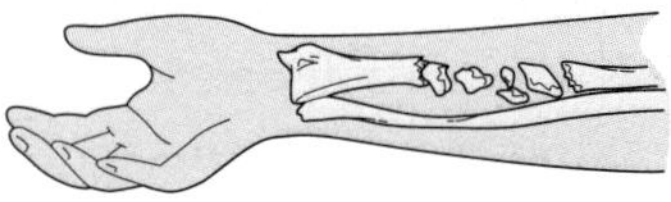	Bone fragments into many pieces	Common in those with conditions causing brittle bones, such as osteogenesis imperfecta	Greenstick 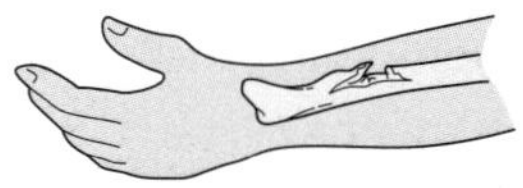	Bone breaks incompletely, much in the way a green twig breaks	Common in children, whose bones have proportionally more organic matrix and are more flexible than those of adults
Compression	Bone is crushed	Common in those with osteoporosis			
Impacted	Broken ends of bone are forced into each other	Commonly results from falls; also common in hip fracture			

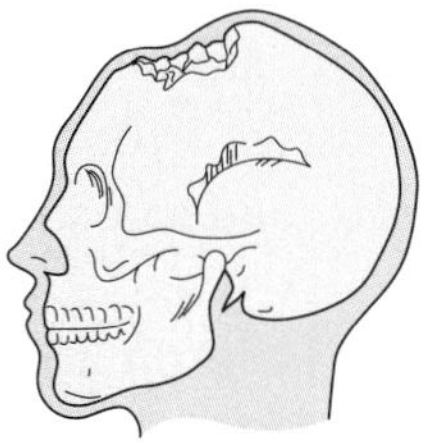

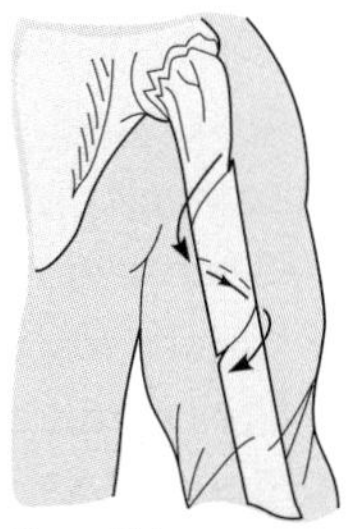

Figure 15.6 Fractures.

(Adapted from Marieb, E. N. (1998). *Human Anatomy and Physiology*, 4th edn. Menlo Park, CA: Benjamin Cummings, p. 180)

especially susceptible to the diseases and disorders discussed in this chapter. The muscles, nerves and bones may also be affected by joint disease.

Arthritis

Arthritis is a term used to describe a wide range of distressing joint diseases, the two most common being degenerative joint disease and rheumatoid arthritis.

Osteoarthritis This means 'inflammation of a joint', but in fact inflammation is rarely present, even though swelling may be, so a better term is degenerative joint disease. Symptoms of degenerative joint disease include persistent joint pain and stiffness. Joints may be swollen and may lose mobility and become deformed to the point of losing function. Commonly affected joints include the lower vertebrae, hips, fingers and knees. Degenerative joint disease is extremely common in older adults, but can also occur in children, where it is termed juvenile idiopathic arthritis or Still's disease. About 1 in 1000 children are affected. Secondary degenerative joint disease is associated with joint injury, trauma or obesity, and so occurs only in one or a few joints.

Muscle tension and fatigue contribute to the aches and pains of degenerative joint disease. The disease in the lower back may pinch a spinal nerve, such as the sciatic nerve, in which case pain radiates down the back and leg. Affected joints lose their range of motion, and associated muscles become weak.

Degeneration occurs at the articular cartilage of the joint. This cartilage caps the bone surface where bone meets another bone in a joint. This cartilage erodes, exposing the underlying bone, which degenerates and leads to new bone deposits in and around the joint. The bone ends thicken and develop sharp irregular bony surface structures called **spicules** and **spurs**. Small joints such as the knuckles enlarge and become knobby (Figure 15.7).

Diagnosis of degenerative joint disease is made principally by X-rays that show the joint damage and a history of the symptoms. There is no cure for degenerative joint disease, but treatment can greatly

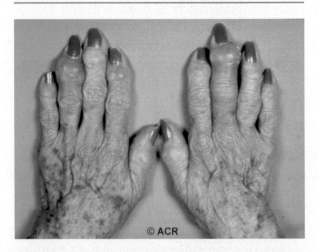

Figure 15.7 Acute gouty arthritis of the finger joints.
(Courtesy of the American College of Rheumatology)

relieve the pain. A combination of rest and mild exercise to maintain range of motion, analgesia and heat applications is generally prescribed. Non-steroidal anti-inflammatory drugs commonly used include aspirin, indomethacin, fenoprofen and ibuprofen. Steroids such as cortisone are sometimes injected into the joint capsule to relieve pain. Surgical replacement of a damaged joint like the hip and knee has become very effective, although factors such as age are important considerations.

Rheumatoid arthritis A less common but more debilitating form of arthritis, rheumatoid arthritis is a chronic and debilitating autoimmune disease. It is a systemic inflammatory disease that affects several joints and the surrounding muscles, tendons and ligaments. Rheumatoid arthritis affects about 0.8% of the UK population, and affects nearly three times more females than males. It is not a disease of older age, and the usual age of onset is between ages 30 and 60. No risk factors have been linked to rheumatoid arthritis and its cause remains unknown, but it appears to be an autoimmune disease. **Rheumatoid factors**, such as anti-immunoglobulins, combine with immunoglobulin in the synovial fluid to form antibody complexes. Neutrophils are attracted to the joint space and cause destruction. The condition is aggravated by stress, and there is a genetic predisposition toward development of the disease.

Symptoms include joint pain and stiffness, particularly on waking. The joints are swollen, red and warm. The same joints are often affected on both sides of the body. The disease, however, is not just one of the joints, but is systemic: the patient experiences fatigue, weakness and weight loss. Rheumatoid arthritis begins with an inflammation of the synovial membrane that lines the joints, particularly the small joints of the hands, feet and wrists. The membrane thickens and extends into the joint cavity, sometimes filling the space with a thickened granulation tissue, called a pannus, which eventually erodes and scars the articular cartilage of the bone ends. When this scar tissue turns to bone, the ends of the bones fuse, a condition called **ankylosis**. The fusion immobilises and deforms the joint. Figures 15.8 and 15.9 illustrate the crippling swan neck deformity and ulnar deviation characteristic of advanced rheumatoid and osteoarthritis in the hands. Rheumatoid nodules may form under the skin, usually near the joints, but they sometimes develop on the white of the eye, too.

Diagnosis is based on physical examination, X-rays showing joint changes, a rheumatoid factor test and synovial fluid analysis. Early diagnosis and a comprehensive treatment programme that includes medicine and exercise can reduce pain and deformity of the joints. Anti-inflammatory drugs are effective, with aspirin (salicylates) and similar drugs being the most commonly used. Other non-steroidal

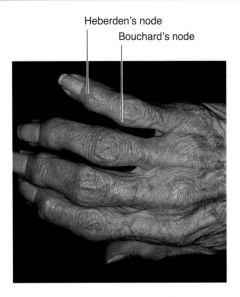

Heberden's node
Bouchard's node

Figure 15.9 Typical joint changes associated with degenerative joint disease.
(Courtesy of the American College of Rheumatology)

anti-inflammatory drugs commonly used include indomethacin, fenoprofen and ibuprofen. Immuno-suppressants such as corticosteroids and methotrexate are now administered in the early stages of the disease. COX-2 inhibitors like Celebrex have also been used. A balance between exercise and rest should be achieved. In an acute phase, the joint should be rested to prevent further inflammation. Physiotherapy can teach patients how to perform range of motion exercises that help preserve joint mobility. Exercises for good posture are directed toward removing stress on weightbearing joints.

Gout Gout affects the joints of the feet, particularly those of the big toe, and sometimes of the hand, fingers, wrist or knee. Gout affects approximately 41 people per 1000 of the UK population. There is some evidence that it may be decreasing very recently. Most are men with an average age of onset of 60 years, but it also affects postmenopausal women. The cause of gout is unknown. It sometimes follows a minor injury or excessive eating or drinking, but there may be no explanation for its occurrence, and heredity may play a role. The pathogenesis of gout is better understood than its cause. Gout attacks are

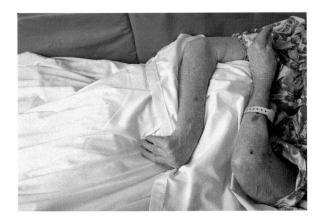

Figure 15.8 Contractures of rheumatoid arthritis.

related to excess uric acid in blood, which results either from a defect in metabolism of purines (a component of nucleic acids), or from abnormal retention of uric acid, or both. The high uric acid level leads to deposits of uric acid crystals in the joints. Uric acid crystals also deposit in the kidneys, stimulating kidney stone formation and irritating the kidney.

The onset of an acute attack of gout is generally sudden. The affected joints exhibit typical signs of inflammation: pain, heat, swelling and redness (see Figure 15.7). Signs and symptoms may last from days to many weeks. Resolution of an acute attack may be followed by symptom-free periods of 6 months to more than 2 years before recurrence. A chronic form of gout also occurs in which a person experiences persistent arthritic pain.

Gout can be diagnosed by microscopic examination of aspirated joint fluid, which reveals needle-like urate crystals. High serum level of uric acid is consistent with gout. X-rays of affected joints may initially appear normal until repeated attacks of chronic gout damage the bone and cartilage at joints.

Acute gout attacks can be treated with rest, application of hot or cold compresses, analgesics, colchicine and corticosteroids. Chronic gout may be treated with colchicine, which prevents acute attacks, and uricosuric agents such as probenecid that promote excretion of uric acid. If diagnosed early and treated properly, the development of chronic gout can be prevented.

Septic arthritis Septic arthritis is a medical emergency. It develops as a result of bacterial infection of a joint. Cartilage and bone destruction may lead to ankylosis and life-threatening septicaemia (bloodborne bacterial infection). Streptococci and staphylococci cause septic arthritis by invading a joint following trauma or surgery. *Neisseria gonorrhoea*, the causative organism of gonorrhoea, may spread to joints via blood from a primary infection site. Antibiotics are required to control the joint infection and to prevent septicaemia.

Bursitis

Bursae are small, fluid-filled sacs located near the joints that cushion and reduce friction on movement. **Bursitis** is an inflammation of these bursae, and it is a very painful condition. The bursae of the shoulder joint are the most frequently affected, although bursitis can develop at any joint. Repeated irritation or injury of a bursa can cause bursitis. Limitation of movement results from the pain of the inflammation. Treatment includes rest, anti-inflammatories and moist heat applications. Steroids are sometimes injected into the joint to reduce the inflammatory response.

Dislocations, sprains and strains

A **dislocation** is a displacement of bones from their normal position in a joint. Dislocations are most common in the shoulder and finger joints, but they can occur anywhere. The dislocation causes pain and reduced mobility at the involved joint. The bone must be reset and immobilised to allow healing of torn ligaments and tendons. Congenital dislocations of the hip result from an improperly formed joint, and they are treated in infancy with a cast or surgery. A subluxation is an incomplete dislocation.

Sprains result from the wrenching or twisting of a joint such as an ankle that injures the ligaments. Blood vessels and surrounding tissues, muscles, tendons and nerves may also be damaged. Swelling and discoloration due to haemorrhage from the ruptured blood vessels occur. A sprain is painful, and the joint should not be used while it is severely inflamed. Immobilisation with a splint or cast might be necessary for more severe sprains. Cold compresses reduce the swelling immediately after the injury, whereas later, heat applications relieve discomfort and speed healing. A 'whiplash' is a sprain in which the cervical (neck) ligaments and tissues are injured. Whiplash injuries are often the result of rear-end motor vehicle accidents.

Strains, also called pulled muscles, result from a tearing of a muscle and/or its tendon from excessive use or stretching. Conditioning and warm-up before exercise minimises the risk of strains. If they occur, strains should be treated with rest, initially with ice to reduce inflammation, and later with warm compresses to encourage blood flow and healing. Severe strains may require many months to heal before safely resuming activity.

Strains and sprains should be treated with caution, as they can conceal the presence of a fracture.

Carpal tunnel syndrome

A painful condition of the hand known as carpal tunnel syndrome (CTS) is fairly common in the UK. About 3 in 100 men and 11 in 100 women develop this at some time in their lives, leading to discomfort and disability. It is an example of a larger class of problems known as repetitive strain injuries (RSIs). Many women report the symptoms during pregnancy, which is attributed to accumulation of fluid within the tissues. Risk factors for CTS include the performance of repetitive manual tasks such as

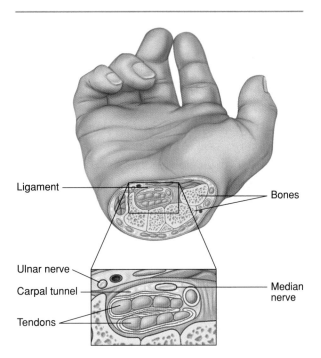

Figure 15.10 Cross-section of the wrist showing tendons and nerves involved in carpal tunnel syndrome.

knitting, driving, typing, computing and piano playing (Figure 15.10). It usually begins as numbness or tingling in the hand but progresses to pain that can radiate up the arm to the shoulder; the pain is most severe at night. Simple tasks requiring finger movements become difficult.

A clinician may diagnose CTS by requiring certain hand manoeuvres. The diagnosis is confirmed by an **electromyogram**. The test measures the velocity of sensory and motor nerve conduction. If electrical impulses are slowed as they travel through the carpal tunnel, compression of the nerve is indicated.

Conservative treatments begin with avoiding the repetitive action where possible, at least temporarily. Immobilising the hand and wrist with a lightweight, moulded plastic splint is often adequate for the inflammation to subside. Injection of a steroidal anti-inflammatory drug into the carpal tunnel is sometimes effective. For some individuals, non-steroidal anti-inflammatory drugs such as aspirin and ibuprofen can reduce symptoms. Surgery may be required to divide the transverse ligament, which is compressing the median nerve. The procedure generally provides permanent relief without affecting hand movement or strength.

DISEASES OF THE MUSCLES

Skeletal muscle moves the body and provides much of the body's heat. Muscle function is intimately associated with nervous system function. Muscles cannot function unless they are stimulated by nerves. In Chapter 13, diseases in which the nerves fail to innervate muscles were discussed. Muscles themselves can also be diseased and lose their ability to contract. Another cause of muscle failure is the improper transmission of the impulse for contraction at the myoneural junction, the site at which a nerve ending sends its signal to a muscle cell.

Muscular dystrophy

The term **muscular dystrophy (MD)** includes several forms of hereditary diseases. The various forms are transmitted differently and affect different muscles, but all forms result in muscle degeneration, which can totally disable the individual. The most common and serious type is Duchenne's, which is caused by a sex-linked gene and affects approximately 1 in every 3500 male births.

Muscular dystrophy can appear at any age, but generally signs appear in the third to fifth year. In Duchenne's muscular dystrophy, a cytoskeletal protein called **dystrophin** is missing. As a result of this defect, muscle fibres die and are replaced by fat and connective tissue. Because neither of these tissues has the ability to contract, skeletal muscles weaken. A severe form can progress rapidly and affect the muscle of the heart, causing death; other forms progress slowly. In the most severe forms of muscular dystrophy, the calf muscles enlarge as a result of fat deposition. The shoulder muscles are weak, which causes the arms to hang limply. A child with this form of muscular dystrophy is very weak and thin and does not usually live to adulthood.

The diagnosis is based on electromyography, which shows weak muscle contractions. Biopsy of muscle shows abnormal muscle fibres: variation in sizes, fat deposits and absence of dystrophin. Immunological and molecular biology techniques can diagnose the disease prenatally as well as at birth.

No cure exists. Treatment includes physical and occupational therapy, exercise and use of orthopaedic appliances.

Myasthenia gravis

Myasthenia gravis is a disorder of the myoneural junction in which the nerves fail to transmit an impulse for contraction to the muscles. Lack of stimulation and use leads to muscle atrophy and muscle weakness. The cause is unknown, but myasthenia gravis may be an autoimmune disease. In some people, particularly those affected at a younger age, the disease can be inherited. Antibodies attach near the myoneural junction and interfere with the actions of acetylcholine or its receptors. Myasthenia gravis is rare, affecting about 1 per 10 000 and occurring more frequently among women than men. No risk factors are known.

 Prevention PLUS!

Carpal tunnel syndrome: an occupational hazard

Carpal tunnel syndrome, caused by damage to the median nerve, is a common problem of data processors, computer users, typists, beauticians and dentists, who often maintain a flexed wrist position. Frequent rest and splinting may help prevent the complications of carpal tunnel syndrome. If surgery is required to relieve pressure on the nerve, a new technique involves a tiny video camera, so the surgeon need only make two tiny incisions in the wrist and palm, each requiring only one stitch. Recovery is therefore faster than with the traditional longer incision, and the patient quickly resumes normal work and activities.

The principal symptoms of this disease are fatigue and the inability to use the muscles. The disease affects the voluntary muscles of the body, including the facial muscles. This renders the person's face expressionless; eyelid control is lost, and even chewing and talking become difficult. The greatest danger in this disease is respiratory failure because the muscles required for ventilation are unable to contract.

Treatment includes drugs that increase acetylcholine levels at the myoneural junction. The thymus gland, which is involved in the immune response, is often enlarged in patients with myasthenia gravis. Removal of this gland often brings about a remission but not a cure.

Tumours of muscle

Muscle tumours are rare, but when they occur, they are usually highly malignant. A malignant tumour of skeletal muscle is a **rhabdomyosarcoma**. The tumour requires surgical removal and the prognosis is poor. The rhabdomyosarcoma metastasises early and is usually an advanced malignancy when it is diagnosed. Muscle malignancy is rare because muscle cells do not continually divide like blood or skin cells.

AGE-RELATED DISEASES

Bones

Osteoblast activity declines with age. Because these cells build bone tissue in response to stress, for remodelling or repair, this results in age-related thinning of bones. In addition, aging bone has more minerals and less protein, making the tissue more brittle. Overall, the total amount of bone declines steadily with age. At menopause, bone loss accelerates, making women more susceptible to osteoporosis and its effects. More than 80% of those with osteoporosis are women, and a majority of women over age 60 have osteoporosis.

Joints

Joint mobility decreases with age because cartilage in movable joints becomes stiffer, ligaments lose flexibility and elasticity, and synovial membranes become fibrous and stiff and produce less synovial fluid. These changes begin at age 20 and become significant by age 30, especially if the joints and muscles are not regularly exercised and stretched. The incidence of arthritis increases with age: while fewer than 20% of young adults have arthritis, 60% of adults over age 60 have some form of arthritis. Most of these cases are degenerative joint disease.

Muscles

Muscles become less sensitive to stimulation with age, meaning that they take longer to contract when stimulated. Recovery following contraction becomes slow, diminishing the ability to sustain repeated contractions and reducing endurance. With age, the number of muscle fibres decreases, and they become shorter and thinner, reducing muscle strength and range of motion. Exercise reduces the rate of these changes and helps maintain muscle mass, strength and flexibility.

> **Resources**
>
> NHS choices: *http://www.nhs.uk/conditions/*
>
> Myasthenia gravis association:
> *http://www.mgauk.org/*
>
> Muscular dystrophy campaign:
> *http://www.musculardystrophy.org/*
>
> Arthritis research campaign (ARC):
> *http://www.arc.org.uk/*

DISEASES AT A GLANCE Musculoskeletal system

DISEASE	AETIOLOGY	SIGNS AND SYMPTOMS	DIAGNOSIS	TREATMENT	PREVENTION	LIFESPAN
Osteomyelitis	Infection by staphylococci	Pain, redness, heat, chills, fever, tachycardia, nausea, weight loss	Bone scan, CT scan, MRI, WBC count	Antibiotics, surgery	Antibiotics for compound fractures or other infected wounds	Any age
Rickets	Vitamin D deficiency in childhood	Deformation of bones, knock-knee, bow-leg, curved spine, nodular swellings at rib ends and joints, enlarged and square head, flaccid muscles	Physical examination, X-ray	Vitamin D-fortified milk, sunlight, cod liver oil	Vitamin D-fortified milk, sunlight, cod liver oil	Children
Osteomalacia	Vitamin D deficiency in adults	Muscular weakness, weight loss, pain in bones, deformation of bones, easily fractured bones	Physical examination, X-ray	Vitamin D-fortified milk, sunshine, cod liver oil, calcium and phosphorus supplements	Vitamin D-fortified milk, sunshine, cod liver oil, calcium and phosphorus supplements	Adults
Osteoporosis	Calcium deficiency, decreased bone density	Decreased height from vertebral compression fractures, curvature of spine, easily fractured bones	X-ray and bone scan	Pain relief, fracture treatment, some medical treatment (oestrogens, calcitonin, bisphosphonates)	Calcium supplements, weightbearing exercises	Postmenopausal women
Paget's disease	Idiopathic, genetic	Enlarged skull, nerve compression curvatures in spine, and deformed legs	Physical examination	Surgical, limited	None	Older men
Bone tumours	Idiopathic; commonly metastatic	Painless lump in bone tissue, fracture without trauma	X-ray, biopsy	Surgery	None	Children and adolescents
Rheumatoid arthritis	Autoimmunity	Pain and stiffness in joints, swollen, red, warm joints, bilateral involvement, exacerbation and remission, rheumatoid nodules, crippling deformities	Physical examination, presence of rheumatoid factor in blood	Mild exercise, anti-inflammatories, steroids	None	Adults
Degenerative joint disease	Idiopathic; may follow joint injury or chronic irritation	Aches, pain, stiffness in joints, limited range of motion, muscle weakness around affected joint, enlarged joints, bone spurs; may involve only one joint	X-ray, history	Pain relief, mild exercise and rest, heat applications, steroids, surgery	None	Adults
Gout	Inherited defect in uric acid metabolism leads to high levels of urate and uric acid deposition in joints	Severe pain, heat, swelling, redness in affected joint; acute onset	Uric acid level in blood, X-ray	Analgesics, hot and cold compresses, colchicine, probenecid	Avoid triggers, which may be dietary	Men over age 40

DISEASES AT A GLANCE Musculoskeletal system (continued)

DISEASE	AETIOLOGY	SIGNS AND SYMPTOMS	DIAGNOSIS	TREATMENT	PREVENTION	LIFESPAN
Septic arthritis	Bacterial infection of joint	Pain, redness, swelling, bone and joint destruction	History, blood and synovial cultures	Antibiotics	Treat infected wounds or other infections with antibiotics to prevent sepsis	Any age
Bursitis	Overuse of joint	Pain at joint, especially during use	Physical examination and history	Moist heat, analgesics, steroids, rest	Reduce or avoid triggering activities	Adults
Carpal tunnel syndrome	Repetitive use of wrist	Numbness and tingling of hand, pain radiating to shoulder, limited finger movement, severe at night	Physical examination, electromyography	Splinting hand and wrist, surgery	Reduce or avoid triggering activities	Adults and adolescents
Muscular dystrophy	Defect in X-linked gene for muscle protein dystrophin	Weakened muscles, muscles may enlarge as fat is deposited; muscles degenerate	Physical examination, serum enzymes, muscle biopsy	Physical therapy, orthopaedic procedures	None; screening helps detect early onset	Onset in young adults
Myasthenia gravis	Autoimmunity interferes with nerve transmission to muscles	Fatigue, muscle paralysis	Antibody level, response to anticholinesterase drugs, electromyography	Thymectomy, anticholinesterase drugs, steroids, immune suppression	None	Onset in young adult women

INTERACTIVE EXERCISES

Cases for critical thinking

1. A 68-year-old woman visits her GP and reports that her back hurts. Physical examination finds kyphosis and that she has lost height since her last visit a few years ago. What is a likely diagnosis for this case? Name two treatment possibilities that the GP might suggest. Name something that might have helped prevent this condition, especially if it had been initiated and applied at an earlier age.

2. A 55-year-old carpenter reports persistent swelling and pain in the knuckles of his right hand. What information do you need to determine the type of joint disease he has?

3. A 20-year-old woman has worsening pain in her leg below the knee. She says she feels 'a little weak and out of sorts' and has stopped her jogging routine. How can you determine whether she has a type of arthritis, a bone infection, a fracture or a joint sprain?

Multiple choice

1. Bones are soft in rickets owing to a
   _____ deficiency.
   a. vitamin A   b. vitamin C
   c. vitamin D   d. vitamin K

2. Osteomalacia affects which of the following?
   a. the joints of young children
   b. the joints of adults
   c. the bones of children
   d. the bones of adults

3. Carpal tunnel syndrome is caused by damage to
   the _____
   a. wrist
   b. fingers
   c. median nerve
   d. forearm muscles

4. Biopsy in addition to electromyography is a
   diagnostic test for _____
   a. gout
   b. sprain
   c. carpal tunnel syndrome
   d. Duchenne's muscular dystrophy

5. _____ is the most common form
   of arthritis.
   a. Rheumatoid arthritis
   b. Degenerative joint disease
   c. Septic arthritis
   d. Gout

6. Ankylosis and immobility result in severe
   _____
   a. rheumatoid arthritis
   b. degenerative joint disease
   c. septic arthritis
   d. gout

7. Colchicine and corticosteroids are used to treat
   acute cases of _____
   a. rheumatoid arthritis
   b. degenerative joint disease
   c. septic arthritis
   d. gout

8. Which of these is *not* caused by calcium
   deficiency?
   a. osteoporosis
   b. osteomalacia
   c. osteogenic sarcoma
   d. rickets

9. Which of these is a type of autoimmune disorder?
   a. rhabdomyosarcoma
   b. Duchenne's muscular dystrophy
   c. myasthenia gravis
   d. osteitis fibrosa cystica

10. Streptococci and staphylococci are associated
    with _____
    a. Pott's disease   b. tuberculosis
    c. osteomyelitis   d. osteoporosis

True or false

_____ 1. Osteomyelitis affects principally children and adolescents.

_____ 2. Women with large bone mass are most prone to osteoporosis.

_____ 3. An osteoma is a malignant bone tumour.

_____ 4. Rheumatoid arthritis is the most crippling form of arthritis.

_____ 5. Osteomyelitis is a local and systemic infection.

_____ 6. Degenerative joint disease is the most common form of arthritis.

_____ 7. Muscular dystrophy is a hereditary disease.

_____ 8. Myasthenia gravis is an infectious disease of the muscles.

_____ 9. Rhabdomyosarcoma is a malignant bone tumour.

_____ 10. There is no cure for degenerative joint disease.

Fill-ins

1. A special form of tuberculosis that affects the vertebral column of children is called _____.

2. A disease of infancy and early childhood in which the bones do not properly ossify, or harden, is called
_____.

3. The word _____ means increased porosity of the bone, which makes the bone abnormally fragile.

4. A very painful condition caused by deposits of uric acid crystals in the joints is called _____.

5. The principle minerals in bone are _____ and _____.

6. Bone is deposited by cells called _____.

7. The _____ membrane becomes inflamed in rheumatoid arthritis.

8. Antibodies against acetylcholine receptors are the cause of _____.

9. Colchicine is an effective treatment for _____.

10. Vitamin D is required for dietary absorption of _____.

Labelling exercise

Use the lines below to label the following images.

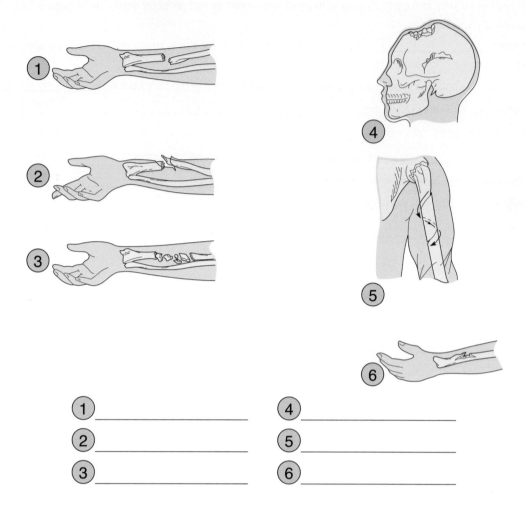

1	_____	4	_____
2	_____	5	_____
3	_____	6	_____

16 DISEASES OF THE INTEGUMENTARY SYSTEM

Macroconidia of the dermatophytic fungus *Epidermophyton floccosum.*
(Courtesy of the CDC/Dr Libero Ajello, 1972)

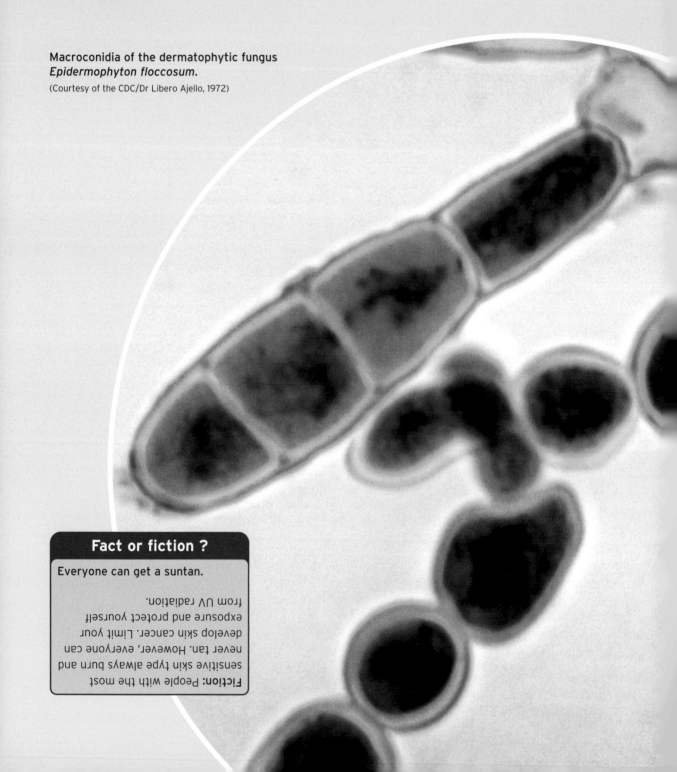

Fact or fiction ?

Everyone can get a suntan.

Fiction: People with the most sensitive skin type always burn and never tan. However, everyone can develop skin cancer. Limit your exposure and protect yourself from UV radiation.

Learning objectives

After studying this chapter, you should be able to:

✦ Describe the normal structure and function of skin

✦ List the aetiology, signs and symptoms, diagnostic tests and treatments for infectious diseases of the skin

✦ Explain hypersensitivity, or immune disorders of the skin

✦ Identify benign tumours of the skin

✦ Compare and contrast the different types of non-melanoma skin cancer

✦ Describe sebaceous gland disorders

✦ Compare and contrast pigment disorders

✦ Define trauma to the skin

✦ List the aetiology, signs and symptoms, diagnostic tests and treatments for age-related diseases of the skin

Disease chronicle

Trench foot

Soldiers in World War 1 suffered from trench foot, a fungal infection that thrived in the skin and tissues of feet damaged by chronic exposure to cold, wet, unsanitary conditions. Although healthy skin can resist fungal infections, soldiers who stood for hours in waterlogged trenches without removing wet socks or boots, found their feet went numb. Reduced circulation caused the skin to turn blue or red and, more importantly, made it difficult to fight infections. Left untreated, gangrene developed and amputation was necessary. British soldiers were ordered to have three pairs of socks with them and to dry their feet and change their socks at least twice per day. Soldiers were also told to cover their dry feet with grease made from whale oil. It is estimated that a battalion at the front used 10 gallons of whale oil every day.

FUNCTIONS OF THE SKIN

Skin is the largest organ in the human body, with a surface area of approximately 2 square metres. The integumentary system includes the skin, hair, nails, and sweat and **sebaceous glands**. The skin is much more than an external body covering; it protects deeper tissue from mechanical, chemical, thermal, ultraviolet and bacterial damage. The skin insulates and cushions the deeper body organs, regulates temperature, senses pain, protects against dehydration, aids in the excretion of urea and uric acid and synthesises vitamin D.

Colour changes on the skin give an indication of malfunction within the body. **Cyanosis**, a bluish colouration of the skin, signals a lack of oxygen and indicates a cardiovascular or pulmonary problem. Jaundice indicates liver disease, bile obstruction or haemolysis of red blood cells, in which case an accumulation of the bilirubin in the blood produces a yellowish discolouration of the skin. An abnormal redness accompanies polycythaemia (see Chapter 7), carbon monoxide poisoning and fever. **Pallor**, or whitening of the skin, may indicate anaemia.

Skin colour, texture and folds identify people as individuals, and anything that disrupts the function or appearance of the skin can have important consequences for physical and mental health.

STRUCTURE OF THE SKIN

Each layer of the skin performs specific tasks. The outermost layer of the skin is the **epidermis** and consists of stratified or layered squamous epithelium. The top portion of the epidermis, the stratum corneum, contains **keratin**, a tough, fibrous protein produced by cells called **keratinocytes**. Keratin protects the skin from harmful substances and prevents water loss. At the bottom of the epidermis are the **melanocytes**, or the cells that produce **melanin**, the dark pigment of the skin that protects the body from the harmful rays of the sun.

The **dermis** lies below the epidermis and is composed of connective tissue that supports blood and lymph vessels, elastic fibres, nerves, hair follicles, sweat glands and sebaceous or oil glands. The subcutaneous tissue lies under the dermis and connects the skin to underlying structures. Adipose tissue or fat cells in the subcutaneous tissue help insulate the body from heat and cold. Figure 16.1 shows the structure of the skin.

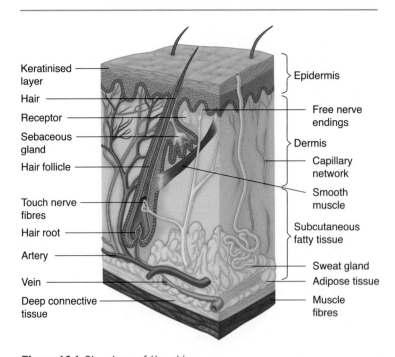

Figure 16.1 Structure of the skin.

DIAGNOSTIC PROCEDURES FOR SKIN DISEASES

Skin diseases are usually identified by visual examination whereas blood and urine tests may be used to rule out underlying diseases. Diagnosis may include microscopic examination of skin scrapings, and cultures, DNA testing or blood tests for antibodies may be used to identify the causative organism in skin diseases.

In hypersensitivity skin disorders, a complete medical history, including prior outbreaks and their locations, may help to identify the allergen. Sensitivity testing or blood tests for antibodies may be used to identify the allergen.

Punch, incisional or total excisional biopsies are used to diagnose benign tumours and non-melanoma skin cancer.

SKIN LESIONS

Skin diseases are identified and classified according to characteristic lesions. **Pruritus** (itching), oedema (swelling), **erythema** (redness) and inflammation usually accompany lesions and are helpful in making a diagnosis. A **macule**, or freckle, is a discoloured spot of the skin whereas a **wheal**, or hive, is a localised elevation in the skin that is often accompanied by pruritus. A **papule**, or pimple, is a solid, elevated area on the skin, while a **nodule** is a larger papule. A **vesicle**, or blister, is a small, fluid-filled sac, and a **bulla** is a larger vesicle. A **pustule** is a small, elevated lesion filled with pus, and an **ulcer**, or erosion, is eating away of the tissue. Figure 16.2 shows various skin lesions.

EPIDERMOID AND PILAR CYSTS

A cyst is a sac that is filled with a fluid or semifluid material. The two most common types occurring underneath the skin surface are epidermoid and pilar cysts. These cysts were previously called sebaceous cysts as they were thought to originate from the sebaceous glands in the skin. Both epidermoid and pilar cysts are smooth, round lumps just beneath the skin surface and their semifluid contents include keratin.

Epidermoid cysts occur in an estimated 1–5% of the population and the sac forms from cells in the epidermis. Epidermoid cysts can affect anyone, but risk factors include age (thirties or forties), gender (men are twice as likely to have epidermoid cysts), a history of acne and traumatic or crushing injury to the skin. They can appear anywhere on the skin, but they develop most commonly on the face, neck, chest and upper back. Pilar cysts occur in an estimated 5–10% of the population and usually occur in clusters on the scalp. The sac forms from cells in the bottom of hair follicles. Pilar cysts can affect anyone but are most common among middle-aged women.

Both epidermoid and pilar cysts do not usually cause any signs or symptoms; however, they may occasionally become infected, leak or form in an uncomfortable place such as in the genital skin folds or beside a nail. Epidermoid and pilar cysts form when there is abnormal cell proliferation which may result from an injury to the skin or damage to a hair follicle or sebaceous gland. The cells that multiply form a sac and produce the keratin that they would normally make on the top layer of the skin, thereby trapping the keratin in the sac. A tendency to form pilar cysts runs in some families but epidermoid cysts are not hereditary, and most occur in healthy people without any apparent reason.

Epidermoid and pilar cysts are diagnosed by visual examination and, if required, they can be removed by excision. Neither epidermoid nor pilar cysts are preventable.

DRUG ERUPTIONS

Adverse drug reactions manifest more often on the skin than in any other organ system and about 2–5% of patients suffer from cutaneous drug eruptions. Although any medication can cause eruptions, the most common types of medications that cause a drug eruption include antibiotics (penicillins), anti-inflammatory medicines (ibuprofen, naproxen or indomethacin), painkillers (codeine or morphine),

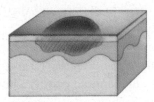

A macule is a discoloured spot on the skin; freckle

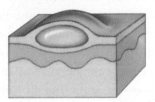

A wheal is a localised, evanescent elevation of the skin that is often accompanied by itching; urticaria

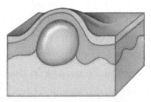

A papule is a solid, circumscribed, elevated area on the skin; pimple

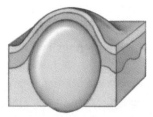

A nodule is a larger papule; acne vulgaris

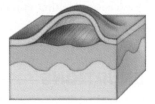

A vesicle is a small fluid-filled sac; blister. A bulla is a large vesicle

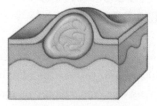

A pustule is a small, elevated, circumscribed lesion of the skin that is filled with pus; varicella (chickenpox)

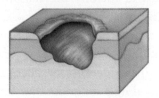

An erosion or ulcer is an eating or gnawing away of tissue; decubitus ulcer

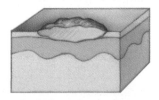

A crust is a dry, serous or seropurulent, brown, yellow, red or green exudation that is seen in secondary lesions; eczema

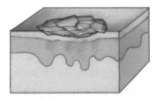

A scale is a thin, dry flake of cornified epithelial cells; psoriasis

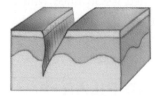

A fissure is a crack-like sore or slit that extends through the epidermis into the dermis; athlete's foot

Figure 16.2 Skin lesions.

anticonvulsants (phenytoin or carbamazepine), chemotherapy drugs, psychotropic medications, diuretics and iodine (especially that found in radiographic contrast dye). Drug eruptions can appear as various types of skin rashes, including pink-to-red papules, wheals, red patches and pustules, or as sensitivity to sunlight. Drug rashes may involve the entire skin surface, or they may be limited to one or a few body parts. Pruritus is common in many drug eruptions. Skin reactions may be serious enough to cause anaphylaxis, shock or death. Therefore a thorough medical history, including current medications, can help diagnose the adverse drug reaction and determine the medication that must be changed.

INFECTIOUS SKIN DISEASES

Bacteria, viruses, fungi and parasites may cause infections of the skin. Normal microbes that reside on the skin, e.g. *Staphylococcus epidermidis*, cause the most common skin infections. Infections from less common microbes may develop in high-risk (immunocompromised or diabetic) individuals and those who reside in nursing homes and hospitals. Most skin infections are not serious unless systemic involvement occurs.

Bacterial skin infections

Impetigo Impetigo is an acute, contagious skin infection usually caused by *Staphylococcus aureus* or *Streptococcus pyogenes* and it affects mainly infants and children. Impetigo affects approximately 1% of children and accounts for approximately one-tenth of all cutaneous problems in paediatric clinics. Two clinical types of impetigo exist: non-bullous and bullous impetigo. The non-bullous type is more common and typically occurs on the face and extremities, initially with vesicles or pustules on reddened skin that eventually rupture to leave the characteristic honey-coloured crust. Bullous impetigo, almost exclusively caused by *S. aureus*, exhibits vesicles with clear, yellow fluid that rupture and leave a golden–yellow crust. Fever and enlarged

lymph nodes may accompany impetigo. Risk factors for contracting impetigo include direct contact with an infected person, contact with a contaminated fomite (an inanimate object that can transmit infectious agents), warm and humid weather, and participation in sports that involve skin to skin contact. Diagnosis is made by visual examination and bacterial culture. The lesions should be washed with soap and water, dried and exposed to air. Impetigo is treated with antibiotics and may be prevented by daily bathing, frequent hand washing and prompt attention to minor wounds.

Erysipelas and cellulitis Erysipelas is a superficial infection of the skin whereas **cellulitis** is a deeper infection that extends to the subcutaneous tissue. *S. aureus* and *S. pyogenes* are the most common pathogens responsible for erysipelas and cellulitis, and these gain acess through a break in the skin. Risk factors for both conditions include circulatory problems, diabetes and trauma to the skin. Mild erysipelas is common, but because it is often self-limited, patients rarely present to the doctor. Cellulitis is a common infection, with an incidence of approximately 2–3 cases per 100 people per year.

Erysipelas and cellulitis infections usually appear on the face or the legs, which generally become swollen, bright red, hot and tender (Figure 16.3). Small vesicles may be present, and fever, chills and swelling of lymph nodes may occur. Diagnosis may include visual examination and bacterial culture; in severe infection antibiotic therapy is required. Prevention of erysipelas and cellulitis includes prompt attention to wounds, moisturisation of the skin and careful trimming of nails.

Folliculitis, furuncles and carbuncles Folliculitis is a superficial infection of the hair follicles characterised by erythema and follicular-based papules and pustules. **Furuncles**, or boils, are a deeper infection of the hair follicle, whereas **carbuncles** are clusters of furuncles. Folliculitis, furuncles and carbuncles are caused by staphylococcus infection.

Folliculitis is common, but because it is often self-limited, patients rarely visit the doctor. This condition commonly occurs in young men and affects

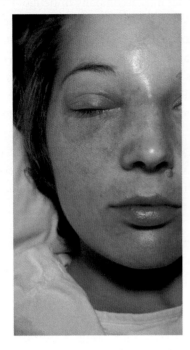

Figure 16.3 Cellulitis indicated by redness and swelling around the eye.

(Courtesy of the CDC/Dr Thomas F. Sellers/Emory University, 1963)

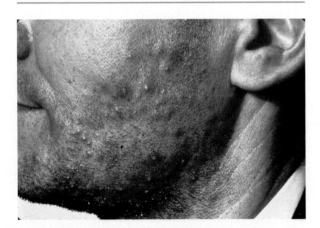

Figure 16.4 The lesions of folliculitis are pustules surrounded by areas of erythema.

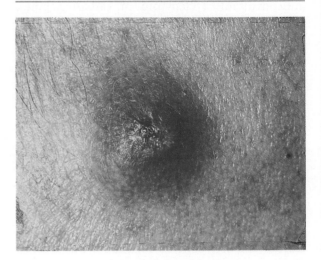

Figure 16.5 A furuncle or boil.

Folliculitis is effectively treated with daily cleansing with antiseptic soap, but in severe cases oral antibiotic therapy may be required. This condition may be prevented by keeping skin clean, dry and free from abrasions or irritation.

Furuncles appear in hair follicles located on the face, neck, breasts or buttocks. The core of the furuncle becomes necrotic and liquefies, forming pus (Figure 16.5). Carbuncles develop and heal more slowly than furuncles; they appear mostly in men and are commonly located on the back of the neck. Risk factors for furuncles and carbuncles include minor trauma to the skin, pre-existing skin disease, poor hygiene and impaired immunity. Diagnosis is based on visual examination and bacterial culture. Furuncles and carbuncles may be treated with application of moist heat, antiseptic skin cleansing, antibiotics and incision and drainage. Keeping skin clean, dry and free from abrasions or irritation may help prevent furuncles and carbuncles.

Viral skin infections

Herpes Herpes is a large family of viruses that cause clusters of fluid-filled vesicles on the skin. Herpes simplex type 1 (HSV-1) causes cold sores or fever blisters (Figure 16.6). Eighty-five per cent of the population has antibody evidence of HSV-1 infection.

thighs, buttocks, head and scalp (Figure 16.4). Risk factors for folliculitis include obesity, trauma to the skin, impaired immunity, long-term antibiotic therapy for acne, living in a warm and humid climate and topical corticosteroid therapy. Diagnosis is based on visual examination and bacterial culture.

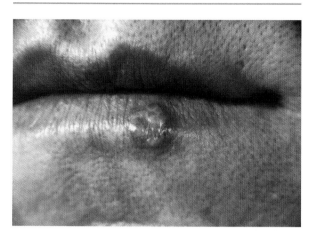

Figure 16.6 Cold sores or fever blisters.
(Courtesy of the CDC/Dr Herrman, 1964)

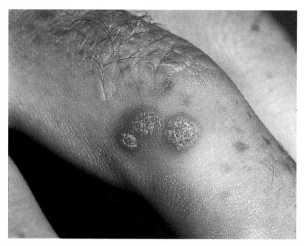

Figure 16.7 Common warts.

The vesicles generally form near the mouth or lips, as in Figure 16.6. Some patients have a burning or tingling sensation that precedes the appearance of vesicles by a few hours or a day or two. The virus goes latent, but a cold, flu, fever, sun exposure, stress, trauma to the skin and changes in the immune system can stimulate a recurrence. HSV-1 is spread from person to person by kissing, close contact with herpetic lesions, or even contact with apparently normal skin that is shedding the virus. Diagnosis may include visual observation of the herpetic vesicles, viral culture and testing for HSV-1 DNA. The outbreaks are usually self-limiting, but antiviral drugs can be used for treatment. Cold sores can be prevented by avoiding contact with HSV-1 and recurrence triggers (e.g. sunlight, stress, fatigue, weakened immune system) and frequent hand washing.

Herpes simplex type 2 causes genital herpes (see Chapter 11 for more information). Herpes varicella zoster causes chickenpox (see Chapter 3 for more information). If an adult develops limited immunity to herpes varicella zoster, the virus may lie dormant for years after recovery from chickenpox. The virus may flare up during periods of stress, disease, trauma or immunosuppression, causing painful vesicles called shingles (see Chapter 13).

Warts Warts, or **verruca vulgaris**, are caused by the human papillomavirus (HPV). HPV infection of keratinocytes causes them to proliferate, forming a benign neoplasm with a rough, keratinised surface. Warts are spread by direct contact with HPV. There are few reliable, population-based data on the incidence and prevalence of non-genital warts. Prevalence probably varies widely among different age groups, populations and periods of time. Prevalence is highest among children and young adults. Warts are most common at sites of trauma, such as the hands and feet, and probably result from inoculation of virus into minimally damaged areas of epithelium. There are several types of warts, including common, plantar, flat, filiform and periungual.

Common warts grow most often on the hands, but they may occur anywhere on the body. Common warts are rough, shaped like a dome, and grey–brown in colour (Figure 16.7). Plantar warts grow inward on the soles of the feet. One observational study of 146 adolescents found that the prevalence of warts on the feet was 27% in those who used a communal shower room and 1.3% in those who used only locker rooms without showers. Plantar warts look like hard, thick patches of skin with dark specks. Pressure on the soles of the feet makes them very painful, and they are often difficult to remove permanently. Flat warts usually grow on the face, arms or legs. They are small (usually smaller than the eraser on the end of a pencil), have flat tops and can be pink, light brown or light yellow. Filiform warts usually grow around the mouth, nose or beard area. They are the same colour as the skin and have growths that look like threads sticking out of them. Periungual warts grow under and around the toenails and fingernails and can affect nail growth. They look like rough bumps with an uneven surface and border.

Warts are diagnosed by visual examination. One study of 1000 children found that two-thirds of warts resolved without treatment within a 2-year period. Warts can be removed by medications, electrocautery, cryosurgery and laser surgery. To prevent HPV infections, avoid touching warts, walking barefoot on warm moist surfaces and incurring trauma to the skin.

Fungal skin infections

Fungi, or **dermatophytes**, that infect the skin tend to live on the dead, top layer of the skin. Superficial fungal infections are among the most common skin diseases, affecting millions of people throughout the world. The estimated lifetime risk of acquiring a dermatophyte infection is between 10% and 20%. Fungal infection may be transmitted through direct contact with infected persons, animals, soil or fomites. Fungi usually reside on moist areas of the body where skin surfaces touch; for example, folds of the breast, groin and toes. Hence obese people, with excessive skin folds, are more susceptible to fungal infections.

Tinea Tinea, or ringworm, is classified by its location on the body (Table 16.1). Tinea corporis, or body ringworm, affects smooth areas of skin on the the arms, legs and body. It is characterised by a pink to reddish rash that sometimes forms round patches with clear areas in the centre (Figure 16.8).

Tinea pedis, or athlete's foot, is the most common type of tinea worldwide. It is characterised by the appearance of scales and fissures on the soles of the feet and between the toes (Figure 16.9). Lesions resulting from this condition usually emit a foul odour. Tinea pedis is highly contagious and is spread by direct contact with contaminated surfaces.

Table 16.1 Ringworm or tinea classification and symptoms.

Tinea	Symptoms
Tinea corporis	Body ringworm – pink to reddish rash sometimes forms round patches with clear areas in the centre
Tinea pedia	Athlete's foot – scales and fissures occur on the soles of the feet and between toes; a foul odour usually accompanies lesions
Tinea cruris	Jock itch – red, ring-like areas with blisters
Tinea capitis	Scalp ringworm – mild, scaly rash or patch of hair loss without a rash
Tinea unguium	Nail fungus – white patches on nails, eventually turn the nail brown; nail thickens and cracks and may be destroyed
Tinea barbae	Barber's itch – deep, inflammatory pustules and crusting around hairs

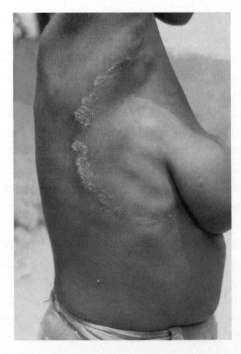

Figure 16.8 Tinea corporis, or body ringworm.
(Courtesy of the CDC/Lucille K. Georg, 1964)

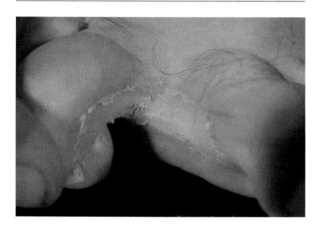

Figure 16.9 Tinea pedia, or athlete's foot.
(Courtesy of the CDC/Dr Lucille K. Georg, 1964)

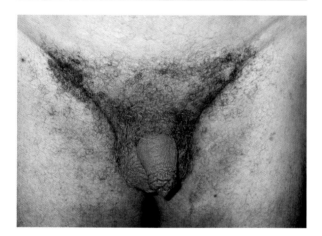

Figure 16.10 Tinea cruris, or jock itch.
(Science Photo Library Ltd/Dr P. Marazzi)

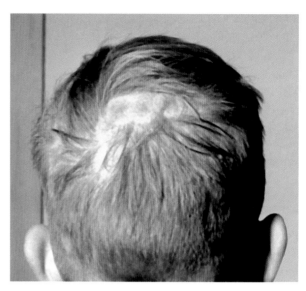

Figure 16.11 Tinea capitis, or scalp ringworm.
(Courtesy of the CDC, 1959)

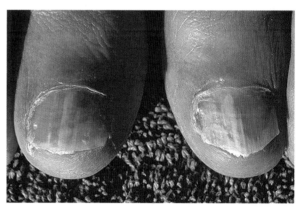

Figure 16.12 Tinea unguium, or nail fungus.
(Courtesy of the CDC/Dr Edwin P. Ewing, Jr, 1997)

Tinea cruris, or jock itch, generally affects the groin and upper and inner thighs. The fungi, which develops more frequently during warm weather, cause red, ring-like areas with vesicles (Figure 16.10). Tinea capitis (Figure 16.11), or scalp ringworm, is highly contagious and most commonly occurs in children. This fungus may produce a mild, scaly rash or a patch of hair loss without a rash.

Tinea unguium, or nail fungus, typically affects toenails and rarely affects fingernails. This fungus is difficult to treat because it resides under the nail. The infection begins at the nail tips, causing white patches and eventually turning the nail brown. The nail thickens and cracks. If left untreated, the fungus may destroy the entire nail and tends to spread to other nails (Figure 16.12).

Tinea barbae causes barber's itch and affects bearded areas of the face and neck. This fungus may produce deep, inflammatory pustules and crusting around hairs (Figure 16.13).

Diagnosis of tinea may include visual examination, scraping the affected area of skin and examining

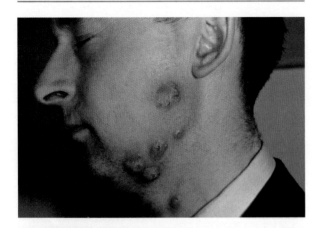

Figure 16.13 Tinea barbae, or barber's itch.
(Courtesy of the CDC, 1975)

the cells under a microscope. Treatment includes keeping the affected area clean and dry and using antifungal medications.

Prevention of tinea includes keeping the skin clean, cool and dry and wearing sandals or shoes at gyms, locker rooms and pools.

Seborrhoeic dermatitis Seborrhoeic dermatitis, or chronic dandruff, is a chronic inflammatory skin disorder generally affecting areas of the head and trunk where sebaceous glands are prominent. The prevalence rate of seborrhoeic dermatitis is 3–5% worldwide. For infants, seborrhoeic dermatitis of the scalp is known as cradle cap. Common signs and symptoms of this condition include dry or greasy scaling of the scalp with variable pruritus. Severe disease may include yellow or red scaling papules. Infants develop thick, yellow-crusted scalp lesions.

The exact cause of seborrhoeic dermatitis is not known, although many factors have been implicated, for example *Pityrosporum ovale* yeast. Although *P. ovale* is a normal flora, the reason that some people develop seborrhoeic dermatitis and others do not remains unclear. It has been suggested that seborrhoeic dermatitis is an inflammatory response to this organism, but this remains to be proven. The fact that seborrhoeic dermatitis responds to antifungal medications suggests yeast involvement. People with neurological conditions frequently develop

seborrhoeic dermatitis, and therefore it has been postulated that it may be caused by increased pooling of sebum resulting from immobility. Increased sebum pooling facilitates growth of *P. ovale*, and consequently seborrhoeic dermatitis.

Seborrhoeic dermatitis may be diagnosed through visual examination and biopsy, which helps to confirm diagnosis as well as exclude other types of dermatitis. There is no known cure for seborrhoeic dermatitis, but its signs and symptoms may be controlled through proper hygiene, frequent cleansing with soap and removing oils from affected areas. Treatment may include medicated shampoo, antifungal medication and corticosteroids.

Candidiasis Candidiasis is the most common fungal infection and is responsible for a variety of diseases. Candidiasis is caused by the fungus *Candida albicans*. *Candida* species are normal flora, ubiquitous fungi found throughout the world and they colonise over 50% of healthy individuals. Usually, *Candida* is kept under control by the normal flora and by the body's immune defences. If the mix of normal flora is changed by antibiotics, the body moisture that surrounds normal flora can also have subtle changes in its acidity or chemistry. This can cause yeast to grow and to stick to surfaces, so that the yeast causes signs and symptoms. *Candida* infections can cause occasional symptoms in healthy people. If a person's immune system is weakened by illness (especially AIDS or diabetes), malnutrition or certain medications such as corticosteroids or anticancer drugs, *Candida* fungi can cause signs and symptoms more frequently. The disease can progress systematically in up to 14% of immunocompromised patients.

Vaginal *Candida* infections are common in pregnant women, diabetics or those who are immunocompromised. During a lifetime, 75% of all women are likely to have at least one vaginal *Candida* infection, and up to 45% have two or more. Women may be more susceptible to vaginal yeast infections after antibiotic therapy or from the use of birth control pills. Signs and symptoms include a white 'cottage cheese'-like discharge from the vagina, accompanied by burning sensation, pruritus and erythema (Figure 16.14). Diagnosis is usually made by visual

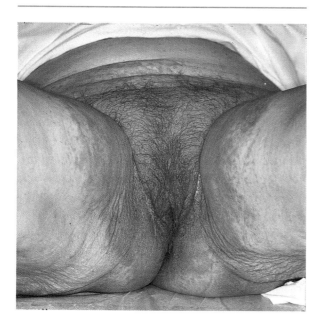

Figure 16.14 Vaginal candidiasis.

examination but may also include microscopic examination and culture. Vaginal candidiasis is effectively treated with vaginal antifungal creams or oral antifungal agents.

Creamy white patches on the tongue or side of the mouth often characterise a *Candida* infection of the mouth, or oral thrush. The patches are often painful and can easily be scraped off. Thrush is common in young healthy children, immunosuppressed adults and diabetics. Diagnosis is usually made by visual examination but may also include microscopic examination and culture. Long-term treatment of oral thrush with topical liquids or oral antifungals is generally required.

Candida can cause skin infections in areas of skin with little ventilation which are unusually moist. Common sites include the nappy area, the hands of people who routinely wear rubber gloves, the rim of skin at the base of the fingernail, especially for hands that are exposed to moisture, areas around the groin and in the crease of the buttocks, and the skin folds under large breasts. Cutaneous candidiasis causes patches of red, moist, weepy skin, sometimes with small pustules nearby. Diagnosis is usually made by visual examination but may also include microscopic examination and culture.

Cutaneous candidiasis can be effectively treated with a variety of antifungal powders and creams. The affected area must be kept clean and dry and protected from chafing.

Prevention of *Candida* infections includes keeping skin clean and dry, using antibiotics exactly as prescribed and following a healthy diet. Diabetics should keep their blood sugar under control.

Parasitic infestations

Pediculosis A **pediculosis**, or louse, infestation is extremely common. Hundreds of millions of cases of louse infestation are reported annually worldwide, with an apparent increase over the past few decades. Lice are ectoparasites that live on the body. The three types of lice that parasitise humans are *Pediculus humanus capitis* (head louse), *Pediculus humanus corporis* (body louse) and *Pthirus pubis* (pubic louse). Lice have claws on their legs that are adapted for feeding and clinging to hair or clothing; they spread from person to person by close physical contact, and overcrowding encourages the spread of lice. Lice are also spread through fomites (e.g. combs, clothes, hats, linens). Lice are blood-sucking insects and feed on humans approximately five times per day for about 35–45 minutes each time. Pruritus, the most common symptom of the infestation, results from the saliva of lice as they penetrate the skin and engorge on human blood. The scratching that follows can open the skin to other invading organisms. Multiple erythematous papules (bites) are usually present.

Pediculus humanus capitis, or head lice, are common among schoolchildren, and, although annoying, these parasites are not dangerous and do not carry epidemic disease. Adult head lice are difficult to see, but their nits (eggs) can be located on the hair shaft. The average lifespan of head lice is 30 days. The female head louse lays as many as 10 eggs per 24 hours, usually at night. The female louse cannot survive for more than 3 days off the human head.

Pthirus pubis, or pubic lice, infest pubic hair of both men and women and are generally spread by sexual contact. The lice do not spread other sexually transmitted infections. The pubic louse gets the nickname of 'crab' from its shorter, broader body and large front claws, which give it a crab-like appearance. Their large claws enable pubic lice to grasp the coarser pubic hairs in the groin, anal and armpit areas. The average life cycle of pubic lice is 35 days. The average female pubic louse lays only one to two eggs per day. Pubic lice cannot survive off the human host for more than 1 day.

Pediculus humanus corporis, or body lice, are most common among underprivileged, transient people. This type of infestation can be prevented with proper grooming and hygiene. Body lice can spread serious disease; the body louse is the vector of typhus, trench fever and relapsing fever. Unlike the head louse and the pubic louse, the body louse does not live on the human body, but prefers cooler temperatures. Body lice live in human clothing, crawling onto the body only to feed, predominantly at night. Body lice lay 10–15 eggs per day some distance from the human body on the fibres of clothing, mainly close to the seams. The adult female body louse, unlike the head louse, can survive as long as 10 days away from the human body without a blood meal.

A diagnosis of any type of pediculosis requires the finding of live specimens of lice and/or a viable nit. Treatment includes use of pediculicidal medication. Washing fomites in temperatures exceeding 131°F (55°C) for more than 5 minutes and machine drying kills nits and lice. Items that cannot be washed in hot water should be dry-cleaned or sealed in a plastic bag for 5 days. Prevention includes proper hygiene and safe sex practices.

Scabies Scabies, commonly called 'the itch', is a contagious skin disease usually associated with poor living conditions. Worldwide, an estimated 300 million cases occur annually. Scabies occurs frequently in homeless populations, and epidemics occur in healthcare facilities and other institutions. No recent published data are available on its incidence in the United States. Scabies is caused by the parasitic mite *Sarcoptes scabiei*. Mites are unable to fly or jump; therefore, transmission is predominantly through direct skin-to-skin contact. Indirect contact through fomites such as infested bedding or clothing is possible, although not usual. Scabies mites can survive up to 4 days off the human body. The female mite burrows into skin folds in the groin, under the breasts and between fingers and toes. As she burrows, she lays eggs in the tunnels, the eggs hatch and the cycle starts again. Intense pruritus is caused by hypersensitivity to the mite. Vesicles and pustules develop, and the tunnels in the skin appear as greyish lines. Scratching opens the lesions to secondary bacterial infection.

The combination of a history of pruritus (especially at night) and a classic rash is adequate for the diagnosis of scabies. Mites seen on microscopic examination of skin scrapings confirm the diagnosis. Treatment includes use of scabicidal medication. Pruritus may persist while treatment is being administered. Washing fomites in temperatures exceeding 131°F (55°C) for more than 5 minutes and machine drying kills scabies and their eggs. Items that cannot be washed in hot water should be dry-cleaned or sealed in a plastic bag for 5 days. Prevention includes proper hygiene.

HYPERSENSITIVITY, OR IMMUNE DISORDERS OF THE SKIN

The skin frequently manifests allergic or hypersensitivity reactions. This fact serves as a basis for the patch tests given to determine specific allergies. Some diseases of the skin develop in atopic people, persons with a genetic predisposition to allergies. Others occur in anyone who has been sensitised to an allergen, such as poison ivy. Emotional stress frequently triggers or exacerbates an allergy-caused skin disease.

Insect bites

Insect bites and stings can produce local inflammatory reactions that may vary in appearance. Acute reactions may appear as hives, whereas more chronic reactions may appear as papules or bullous.

See Chapter 2 for more information on allergy to insect bites.

Urticaria (hives)

Urticaria, or hives, results from a vascular reaction of the skin to an allergen. Urticaria is a common skin condition that affects 15–25% of the population at some point in their lives. The word *urticaria* is derived from a Latin word that means 'plants covered with stinging nettles'. The lesions are wheals, rounded elevations with red edges and pale centres. Urticaria is a rash of smooth, raised, pink or reddish wheals that comes on suddenly. Wheals usually appear first on the covered areas of the skin such as the trunk and upper parts of the arms and legs, and appear in batches. Each wheal may last from a few minutes up to 6 hours. The allergic response causes damage to mast cells, which then release histamine. Histamine causes blood vessels to dilate and become more permeable. Blood proteins and fluid ooze out of the capillaries into the tissues and result in oedema. This irritation to the tissues causes intense pruritus.

At least half of the time, the specific cause of urticaria cannot be determined. Some of the most common triggers are allergies to food, medications, cosmetics, soap and detergent; viral infections; insect stings and bites; transfusion of blood or blood products; emotional and physical stress; and physical agents such as sunlight, heat, cold, water and pressure. Risk factors include a previous case of urticaria, a previous allergic reaction and family members who have urticaria. Urticaria is diagnosed by visual examination and is generally treated with corticosteroids, antihistamines and calamine lotion applied topically to reduce pruritus. If the cause of the allergic reaction can be determined, the allergen should be avoided. Reducing emotional and physical stress may also help.

Dermatitis

Dermatitis is a broad term covering many different disorders that all result in a rash accompanied by pruritus and erythema.

Allergic contact dermatitis This is a localised inflammation of the skin caused by contact with an allergen. There are an estimated 13.6 cases of allergic contact dermatitis per 1000 people. Allergic contact dermatitis is a type I hypersensitivity triggered by allergen binding to IgE on mast cells, which produces local severe inflammation (see Chapter 2). Unlike most allergic reactions, the trigger is external rather than internal. Initial exposure does not cause a rash; however, it sensitises the skin so that it will react to the next exposure. Common plant allergens that cause allergic contact dermatitis include poison ivy, poison oak and poison sumac. Many other substances can cause allergic contact dermatitis, including hair products, the metal nickel which is found in jewellery and belt buckles, tanning agents in leather, latex rubber and citrus fruit, especially the peel. Fragrances in soaps, shampoos, lotions, perfumes and cosmetics can also cause a reaction (Figure 16.15). Even certain medications applied to the skin can cause the condition. Allergic contact dermatitis is usually confined to the area where the trigger actually touched the skin. A rash accompanied by erythema is the usual reaction, but sometimes the rash does not appear for 1–2 days after the exposure. Pruritus and burning may accompany the rash.

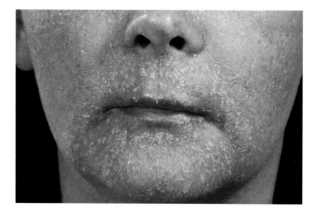

Figure 16.15 Allergic contact dermatitis, a type I hypersensitivity.
(Science Photo Library Ltd/St Bartholomews Hospital)

Allergic contact dermatitis is diagnosed by visual examination. Treatment may include corticosteroids and antihistamines. Allergic contact dermatitis can be prevented by avoiding contact with the allergen. If contact does occur, the material should be washed off immediately with soap and water. If circumstances risk ongoing exposure, gloves and protective clothing may be helpful. Barrier creams are also available that can block certain substances, such as poison ivy, from contacting the skin.

Atopic dermatitis Atopic dermatitis, also known as eczema, is one of the most common skin diseases, affecting 10–15% of children. In half of these children, atopic dermatitis will be gone by the teenage years. Doctors do not know what causes atopic dermatitis, but people who have it usually have many allergic disorders, particularly asthma, hay fever and food allergies. The relationship between atopic dermatitis and these disorders is not clear because atopic dermatitis is not an allergy to a particular substance. Many conditions can make atopic dermatitis worse, including emotional stress, changes in temperature or humidity, bacterial skin infections and contact with irritating clothing. In some infants, food allergies may provoke atopic dermatitis.

In babies, atopic dermatitis primarily affects the face, neck, ears and torso. It also appears on the tops of feet or the outside of the elbows. Atopic dermatitis in older children, teenagers and adults usually involves the skin inside the creases of the inward bend of the elbow, as well as the knee, ankle or wrist joints, the hands and upper eyelids. Atopic dermatitis appears as irritated, red, dry, crusted patches on the skin (Figure 16.16). If the skin becomes infected, it may develop a weeping look. Scratching causes more irritation and increases the risk of infection.

Atopic dermatitis may be diagnosed by visual examination. Atopic dermatitis is treated with corticosteroids. There is no way to prevent the condition.

Rosacea

Rosacea is an inflammatory skin disease that causes facial erythema. Rosacea affects 1 in 10 people in

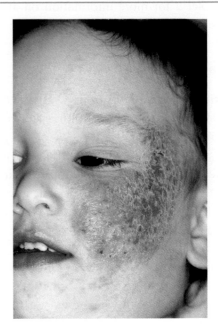

Figure 16.16 Atopic dermatitis.
(ISM/Phototake NYC)

the UK, an estimated 14 million people in the United States and over 45 million worldwide. Although rosacea can affect all segments of the population, individuals with fair skin who tend to flush or blush easily are believed to be at greatest risk. The disease is more frequently diagnosed in women; studies have shown that women are affected about two to three times more frequently than men. However, men have more severe signs and symptoms.

The primary signs of rosacea include flushing, persistent erythema, papules and pustules, and telangiectasias (tiny blood vessels dilate and become more visible through the skin) (see Figure 16.17). Left untreated, rosacea tends to be progressive; however, in most people rosacea is cyclic. In severe cases the nose may grow swollen and bumpy from excess tissue. This condition, called rhinophyma, gave the late comedian W.C. Fields his trademark bulbous nose. Rhinophyma occurs mainly in men. Ocular problems, including burning and grittiness, occur in at least 50% of patients with rosacea. If untreated, a serious complication that can damage the cornea, rosacea keratitis, may occur, resulting in visual impairment.

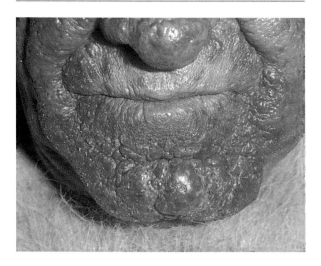

Figure 16.17 Rosacea.

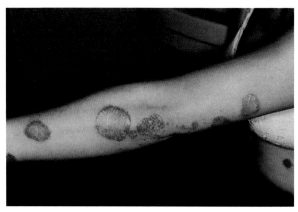

Figure 16.18 Plaque psoriasis.
(Courtesy of the CDC/Dr N. J. Fiumara, 1976)

Although the exact cause of rosacea is unknown, a number of factors can aggravate it or make it worse by increasing blood flow to the surface of the skin. Some of these include hot foods or beverages, spicy foods, alcohol, temperature extremes, sunlight, stress, anger or embarrassment, strenuous exercise, wind, hot baths or saunas, skin care products and drugs that dilate blood vessels.

Diagnosis of rosacea is based on visual examination; there is no cure. The first step in treatment and for prevention is avoidance of rosacea triggers. Treatment may include antibiotics and topical vitamin A derivatives (retinoid). Telangiectasias can be treated with laser surgery.

Psoriasis

Psoriasis is a chronic skin disease characterised by scaling and inflammation. Psoriasis affects an estimated 2–3% of the population in the UK and worldwide. Psoriasis occurs in all age groups and equally in men and women. Psoriasis is characterised by rapidly multiplying skin cells occurring up to 10 times faster than normal. As underlying cells reach the skin's surface and die, their sheer volume causes raised, red patches covered with white scales. Psoriasis typically occurs on the knees, elbows and scalp, and can also affect the torso,

palms and soles of the feet. There are many forms of psoriasis, including plaque, guttate, pustular, inverse and erythrodermic psoriasis.

The most common type of psoriasis is plaque psoriasis. Approximately 9 out of 10 people with psoriasis have plaque psoriasis. In plaque psoriasis, lesions have a reddened base covered by silvery scales (Figure 16.18). Plaque psoriasis may be caused by an abnormal immune system that produces too many T cells in the skin. These T cells trigger the inflammation and excessive skin cell reproduction, leading to inflammation and flaking of skin. Plaque psoriasis may worsen and then improve. Conditions that may cause flare-ups include changes in climate, infections, stress and dry skin.

Diagnosis of psoriasis is based on visual examination. Biopsy may be used to confirm the diagnosis and rule out other skin conditions. There is no cure for psoriasis, nor is it preventable. Three basic categories of treatment are used. Topical or external treatments include steroids, coal tar and anthralin. Phototherapy, which employs lasers and UV light, is generally used for patients with moderate to severe psoriasis who are not responding to topical treatments or who have disease too extensive for topical treatment. Systemic drugs, including the organ transplantrejection drug cyclosporin, the cancer drug methotrexate and oral retinoids, are usually reserved for patients with moderate to severe psoriasis.

BENIGN TUMOURS

Nevus (mole)

A **nevus** is a small, dark skin growth that develops from pigment-producing cells or melanocytes. Most people have between 10 and 40 nevi. Although the typical nevus is a plain, brown spot, nevi come in a wide variety of colours, shapes and sizes. It is unknown why nevi develop or what purpose they serve, if any.

The nevi themselves are usually harmless, but they can become malignant. Nevi should be examined by a physician if they are painful, itching or burning, oozing or bleeding, inflamed, scaly or crusty, or suddenly different in size, shape, colour or elevation.

Diagnosis of nevi may include visual examination and biopsy. Nevi can be removed by excision or cryosurgery. There is no way to prevent nevi, but the best way to catch potential problems at an early stage is to become familiar with the location and pattern of the nevi. Skin should be examined carefully on a regular basis.

Haemangioma

Haemangioma is a benign tumour made of small blood vessels that form a red or purple birthmark. Haemangiomas are present in 62 of every 1000 newborns. At the age of 1 year, the prevalence is 120 per 1000 children. The cause of haemangiomas is unknown, and there is no way to prevent the condition. Haemangiomas are diagnosed by visual examination and biopsy.

 Prevention PLUS!

Examining your skin

It is important to check your own skin, preferably once a month. A self-examination is best done in a well lit room in front of a full length mirror. You can use a hand-held mirror for areas that are hard to see. A spouse, close friend or family member may be able to help you with these examinations, especially for those hard-to-see areas like the lower back or the back of your thighs. The first time you inspect your skin, spend a fair amount of time carefully going over the entire surface. Learn the pattern of moles, blemishes, freckles and other marks on your skin so that you'll notice any changes next time. Any trouble spots should be seen by a doctor.

Follow these step-by-step instructions to examine your skin.

Face the mirror

Check your face, ears, neck, chest and belly. Women will need to lift breasts to check the skin underneath. Check the underarm areas, both sides of your arms, the tops and bottoms of your hands, in between your fingers and fingernail beds.

Sit down

Check the front of your thighs, shins, tops of your feet, in between your toes and toenail beds. You will need a hand mirror for your thighs, back and scalp. Now look at the bottoms of your feet, your calves and the backs of your thighs, first checking one leg and then the other. Use the hand mirror to check the buttocks, genital area, lower back, upper back and the back of the neck. It may be easier to look at your back in the wall mirror using a hand mirror. Use a comb or hair dryer to part your hair so that you can check your scalp.

Source: The American Cancer Society.

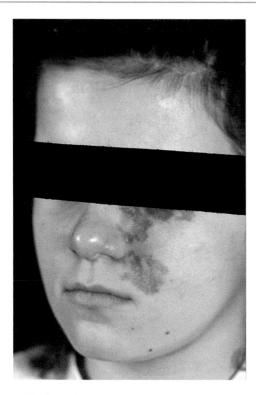

Figure 16.19 Port-wine haemangioma.
(© Custom Medical Stock Photo)

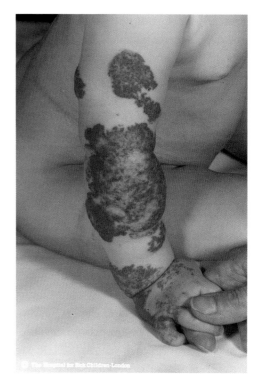

Figure 16.20 Strawberry haemangioma.
(© NMSB/Custom Medical Stock Photo)

Port-wine stain (Figure 16.19) is a dark red to purple birthmark that occurs in 3 of every 1000 infants. Port-wine stain can appear anywhere on the body, and most are readily visible at birth. Port-wine stain can be flat or slightly raised and is usually permanent. Laser treatment can reduce colour and improve skin texture.

Strawberry haemangioma (Figure 16.20) is a strawberry red, rough, protruding lesion on the face, neck or trunk and is seen in approximately 0.5% of infants. The tumour may be present at birth or a few weeks after birth. Strawberry haemangioma will grow, start to fade and turn grey in colour, usually disappearing between the ages of 5 and 10. Surgery to remove the haemangioma might be necessary depending on size and location of the tumour. Other treatments may include compression and massage, steroids, X-ray therapy, laser therapy, cryotherapy or injection of hardening agents.

Cherry haemangioma (Figure 16.21) is a small, red, dome-shaped tumour that appears most frequently after age 40. More than 70% of people age 70 or older have cherry haemangiomas. Cherry

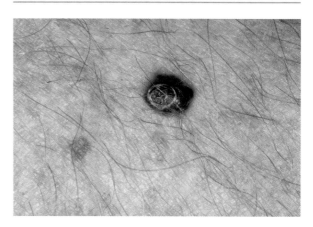

Figure 16.21 Cherry haemangioma.
(Science Photo Library Ltd/Dr P. Marazzi)

haemangiomas can occur almost anywhere on the skin, but are most common on the torso. When they first occur, cherry haemangiomas are about the size of a pinhead and do not protrude above the surface of the skin. However, some grow to one-quarter of an inch across or more and become spongy and dome-shaped. Cherry haemangiomas can be removed by electrosurgery, cryosurgery or laser or simply left alone.

NON-MELANOMA SKIN CANCER

Although registration of this condition remains inconclusive, with an approximate figure of 81 600 cases recorded in 2006, Cancer Research UK estimates that about 100 000 people develop non-melanoma skin cancer each year in the UK. Men are about twice as likely to develop these cancers as women. The number of these cancers has been increasing. Perhaps this is because of a combination of increased detection, more sun exposure and aging of the population. (Melanoma is discussed in Chapter 4.)

Basal cell carcinoma

The most common skin cancer is **basal cell carcinoma**, a slowly growing and generally non-metastasising tumour. Basal cell carcinoma begins in the lowest layer of the epidermis, called the basal cell layer. Cancer Research UK estimates that approximately 75% of all skin cancers are basal cell carcinomas. Basal cell carcinoma usually develops on sun-exposed areas, especially the head and neck. The lesion begins as a pearly nodule with rolled edges that may bleed and form a crust (Figure 16.22). Ulceration occurs and size increases if basal cell carcinoma is not treated.

Risk factors for basal cell carcinoma include ultra-violet (UV) light exposure, fair skin, male gender (men are twice as likely as women to develop basal cell carcinoma), exposure to certain chemicals (e.g.

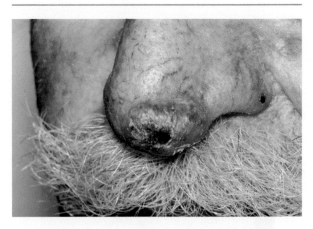

Figure 16.22 Basal cell carcinoma.
(Science Photo Library Ltd/Dr P. Marazzi)

arsenic, industrial tar, coal, paraffin, certain types of oil), radiation exposure and previous skin cancer. UV radiation damaging DNA is the cause of basal cell carcinoma. Diagnosis of basal cell carcinoma includes visual examination and biopsy. Basal cell carcinoma may be treated by surgery, chemotherapy or radiation therapy. The best way to prevent basal cell carcinoma is to limit exposure to UV radiation. Examining the skin on a regular basis can help find cancer early.

Squamous cell carcinoma

Squamous cell carcinoma is more serious than basal cell carcinoma because it grows more rapidly, infiltrates underlying tissues and metastasises through the lymphatic system. This cancer develops in any squamous epithelium of the body, including the skin or mucous membranes lining a natural body opening. Cancer Research UK estimates that there are 10 000 cases per year in the UK. Squamous cell carcinoma is responsible for around 20% of non-melanoma skin cancers. Squamous cell carcinoma is a malignancy of the keratinocytes in the epidermis of people who have been excessively exposed to the sun. It commonly appears on sun-exposed areas of

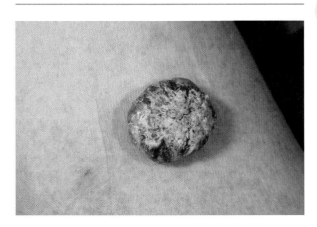

Figure 16.23 Squamous cell carcinoma.
(Bart's Medical Library/Phototake NYC)

the body such as the face, ears, neck, lips and back of the hands. The lesion is a crusted nodule that ulcerates and bleeds (Figure 16.23).

Risk factors for squamous cell carcinoma include UV light exposure, fair skin, male gender (men are three times more likely than women to develop squamous cell carcinoma), exposure to certain chemicals (e.g. arsenic, industrial tar, coal, paraffin and certain types of oil), radiation exposure and previous skin cancer. UV radiation damaging DNA is the cause of squamous cell carcinoma. Diagnosis of squamous cell carcinoma includes visual examination and skin biopsy. Squamous cell carcinoma may be treated by surgery, chemotherapy or radiation therapy. The best way to prevent squamous cell carcinoma is to limit exposure to UV radiation. Examining the skin on a regular basis can help find cancer early.

SEBACEOUS GLAND DISORDERS

Acne (vulgaris)

Acne affects more than 85% of teenagers in the UK. There are two types of acne: non-inflammatory acne and inflammatory acne. Several factors contribute to acne development, including abnormal exfoliation of skin, bacteria, hormones and possibly genetics.

Acne begins in the sebaceous hair follicles. Each hair follicle is connected to a sebaceous gland that secretes sebum, an oily substance that lubricates hair and skin. Old skin cells are exfoliated to prepare for new skin. If old skin cells are not shed or are shedn unevenly, they may clump and form a plug (or comedo) that traps sebum and bacteria inside the hair follicle. Non-inflammatory acne includes closed comedones (whiteheads) and open comedones (blackheads).

If there is a break in the follicle wall (forming a papule), inflammation is triggered and inflammatory acne develops. Pustules form as white blood cells make their way to the surface of the skin. If the hair follicle totally collapses, a nodule is formed. Severe chronic acne, as seen in Figure 16.24, can lead to disfiguring and scarring. Acne is diagnosed by visual examination.

Treatment for acne may include topical antibiotics and antibacterials (benzoyl peroxide), retinoids (Retin-A), oral antibiotics and oral contraceptives. Often, a combination of such products is required to achieve optimal results. Isotretinoin (Accutane) may be used to treat severe acne or acne that does not respond to other treatments. Isotretinoin is associated with severe birth defects if pregnancy occurs during

 Prevention PLUS!

Limiting UV exposure

The most important way to lower the risk of basal and squamous cell carcinoma is to limit your exposure to UV radiation. Practise sun safety when you are outdoors. Wear protective clothing and a hat with at least a 5–8-cm brim. Use sunscreen and lip balm with an SPF of 15 or higher. Wear sunglasses to protect your eyes and the skin around your eyes.

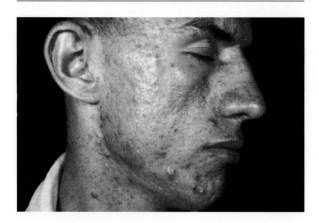

Figure 16.24 Severe acne.
(© Custom Medical Stock Photo)

the course of treatment or within several weeks of concluding treatment. Isotretinoin may increase the levels of triglycerides and cholesterol in the blood and may increase liver enzyme levels.

Prevention of acne includes not overcleansing the skin, not using harsh scrubs, avoiding products with high concentrations of alcohol, and keeping the hands away from the face.

PIGMENT DISORDERS

The main skin pigment, melanin, is interspersed among other cells in the epidermis. Skin colour varies from light to dark depending on the number of melanocytes present. Melanin production normally increases with exposure to sunlight, causing tanning. Hypopigmentation is caused by an abnormally low amount or absence of melanin. The skin may be pale white to various shades of pink caused by blood flowing through it. Hyperpigmentation is caused by an abnormally high amount of melanin.

Albinism

Albinism is a group of genetic conditions that cause a lack of pigment. Albinism affects people from all races. About 1 in 17 000 people has some type of albinism, although up to 1 in 70 is a carrier of albinism genes. People with albinism have visual

issues, including rapid eye movements, eyes that do not track properly, photophobia, decreased visual acuity or even functional blindness.

Ocular albinism affects only the eyes. People with ocular albinism usually have normal or only slightly lighter than normal skin. However, examination of the eye will show that there is no pigment in the retina. Ocular albinism is X-linked recessive.

Oculocutaneous albinism affects both the skin and the eyes. Common signs of oculocutaneous albinism include absence of pigment from the hair, skin or iris of eyes. Oculocutaneous albinism is autosomal recessive.

Albinism may be diagnosed based on the appearance of the skin, hair and eyes and genetic testing. Treatment includes improving vision, protecting eyes from bright light, and protecting the skin and eyes from the sun.

Vitiligo

Vitiligo is a loss of melanin resulting in white patches of skin. An estimated 1% of the world's population have vitiligo. Although any part of the body may be affected by vitiligo, depigmentation usually develops first on sun-exposed areas of the skin (Figure 16.25). Vitiligo affects both sexes and all races but is often more noticeable and more disfiguring in people

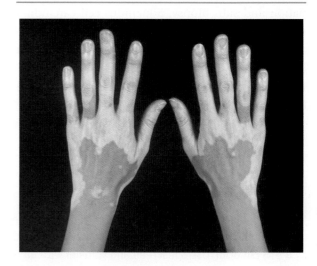

Figure 16.25 Vitiligo.
(Science Photo Library Ltd/CMSP)

with darker skin. Vitiligo usually starts as small areas of pigment loss that spread and become larger with time. The white patches are usually well demarcated and may cover large parts of the body. The cause of vitiligo is unknown, and there is no cure. Possible risk factors include immune system disorders, heredity, sunburn and emotional distress.

Diagnosis is based on visual examination. Small areas of skin may be covered with tinted make-up, and sunscreen should always be applied to the skin to prevent sunburn. Treatment options include corticosteroids, Psoralen (contains chemicals that react with UV light to cause darkening of the skin), UV light therapy, depigmentation therapy and surgical therapies. There is no way to prevent vitiligo.

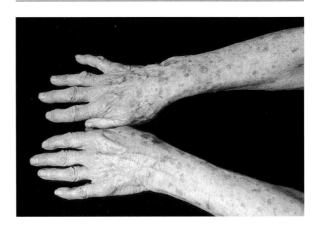

Figure 16.26 Lentigo.
(Science Photo Library Ltd/Zuber/CMSP)

Ephelides and lentigines

Ephelides, also known as macules or freckles, refer to flat spots that are red or light brown and typically appear during the sunny months and fade in the winter. They occur most often in people with light complexions. Ephelides are genetic and are related to the presence of the melanocortin-1 receptor gene variant, which is dominant. Ephelides can also be triggered by long exposure to sunlight. Ephelides are predominantly found on the face, although they may appear on any skin exposed to the sun. The regular use of sunscreen helps suppress the appearance of ephelides.

Lentigines are a type of freckle that develops in older adults and are often called liver spots or age spots. Lentigines are small, brown lesions occurring on the face, neck and back of the hands (Figure 16.26). Lentigines are not caused by aging but by excessive sun exposure. Ephelides and lentigines pose no medical risks. Diagnosis is based on visual examination. Treatment may include bleaching creams, retinoids, cryosurgery and laser treatment. Protecting the skin from sunlight is the best way to prevent ephelides and lentigines.

Melasma

Melasma, also known as chloasma or pregnancy mask, is characterised by patches of darker skin on the face, especially over the cheeks. The cause of melasma remains unknown but it is believed to be caused by an increase in the production of melanin. What causes the increased production of melanin is not known. Possible triggers include hormones, prolonged sun exposure, use of birth control pills and certain medications like tetracycline and antimalarial drugs. Melasma is diagnosed by visual examination. Treatment may include bleaching creams, chemical peels or laser treatment. Protecting skin from the sun is key to preventing melasma.

SKIN TRAUMA

Lacerations are cuts in the skin caused by a sharp object. **Abrasions**, or scrapes, result from wearing away the upper layer of skin by friction; they are red, raw and painful, and bleeding is minimal. **Punctures** are injuries caused by a pointed object piercing or penetrating the skin, with minimal bleeding. A possible complication of puncture is tetanus; the puncture creates the anaerobic environment preferred by the bacteria. Sutures or glue may be needed to close skin that has been split open or is gaping.

Contusions, or bruises, are caused when blood vessels are damaged or broken as a result of a blow to the skin. Blood leaks out of the damaged vessels into the surrounding tissues. A purplish, flat bruise that occurs when blood leaks out into the top layers of skin is known as an **ecchymosis**. In an **avulsion**, a portion of the skin has been torn away or is barely attached. Crushing injuries result when a body part is subjected to a high degree of force or pressure, usually after being squeezed between two heavy objects. Haemorrhage, contusions, lacerations and fractures are possible complications of a crushing injury.

Pressure sores or decubitus ulcers

Pressure sores, or decubitus ulcers, usually occur in skin overlying bony projections such as the hips, heels, elbows and ankles. Constant pressure against the skin reduces the blood supply to that area, and the affected tissue dies. At-risk patients can develop a pressure sore within 2–6 hours of the onset of pressure. An estimated 412 000 people in the UK develop a pressure sore each year, and 70% of pressure sores occur in patients older than 70 years, probably owing to a decrease in adipose tissue and reduced mobility. The incidence of pressure sores in hospitalised patients with acute illness is between 4 and 10%, whereas the prevalence rate is nearly doubled in residents of long-term care facilities such as nursing homes.

The hip and buttock regions account for 67% of all pressure sores. The lower extremities account for an additional 25%. The remaining 10% or so may occur in any location that experiences long periods of uninterrupted pressure. No surface of the body can be considered immune to the effects of pressure.

Risk factors for pressure sores include impaired mobility, skin atrophy, chronic conditions such as diabetes or vascular disease that prevent areas of the body from receiving proper blood flow, sensory loss, malnourishment, mental disability, older age and urinary or bowel incontinence.

Pressure sores are categorised by severity. There are four stages, ranging from intact red or discoloured skin to full-thickness loss of skin and subcutaneous tissue that extends into muscle or bone. Figure 16.27 shows a patient with several pressure sores.

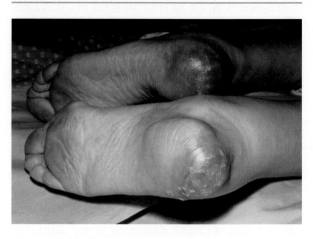

Figure 16.27 Pressure sores.
(Science Photo Library Ltd/Mike Devlin)

Diagnosis is based on visual examination and may include bacterial culture if the sore is infected. The first step in treatment is eliminating the pressure. Specialised support surfaces and pressure reduction devices have been shown to reduce pressure. Regardless of support surface or device, turning and repositioning the patient remain the cornerstones of prevention and treatment. This should be performed every 2 hours, even in the presence of a specialty surface or bed.

Corns and calluses

Corns and **calluses** are areas of the skin that have grown thick in response to repeated pressure and friction and form to protect the skin. Calluses (tyloma) involve thickening of skin without distinct borders and usually form on feet and hands over bony spots. Calluses vary in colour from white to grey–yellow, brown or red and may be painless, tender, or may throb or burn.

When a callus develops a mass of dead cells in its centre (glassy core), it becomes a corn (heloma). Corns have distinct borders and usually form on the feet. Corns may be hard or soft and are usually painful. Causes of calluses and corns include ill-fitting shoes or socks, not wearing shoes or socks, manual labour, bony prominences on the feet and biomechanical or gait abnormalities.

Diagnosis may include visual examination, biopsy and X-rays. Treatment may include shaving or cutting off the hardened area on the skin, removing the corn or callus by medication or surgery, or surgically removing areas of protruding bone where corns and calluses form. Prevention includes wearing gloves to protect hands, making sure shoes and socks fit properly and do not rub, surgically correcting bony abnormalities, and keeping hands and feet moisturised.

Burns

A burn is damage to the body's tissues caused by heat, chemicals, electricity, sunlight or radiation. Thermal burns are the most common. When tissues are burned, fluid leaks into the tissue from the blood vessels, causing oedema and pain. In addition, damaged skin and other body surfaces are easily infected because they can no longer act as a barrier against invading organisms. More than 250 000 people in the UK require treatment for burns each year, and over 200 die annually as a result of burns or scalds. In 50% of cases, burns occur in the kitchen, with the incidence highest in children under the age of 5 and those over 70 years old.

The extent of damage depends on surface temperature and contact duration. Burns are classified according to the depth of skin involved. First-degree or superficial burns affect the epidermis. The epidermis is red, swollen and painful (Figure 16.28). First-degree burns heal in approximately 1 week and do not scar.

Second-degree, or partial thickness, burns affect the epidermis and the dermis. The epidermis is extremely red and blistered, and the area is very painful (Figure 16.29). Second-degree burns heal in a few weeks; some scarring and depigmentation may occur. Treatment includes antibiotic cream and pain relievers.

Third-degree, or full thickness, burns affect the epidermis, dermis and subcutaneous tissue (Figure 16.30). The skin may appear white or black with a leathery appearance. The nerve endings are destroyed, so the burned area will not be painful. The patient may go into shock owing to loss of

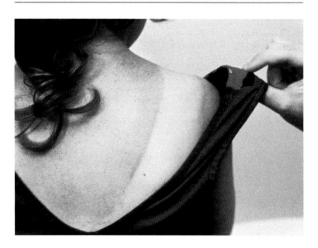
Figure 16.28 First-degree burn.

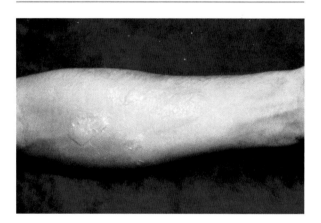
Figure 16.29 Second-degree burn.

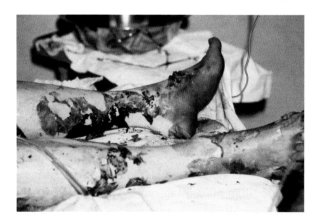
Figure 16.30 Third-degree burn.

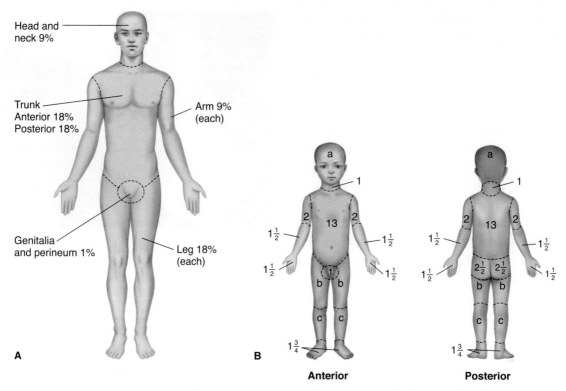

Relative percentage of body surface area (% BSA) affected by growth

			Age		
Body part	0 yr	1 yr	5 yr	10 yr	15 yr
a = $\frac{1}{2}$ of head	$9\frac{1}{2}$	$8\frac{1}{2}$	$6\frac{1}{2}$	$5\frac{1}{2}$	$4\frac{1}{2}$
b = $\frac{1}{2}$ of 1 thigh	$2\frac{3}{4}$	$3\frac{1}{4}$	4	$4\frac{1}{4}$	$4\frac{1}{2}$
c = $\frac{1}{2}$ of 1 lower leg	$2\frac{1}{2}$	$2\frac{1}{2}$	$2\frac{3}{4}$	3	$3\frac{1}{4}$

Figure 16.31 Determining the extent of a burn: (A) rule of nines (adult); (B) Lund–Browder chart (children).

fluids. Treatment may include antibiotics, IV fluids, pain relievers, surgical debridement and grafting. Severe third-degree burns cause extensive scarring.

To determine the severity of a burn, doctors estimate what percentage of the body's surface has been burned. For adults, doctors use the rule of nines. This method divides almost all of the body into sections of 9% or 18% (Figure 16.31). Burns that involve more than 90% of the body surface, or more than 60% in an older person, are usually fatal. For children, doctors use charts that adjust these percentages according to the child's age (Lund–Browder charts; Figure 16.31). Adjustment is

needed because different areas of the body grow at different rates.

Hypothermia and frostbite

Hypothermia is an abnormally low body temperature resulting from prolonged exposure to cold air or water. Hypothermia occurs when more heat escapes from the body than the body can produce. Approximately 400 people above age 65 die annually in the UK of hypothermia. Signs and symptoms of hypothermia include shivering (the body is attempting to generate heat), cold and pale skin, lack of coordination, disorientation, and decreased heart rate, respiration rate and blood pressure that can lead to loss of consciousness or death. Diagnosis is based on body temperature. Risk factors for hypothermia include age (young or old), living in a cold climate and alcohol use. Rewarming is the main treatment. Prevention includes dressing appropriately for the weather by wearing dry, loose-fitting, layered clothing that wicks moisture away from skin. It is important to wear a hat; 30–50% of body heat is lost through the head. Alcohol should be avoided because it causes the blood vessels in the skin to dilate, reducing circulation.

Frostbite is damage to the skin caused by freezing owing to prolonged exposure to cold conditions. Freezing causes formation of ice crystals within cells, rupturing and destroying the cells. Signs and symptoms of frostbite may include pain, tingling, numbness, eventual loss of sensation, blistering and tissue death.

Risk factors for frostbite include age (young or old), living in a cold climate, alcohol use, smoking and circulatory problems. Diagnosis of frostbite is based on visual examination. Treatment may include rewarming, pain medication, antibiotics and anti-inflammatory medication. Tissue affected by severe frostbite may require surgery or amputation.

Prevention includes dressing adequately for the weather by wearing loose-fitting, layered clothing, keeping clothes dry, refraining from smoking and avoiding alcohol.

AGE-RELATED DISEASES

The structure and function of skin changes with age. Skin loses some of its elasticity with age owing to a decrease in elastic fibres, and the skin appears wrinkled and saggy. Touch sensation of the skin decreases with aging, making burns and frostbite more likely. Stem cell production declines with aging, causing slower epidermal cell reproduction and thinner, more translucent skin that is more prone to injury and infection and retains less water. Migration of cells to the top of the epidermis slows. As a result, skin heals more slowly; healing time

may be more than twice as long in the elderly as in younger people. This longer healing time increases the risk of secondary infections. A decrease in the blood supply to the dermis and a decrease in sweat production lead to impaired thermoregulation. The elderly have an increased risk for hypothermia. The number of macrophages and other cells of the immune system decrease and these cells are less efficient, increasing the risk of infection. Melanocyte number and activity declines with aging, causing the skin to become paler and the hair to turn grey or white. This also causes an increased susceptibility to sunburn and skin cancer. In addition, selected melanocytes increase their production in areas exposed to the sun, resulting in lentigines. Sebaceous gland activity decreases, as does sebum production. The skin becomes dry and flaky. Hair becomes brittle, thin and may be lost. Vascularity and circulation decrease in the subcutaneous tissue, causing drugs that are administered in this manner to be absorbed slowly. Vascular supply to the nails and hair decreases, resulting in slowed growth. Nails become dull, brittle, hard and thick and become difficult to trim.

Seborrhoeic keratosis is a benign overgrowth of epithelial cells. Seborrhoeic keratoses are the most common benign tumour in older individuals. Most people develop at least one seborrhoeic keratosis at some point in their lives. A seborrhoeic keratosis has a characteristic 'pasted on' look and typically appears on the head, neck or trunk of the body. Seborrhoeic keratoses range in colour from light tan to black, are round to oval-shaped, are flat or slightly elevated with a scaly surface, and range in size from very small to more than 1 inch across (Figure 16.32). Seborrhoeic keratosis may cause pruritus. The exact cause of the condition is unknown. They tend to run in some families, so genetics may play a role. UV light may also play a role in their development. Diagnosis is made by visual examination; a biopsy may be performed to rule out skin cancer. Treatment of seborrhoeic keratoses is not usually necessary; however, they can be removed by cryosurgery, curettage or electrocautery.

Actinic keratosis, also known as solar keratosis, is a precancerous skin condition caused by exposure

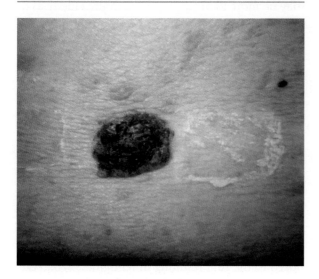

Figure 16.32 Seborrhoeic keratosis.
(Courtesy of the CDC/Dr Steve Kraus, 1981)

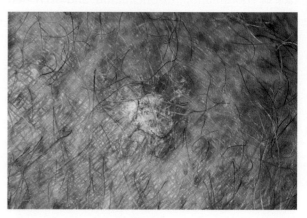

Figure 16.33 Actinic keratosis.
(Science Photo Library Ltd/Dr P. Marazzi)

to UV radiation. The prevalence of actinic keratosis increases dramatically with age. Multiple wart-like lesions develop on areas of the body exposed to the sun such as the face, arms and legs (Figure 16.33). Actinic keratoses are small (usually less than one-quarter of an inch) rough spots that may be pink–red or flesh-coloured. If actinic keratosis is not treated, 10–15% may develop into squamous cell carcinoma. Even though most actinic keratoses do not become cancers, they are a warning that the skin has suffered sun damage and should be checked regularly. Diagnosis of actinic keratosis is made by visual examination and may include biopsy.

Treatment of actinic keratosis may include surgery, acid chemical peels and topical chemotherapy. The best way to prevent actinic keratosis is to limit exposure to UV radiation.

Resources

The National Organization for Albinism and Hypopigmentation: *www.albinism.org*

The National Psoriasis Foundation: *www.psoriasis.org*

The National Rosacea Society: *www.rosacea.org*

NICE Clinical Guideline. *Skin Tumours Including Melanoma*. February 2006: *www.nice.org.uk*

NICE Clinical Guideline. *Referral for Suspected Cancer*. June 2005: *www.nice.org.uk*

DISEASES AT A GLANCE Integumentary system

DISEASE	AETIOLOGY	SIGNS AND SYMPTOMS	DIAGNOSIS	TREATMENT	PREVENTION/ LIFESPAN
Epidermoid and pilar cysts	Abnormal cell proliferation	Smooth, round lump just beneath the skin surface	Visual examination	Removal by excision if required	None
Impetigo	*S. pyogenes, S. aureus*	Vesicles and pustules that rupture forming a crust, fever, swollen lymph nodes	Visual examination, bacterial culture	Antibiotics	Proper hygiene
Erysipelas, cellulitus	*S. pyogenes, S. aureus*	Swollen, bright red, hot and tender area of the skin, small vesicles, fever, chills, swelling of lymph nodes	Visual examination, bacterial culture	Self-limiting, antibiotics	Prompt attention to wounds, moisturising the skin, careful trimming of nails
Folliculitis	Staphylococci	Erythema, follicular-based papules and pustules	Visual examination, bacterial culture	Self-limiting, daily cleansing with antiseptic soap, antibiotics	Keep skin clean, dry and free from abrasions or irritation
Furuncles, carbuncles	Staphylococci	Furuncles – large, tender, swollen, pus-filled lesion Carbuncles – cluster of furuncles	Visual examination, bacterial culture	Moist heat, antiseptic skin cleansing, antibiotics, incision and drainage	Keep skin clean, dry and free from abrasions or irritation
Herpes	Herpes virus family	Small, fluid-filled, painful vesicles	Visual examination, viral culture, DNA testing	Self-limiting, antiviral drugs	Avoid contact with HSV-1, frequent hand washing, avoid recurrence triggers
Warts	Human papillomavirus	Benign neoplasms with rough, keratinised surface	Visual examination	Removal by medication, electrocautery, cryosurgery, laser surgery	Avoid touching warts, walking barefoot on warm moist surfaces, trauma to the skin
Tinea	Fungi	Mild scales, rash, fissures	Visual examination, microscopic examination of skin scrapings	Keeping area clean and dry, antifungal medication	Keep skin clean, cool and dry; wear sandals or shoes at gyms, locker rooms and pools
Seborrhoeic dermatitis	Unknown	Adults – dry or greasy scaling with variable pruritus Infants – thick, yellow-crusted scalp lesions	Visual examination, biopsy	Medicated shampoo, antifungal medication, corticosteroids	None
Candidiasis	*Candida albicans, Candida tropicalis, Candida parapsilosis, Candida guilliermondi, Torulopsis glabrata*	Vaginal – white cottage-cheese discharge, burning, pruritus, erythema Oral – creamy white, painful patches Cutaneous – patches of red, moist, weepy skin	Visual examination, culture	Antifungal medication	Keeping skin clean and dry, proper use of antibiotics, healthy lifestyle, controlling blood sugar
Pediculosis	*Pediculus humanus capitis, Pediculus humanus corporis, Pthirus pubis*	Pruritus, multiple erythematous papules	Finding lice or nits	Pediculocidal medication	Proper hygiene, safe sex practices
Scabies	*Sarcoptes scabiei*	Pruritus, vesicles, pustules, greyish lines (tunnels)	Pruritus, rash, microscopic examination of skin scrapings	Scabicidal medication	Proper hygiene

DISEASES AT A GLANCE Integumentary system (continued)

DISEASE	AETIOLOGY	SIGNS AND SYMPTOMS	DIAGNOSIS	TREATMENT	PREVENTION/ LIFESPAN
Urticaria (hives)	Hypersensitivity	Wheals with rounded elevations and pale centres, pruritus	Visual examination	Corticosteroids, antihistamines, calamine lotion	Avoid allergen, reduce emotional and physical stress
Allergic contact dermatitis	Type 1 hypersensitivity	Rash with erythema, pruritus, burning	Visual examination	Corticosteroids, antihistamines	Avoid allergen
Atopic dermatitis	Unknown	Red, dry, crusted patches on the skin	Visual examination	Corticosteroids	None
Rosacea	Unknown	Flushing, persistent erythema, papules, pustules, telangiectasias	Visual examination	Antibiotics, retinoid, laser surgery	Avoid triggers
Psoriasis	Hereditary; too many T cells trigger inflammation	Red lesions with silvery scales	Visual examination, biopsy	Steroids, coal tar, anthralin, phototherapy, cyclosporin, methotrexate, oral retinoids	None
Nevus (mole)	Benign tumour	Small, dark skin growth	Visual examination, biopsy	Cryosurgery, excision	Be familiar with pattern and location of nevi, examine skin on a regular basis
Haemangioma	Benign tumour	Red or purple birth marks	Visual examination, biopsy	Electrosurgery, cryosurgery, laser surgery	None; aging plays a role in cherry haemangioma
Basal cell carcinoma	UV radiation damaging DNA	Pearly nodule with rolled edges may bleed, form crust	Visual examination, biopsy	Surgery, chemotherapy, radiation	Limit UV radiation exposure, examine skin on a regular basis
Squamous cell carcinoma	UV radiation damaging DNA	Crusted nodule, ulcerates and bleeds	Visual examination, biopsy	Surgery, chemotherapy, radiation	Limit UV radiation exposure, examine skin on a regular basis
Acne (vulgaris)	Abnormal skin exfoliation, bacteria, hormones, genetic factors	Comedones, papules, pustules, nodules	Visual examination	Topical antibiotics and antibacterials, retinoids, oral antibiotics, oral contraceptives, isotretinoin	Avoid overcleansing the skin and using harsh scrubs, avoid products with high concentrations of alcohol, keep the hands away from the face
Albinism	Hereditary	Absence of melanin	Visual examination, genetic testing	Improving vision, protecting eyes from bright light, protecting the skin and eyes from the sun	None
Vitiligo	Unknown	White, well demarcated areas of skin without melanin	Visual examination	Corticosteroids, psoralen, UV light treatment, depigmentation therapy, surgical therapy	None
Ephelides, lentigines	Hereditary, sun exposure	Red or brown macule	Visual examination	Bleaching creams, retinoid, cryosurgery, laser treatment	Protection from the sun

DISEASES AT A GLANCE Integumentary system (continued)

DISEASE	AETIOLOGY	SIGNS AND SYMPTOMS	DIAGNOSIS	TREATMENT	PREVENTION/ LIFESPAN
Melasma	Unknown	Patches of darker skin over the cheeks	Visual examination	Bleaching cream, chemical peels, laser treatment	Protection from the sun
Pressure sore (decubitus ulcer)	Constant pressure decreases blood flow and the skin dies	Reddened area, abrasion, vesicle, superficial ulceration, deep erosion	Visual examination, bacterial culture	Eliminate pressure	Turn and reposition patients every 2 hours, use specialised support surfaces
Corns and calluses	Repeated pressure and friction	Areas of skin that grow thick	Visual examination, biopsy, X-ray	Shaving or cutting off the hardened area on the skin, removal by medication or surgery, surgically removing areas of protruding bone	Wear gloves to protect hands, make sure shoes and socks fit properly and do not rub, surgically correct bony abnormalities, and keep hands and feet moisturised
Burns	Heat, radiation, sunlight, chemicals, electricity	First-degree - red, swollen, painful Second-degree - extremely red, blistered, painful Third-degree - white or black skin with a leathery appearance, no pain in the burned area	Visual examination	First-degree - none Second-degree - antibiotic cream, pain relievers Third-degree - IV fluids, antibiotics, pain relievers, surgical debridement, grafting	Avoid excessive exposure to heat, radiation, sunlight, chemicals and electricity
Hypothermia, frostbite	Prolonged exposure to cold air or water	Hypothermia - shivering, cold and pale skin, lack of coordination, disorientation, decrease in heart and respiratory rates and blood pressure, loss of consciousness Frostbite - pain, numbness, tingling, loss of sensation, blistering, tissue death	Hypothermia - body temperature Frostbite - visual examination	Hypothermia - rewarming Frostbite - rewarming, pain medication, antibiotics, anti-inflammatory medication, surgery	Hypothermia - dress appropriately for the weather in loose layers, hat, keep clothing dry, avoid alcohol Frostbite - dress appropriately for weather in loose layers, keep clothing dry, avoid alcohol, do not smoke
Seborrhoeic keratosis	Unknown	Benign lesions with pasted-on look, flat or slightly elevated with a scaly surface, range in size, pruritus	Visual examination, biopsy	Not usually necessary, cryosurgery, curettage, electrocautery	None; aging plays a role
Actinic keratosis	UV radiation	Multiple wart-like lesions	Visual examination, biopsy	Surgery, acid chemical peels, topical chemotherapy	Limit UV radiation exposure; aging plays a role

INTERACTIVE EXERCISES

Cases for critical thinking

1. A 4-year-old girl has red lesions with a honey-coloured crust under her nose and on her cheek. According to her mother, the lesions appeared shortly after she developed a cold. On examination, the doctor notes that the girl's lymph nodes are still swollen. What is your diagnosis? What is the cause? What is the treatment?

2. A 25-year-old man complains of intense jock itch. On examination, the doctor observes raised lesions on his penis and red circular patches on his groin. The patient lives in a hotel, and his hygiene is poor. What are the possible causes for this rash? What diagnostic tests should the doctor order?

3. A 39-year-old woman who plays tennis for hours a day during the spring and summer notices a lesion on her ear that bleeds. What are the possible diagnoses? What diagnostic tests should be ordered?

4. Fifteen-year-old Jamie has a bad case of acne. According to his mother, Jamie's acne is from too much late-night TV, frozen pizza and cheddar popcorn. What factors contribute to acne? What treatments are available? Can acne be prevented?

5. Ray has small, painful vesicles near his mouth. What is your diagnosis? How did Ray become infected? What treatments are available?

6. Jemima joined a gym to get in better shape. Since she has been working out at the gym, she has noticed hard, thick patches of skin with dark specks on the sole of one of her feet. They are very painful. What is your diagnosis? What is the cause? What is the treatment?

Multiple choice

1. Bacterial infections on the skin may be caused by _____
   a. tinea
   b. herpes simplex
   c. staphylococci
   d. candida

2. A discoloured spot of the skin is a _____
   a. nodule
   b. macule
   c. wheal
   d. cyst

3. A sac filled with a fluid or semifluid material is a _____
   a. nodule
   b. cyst
   c. wheal
   d. macule

4. The outermost layer of the skin is the _____
   a. epidermis
   b. subcutaneous tissue
   c. dermis
   d. keratin

5. In pallor, the skin appears _____
   a. blue
   b. red
   c. white
   d. brown

6. The _____ lies under the dermis and connects the skin to underlying structures.
   a. epidermis
   b. dermis
   c. subcutaneous tissue
   d. stratum corneum

7. Solid elevated areas of the skin are called _____
   a. pustules
   b. macules
   c. papules
   d. nodules

8. Folliculitis is an inflammation of _____
   a. sebaceous glands
   b. sweat glands
   c. hair follicles
   d. furuncles

9. Pediculosis is a _____ infection.
   a. parasitic
   b. bacterial
   c. viral
   d. fungal

10. _____ is the oily fluid that is released through the hair follicles.
   a. Macula
   b. Keratin
   c. Sebum
   d. Wheals

True or false

_____ **1.** Impetigo is caused by a virus.

_____ **2.** Basal cell carcinoma metastasises rapidly.

_____ **3.** Cold sores are caused by a bacterial infection.

_____ **4.** Seborrhoeic dermatitis is a malignant skin tumour.

_____ **5.** Warts are caused by bacteria.

_____ **6.** A mole is a nevus.

_____ **7.** Ringworm is a viral infection.

_____ **8.** Erythema is whitening of the skin.

_____ **9.** The cause of seborrhoeic dermatitis is unknown.

_____ **10.** Rosacea is caused by fungus.

Fill-ins

1. _____ is the dark pigment of the skin that protects the body from the harmful rays of the sun.

2. _____ is a tough, fibrous protein that protects the skin from harmful substances.

3. The _____ is composed of connective tissue that supports blood and lymph vessels and elastic fibres.

4. _____ is a large family of viruses that cause clusters of fluid-filled vesicles on the skin.

5. _____ is a contagious skin disease usually associated with poor living conditions.

6. _____ is a chronic skin disease characterised by scaling and inflammation.

7. _____ are caused when blood vessels are damaged or broken as a result of a blow to the skin.

8. _____ is a benign tumour made of small blood vessels that form a red or purple birthmark.

9. _____ is loss of melanin resulting in white patches of skin.

10. _____ _____ causes scales and fissures on the soles of the feet and between toes.

Labelling exercise

Use the lines below to label each photo.

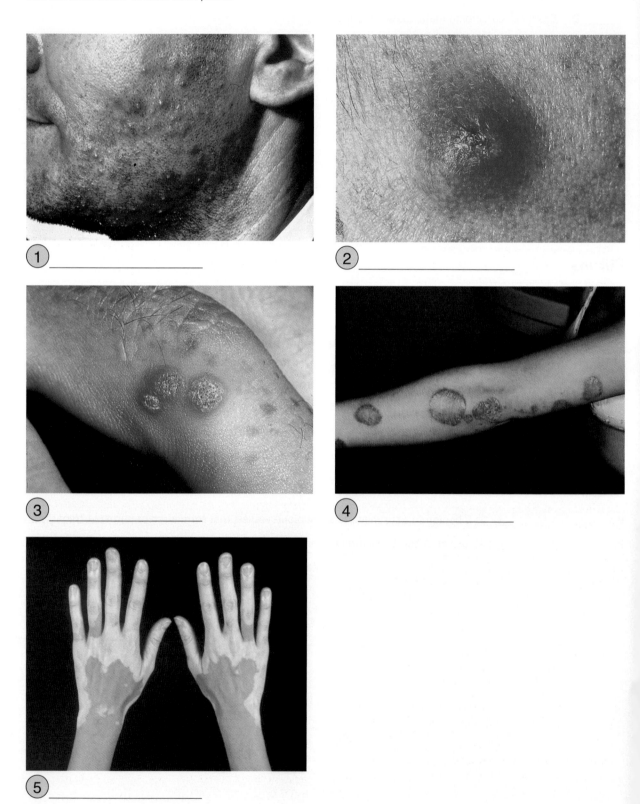

1 _____

2 _____

3 _____

4 _____

5 _____

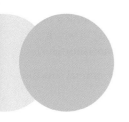

Appendix A GLOSSARY

Abruptio placentae (plass-en-tay) Premature separation of the placenta from the uterus prior to or during birth.

Acetylcholine (uh-**seat**-isle-**coe**-lean) Neurotransmitter between neurons in the brain and spinal cord, also between a neuron and a voluntary skeletal muscle.

Achlorhydria (**ay**-clor-high-dree-ah) A condition in which hydrochloric acid is absent in the stomach.

Achondroplasia (a-con-droe-play-see-ah) An autosomal dominant disorder of defective cartilage formation in the fetus.

Achondroplastic dwarfism (a-con-droe-plastic) A condition caused by defective cartilage formation that results in improper bone development.

Acidosis (a-sid-oh-siss) The condition in which the production of acids lowers the body's pH.

Acne (**ak**-nee) Blackheads, pimples and pustules that result from hormonal changes occurring most often during puberty.

Acne rosacea (**ak**-nee rose-ace-see-uh) Tiny pimples and broken blood vessels on the cheeks, chin and nose of some fair-skinned people.

Acquired immunodeficiency syndrome (AIDS) The deadly disease caused by HIV that destroys an individual's immune system, making the victim remarkably susceptible to infection.

Acrodermatitis enteropathica (ack-row-derm-ma-tie-tiss **enter**-row-**pa**-thicker) A rare autosomal recessive disorder that results in defective malabsorption of zinc.

Acromegaly (ack-**row**-meg-ally) The condition that results from excessive production of growth hormone after puberty.

Actinic keratosis (ack-tin-**ick** kera-**toe**-siss) Wart-like lesions found on areas of the body that receive excessive sun exposure.

Activated lymphocytes (**limf**-oh-sites) White blood cells that have been stimulated by antigens that include B and T cells.

Active immunity A type of artificial immunity; the person is given a vaccine or toxoid as the antigen, and he or she forms antibodies to counteract it.

Acute A disease that has a sudden onset and a short duration.

Adenocarcinoma (a-**dee**-know-**car**-sin-oh-mah) A cancerous glandular tumour.

Adenohypophysis (a-**dee**-know-high-**poff**-y-siss) The anterior and larger portion of the hypophysis; it is glandular and maintains direct communication with the hypothalamus of the brain.

Adenoma (aden-**oh**-mah) A benign tumour of glandular tissue that often develops in the breast, thyroid gland or mucous glands of the intestinal tract.

Adhesion (add-**hee**-shun) Condition caused by connective tissue fibres that anchor adjacent structures together; a kinking of the intestine.

Adipose (add-i-pose) Fat tissue.

Adrenaline (ad-**ree**-nal-in) A hormone of the sympathetic nervous system; the most vital therapy in treatment of allergies and can be self-injected in an emergency.

Adrenal virilism (ad-**ree**-nal vye-rall-**is**-m) Expression of secondary male sexual characteristics in females caused by a testosterone-secreting adrenal gland neoplasm.

Adrenocorticotropic hormone (ACTH) (add-ree-**know**-caught-ik-oh-**trow**-pic) The tropic hormone that affects the adrenal cortex.

Adult or (acute) respiratory distress syndrome (ARDS) Condition characterised by the development of sudden breathlessness within hours to days of an inciting event such as trauma, sepsis (micro-organisms growing in a person's blood) or drug overdose.

Aetiology (ee-tee-all-oh-jee) The cause of a disease.

Affect Emotional state or feeling tone used to describe one's emotional expression.

Agglutinate (agg-**loo**-tin-ate) Clumping or aggregation, as occurs in some antibody–antigen reactions.

Albinism An autosomal recessive disorder in which no melanin is formed, causing a person to have white hair, pale skin and pink eyes.

Albuminuria (al-bue-**min**-you-**ree**-a) The presence of the plasma protein albumin in urine.

Aldosterone (al-**doss**-ter-ohn) The principal hormone from the adrenal cortex that causes sodium retention and potassium secretion by the kidneys.

Alleles (al-ee-alls) Alternative forms of a gene.

Allergens Agents that initiate an allergic response.

Allergy Abnormal immunological response to allergens such as pollens, dust, animal dander and certain foods.

Alpha cells Glucagon-secreting cells of the endocrine pancreas.

Alpha-fetoprotein Fetal protein found in maternal blood and sometimes detected in adults with various cancers.

Alveoli (al-**vee**-oh-lye) Small air sacs in the lungs where gas exchange occurs.

Alzheimer's disease (altss-**high**-mers) A common form of dementia that generally affects people after age 65.

Amenorrhea (a-**men**-oh-ree-ah) The absence of menstruation.

Amniocentesis (am-knee-**oh**-sen-tee-siss) A diagnostic test for hereditary diseases performed on fetal cells withdrawn from amniotic fluid.

Amoeboid (am-**ee**-boid) A type of protozoa that moves with pseudopodia.

Amygdala (am-**igg-dull**-uh) Almond-shaped structure located deep within the brain.

Amylase (ami-**laze**) A digestive enzyme that breaks down carbohydrates.

Amyotrophic lateral sclerosis (ALS) (ay-my-**trow**-fick lat-er-all **skler**-oh-siss) Also known as Lou-Gehrig's disease; a chronic, terminal, degenerative disease of the motor nervous system.

Anaemia (a-**nee**-mee-ah) A condition caused by a reduction of oxygen-carrying haemoglobin.

Analgesics Medications that reduce pain.

Anaphylactic shock (anna-fill-**ack**-tick) A severe inflammation brought on by a severe antigen-antibody reaction such as occurs in an incompatible blood transfusion.

Anaphylaxis (anna-fill-**ack**-siss) The condition of anaphylactic shock, a life-threatening state in which blood pressure drops and airways become constricted.

Anatomy (**anna**-toe-me) Study of the normal structure of the body.

Androgen (an-drow-**jen**) The sex hormone in males.

Androgenital syndrome (an-drow-**jen**-it-all) A form of hyperadrenalism caused when the male hormone is secreted in excess.

Aneurysm (an-you-**riz**-um) A localised dilatation caused by a weakening in the wall of a blood vessel.

Angina pectoris (an-**jye**-nah peck-**tor**-iss) The temporary chest pain or sensation of chest pressure caused by transient oxygen insufficiency.

Angiocardiography (an-**jee**-oh-card-ee-**ogg**-raff-ee) An X-ray of the heart and great vessels in which a contrast indicator (dye) is injected into the cardiovascular system.

Angioma (an-jee-**oh**-ma) A type of benign tumour composed of blood vessels, such as red birthmark or 'port-wine' stain.

Angioplasty (an-jee-oh-**plar**-stee) A procedure by which a balloon-tip catheter is inserted into the coronary arteries and expanded to break and crush plaque build-up.

Ankylosis (an-key-**low**-siss) Scar tissue formation at bone ends that can turn to bone, causing the ends to fuse.

Anorexia (an-oh-**rex**-ee-ah) A loss of appetite.

Anorexia nervosa (an-oh-**rex**-ee-ah ner-**voe**-sah) A disease of psychoneurotic origin in which an aversion to food leads to emaciation and malnutrition; found to be most common in teenage girls.

Antibiotic resistance (**an**-tea-by-**o**-tick) Resistance arising when bacteria adapt to antibiotics and the adaptation becomes common in the bacterial population, rendering the antibiotics ineffective.

Antibiotics Drugs used to treat bacterial infections.

Antibodies (an-tea-bod-eez) Proteins secreted by plasma cells that aid in defence against infectious agents.

Anticoagulant (an-tea-coe-**agg**-you-lant) Medication used to prevent intravascular clotting.

Antidiuretic hormone (ADH) (an-tea-dye-you-**ret**-ik) One of two hormones secreted by the posterior pituitary (neurohypophysis).

Antigen (**an**-tea-jenn) A substance, usually foreign to the body, which triggers the immune response.

Antihistamine (**an**-tea-**hiss**-toe-mean) A drug to counteract the unpleasant effects caused by the release of histamines in the body due to allergies; has a drying effect on the mucous membranes of the mouth and throat.

Antitussive (an-tea-**tuss**-iv) A substance administered to suppress a cough.

Anuria (an-you-**ree**-ah) The total stoppage of urine production.

Anxiety disorder General term for disorders in which the primary feature is abnormal or inappropriate anxiety that interferes with daily work, school, recreational and family activities. Subtypes include panic disorder, generalised anxiety disorder, phobic disorders, social phobia, obsessive compulsive disorder and post-traumatic stress disorder.

Aorta (ay-**or**-tah) The largest artery in the body; carries blood away from the heart to the arteries.

Aortic stenosis (ay-**or**-tick sten-oh-siss) The narrowing of the valve leading into the aorta.

Aphasia (ay-**faze**-ee-uh) Loss of speech.

Aphonia (ay-**phone**-ee-uh) Inability to produce sounds from the larynx.

Aplasia (ay-**play**-zee-uh) Developmental failure leading to the absence of a structure or tissue.

Apnoea (app-**knee**-uh) Temporary cessation of breathing.

Apoptosis (ay-pop-**toe**-siss) Cell death or cell deletion by fragmentation into membrane particles, which are phagocytosed by other cells.

Arrhythmia (ay-**rith**-mee-**uh**) A deviation from the normal rhythm of the heartbeat.

Arterial blood gas (ABGs) A blood test that is performed to determine the concentration of oxygen, carbon dioxide and bicarbonate, as well as the pH of the blood.

Arteriosclerosis (ar-tee-ree-oh-skler-**oh**-sis) Progressive hardening of blood vessels, especially arteries.

Arthritis (arth-**rye**-tiss) The inflammation of a joint.

Ascites (ay-**sigh**-teeze) Fluid that develops as a result of liver failure and accumulates in the peritoneal cavity.

Aspermia (ay-**sperm**-ee-uh) Caused when there is no formation or emission of sperm because of the absence of the gonadotrophic hormones in a male before puberty.

Asthma (**ast**-mah) A disease caused by increased responsiveness of the tracheobronchial tree to various stimuli, which tends to cause dyspnoea and wheezing.

Astigmatism (ay-**stig**-mat-is-um) Caused by the front surface of the eye, the cornea, having an irregular curvature or the lens having irregularities.

Astrocytoma (ass-trow-sigh-**toe**-mah) Basically benign, slow-growing tumours of the brain.

Atelectasis (at-el-leck-**ta**-siss) A state in which the lung, in whole or in part, is collapsed or without air.

Atherosclerosis (at-her-oh-scler-**row**-sis) The accumulation of fatty material under the inner lining of the arterial wall.

Atresia (a-**tree**-see-ah) The absence or closure of a normal body opening or tubular structure.

Atrophic (ay-**trow**-fick) A degenerating, wasting condition.

Atrophy (**at**-row-fee) The decrease in size or function of an organ.

Attention deficit hyperactivity disorder (ADHD) Neurobiological disorder characterised by prominent symptoms of inattention, hyperactivity and impulsivity.

Aura (orr-ah) A warning signal such as the symptoms that precede an epileptic seizure.

Auscultation (oss-ull-**tay**-shun) Listening with a stethoscope for sounds within the body, such as heart valve sounds or the lungs, during an examination.

Autistic disorder Developmental disorder of reciprocal language and social interactions, with stereotypical behaviour.

Autoantibodies (aw-toe-**an**-tea-bod-ee) Antibodies produced against self-antigens.

Autoimmune diseases Failure of immune tolerance; activated T cells and antibodies attack the body's own tissue.

Autosomes (aw-toe-**zomes**) Name for 44 of the 46 chromosomes; does not include the sex hormones.

B lymphocytes (B-**limf**-oh-sights) Lymphocytes that produce antibodies in cell-mediated immunity.

Bacilli (bass-**ill**-eye) Rod-shaped bacterial cells.

Bacteria (back-**tear**-ee-uh) A single-celled organism with simple structure and lacking a nucleus.

Bartholin's gland Mucus-secreting glands situated at the vaginal entrance.

Basal cell carcinoma Most common form of skin cancer.

Basal ganglia (basal nuclei) Nerve cell bodies deep within the white matter of the brain, which help control position and unconscious movements.

Basophil (**bay**-so-fill) A type of white blood cell that promotes inflammation and participates in allergic responses.

Benign (ben-**ine**) A non-cancerous neoplasm or tumour.

Benign prostatic enlargement (ben-**ine** pross-**ta**-tick) Enlargement of the prostate gland in older men.

Beri beri (berry-berry) A thiamine deficiency; includes dry or wet syndromes, cerebral beri beri and Wernicke–Korsakoff syndrome.

Beta cells Insulin-secreting cells of the endocrine pancreas.

Beta human chorionic gonadotrophin (corry-on-ick go-nad-oh-**trow**-phin) Hormone secreted during pregnancy.

Bile Substance secreted by the liver and necessary for fat digestion; consists of water, bile salts, cholesterol and bilirubin.

Biliary calculi (bill-ee-**ah**-ree cal-cue-**lie**) Gallstones; consist mainly of cholesterol, bilirubin and calcium.

Biliary cirrhosis (bill-ee-**ah**-ree sir-**oh**-siss) A form of cirrhosis resulting from cholecystitis.

Bilirubin (billy-**rue**-bin) A coloured pigment produced when haemoglobin breaks down.

Binary fission Process in which bacteria reproduce by splitting in half.

Binge Eating excessive amounts of food within a restricted period of time.

Biopsy Procedure in which a small sample of a tissue is surgically removed and examined microscopically for abnormalities.

Bipolar disorder Mood disorder associated with shifts from depression to mania. Includes three subcategories: bipolar I, bipolar II and cyclothymic disorder.

Blunted conduct Dull behaviour bearing no relationship to social signals; may occur in persons with schizophrenia.

Bowman's capsule A sac containing the glomerular capillaries; also called glomerular capsule.

Bradycardia (brad-ee-**card**-ee-ah) Heart rate of 60 beats per minute or less.

Bradykinesia (brad-ee-kin-**ee**-see-uh) Slowness of movement.

Bradykinin (brad-ee-**kine**-in) Substance released by damaged tissue that promotes inflammation.

Bronchi (**brong**-kye) Passageways that lead from the trachea to the lungs.

Bronchioles (**brong**-kee-olz) Small soft tissue tubules with smooth muscle wrappings that connect small bronchi to alveolar structures.

Bronchitis (brong-**kye**-tiss) Inflammation of the bronchi; may be acute or chronic.

Bronchogenic carcinoma (brong-coe-**jen**-ick car-sin-**oh**-ma) Most common type of lung cancer that arises from the bronchial tree.

Bronchopneumonia (brong-coe-new-**mow**-knee-ah) Type of pneumonia that may develop as a result of small bronchi becoming obstructed because of infection or aspirated gastric contents.

Bulbourethral glands (bulb-oh-you-**ree**-thrall) A pair of glands that secrete into the urethra as it enters the penis.

Bulimia nervosa (bull-**ee**-me-ah) Eating disorder characterised by episodes of excessive eating (binging), followed by purging, either through intentional vomiting or use of laxatives.

Bundle of His (hiss) The specialised tissue in heart muscle capable of sending the impulse for contraction to the ventricles.

Bursa (**ber**-sah) Sac of fluid situated near the joint to reduce friction on movement.

Bursitis (ber-**sigh**-tiss) Inflammation of the bursa.

Cachexia (kuh-**kex**-ee-ah) Condition caused when a patient becomes weak and emaciated in appearance owing to the rapid growth of a malignant tumour; also accompanies many chronic diseases like cancer, HIV/AIDS and tuberculosis.

Calcium Mineral essential for bone and tooth structure and for cell physiology.

Capsid Protein coat of viruses.

Carbuncles Clusters of boils.

Carcinogens (car-**sin**-oh-**jens**) Various chemicals that promote cancer development.

Carcinoma (car-sin-**oh**-mah) Type of cancer affecting epithelial tissues, skin and mucous membranes lining body cavities, or glandular tissue such as the breast, liver or pancreas.

Carcinoma in situ Premalignant lesion, the earliest stage of cancer in which the underlying tissue has not yet been invaded.

Cardiac catheterisation Procedure in which a catheter is passed into the heart through appropriate blood vessels to sample the blood in each chamber for oxygen content and pressure.

Cardiac cycle The alternate contraction and relaxation of atria and ventricles.

Cardiac sphincter (sf-**ink**-ter) Muscular gateway between the oesophagus and stomach.

Cardiogenic shock The result of extensive myocardial infarction; often fatal, but drugs to combat it are sometimes effective.

Cardiopulmonary resuscitation (CPR) Pertains to both heart and lung assistance by trained personnel to compress the chest rhythmically and breathe into victim's airway until medical services can be provided.

Carotene A plant pigment from which vitamin A is derived.

Caseous The term used to describe soft and cheese-like lung tissue in tuberculosis.

Casts Moulds of kidney tubules consisting of coagulated protein and blood.

Cataracts (**kat**-ah-rakts) Clouding of the eye lens to the point of opacity.

Catatonia (**kat**-a-tone-**ee**-ah) Motor disturbance that may occur in persons with schizophrenia.

Cell walls A rigid layer of organic material surrounding delicate cell membranes of bacteria.

Cell-mediated immunity Protection from infection provided by T cells.

Cellulitis Spreading skin infection caused by streptococci.

Cerebrospinal (sir-ree-brow-**spy**-nal) A term pertaining to the brain and spinal cord; cerebrospinal fluid bathes these organs.

Cerebrovascular accident (CVA) A stroke.

Chancre (cank-uh) An ulceration on the genitals in the primary stage of syphilis.

Chemotaxis (key-mow-**tax**-siss) The attraction of white blood cells to the site of inflammation.

Chemotherapy Systemic administration of medications to kill malignant cells.

Chlamydial infection (cla-**midd**-ee-all) Sexually transmitted disease caused by *Chlamydia trachomatis*.

Cholecystectomy (koh-lee-sis-**teck**-toe-me) The surgical removal of the gallbladder.

Cholelithiasis (koh-lee-lith-**eye**-ah-sis) The formation or presence of gallstones.

Cholesterol A fatty substance found in animal cell membranes.

Choriocarcinoma (core-ee-oh-car-sin-**oh**-ma) Malignant tumour of the placenta.

Chorionic gonadotrophin hormone (core-ee-**on**-ick go-nad-oh-trow-phin) The hormone that indicates a positive pregnancy test.

Chorionic villus sampling Genetic test involving the removal of cells from the villi through the cervix.

Chromosome A molecule of DNA found in the human cell. Each human cell contains 46 chromosomes divided into 23 pairs.

Chronic A disease that may begin insidiously and be long-lived.

Chronic fatigue syndrome A disease that produces flu-like symptoms, including severe and persistent fatigue, muscle and joint pain and fever.

Chronic obstructive pulmonary disease (COPD) The term used to describe a number of conditions, including chronic bronchitis and emphysema, in which the exchange of respiratory gases is ineffective.

Chronic ulcerative colitis A serious inflammation of the colon, the origin of which is unknown.

Chymotrypsin (chime-oh-**trip**-sin) A digestive enzyme that digests protein.

Cilia (**sill**-ee-ah) The hair-like projections found in the mucous membrane that lines the respiratory tract.

Ciliates A type of protozoa that moves using hair-like cilia.

Cirrhosis (si-**row**-siss) A chronic destruction of liver cells and tissues with a nodular, bumpy regeneration.

Coarctation (kow-arc-**tay**-shun) A narrowing, or stricture, of the aorta that provides blood to the entire body.

Cocci (cock-eye) Spherical bacterial cells.

Collagen A fibrous protein found in connective tissues, causing wounds to heal poorly.

Colostomy An artificial opening in the abdominal wall with a segment of the large intestine attached.

Communicable An infectious disease transmitted from human to human.

Comorbid The occurrence of two or more concurrent illnesses or conditions.

Compact bone Dense bone tissue surrounding most bones.

Complications Conditions that develop in a patient already suffering from a disease.

Compression sclerotherapy (sklair-**oh**-therapy) A treatment for varicose veins in which a strong saline solution is injected into specific sites within the vessel tract.

Computerised tomography (CT scan) A diagnostic imaging technique used to make diagnosis and determine the location of lesions or growths inside the body.

Concussion A transient disorder of the nervous system resulting from a violent blow on the head or from a fall.

Conduct disorder Disruptive behaviour disorder diagnosed in children.

Cone biopsy Procedure in which a cone-shaped wedge of abnormal tissue is removed from the cervix and examined under a microscope.

Congenital diseases Diseases that appear at birth or shortly after but are not caused by genetic or chromosomal abnormalities.

Conjunctiva (kon-**junk**-tye-vah) The membrane that lines the eyelids and covers the eyeball.

Conn's syndrome A form of hyperadrenalism in which aldosterone is excreted in excess.

Contagious An infectious disease transmitted from human to human.

Continuous positive airway pressure (CPAP) Nasal CPAP delivers air into the airway through a specially designed nasal mask or pillow; the flow of air creates enough pressure when inhaled to keep the airway open.

Contusion An injury to tissue without a breaking of the skin at the site of the trauma; also called a bruise.

Cor pulmonale (**kor** pull-mun-**ah**-lee) A serious heart condition in which the right side of the heart fails as a result of longstanding chronic lung disease.

Coronary arteriography (ah-tear-ee-**og**-raff-ee) The selective injection of contrast material into coronary arteries for a film recording of blood vessel action.

Corpus luteum (**kor**-pus-loo-tea-um) The structure that develops from the ovarian follicle after ovulation.

Cortisol The principal hormone in the group of steroid hormones, also known as hydrocortisone; stress increases production of cortisol.

Cortisone A hormone of the adrenal gland that has anti-inflammatory properties.

C reactive protein An actue phase protein which binds to some bacteria, acting as a marker of acute infection when measured in blood tests.

Creatinine (cree-**at**-eh-neen) Nitrogen-containing waste products of protein metabolism.

Cretinism (kret-in-**is**-um) A congenital thyroid deficiency in which thyroxine is not synthesised.

Cri du chat syndrome (**cree** duh shat) A hereditary disease resulting from the deletion of part of the short arm of chromosome 5; the name comes from the characteristic cat-like cry.

Crohn's disease (**krones**) An inflammatory disease of the intestine in which the intestinal walls become thick and rigid.

Croup Characterised by a loud cough that resembles the barking of a seal, difficulty breathing, and a grunting noise or wheezing during breathing.

Cryosurgery (cry-oh) A technique that uses extreme cold to freeze and destroy skin conditions and tumours.

Cryptorchidism (kript-**ork**-id-ism) The failure of the testes to descend from the abdominal cavity, where they develop during fetal life, to the scrotum.

CT scan Computed tomography scan; 3-D computer-aided X-ray.

Cushing's syndrome A condition resulting from excessive levels of glucocorticoid hormones.

Cyanosis (sign-ah-**noh**-siss) A bluish colour of the skin and the mucous membranes owing to insufficient oxygen in the blood.

Cyclins Cell cycle proteins.

Cyst (sist) A sac or capsule containing fluid; usually harmless.

Cystic fibrosis (sis-tick fye-**broe**-siss) A disease that affects all the exocrine glands of the body, the glands of external secretion usually affecting children.

Cystitis (sis-**tie**-siss) An inflammation of the urinary bladder, commonly called a bladder infection.

Cystocele (sis-**toe**-seal) Urinary bladder is displaced into the vagina.

Cystoscope (sis-**toe**-scope) An endoscope (lighted scope) through which the interior of the urinary bladder is made visible for observation.

Cytotoxic T cells T cells, often called *killer cells* because of their capability to kill invading organisms.

Decubitus ulcers (dee-**kyoo**-bih-tus **ul**-sir) Bedsores that typically occur on the bony areas of the body.

Defibrillator A machine that delivers electrical shocks used to re-establish normal heart rhythm.

Delirium tremens A medical emergency caused by heavy drinking over a long period of time; may occur after withdrawal from heavy alcohol intake.

Delusion False beliefs associated with various mental illnesses.

Dementia Organic loss of intellectual functions.

Deoxyribonucleic acid (DNA) (dee-**ox**-ee-**rye**-bow-new-clee-ick Asid) The blueprint for protein synthesis within the cell.

Dermatitis (der-ma-**tie**-tiss) A non-contagious skin disorder.

Dermatophytes (der-**mat**-oh-fights) Fungi that infect the skin and tend to live on the dead, top layer.

Desensitise A procedure for causing tolerance to allergens so that they do not trigger allergic reactions.

Diabetes insipidus A disease that results from a deficiency of ADH.

Diabetes mellitus An endocrine disease in which the beta cells fail to secrete insulin or target cells fail to respond to insulin.

Diabetic nephropathy A kidney disease resulting from diabetes mellitus.

Diagnosis (dye-ahg-**noh**-siss) The determination of the nature of a disease based on many factors, including signs, symptoms and, often, laboratory results.

Diaphragm (**dye**-uh-fram) Primary muscle for inspiration that divides the thorax and abdominopelvic cavities.

Diastole (dye-**ass**-toe-lee) The period of the heartbeat when the heart relaxes and fills with blood.

Diethylstilbestrol (DES) (dye-thile-still-**best**-roll) A synthetic hormone used in the 1950s and early 1960s to prevent spontaneous abortion.

Discoid The mild form of lupus erythematosus in which red, raised, itchy lesions develop.

Disease (dih-**zeez**) A state of functional disequilibrium that may be resolved by recovery or death.

Disinfection Reducing the risk of infection or contamination.

Diuretic (dye-you-**ret**-ik) A substance that causes the kidneys to excrete water; can be administered as a drug to lower blood pressure.

Diverticula (dye-ver-**tick**-you-lar) Little pouches or sacs formed when the mucosal lining pushes through the underlying muscle layer.

Diverticulitis (dye-ver-**tick**-you-**lie**-tiss) Inflammation of the diverticula, usually occurring in the colon or small intestines.

DNA repair genes Also known as caretaker genes, these are genes responsible for the repair of errors in normal DNA replication.

Dominant A gene that is expressed when inherited.

Dopamine (dope-**er**-mean) A neuronal transmitter substance.

Doppler echocardiography Instrument that uses echoes of moving blood columns to produce images of the vessel wall outline; the velocity of the blood is measured and the degree of carotid stenosis is determined.

Down's syndrome Chromosomal disorder that causes cognitive impairment; also called trisomy 21.

Duodenal ulcers (dew-oh-**dean**-all) Ulcers of the small intestine caused by an excessive secretion of hydrochloric acid and *Helicobacter pylori* infection.

Duodenum (dew-oh-**dean**-um) First section of the small intestine; receives digested material from the stomach.

Dysentery (diss-**un**-tree) An acute inflammation of the colon, a colitis.

Dysmenorrhoea (diss-men-or-ree-er) Painful or difficult menses.

Dyspareunia (diss-par-rune-ee-ah) Painful sexual intercourse.

Dysphagia (diss-**fage**-ee-ah) Difficult or painful swallowing.

Dyspnoea (disp-near) Air hunger resulting in laboured or difficult breathing.

Dysthymia (diss-**thigh**-me-ah) Chronic, persistent depression for a period of at least 2 years.

Dystrophin (diss-**trow**-fin) A skeletal protein that is missing in Duchenne's muscular dystrophy.

Dystrophy (diss-**trow**-fee) Muscle degeneration that disables an individual.

Dysuria (diss-**yur**-ee-ah) Painful urination.

Ecchymoses (eck-ee-**mow**-sees) Haemorrhagic spots that develop on the skin and in mucous membranes, causing discolouration.

Echocardiography A non-invasive procedure (ultrasound cardiography) that utilises high frequency sound waves to examine the size, shape and motion of heart structures.

Eclampsia (ee-**clamp**-see-ah) Convulsions and coma that follow untreated pregnancy-induced hypertension.

Ectopic pregnancy A pregnancy in which the fertilised ovum implants in a tissue other than the uterus, most commonly in the Fallopian tubes.

Eczema (ex-ma) A non-contagious inflammatory skin disorder.

Electrocardiogram (ECG) An electrical recording of the heart action that aids in the diagnosis of coronary artery disease, myocardial infarction, valvular heart disease and some congenital heart diseases.

Electroencephalogram (EEG) (ee-lek-trow-**en**-keffa-low-gram) A recording of brain waves.

Electrolyte balance The proper balance of salts, like potassium and calcium.

Electromyography (EMG) (ee-lek-trow-my-**og**-ruf-ee) A diagnostic procedure to establish the presence or extent of disease or nerve damage.

Embolism (em-boll-**is**-um) A circulating blood clot.

Emphysema (em-fuh-**see**-muh) A crippling, non-contagious disease of chronic lung obstruction and destruction.

Encephalin (en-**keff**-al-in) Naturally occurring molecules in the brain that attach to special receptors in the brain and spinal cord to stop pain messages. These are the same receptors that respond to morphine and other opioid analgesics.

Encephalitis (en-**keff**-al-eye-tiss) The inflammation of the brain and meninges, caused by a viral infection.

Encephalomyelitis (en-**keff**-al-oh-my-**lie**-tiss) Acute inflammation of the brain and spinal cord.

Endarterectomy (end-ah-ter-**eck**-toe-me) A common surgical procedure used to treat a blockage in an artery by removing the thickened area of the inner vascular lining.

Endemic Describes a disease that is always present at low levels in a population.

Endocarditis (end-oh-card-**eye**-tiss) Inflammation within the heart.

Endocardium (end-oh-**card**-ee-um) A smooth delicate membrane that lines chambers of the heart.

Endogenous (en-**dodge**-in-uss) Originating or produced within an organism, tissue or cell.

Endometriosis (end-oh-me-tree-**oh**-siss) Condition in which endometrial tissue from the uterus becomes embedded elsewhere.

Endorphins (en-**door**-fins) Naturally occurring molecules made up of amino acids, the building blocks of proteins. Endorphins attach to special receptors in the brain and spinal cord to stop pain messages. These are the same receptors that respond to morphine and other opioid analgesics.

Endoscope An instrument consisting of a hollow tube with a lens and light system used to view the inner surface of the digestive tract.

Endoscopic sclerotherapy A procedure used to guide a retractable needle device through an area such as the oesophagus to seal off vessels such as oesophageal varices with a hardening agent.

Endoscopy Imaging technique using flexible tubing mounted with camera and surgical tools.

Endospores Structures produced by bacteria and formed to cope with harsh environmental conditions.

Endotoxins A bacterial toxin that is only released when the bacterial cells are damaged. Toxins can cause damage to other animal species and can cause some disease.

Enuresis (en-yure-**ee**-sis) Commonly called bed-wetting; a disorder of elimination that involves the voluntary or involuntary release of urine into bedding, clothing or other inappropriate places.

Eosinophilia-myalgia syndrome (ee-oh-**sin**-oh-fee-lee-ah my-**al**-jar) Multisystem disease with pain, fatigue and elevations of circulating blood eosinophils.

Eosinophils (ee-oh-**sin**-oh-filz) White blood cells that kill parasites and are involved in allergic responses.

Ephelides Freckles.

Epidemic The occurrence of a disease in unusually large numbers over a specific area.

Epidemiological studies Population-based studies.

Epididymis (epi-**did**-ee-miss) A coiled tube that lies along the outer wall of the testis and leads into the vas deferens.

Epididymitis (epi-**did**-ee-**my**-tiss) Inflammation of the epididymis.

Epidural (ep-ee-**dure**-all) A haemorrhage between the dura mater and the skull.

Epilepsy A group of uncontrolled cerebral discharges that recur at random intervals.

Epinephrine (ep-ee-**neff**-rinn) The hormone secreted by the adrenal medulla in emergency situations or during periods of high stress; also used as a drug to dilate bronchioles in some asthma attacks. Also called adrenaline.

Erectile dysfunction The inability of a man to obtain an erection of sufficient strength for sexual activity.

Erysipelas (err-ee-**sip**-eh-luss) An inflammatory skin infection caused by streptococcus bacteria. Most commonly, the infections appear on the face, arm or leg.

Erythema (eh-ree-**thee**-ma) A reddened area of skin.

Erythematous (eh-ree-**them**-at-us) An area of skin reddened by congested blood vessels resulting from injury or inflammation.

Erythrocytes (eh-**rith**-roh-sights) Red blood cells.

Erythropoiesis (eh-**rith**-roh-poy-**ee**-sis) The process of red cell formation that takes place in the red marrow of flat bones such as the sternum, hip bones, ribs and skull bones.

Erythropoietin (eh-**rith**-roh-poy-**ee**-tin) A hormone synthesised principally by the kidney that stimulates red blood cell development.

Essential trace minerals Minerals required in the diet in very low amounts.

Exacerbation The period of a chronic disease when signs and symptoms recur in all their severity.

Exocrine glands The glands of external secretion. They secrete mucus, perspiration and digestive enzymes.

Exophthalmia (ex-op-**thal**-me-ah) The condition in which the eyeballs protrude outward, characteristic of a person with Graves' disease.

Exotoxins A bacterial toxin released by some bacterial cells.

Extradural A haemorrhage between the dura mater and the skull.

Familial hypercholesterolaemia (high-per-coll-est-erol-lee-me-ah) An autosomal dominant disorder caused by a mutation in the gene encoding the receptor for low density lipoproteins.

Familial polyposis A hereditary disease in which numerous polyps develop in the intestinal tract.

Female arousal-orgasmic dysfunction Lack of sexual desire or response in a female.

Fibrillation Quivering or spontaneously uncoordinated contraction of muscle fibres, such as heart ventricles.

Fibrin (fye-**brinn**) A plasma protein essential for blood clotting.

Fibroblasts (fye-bro-blasts) Connective tissue cells that produce fibres to aid in healing damaged tissue.

Fibrocystic disease (fye-bro-**siss**-tick) The formation of numerous fluid-filled lumps in the breast.

Fimbriae (**fim**-bree-ay) Finger-like projections at the outer ends of the Fallopian tubes, which propel ova into the tube.

Flagella Whip-like cell appendages used for locomotion.

Flagellates A type of protozoa that moves using whip-like appendages called flagella.

Flatus Intestinal gas.

Flatworm A worm-like animal that has a flattened body.

Fluoroscopy (floor-**oss**-cop-ee) A diagnostic procedure that permits visualisation of the lungs and diaphragm during respiration.

Folliculitis (foll-**ick**-you-light-iss) Inflammation of hair follicles caused by staphylococci.

Foramen ovale A small opening that allows blood from the right side of the heart to enter the left side directly, bypassing the non-functional fetal lungs.

Fragile X syndrome A sex-linked disorder associated with mental retardation. It is identified by a break or weakness on the long arm of the X chromosome.

Free radicals The molecules that may cause disease by injuring cells.

Friable Easily broken nodules or vegetations.

Fulminating Having a rapid or severe onset.

Functional Condition is one in which there is no organic change.

Furuncles (fern-ickles) Large, tender, swollen raised lesions, boils, caused by staphylococci.

Galactosaemia (galacto-**seem**-ee-ah) An autosomal recessive disorder in which the enzyme necessary to convert galactose, a sugar derived from lactose in milk, to glucose is lacking.

Gamma-aminobutyric acid (GABA) (gamma-a-**mee**-no-bue-**Tirrick**) Inhibitory neurotransmitter associated with various mental illnesses, sleep, mood and behaviour.

Gangrene Condition in which bacteria infects and destroys dead tissue.

Gastric ulcers Ulcers of the stomach.

Gastritis Inflammation of the stomach caused by irritants such as aspirin, excessive coffee, tobacco, alcohol or an infection.

Gastro-oesophageal reflux disease (gastro-eh-**soff**-ah-jeel) Regurgitation of acidic stomach contents into the oesophagus.

Gastroscopy A procedure in which a camera is attached to a gastroscope, and the entire inner stomach is photographed.

Genes Found in chromosomes; each is responsible for the synthesis of one protein.

Genital herpes Sexually transmitted infection caused by herpes simplex virus type 2.

Genital warts Sexually transmitted infection caused by the human papillomavirus.

Gigantism Usually the result of a tumour of the anterior pituitary.

Glioblastomas (gly-oh-blast-**oh**-mah) Highly malignant, rapid-growing tumours of the brain.

Glioma (gly-**oh**-mah) A sarcoma of neuroglial tissue or glial cells.

Glomerular capsule (glom-er-**roo**-lar cap-sule) Structure surrounding the glomerular capillaries of the nephron.

Glomerulonephritis (glom-er-**roo**-low-**neff**-right-iss) A degenerative inflammation of the glomerulus of a nephron, which usually follows a prior streptococcal infection.

Glomerulus (glom-er-**roo**-luss) A tuft of capillaries situated inside the glomerular capsule of a nephron.

Glucagon A hormone that works antagonistically to insulin and is released when the blood sugar level falls below normal.

Glucocorticoids (glue-co-**caught**-ee-coids) The group of steroid hormones that helps regulate carbohydrate, lipid and protein metabolism.

Glycogen (**gly**-co-jin) A form of glucose that is stored in the liver and muscle.

Glycosuria (gly-**koss**-yure-ear) The condition in which excess glucose is excreted in the urine, a major sign of diabetes mellitus.

Gonadotrophins (go-nad-oh-**trow**-fins) Hormones of the anterior pituitary that regulate sexual development and function.

Gonorrhoea (**gone**-oh-rear) Sexually transmitted infection caused by *Neisseria gonorrhoeae*.

Gout Often called 'gouty arthritis', it affects the joints of the feet, particularly those of the big toe and is very painful.

Graafian follicles Ovarian follicles stimulated by a pituitary gonadotrophic hormone at the beginning of each monthly cycle so that they begin to grow and develop.

Gram stain The staining technique that permits the identification of bacteria.

Grandiose delusion A false belief of having special power, influence or wealth.

Gynaecomastia (guy-nay-coe-**mass**-tee-ah) A condition in which the breasts become enlarged.

Haemangioma (he-man-**gee**-ohm-ah) Benign tumour made of small blood vessels that forms a red or purple birthmark.

Haematemesis (hema-**temma**-siss) Vomiting of blood.

Haematocrit (he-**mat**-oh-crit) The ratio of red blood cell volume to whole blood.

Haematoma (he-mat-**oh**-ma) A bruise caused by an injection.

Haematuria (he-mat-**yure**-ree-ah) Blood in the urine.

Haemodialysis (he-mow-die-**al**-ee-siss) Treatment for kidney failure; blood removed from the body is cleansed of metabolic waste, restored to physiological balance and returned to the body.

Haemoglobin (he-mow-**gloh**-binn) A protein containing iron; serves as the oxygen carrier protein that enables red blood cells to carry oxygen from the lungs to all body tissues.

Haemolyse (he-mow-lies) Lysis of erythrocytes.

Haemolysis (he-mow-**lie**-siss) The rupture of red blood cells.

Haemolytic streptococci (he-mow-lit-ick strep-toe-**cock**-eye) A type of bacteria that cause a variety of infectious diseases, including infections of throat, skin, ear and heart valves.

Haemophilia (he-mow-**fill**-ee-ah) Sex-linked inherited coagulation disorder caused by a deficiency of clotting factors.

Haemoptysis (he-**mop**-tiss-iss) Coughing blood.

Haemorrhage (hem-or-idge) A large loss of blood in a short period of time, either internally or externally.

Haemorrhoids (hem-or-oids) Varicose veins of the rectum or anus.

Haemostasis (he-mow-**stay**-siss) Reduced blood flow.

Hallucination Disturbance in sensory perception in sight, sound, touch or smell.

Health A state of relative equilibrium in which the body's many organ systems function adequately and are free from disease.

Heart block Impulses are prevented from flowing from the atria to the ventricles because of a damaged route (e.g. MI), and thus the heart rate and ECG are altered.

Heart murmurs Characteristic sounds of the heart that indicate the presence of valve defects.

Helicobacter pylori A bacterium associated with ulcers.

Helper T cells T cells that help the immune system by increasing the activity of killer cells and stimulating the suppressor T cells.

Hemiplegia (hemmy-**plee**-jee-ah) Paralysis on one side of the body.

Heparin An anticoagulant.

Hepatic coma Develops in the final stages of advanced liver disease; it is caused by an accumulation of ammonia in the blood, which has a toxic effect on the brain and may cause death.

Hepatocarcinoma (hep-at-oh-car-sin-**oh**-ma) Cancer of the liver.

Hepatomegaly (hep-at-oh-**meg**-al-ee) Enlarged liver.

Hereditary haemorrhagic telangiectasia (hem-or-a-jick-tell-**an**-jee-eck-**tay**-see-ah) Abnormal dilatation of small vessels causing the appearance of red–violet lesions on the face, lips and oral and nasal mucosa.

Hermaphrodites (herm-**aff**-row-dites) Individuals who have both testes and ovaries.

Heterozygous (hetta-row-**zye**-goats) A person having two different alleles of a certain gene.

Hiatal hernia The protrusion of part of the stomach through the diaphragm at the point where the oesophagus joins the stomach.

High density lipoproteins (HDL) (lie-poe-proteins) The smallest lipoprotein particles containing the smallest amount of triglycerides; 'good' cholesterol.

Hippocampus Structure of the brain that processes and stores information to memory.

Hirsutism (hers-**ute**-ism) Condition in which excess hair develops on the face of a woman.

Histamine (**hist**-ar-mean) Released by basophils. Histamine dilates blood vessels and increases blood flow to damaged tissue. Allows protein molecules to leak out of blood vessels into the surrounding tissue. This produces redness and swelling.

Histology The study of cells.

Hodgkin's disease A type of lymphoma, distinguished by the presence of characteristic Reed–Sternberg cells in affected lymph nodes.

Homeostasis (hoh-mee-oh-**stay**-siss) State of equilibrium of the internal environment of the body, including fluid balance, acid–base balance, temperature, metabolism, etc. to maintain a steady state within the body.

Homozygous (homo-**zye**-gus) A person having the same two alleles of a particular gene.

Hordeolum (hord-ee-**oh**-lum) An infection of the sebaceous gland of the eyelid.

Horizontal transmission The route by which an infectious disease is transmitted directly from an infected human to a susceptible human.

Hormones (**hor**-moans) Chemical messengers secreted by endocrine glands.

Human chorionic gonadotrophin (HCG) Hormone secreted by the chorionic villi after implantation of the fertilised ovum in the uterus.

Human immunodeficiency virus (HIV) The causative agent of AIDS; a retrovirus – that is, it carries its genetic information as RNA rather than DNA.

Human papillomavirus (HPV) (pap-ill-**oh**-ma-virus) The type of virus responsible for genital warts that seems to be the causative agent in uterine cervical carcinoma.

Humoral immunity Protection from infection provided by antibodies.

Huntington's chorea (**kor**-ear) A progressive degenerative disease of the brain that results in the loss of muscle control.

Hydatidiform mole (high-dat-**tidi**-form) A benign tumour of the placenta, consisting of multiple cysts and resembling a bunch of grapes.

Hydrocephalus (high-drow-**keff**-al-us) The accumulation of cerebrospinal fluid in the brain.

Hydrocortisone (high-drow-**caught**-is-own) Anti-inflammatory agent.

Hydrolithotripsy (high-drow-**lith**-oh-trip-see) A procedure using sonic vibrations to crush kidney stones while the patient is immersed in a tank of water.

Hydronephrosis (high-drow-**neff**-row-siss) A condition when the kidney is extremely dilated with urine.

Hydroureters (high-drow-yure-**eat**-ers) The condition caused when the ureters above a kidney obstruction dilate.

Hymen A membranous fold that partly or completely closes the vaginal opening.

Hyperactive The term used to describe when a gland produces an excessive amount of its secretion.

Hyperaemia Increased blood flow to an injured area, causing heat and redness associated with inflammation.

Hypercalcaemia (high-per-cal-**see**-me-er) A condition in which too much calcium occurs in the blood.

Hyperemesis gravidarum (high-per-em-ee-sis grav-id-ar-um) Excessive vomiting during pregnancy.

Hyperglycaemia (high-per-gly-**see**-me-ah) A condition resulting from deposits of calcium in organs such as kidneys, heart, lungs and the walls of the stomach.

Hyperkalaemia (high-per-cal-**ee**-me-ah) An excess of potassium, which causes muscle weakness and can slow the heart to the point of cardiac arrest.

Hypernephroma (high-per-neff-**row**-ma) Carcinoma of the kidney; causes enlargement of kidney and destroys the organ.

Hyperpituitarism (high-per-pit-**you**-it-air-ism) Condition associated with hypersecretion of the pituitary, usually manifested as the effects of excessive growth hormone, which retards the normal closure of bones at puberty.

Hypersensitivity An abnormal immune response and sensitivity to allergens such as pollens, dust, dog hair and certain foods.

Hypertension High blood pressure (diastolic greater than 95 mmHg).

Hypertrophy Abnormal enlargement of an organ.

Hypoactive When a gland fails to secrete its hormone or secretes an inadequate amount.

Hypoalbuminaemia (high-poh-al-bue-**meen**-ee-me-ah) An albumin deficiency.

Hypochromic (high-poh-**crow**-mick) Red blood cells appear lighter than normal, caused by an iron deficiency.

Hypophysis (high-**poff**-i-siss) Another name for the pituitary gland; has two parts, each of which acts as a separate gland.

Hypothalamus (high-poh-**thal**-a-muss) The homeostatic centre for the body, located just superior to the pituitary; controls thirst, temperature and other functions, as well as release of pituitary hormones.

Hypovolaemic shock (high-poh-vol-**ee**-mick) Results from fluid volume loss after severe haemorrhage or loss of plasma in burn patients.

Hypoxia (high-**pox**-ee-ar) Decreased concentration of oxygen in the blood owing to low oxygen availability or blockages that prevent oxygen diffusing into the bloodstream.

Hysterectomy Surgical removal of the uterus.

Icterus Jaundiced, yellow colouration.

Idiopathic Describes a disease for which the cause is not known.

Idiopathic hypereosinophilic syndrome (high-per-eh-oh-**sin**-oh-**fill**-ick) Mulitsystem disease associated with persistent increases in blood eosinophils.

Immunity The ability of the body to defend itself against infectious agents, foreign cells and abnormal body cells.

Immunoglobulin (im-yune-oh-**glob**-you-lin) Antibodies.

Impetigo An acute, contagious skin infection common in children, most frequently affecting face and hands.

Impotence Inability to achieve and maintain an erection sufficient for sexual intercourse (more commonly known as erectile dysfunction).

In situ In position; not disturbing surrounding tissues.

Incidence The number of new cases of a disease in a population.

Incontinence Inability to retain urine or faeces owing to loss of sphincter control or because of cerebral or spinal lesions.

Infarct (in-**farkt**) Dead tissue that occurs owing to lack of blood flow in any organ or area, such as a coronary blockage in a heart vessel.

Infectious diseases Diseases caused by pathogenic micro-organisms.

Infestations Infections involving worm-like animals called helminths.

Inflammatory exudate (**ex**-you-date) Fluid composed of plasma and white cells that escape from capillaries.

Influenza A viral infection of the upper respiratory system.

Initiation The first stage of cancer in which there is a genetic change in a cell, an altering of the DNA by some agent, chemical, radiation or an oncogenic virus.

Insulin A hormone that is secreted when the blood sugar level rises.

Insulin shock Hypoglycaemic shock that results from too much insulin, not enough food or excessive exercise.

Interferon (in-ter-**fear**-on) A group of substances that stimulates the immune system.

Interleukins A term for chemicals produced by leukocytes, also referred to as cytokines.

Intrapleural pressure (in-tra-**plur**-al) The pressure within the pleural cavity.

Intravenous pyelogram (in-tra-venus **pie**-low-gram) Allows the visualisation of the urinary system by means of contrast dyes injected into the veins, followed by an X-ray examination.

Intrinsic factor Produced in the stomach, it carries vitamin B_{12} to the small intestine, where it is absorbed into the bloodstream.

Intussusception (in-tuss-suss-**sep**-shun) A type of organic obstruction in which a segment of intestine telescopes into the part forward of it.

In vitro research Research conducted in a laboratory.

Irritable bowel A functional condition of the colon with diarrhoea, constipation, abdominal pain and gas.

Irritable colon A functional disorder of the colon that results in diarrhoea and cramping.

Ischaemia (iss-skee-me-ah) A deficiency of blood supply to any organ.

Isolation Keeping an infected person in the hospital or staying at home in bed when suffering from a disease as a way of controlling the transmission of infectious diseases.

Jaundice A yellow–orange discolouration of the skin, tissues and the whites of the eyes caused when bilirubin (an orange pigment) accumulates in the plasma.

Kaposi's sarcoma Purple neoplasm of the lower extremities.

Karyotype (carry-oh-type) The normal chromosomal composition of the nucleus of the cell that is characteristic of each species.

Keloid (key-loid) The healing that occurs after surgery or a severe burn, consisting of a hard, raised scar.

Keratin (**care**-ah-tin) Protein in the epidermis produced by cells called keratinocytes; protects the skin from harmful substances.

Ketone bodies (key-tone) Substances produced in diabetics' blood when insulin levels are low.

Kidney dialysis Treatment for kidney failure; removes metabolic waste from blood and restores it to physiological balance.

Klinefelter's syndrome (Cline-felt-ers) A condition in which there is an extra sex chromosome resulting in a karyotype of 47XXY.

Kupffer cells (cup-fur) Specialised cells that line the blood spaces within the liver. They engulf and digest bacteria and other foreign substances, thus cleansing the blood.

Kwashiorkor (quosh-ick-or) Protein-calorie malnutrition that results from early weaning from breast milk.

Laparoscopy A procedure in which an illuminated tube is inserted through a small incision or opening; used to diagnose endometriosis.

Larynx (la-rinks) The voice box located at the entrance of the trachea.

Latent infection A condition caused when viruses insert themselves in cells and do not reproduce.

Legionnaire's disease A lung infection caused by the bacterium *Legionella pneumophila*; characterised by flu-like symptoms.

Leiomyomas (leo-my-**oh**-mars) Benign tumours of the smooth muscle of the uterus, known as fibroid tumours.

Lesion (**lee**-shun) An abnormal tissue structure or function. May be the result of a wound, injury or pathological condition.

Lethargy A condition of drowsiness.

Leucocytes (loo-koh-**sights**) White blood cells. There are five different types of mature leucocytes: neutrophils, eosinophils, basophils, lymphocytes and monocytes.

Leucocytosis (loo-koh-**sigh**-tow-siss) The excessive production of white cells.

Leucorrhoea (loo-**koh**-re-ah) White, foul-smelling vaginal discharge.

Leukaemia (loo-**key**-me-uh) A cancer of white blood cells in which the bone marrow produces a large number of abnormal white blood cells.

Ligament The substance that holds bones together.

Lipase A digestive enzyme that breaks down lipid or fat.

Lipoma Tumour that develops in adipose or fat tissue.

Lipoprotein A water-soluble lipid fat. It is packaged into particles that contain blood proteins, which do mix with water.

Lithotripsy (**lith**-oh-trip-see) A procedure using sonic vibrations to crush kidney stones; the patient is not immersed in water for the procedure.

Low density lipoproteins (LDL) The larger lipoprotein particles containing triglycerides; 'bad' cholesterol.

Lumbar puncture Procedure in which a hollow needle is inserted into the spinal canal between vertebrae near the L4, or lumbar region, to obtain and analyse cerebrospinal fluid; also known as a spinal tap.

Lumen The inner space of a hollow organ such as a blood vessel or intestine.

Lumpectomy Surgery to remove only the tumour from the breast.

Lymphadenopathy (limf-**add**-en-opathy) Enlarged lymph nodes.

Lymphatic system (limf-**at**-ik) An important part of the body's immunity, it consists of nodes, organs and a complex network of thin-walled capillaries carrying lymph fluid to help to maintain the internal fluid environment of the body.

Lymphocytes (limf-oh-sites) A type of white blood cell consisting of T lymphocytes and B lymphocytes.

Lymphocytic (limf-oh-**sit**-ick) The type of leukaemia that results from cancer of the lymphocytic stem cells, found in both the bone marrow and the lymph nodes.

Lymphoma (limf-oh-ma) Malignancy of the lymphatic system.

Lyse (lies) The infecting of cells by viruses.

Macular Flat lesions on the skin.

Magnetic resonance imaging (MRI) A diagnostic imaging technique that uses the behaviour of protons when placed in powerful magnetic fields to make images of organs and tissues.

Major depression Mood disorder associated with sadness, hopelessness and despair.

Malabsorption The inability of a person to absorb substances from the small intestine.

Malignancy (ma-**lig**-nan-see) A cancerous tumour that can invade and destroy nearby tissue, and that may metastasise to other organs or parts of the body.

Malignant (ma-**lig**-nant) Term used to describe a neoplasm or tumour that spreads and possibly causes death.

Malignant melanoma (ma-**lig**-nant-mella-**no**-ma) The most serious skin cancer; arises from the melanocytes.

Malnutrition Suboptimal supply of nutrients that results in decreased tissue mass and energy stores needed for proper growth and development.

Mammography Diagnostic X-ray for breast tissue that can detect even small, early cancers.

Mania An overly energetic elevated or irritable mood.

Marasmus Protein-calorie malnutrition caused by near starvation.

Marfan syndrome An autosomal dominant disorder that results from the dysfunction of the gene that codes for the connective tissue protein fibrillin.

Mast cells Cells found in connective tissue; they contain heparin, serotonin, bradykinin and histamine.

Mastectomy Surgery to remove the breast due to cancer.

Mastoiditis (mass-toid-**eye**-tiss) Inflammation of the air cells in the mastoid process of the temporal bone.

Medullary cavity (me-**dull**-lah-ree) A hollow cavity found in the long bones of the arms and legs that is filled with yellow bone marrow primarily consisting of fat.

Melaena (mell-**ee**-na) Stool with a dark, tarry appearance caused by blood from the upper part of the digestive tract.

Melanin (**mell**-an-in) The dark pigment of the skin that protects the body from the harmful rays of the sun.

Melanocytes (mell-**an**-oh-sights) Cells at the bottom of the epidermis that produce melanin.

Melanoma Skin cancer.

Melasma Patches of dark skin on the cheeks that develop owing to hormonal changes.

Memory cells B lymphocytes that do not become plasma cells but remain dormant until reactivated by the same antigen.

Menarche (men-are-shay) The onset of menstruation, signalling the start of a woman's reproductive years; occurs generally between ages 10 and 15.

Meninges (men-**in**-jeez) Three coverings that protect the delicate nerve tissue of the spinal cord and brain.

Meningioma (men-**in**-jee-oh-ma) A benign tumour that occurs in the membranes that surround the brain.

Meningitis (men-in-**jye**-tiss) An acute inflammation of the first two meninges that cover the brain and spinal cord.

Meningocele (men-**in**-jo-seal) A form of spina bifida noticeable at birth; the spinal cord is not involved in this defect.

Meningomyelocele (men-**in**-jo-**my**-low-seal) A form of spina bifida in which the nerve elements protrude into the sac and are trapped, thus preventing proper placement and development.

Menopause The cessation of menstrual periods, the ending of a woman's reproductive years; usually begins in the late 40s or early 50s.

Menorrhagia (men-or-**rage**-ee-ah) Excessive or prolonged bleeding during menstruation.

Mesothelioma (me-so-thee-lee-**oh**-ma) Cancer of the membrane that covers and protects most of the internal organs of the body.

Metastasis (meh-**tass**-ta-siss) The spread of cancer to distant sites within the body.

Metastasise (meh-**tass**-ta-size) To invade by metastasis.

Metrorrhagia (metro-**rage**-ee-ah) Bleeding between menstrual periods or extreme irregularity of the cycle.

Mineralocorticoids (mineral-oh-caught-ee-coids) A group of steroid hormones that regulate salt balance in the body.

Mitral stenosis Occurs when the mitral valve opening is too small and the cusps that form the valve become rigid and fuse together.

Mitral valve The valve between the left atrium and left ventricle; it has two flaps, or cusps, that meet when the valve is closed.

Mixed cancers Cancer consisting of cells of different origins or tissue types.

Monocyte (mono-site) A type of white blood cell that aids in clearing pus.

Morbidity The number who become sick or disabled from a disease per 100 000 within a population.

Mortality The number who die from a disease per 100 000 who have the disease within a population.

Mucosa Secretes excessive mucus, causing a runny nose and congestion.

Mucus Secretions from the mucous membranes; can be thick or watery.

Mutagens Chemicals introduced to the lungs by cigarette smoking.

Mutations Changes in DNA structure that may be inherited and cause disease.

Myasthenia gravis (my-as-**thee**-nee-ah graa-viss) An autoimmune neuromuscular disorder characterised by muscular fatigue that develops with repetitive muscle use and improves with rest.

Mycelia (my-**see**-lee-ah) Filaments in fungi specialised for absorption of nutrients.

Mycoses (my-**coe**-sees) Infectious diseases caused by fungi.

Myelin (**my**-lin) A lipid covering that insulates the fibres of sensory and motor neurons.

Myelocele (**my**-low-seal) The most severe form of spina bifida.

Myelogenous (my-**lodge**-en-uss) The type of leukaemia in which the cancer originates in the bone marrow.

Myelomonocytic leukaemia (my-low-mono-**sit**-ick) A type of myelogenous leukaemia of malignant monocytes.

Myocardial infarction A heart attack.

Myocardium The cardiac muscle found in the chamber walls of the heart.

Myoma A tumour of the muscle that develops in smooth or involuntary muscle.

Myopia (my-**oh**-lee-ah) A visual defect in which distant objects appear blurred because their images are focused in front of the retina rather than on it.

Myxoedema (mix-oh-**dee**-ma) The condition of severe hypothyroidism, an inadequate level of thyroxine.

Natural killer cells A type of leucocyte that destroys cells with abnormal membranes.

Nebuliser A device used to administer medication in a liquid mist to the airways.

Necrotic (neh-**kroh**-tick) Dead tissue caused by lack of blood flow to the area.

Negative feedback Homeostatic control mechanism.

Neoplasm A mass of new cells that grows in a haphazard fashion with no useful function; a tumour.

Nephron (**neff**-ron) The functional unit of the kidney.

Neurofibrillatory tangle Abnormal collection of protein in the brain associated with Alzheimer's disease.

Neurogenic bladder (new-row-**jen**-ic) A condition in which the nerves of the urinary system don't work properly when the bladder is full and may allow urine leakage.

Neurogenic shock (new-row-**jen**-ic) Condition caused by generalised vasodilatation resulting from decreased vasomotor tone.

Neuron (**new**-ron) Nerve cell.

Neurotransmitter (new-row-**trans**-mit-ter) Chemical messengers that communicate in the synapse between nerve cells, or neurons.

Neutropenia (new-trow-**pee**-near) A reduction of circulating neutrophils, or white blood cells.

Neutrophils (**new**-trow-**fills**) White blood cells that fight against invading agents or injury.

Nevus (knee-vuss) A small, dark skin growth that develops from pigment-producing cells, or melanocytes; a benign tumour.

Nitroglycerin (night-row-**gliss**-er-in) Medication used to dilate coronary arteries, permitting adequate blood flow.

Nocturia Urination at night, especially when excessive.

Non-communicable Infectious diseases that are not transmitted directly by humans.

Non-disjunction The failure of two chromosomes to separate as the gametes, either the egg or the sperm, are being formed.

Non-specific defences Defences that are effective against any foreign agent that enters the body.

Norepinephrine (nor-ep-ee-**neff**-rinn) Neurotransmitter of the sympathetic nervous system. Controls the fight or flight response. Also secreted by the adrenal medulla in response to stimulation by nerves of the sympathetic nervous system. Also called noradrenaline.

Notifiable diseases Diseases under surveillance that must be reported by physicians to the Centres for Disease Control and Prevention.

Nucleic acid analogues (**new**-clee-ick) Antiviral medications.

Nutrient Chemical compound consumed in food that is required for vital cellular processes.

Nystagmus (nye-**stag**-muss) Involuntary, rapid movement of the eyeball, characteristic of multiple sclerosis.

Obesity A nutritional disorder in which an abnormal amount of fat accumulates in adipose tissue.

Obesity-hypoventilation syndrome Also called Pickwickian syndrome, a condition of recurrent episodes of apnoea during sleep caused by airway occlusion owing to excess weight or obesity.

Obstructive sleep apnoea syndrome Respiratory complication often associated with obesity.

Occult blood Blood detected in stool by means of a chemical test but not apparent to the naked eye.

Oedema (uh-dee-muh) Swelling caused by leakage of plasma into tissues.

Oesophageal varices (eh-soff-ah-jeel vara-seas) Varicose veins of the oesophagus.

Oesophagitis (eh-soff-ah-jye-tiss) Inflammation of the oesophagus caused by acid reflux.

Oestrogen The sex hormone in females.

Oliguria (olly-go-rea) A reduced production of urine.

Oncogene (on-coe-jean) Any gene having the potential to induce a cancerous transformation.

Oppositional defiant disorder Disruptive behaviour disorder diagnosed in childhood.

Orchitis (or-kite-iss) Inflammation of the testes; can follow an injury or viral infection such as mumps.

Organic obstructions A material blockage that prevents the contents of the intestinal tract from moving forward.

Ossification (oss-siff-i-cay-shun) Process by which bone tissue is formed. Also known as osteogenesis.

Osteitis fibrosa cystica (ost-ee-eye-tiss fye-bro-sir sis-tick-er) In this disease, fibrous nodules and cysts form in the bones, which become very porous and decalcified.

Osteoarthritis (oss-tee-oh-arth-rye-tiss) The most common form of arthritis, a chronic disease that accompanies aging and may affect only one joint.

Osteoblasts A cell that works within the bone to form bone tissue.

Osteoclasts A cell that works within the bone and reabsorbs bone.

Osteocytes (oss-tee-oh-sites) Mature cells in bone tissue.

Osteogenic sarcoma A primary malignancy of the bone.

Osteoma The most common benign tumour of the bone.

Osteomalacia (oss-tee-oh-may-lay-she-ah) A bone disease in adults caused by the lack of vitamin D, which results in a softening of the bones.

Osteomyelitis (oss-tee-oh-my-light-iss) An inflammation of the bone, particularly of the bone marrow in the medullary cavity and in the spaces of spongy bone.

Osteoporosis (oss-tee-por-os-sis) The increased porosity of the bone.

Outbreak The sudden occurrence of a disease, in unexpected numbers in a limited area, which then subsides.

Oxytocin (ock-see-toh-sin) One of two hormones secreted by the posterior pituitary; it causes smooth muscle, particularly that of the uterus, to contract and initiates milk secretions.

Paget's disease (pa-jets) A rare cancer involving inflammatory changes that affect the nipple and the areola.

Pallor Whitening of the skin.

Pancreatic islets (pan-kree-ah-tick) Endocrine cells of the pancreas.

Pancreatitis (pan-kree-ah-tye-tiss) A potentially life-threatening inflammation of the pancreas.

Pandemic Describes an epidemic that has spread to include several large areas worldwide.

Papanicolaou (Pap) test Screening test for cervical cancer based on observations of cells obtained in biopsies of the cervix.

Papilloma Also known as a polyp; an epithelial tumour that grows as a projecting mass on the skin or from an inner mucous membrane. The common wart is an example.

Pap smear A diagnostic technique for identifying cancer in the cervix by scraping cells from the cervix and examining them microscopically.

Papular Raised lesions on the skin.

Paraesthesia (paras-these-ee-ar) Numbness, burning or tingling sensation resulting from nerve injury.

Paralytic obstructions Caused when the contents of the intestinal tract are unable to move forward owing to a decrease in peristalsis, preventing propulsion of intestinal contents.

Parathormone The hormone secreted by the parathyroids.

Paresis (pa-ree-siss) A general paralysis associated with organic loss of brain function; results in death if untreated.

Passive immunity Immunity transmitted through doses of preformed antibodies from immune serum of an animal, usually a horse. This type of immunity is short-lived but acts immediately.

Patent ductus arteriosus (PDA) (duck-tuss art-ear-ee-oh-suss) A common congenital disease in which the ductus arteriosus remains open and blood intended for the body flows from the aorta to the lungs, overloading the pulmonary artery.

Pathogen (path-oh-jenn) Micro-organism that causes disease.

Pathogenesis The source or cause of an illness or abnormal condition and its development.

Pathology (path-all-oh-jee) Study of the characteristics, causes and effects of disease.

Pathophysiology Study of the physiological processes leading up to disease.

Pediculosis (ped-ick-you-low-siss) Louse infestations that are classified into three categories: head lice, pubic lice and body lice.

Pellagra Niacin deficiency.

Pelvic inflammatory disease (PID) Inflammation of the female reproductive organs owing to bacterial, viral, fungal or parasitic invasion.

Peptic ulcers Ulcers of the stomach and small intestine due, in part, to the action of pepsin, a proteolytic enzyme secreted by the stomach.

Perforation An ulcer that breaks through the intestinal or gastric wall, causing sudden and intense abdominal pain.

Pericardium The double membranous sac that encloses the heart.

Periosteum (pair-ee-oss-tee-um) A highly vascular layer of fibrous connective tissue that covers the surface of bones.

Peristalsis Muscle contractions that propel food during the digestive process.

Peritoneal dialysis Treatment for kidney failure; fluid added to the peritoneal cavity draws metabolic waste from the blood and restores it to physiological balance.

Peritonitis Inflammation of the lining of the abdominal cavity. Usually results when the digestive contents enter the cavity, because this material contains numerous bacteria.

Pernicious anaemia (per-nish-us) Anaemia caused by a vitamin B_{12} deficiency.

Persecutory delusion False belief that one is being followed, watched or plotted against.

Personality disorder Mental disturbance characterised by inflexible patterns of behaviour that affect interpersonal relationships. Includes three major categories or clusters based on symptoms: paranoid, schizoid (cluster A); antisocial, borderline, histrionic, narcissistic (cluster B); and avoidant, dependent, obsessive compulsive (cluster C).

Petechiae (per-teak-ee-eye) Tiny red or purple spots caused by minute blood vessels that rupture in the skin.

Phaeochromocytoma (fee-oh-crow-mow-site-oh-mah) A neuroendocrine tumour of the adrenal gland.

Phagocyte (fag-oh-site) Leucocytes that take in and destroy foreign material.

Phagocytosis (fag-oh-sigh-toe-sis) White blood cells taking in and destroying foreign material.

Pharyngeoplasty (farin-jee-oh-plar-stee) Surgical removal of the uvula to alleviate obstructive sleep apnoea.

Pharynx (fa-rinks) The throat.

Phenylketonuria (PKU) (fee-nile-key-tone-yure-ea) Caused by an autosomal recessive allele that lacks a specific enzyme that converts one amino acid, phenylalanine, to another, tyrosine.

Phlebitis (fleb-eye-tiss) An inflammation of a vein, usually in the leg.

Phosphate Compound containing phosphorus essential for bone and tooth structure as well as cell physiology.

Physiology (fiz-ee-all-oh-jee) Study of the normal function of the body.

Pipe stem colon Term used to describe the colon in patients suffering from chronic ulcerative colitis; colon appears straight and rigid.

Placenta The interdigitation of embryonic and maternal tissue.

Placenta praevia Abnormal positioning of the placenta in the lower uterus, often near the cervical opening.

Plantar warts Painful warts that form on the soles of the feet.

Plaque Fatty deposits in the walls of arteries.

Plasma cells Cells that develop from B cells and produce antibodies.

Platelets Clotting elements of blood.

Pleura (pler-ra) A double membrane consisting of two layers that encases the lungs.

Pleural cavity (pler-ral) The space between the two layers of the pleura containing a small amount of fluid that lubricates the surfaces, preventing friction as the lungs expand and contract.

Pleurisy (pler-ris-ee) The inflammation of the pleural membranes occurring as a complication of various lung diseases like pneumonia or tuberculosis.

Pneumoconiosis (new-mow-coe-knee-oh-sis) A lung disease caused by the inhalation of a variety of organic or inorganic dusts or chemical irritants, usually over a prolonged period of time.

Pneumonia (new-mow-knee-ah) An acute inflammation of the lung in which air spaces in the lungs become filled with an inflammatory exudate.

Pneumothorax (new-mow-thor-axe) A collection of free air in the chest outside the lung.

Poliomyelitis (po-leo-my-light-iss) An infectious disease of the brain and spinal cord caused by a virus.

Polydactyly (poly-dac-tilly) An autosomal dominant disorder that causes extra fingers or toes.

Polydipsia (poly-dip-see-ah) Extreme thirst.

Polymorphs White blood cells specialised to fight against invading agents or injury.

Polyp Benign epithelial tumour.

Polysomnography (poly-som-nog-raphy) Used in a sleep study to measure sleep cycles and stages by recording brain waves (EEG), electrical activity of muscles and eye movement.

Polyuria (poly-yure-ee-ah) The excessive production of dilute urine.

Postpartum depression Subcategory of depression that occurs 2 weeks to 6 months following the birth of a child.

Premature ejaculation Ejaculation during foreplay or immediately after beginning intercourse.

Premenstrual dysphoric disorder (dis-forrick) Subcategory of depression with cyclical symptoms prior to menstruation.

Premenstrual syndrome (PMS) Emotional, physical and behavioural symptoms that are associated with the menstrual cycle.

Prevalence The number of existing cases of a disease.

Primary atypical pneumonia Also known as 'walking pneumonia', it is caused by a variety of micro-organisms, including viruses and an unusual bacterium called *Mycoplasma pneumoniae.*

Primary follicle A single layer of cells that surround each ovum.

Proctoscope An instrument consisting of a hollow tube with a lighted end used by physicians to observe the lining of the colon.

Prognosis (prog-noh-siss) The predicted course and outcome of a disease.

Progression The third stage of cancer development.

Prolapse A falling or dropping down of an organ or internal structure, such as the uterus or rectum.

Promotion The second stage of cancer development in which altered cells proliferate and resemble benign neoplasms, which can either regress to normal appearing tissue or evolve into cancer.

Prostaglandins A group of hormone like substances found in a wide variety of regions of the body including the uterus, lungs and brain. They have a wide variety of functions such as inflammation and in reproduction.

Prostate Produces alkaline fluid to help neutralise vaginal pH.

Prostatitis (pross-ta-tye-tiss) Inflammation of the prostate.

Prothrombin (pro-throm-bin) An enzyme synthesised by the liver with the aid of vitamin K that initiates the chain reaction in the blood coagulation process.

Pruritis (pure-eye-tiss) Itching that accompanies many skin diseases.

Pseudopodia (sue-dow-po-dee-ah) Cell membrane extensions used for locomotion of phagocytosis.

Psoriasis (sore-rye-a-siss) A superficial, recurring idiopathic skin disorder characterised by an abnormal rate of epidermal cell production and turnover.

Psychiatric Pertaining to mental health.

Psychiatry Medical field that studies and treats mental illness.

Psychology Study of human behaviour.

Puerperal mastitis (perp-er-al) Bacterial infection of the breast after birth.

Puerperal sepsis An infection of the endometrium after childbirth or an abortion.

Puerperium (pue-per-ee-um) The time period after childbirth when the endometrium is open and particularly susceptible to infection.

Pulmonary oedema A build-up of fluid in the lungs, causing shortness of breath.

Pulmonary stenosis The first cause of cyanosis in which the valve opening that leads into the pulmonary artery is too small and an inadequate amount of blood reaches the lungs to be oxygenated.

Purging Self-induced, wilful elimination of consumed food by vomiting or misuse of laxatives or diuretics.

Purkinje fibres (per-**kin**-jee) The specialised heart tissue that conducts the impulse for contraction to the myocardium of the ventricles.

Purpura Small haemorrhages into the tissue beneath the skin or mucous membranes.

Purpura simplex A condition of easy bruising.

Pustules Lesions containing pus.

Pyelitis (pie-**light**-iss) An inflammation of the renal pelvis, the juncture between the ureter and the kidney, caused by *E. coli* or other pus-forming bacteria.

Pyelonephritis (pie-low-neff-**right**-iss) A suppurative inflammation of the kidney and renal pelvis.

Pyloric sphincter (pye-**lor**-ik **sfink**-ter) The sphincter muscle through which food passes from the stomach into the small intestine.

Pyloric stenosis A congenital obstruction of the intestinal tract.

Pyogenic Bacteria that cause the formation of pus.

Pyuria This condition is caused when abscesses in the kidney rupture and pus enters the renal pelvis and then appears in urine.

Quarantine The separation of persons who may or may not be infected from healthy people until the period of infectious risk is passed.

Rabies An infectious disease of the brain and spinal cord caused by a virus that is transmitted by the saliva, urine or faeces of an infected animal.

Rales Abnormal respiratory sounds detected with a stethoscope.

Raynaud's disease The condition in which small arteries or arterioles in the fingers and toes constrict.

Recessive Term used to describe an allele that manifests itself when the person is homozygous for the trait.

Rectocele (recto-**seal**) Protrusion of the rectum into the vagina.

Reflux The backflow of the acid contents of the stomach causing inflammation of the oesophagus.

Regional enteritis An inflammatory disease of the intestine that most frequently affects young adults, particularly females.

Regurgitation Passage of stomach contents into the oesophagus.

Relapse Occurs when a disease returns weeks or months after its apparent cessation.

Remission The period of a chronic disease when signs and symptoms subside.

Renal pelvis (ree-nal **pell**-vis) The juncture between the kidneys and the ureters; final urine from all collecting ducts empties here.

Renin (**ree**-nin) Secreted by cells that convert angiotensinogen to angiotensin, an active enzyme to help elevate blood pressure.

Reservoirs The sources of a pathogen and a potential source of disease.

Respiratory epithelium A mucous membrane that lines the entire respiratory tract.

Resuscitation Assisting or reviving respiration to a person with a myocardial infarction.

Reticulocyte (reh-**tick**-you-low-site) The late stage of erythrocyte development.

Reye's syndrome A potentially devastating neurological illness that sometimes develops in young children after a viral infection.

Rh factor Antigen on erythrocyte, used for blood typing.

Rhabdomyosarcoma (rab-doh-my-oh-sar-coma) A malignant tumour of the skeletal muscle.

Rheumatoid factor (**roo**-ma-toid) Antibodies in blood associated with rheumatoid arthritis.

Rhodopsin (rod-**op**-sin) The pigment that absorbs light in the rods of the retina.

Rickets A disease of infancy and early childhood in which the bones do not properly ossify, or harden, generally caused by a vitamin D deficiency.

Roundworm A worm-like animal that is relatively round in cross-section.

Salpingitis (sal-pin-**jye**-tiss) An inflammation of the Fallopian tubes.

Sarcoma A less common type of cancer that spreads rapidly and is highly malignant.

Scabies A contagious skin disease associated with poor living conditions.

Schizophrenia Mental illness characterised by social withdrawal, delusions, hallucinations and unpredictable behaviour.

Scleroderma (sklare-oh-der-ma) A chronic, progressive autoimmune disorder of the skin.

Sclerosis (sklare-oh-siss) An abnormal hardening of a tissue.

Sclerotherapy Use of sclerosing or hardening agents to treat diseases like haemorrhoids or oesophageal varices.

Scurvy Disease caused by vitamin C deficiency.

Seasonal affective disorder Subcategory of major depression associated with decreased sunlight exposure during the winter months.

Sebaceous glands (seb-ay-shuss) Oil glands located within the dermis.

Seborrhoeic dermatitis (seb-or-ree-ick) The excessive secretion of sebum from the sebaceous glands; chronic dandruff.

Seborrhoeic keratosis Benign overgrowth of epithelial cells common in older adults.

Sebum Oily fluid released through the hair follicles.

Secondary pneumonia A pneumonia that develops as a secondary disorder from other diseases that weaken the lungs or the body's immune system.

Seizures An uncontrolled nervous system activity manifested by uncoordinated motor action.

Seminal vesicle Produces fructose to nourish sperm.

Seminiferous tubules Highly coiled tubules contained within the testes in which sperm develop.

Septic embolism An embolism that contains infected material from pyogenic bacteria.

Sequela (see-kway-lar) The aftermath of a particular disease, such as permanent damage to the heart after rheumatic fever.

Serotonin One of many neurotransmitters involved in regulating mood, emotions and behaviour.

Serum Liquid portion of the blood.

Sex-linked inheritance Diseases transmitted on the sex chromosomes.

Shingles An acute inflammation of nerve cells caused by the chickenpox virus, herpes zoster.

Sickle cell anaemia An autosomal recessive disorder, in which haemoglobin is abnormal, resulting in deformed, sickle-shaped red blood cells.

Signs The objective evidence of disease observed on physical examination, such as abnormal pulse or fever.

Sinoatrial node (sign-noh-at-tree-al) The pacemaker of the heart, it is a small patch of tissue that initiates the heartbeat.

Skeletal muscle (skell-ee-tal) Striated muscle attached to bone and that is under conscious control.

Somatic False belief that something physical is occurring in one's body.

Somnoplasty A controlled delivery process of radiofrequency energy; the tissue is heated in a limited area to trim or reduce its size.

Spastic colon (irritable colon) A functional condition of the colon with diarrhoea and cramping.

Specific defences Defences that are effective against particular identified foreign agents.

Spider veins Small, dense, red networks of veins close to the skin surface.

Spina bifida A condition in which one or more vertebrae fail to fuse, leaving an opening in the vertebral canal. The word *bifid* means a cleft, or split into two parts, which is the condition of the vertebra in spina bifida.

Spirilla Spiral-shaped bacterial cells.

Spirochaetes (spy-row-keats) Corkscrew-shaped bacterial cells.

Spirometer A simple instrument used to measure the movement of air in and out of the lungs.

Spirometry A diagnostic procedure that measures and records changes in gas volume in the lungs, determining ventilation capacity and flow rate.

Splenomegaly An enlarged spleen.

Spongy bone Bone tissue with blood-filled spaces; found at ends of bones or in flat bones like those of the skull.

Spores Microscopic fungal reproductive structures that can induce allergies.

Sporozoans A form of protozoa; a single-celled, immobile, eukaryotic micro-organism.

Sprain The result of the wrenching or twisting of a joint such as an ankle that injures the ligaments.

Spurs Spicules of abnormal new bone development.

Squamous cell carcinoma A malignancy of the keratinocytes in the epidermis.

Staghorn calculus A kidney stone that becomes so large it fills the renal pelvis completely, blocking the flow of urine.

Staging Method used to establish the extent of disease, particularly cancer.

Standard precautions Precautions such as gloves required of medical personnel when handling patients or bodily fluids.

Stasis Slow blood flow that may lead to thrombosis or cause infection; slow urine flow that may promote kidney stones.

Status asthmaticus Life-threatening form of an asthma attack.

Stenosis Constriction or narrowing of a passage or orifice.

Stent Rigid structure surgically inserted into arteries to hold them open.

Stomatitis Inflammation of the lining of the mouth often caused by bacteria or fungi.

Strabismus The condition of crossed eyes.

Strains Pulled muscles that result from a tearing of a muscle and/or its tendon from excessive use or stretching.

Streptococci A type of bacterium associated with infections of the ear, throat, skin and heart valves.

Stridor (stry-door) High-pitched breath sound.

Stroke Common term to describe cerebral haemorrhages and blood clot formation within cerebral blood vessels.

Stye A red, tender bump on the eyelid that is caused by an acute infection of the oil glands of the eyelid.

Subarachnoid (sub-ah-rak-noyd) A tear in the surface membrane of the brain, caused by a skull fracture.

Subdural (sub-dure-al) A haemorrhage under the dura mater, from large venous sinuses of the brain rather than an artery.

Substance use disorders Includes alcohol and drug abuse and addiction.

Suppressor T cells The type of T cell that controls the immune response.

Suppurative A type of inflammation associated with pus formation.

Symptom An indication of disease perceived by the patient, such as pain, dizziness and itching.

Syncope (sin-co-pee) Fainting caused by insufficient blood supply to the brain.

Syndrome (sin-drohm) Combination of symptoms.

Synovial fluid (sigh-no-vee-al) Lubricating and shock-absorbing fluid found within joints.

Synovial membrane (sigh-no-vee-al) The membrane that lines the joints.

Syphilis (siff-ill-iss) Sexually transmitted disease caused by *Treponema pallidum*.

Systemic lupus erythematosus (SLE) (erith-em-a-toe-sis) An autoimmune disease that not only affects the skin but causes the deterioration of collagenous connective tissue.

Systole (siss-toe-lee) The period of the heartbeat when the heart contracts and pumps the blood.

T lymphocytes (T limf-oh-sights) Provide cell-mediated immunity and are processed by the thymus gland.

Tachycardia (tacky-card-ee-uh) Heart rate of 100 beats per minute or more.

Tachypnoea (tack-ip-knee-ah) Rapid respiration rate.

Tay-Sachs An autosomal recessive disorder caused by the absence of the Hex A enzyme.

Tendons Connective tissue that attaches skeletal or voluntary muscles firmly to bones.

Terminal A disease ending in death.

Tetanus toxoid A type of immunisation that protects from the disease tetanus.

Tetany (tet-an-ee) A sustained muscular contraction.

Tetralogy of Fallot One of the most serious congenital defects consisting of four (*tetra*) abnormalities.

Thalassaemia Group of inherited blood disorders in which there is deficient synthesis of one or more alpha or beta chains required for proper formation and optimal performance of the haemoglobin molecule.

Thrombi (throm-bye) Blood clots.

Thrombocytopenia (throm-boh-sigh-toh-pee-nee-ah) A disease of platelets resulting in gastrointestinal and urogenital haemorrhages as well as severe nosebleeds.

Thrombolytic (throm-boh-**lit-**ick) Agents that dissolve blood clots.

Thrombophlebitis (throm-boh-**fleb-**eye-tiss) Thrombus formation in deep veins.

Thrombosis The forming of blood clots on blood vessel walls.

Thrombus (throm-buss) A blood clot that forms in a blood vessel.

Thyroxine One of the thyroid hormones.

Tic Sudden, rapid, involuntary stereotyped movement or vocalisation.

Tinea Fungal skin infection.

Toxic shock syndrome (TSS) Caused by infection with *Staphylococcus aureus*.

Toxoid A chemically altered toxin that stimulates an immune response.

Trachea (track-ee-uh) The 'windpipe', which connects the larynx to the primary bronchi of the lungs.

Tracheostomy Emergency procedure to maintain airway by cutting a hole in the trachea.

Trachoma A chronic contagious form of conjunctivitis causing hypertrophy of the conjunctiva.

Transformation A change from one tissue to another.

Tremor A shakiness, particularly of the hands.

Trichomonas vaginalis A parasite that can be transmitted by sexual intercourse; one causative agent of vaginitis.

Trichomoniasis (try-coe-moan-ee-ay-siss) Sexually transmitted disease caused by the protozoan *Trichomonas vaginalis*.

Tricuspid valve The valve between the right atrium and right ventricle. It has three cusps.

Triglycerides (try-gliss-er-ides) A lipid fat that is not water-soluble and therefore cannot mix with blood plasma.

Tri-iodothyronine (try-eye-oh-doh-**thigh-**row-neen) A thyroid hormone.

Trisomy 21 The condition of having three, rather than two, copies of chromosome 21; causes Down's syndrome.

Tubercles Lesions that are formed when tissue infected with tuberculosis heals with fibrosis and calcification, walling off the bacteria for months or many years.

Tuberculosis (TB) (tue-ber-cue-low-sis) A chronic infectious disease characterised by necrosis of vital lung tissue, which can affect other body systems as well.

Tumour A mass of new cells that grows in a haphazard fashion with no control or useful function.

Tumour marker Abnormal levels or substances found in the blood of cancer patients; used to monitor the presence of cancer and the extent of disease.

Tumour necrosis factor (TNF) A cytokine produced by leukocytes which has multiple functions in the immune response, believed to play a role in cachexia.

Turner's syndrome The condition caused when one of the sex chromosomes is missing, resulting in a karyotype of 45XO.

Ultrasound Imaging technique utilising low frequency sound waves.

Ultrasound cardiography Shows the anatomy of arteries, particularly the carotid bifurcation and the internal carotid artery.

Upper respiratory infections Disorders of the nose and throat, including common infections and allergies.

Uraemia A toxic condition of blood; the end result is kidney failure.

Urea Nitrogen-containing waste products formed in the liver.

Ureter (you-ree-ter) Muscular tube that passes urine from the kidney to the urinary bladder.

Ureterocele (you-ree-ter-seal) Cyst-like dilatation of the ureter near its opening to the urinary bladder.

Urethra (you-ree-thrah) The single tube through which urine empties to the outside from the urinary bladder.

Urethritis (you-rith-rye-tis) Inflammation of the urethra.

Urinalysis A simple diagnostic procedure that examines a urine specimen physically, chemically and microscopically.

Urinary calculi Stones formed primarily in the kidney when certain salts in the urine form a precipitate and grow in size.

Urticaria Known as hives, results from a vascular reaction of the skin to an allergen.

Uterine prolapse Uterus dropping downward into the vagina.

Uvula Soft structure hanging from free edge of the soft palate in midline above the root of the tongue.

Uvulopalatopharyngoplasty (UPPP) (you-view-low-pal-at-oh-farr-in-go-plasty) A procedure that removes excess tissue in the throat (uvula and pharynx) to make the airway wider.

Vaccine A low dose of dead or deactivated bacteria or virus that stimulates an immune response.

Valvular insufficiency Occurs when a valve opening is too large and does not prevent backflow.

Vas deferens A duct that passes through the inguinal canal into the abdominal cavity of males.

Vascular dementia Degenerative memory disorder most often caused by physical insults to the brain.

Vasopressin One of two hormones secreted by the posterior pituitary (neurohypophysis); also called antidiuretic hormone.

Vectors Animals that transmit pathogenic micro-organisms to humans.

Vegetations Small nodular structures composed of bacteria and clots that form along the edge of cusps in a valve opening.

Venae cavae (veena-cave-a) The two largest veins of the body.

Ventricular fibrillation Occurs when a series of uncoordinated impulses spread over the ventricles, causing them to twitch or quiver rather than contract.

Verruca vulgaris Warts caused by viruses affecting the keratinocytes of the skin, causing them to proliferate.

Vertical transmission The route by which an infectious disease is transmitted from one generation to the next.

Vesicles (vee-sickles) Small, blister-like eruptions on the skin.

Vibrios Comma-shaped bacterial cells.

Vitiligo A loss of melanin resulting in white patches of skin, which are usually well demarcated and may cover large parts of the body.

Voluntary muscle Striated muscle attached to bone and that is under conscious control.

Volvulus A condition in which the intestine is twisted on itself.

Wernicke's encephalopathy (were-nicks en-keff-al-opathy) A brain disease, often associated with chronic alcoholism, in which the patient becomes mentally confused and disorientated and may suffer delirium tremens.

Wheals Rounded elevations on the skin known as lesions, with red edges and pale centres; extremely pruritic, or itchy.

Wheezing The sound of laboured breathing as a result of narrowed tubes in the lungs.

Wilms' tumour A malignant tumour of the kidney that develops in very young children.

Appendix B
ANSWERS TO INTERACTIVE EXERCISES

Chapter 1
INTRODUCTION TO DISEASE

Cases for critical thinking

1. Abnormally high red blood cell counts can and do occur in well trained athletes. Athletes develop increased cardiovascular efficiency and produce more red blood cells. Their hearts can handle the slightly increased viscosity of the blood and thus higher red blood cell levels may not be a sign of disease.
2. No. Many diseases share these symptoms. A simple history can determine if she ate recently or if she is under stress, depressed or anxious, and a blood test can determine sugar levels and the presence of diabetes. The physician can consult a blood test to determine anaemia or other blood disorders. A physical examination can determine whether she has hypertension. Cardiovascular abnormalities can be determined with a physical examination or with imaging techniques. In short, several diseases can explain these symptoms.
3. Many of the diseases are chronic. Education, screening, early diagnosis and treatment and reduction of risk factors should have an impact on the prevalence of the diseases. Accidents are a significant cause of death. By applying the science of epidemiology to accidents, perhaps prevention can reduce mortality from accidents as well.

Multiple choice

1. a. sign
2. a. acute
3. d. aetiology
4. a. homeostasis
5. b. exacerbation

True or false

1. False
2. True
3. False
4. True
5. True

Fill-ins

1. prognosis
2. lesions
3. idiopathic
4. relapse
5. remission

Chapter 2
IMMUNITY AND THE LYMPHATIC SYSTEM

Cases for critical thinking

1. Antiserum containing preformed antibodies is given to act immediately, providing short-lived immunity.
2. Since identical twins have identical DNA, rejection of the organ is not an issue.
3. The bites happened after the women died because trauma is a trigger for inflammation and the bites were not inflamed.
4. Active immunity. The polio virus will trigger antibody production in the body. The baby will develop specific immunity against the virus.
5. IgA provides localised protection at mucosal surfaces like the respiratory system.
6. Helper CD4 T lymphocytes help the immune system in many ways. They increase the activity of cytotoxic T lymphocytes, they stimulate B lymphocytes and they secrete lymphokines that increase the response of other types of lymphoid cells.

Multiple choice

1. a. preformed antibodies
2. d. memory lymphocytes
3. a. humoral immunity
4. d. all of the above
5. a. antigen
6. c. plasma
7. d. IV
8. a. IgE
9. c. helper or CD4 lymphocytes
10. d. helper cells

True or false

1. False
2. False
3. False
4. True
5. False
6. False
7. True
8. True
9. False
10. False

Fill-ins

1. pyogenic
2. Interferon
3. antigen
4. vaccine
5. Non-specific
6. histamine
7. M
8. Natural killer
9. human immunodeficiency virus (HIV)
10. passive

Chapter 3
INFECTIOUS DISEASES

Cases for critical thinking

1. Influenza is transmitted in respiratory droplets generated by coughing and sneezing. Isolation of flu patients would help decrease the transmission of the disease. Encouraging people to cover their noses and mouths when they sneeze or cough would also help decrease transmission. To control the spread of malaria we must control the vector, the mosquito.
2. Viruses do not have the targets of antibiotics – cell walls and membranes, metabolic and protein synthesis machinery. If antibiotics are used for viral infections, bacterial populations will be more likely to evolve resistance to those antibiotics.
3. Vaccines prevent disease, and prevention is a very effective method for controlling infectious disease.
4. Whooping cough is caused by *Bordetella pertussis*. The bacteria are spread by direct contact with respiratory droplets. Antibiotics would be the treatment for this bacterial infection. There is a vaccine; whooping cough is part of the diphtheria, tetanus, pertussis vaccine.
5. Chickenpox is caused by the varicella zoster virus. The virus is spread by direct contact, droplet transmission and airborne transmission. Treatment is supportive and may include treatments to control scratching, pain relievers and fever reducers. A vaccine is available for varicella zoster.
6. Diphtheria. Diagnosis is based on throat culture. Antibiotics would be the treatment for this bacterial infection.

Multiple choice

1. c. capsule
2. c. endospores
3. c. plasmid
4. c. binary fission
5. d. protozoa
6. c. rubella virus
7. a. *Bordetella pertussis*
8. b. capsid
9. a. *Enterobius vermicularis*
10. d. needlestick

True or false

1. False
2. False
3. False
4. True
5. True
6. True
7. False
8. True
9. False
10. False

Fill-ins

1. normal flora
2. Re-emerging
3. rubeola
4. Nosocomial
5. horizontal
6. glycocalyx
7. Fimbriae
8. Prions
9. paramyxovirus
10. varicella zoster

Labelling exercise

1. Trypanosome
2. Amoeba
3. *Plasmodium*
4. Tapeworm
5. Liver fluke
6. *Ascaris*

Chapter 4
CANCER

Cases for critical thinking

1. Diagnostic procedures used to rule out lung cancer include a chest X-ray, sputum analysis, bronchoscopy with a biopsy and PET scan. Historical information should include the following.
   - have you smoked? (Smoking is the single most preventative cause of lung cancer.)
   - how many packs of cigarettes per day/week?
   - how many years have you smoked?
   - what type of work do you do?
   - is it in a factory? (Potential for industrial chemicals also to cause symptoms of lung cancer.)

   Ask about history of cancers in other parts of the body. The lung is a common site for cancer metastases. Is there a history of asthma, bronchitis, pneumonia? Is there a history of hoarseness of the voice?
2. Risk factors for breast cancer include age, female gender, genetics, overweight and obesity, postmenopausal hormone replacement therapy, physical inactivity and consumption of alcohol. Mammography, breast ultrasound and biopsy are common diagnostic tests and procedures. The definitive test for breast cancer is a biopsy.

Multiple choice

1. c. mutation
2. c. DNA repair genes
3. a. tobacco use
4. d. colorectal
5. b. cervical
6. b. age (greater than 65 years)
7. d. germ
8. c. cigarette smoking
9. b. Reed–Sternberg
10. d. 10

True or false

1. False
2. True
3. True
4. True
5. True
6. False
7. True
8. False
9. True
10. True

Fill-ins

1. Sunlight
2. hepatitis B and hepatitis C
3. surgery
4. *Helicobacter pylori*
5. Hepatocellular
6. Pap
7. lymphomas
8. melanocytes
9. thyroid
10. glial

Labelling exercise
1. Stomach cancer
2. Colon cancer
3. Liver cancer
4. Malignant melanoma

Chapter 5
GENETICS AND DISEASE

Cases for critical thinking
1. Turner's and Klinefelter's syndromes involve non-disjunction of an X sex chromosome, and either an egg or a sperm donate an X sex chromosome. XXY involves non-disjunction of a Y sex chromosome; only the sperm donates a Y sex chromosome.
2. 50%
3. 50% of male children have haemophilia A. 0% of female children have haemophilia A but 50% will be carriers.
4. Haemochromatosis. Blood donation throughout normal life expectancy would reduce iron levels.

Multiple choice
1. d. both are autosomal dominant traits
2. b. 46
3. a. recessive
4. c. men have one X chromosome
5. c. red and green
6. b. autosomal recessive
7. b. 50
8. c. 50
9. c. heterozygous
10. c. autosomes

True or false
1. True
2. True
3. False
4. False
5. False
6. False
7. False
8. True
9. True
10. False

Fill-ins
1. Congenital
2. Hermaphrodites
3. Dominant
4. Genes
5. Alleles
6. Polydactyly
7. Non-disjunction
8. 23
9. phenylketonuria (PKU)
10. gene therapy

Chapter 6
DISEASES OF THE CARDIOVASCULAR SYSTEM

Cases for critical thinking
1. The heart or vascular diseases that should be considered for this patient include atherosclerosis, coronary heart disease and myocarditis.
2. The heart diseases that should be considered for this patient include coronary heart disease, shock and myocarditis.
3. Smoking increases risk of atherosclerosis, chronic venous insufficiency and cardiac arrhythmia. Diabetes increases risk of atherosclerosis, hypercholesterolaemia, peripheral artery disease and coronary heart disease.

Multiple choice
1. c. light-headedness
2. a. filling phase of the heart
3. d. LDL
4. b. carotid artery
5. a. atherosclerosis
6. b. angioplasty
7. b. between the left atrium and the left ventricle
8. d. sinoatrial node
9. a. myocarditis
10. c. autoimmune

True or false
1. True
2. True
3. False
4. False
5. True
6. False
7. True
8. False
9. False
10. False

Fill-ins
1. thrombosis
2. atherosclerosis
3. Restrictive cardiomyopathy
4. Stenosis
5. rheumatic fever
6. ventricle
7. ectopic pacemaker
8. automated external defibrillator
9. tetralogy of Fallot and transposition of the great arteries
10. coronary

Labelling exercise
1. Superior vena cava
2. Right pulmonary artery
3. Right pulmonary veins
4. Right atrium
5. Tricuspid valve
6. Chordae tendineae
7. Inferior vena cava
8. Aorta
9. Left pulmonary artery
10. Pulmonary semilunar valve
11. Left pulmonary veins
12. Left atrium
13. Bicuspid (mitral) valve
14. Aortic valve
15. Left ventricle
16. Right ventricle

Chapter 7
DISEASES OF THE BLOOD

Cases for critical thinking

1. Anaemia should be considered with this patient. A blood test and health history will help confirm the diagnosis.
2. Thrombocytopenia, impaired synthesis of clotting factors and vitamin K deficiency are to be considered. Symptoms to look for include prolonged bleeding, petechiae and ecchymosis. Diagnostic tests include blood tests and bone marrow testing.

Multiple choice

1. d. haemoglobin
2. a. erythropoiesis
3. a. vitamin B_{12}
4. d. 50
5. c. haemoglobinopathy
6. b. thalassaemia
7. a. polycythaemia vera
8. d. Idiopathic thrombocytopenic purpura
9. c. Haemophilia A
10. b. Neutropenia

True or false

1. True
2. False
3. True
4. False
5. True
6. True
7. False
8. True
9. True
10. True

Fill-ins

1. leucocytes
2. erythrocytes
3. haemoglobin S
4. platelets
5. alpha thalassaemia major and beta thalassaemia major
6. iron deficiency
7. megaloblastic anaemia
8. 90–120
9. polycythaemia vera
10. thrombin

Labelling exercise

1. Ecchymosis
2. Petechiae

Chapter 8
DISEASES OF THE RESPIRATORY SYSTEM

Cases for critical thinking

1. In this case he should have a chest X-ray to determine if he has pneumonia and what type. A sputum sample can help identify bacteria.
2. These symptoms are typical of emphysema. It may have been triggered by years of exposure to irritating minute airborne particles at the grain mill.
3. Sara should be able to pursue track and enjoy running, because asthma can be managed with medicine and by avoiding triggers.

Multiple choice

1. d. emphysema
2. c. asthma
3. b. emphysema
4. c. tuberculosis
5. c. asthma
6. a. pneumonia
7. b. emphysema
8. d. bacteria
9. b. infant respiratory distress syndrome (IRDS)
10. c. pleurisy

True or false

1. True
2. False
3. False
4. True
5. False
6. False
7. False
8. True
9. False
10. False

Fill-ins

1. Mantoux skin
2. atelectasis
3. cigarette smoking
4. spirometry
5. viruses
6. pleurisy
7. lobar
8. emphysema
9. cystic fibrosis

Labelling exercise

1. Pharynx
2. Tonsil
3. Larynx
4. Trachea
5. Frontal sinus
6. Ethmoid sinus
7. Eustachian tube
8. Maxillary sinus

Chapter 9
DISEASES OF THE GASTROINTESTINAL SYSTEM

Cases for critical thinking

1. Gastro-oesophageal reflux disease (GORD) produces these symptoms. History should reveal a pattern of pain that follows meals and occurs at night or when prone. A physical examination can rule out little, but endoscopy can reveal abnormalities at the junction of the stomach and oesophagus, such as a hiatus hernia. Treatment involves behaviour changes such as taking smaller meals and avoiding food an hour before sleeping. Serious cases require surgical repair of the hernia.
2. Cholelithiasis (gallstones) causes these symptoms. If bile flow to the small intestine is blocked, dietary fat remains undigested and is not absorbed from the intestines. As

a result, fat appears in the faeces. Following a high fat meal the gallbladder secretes bile into the small intestine. Gallstones lodge in the bile ducts and cause pain in the upper right abdomen.

3. In cirrhosis, normal liver tissue is replaced by scar or fat tissue, which does not function as normal liver tissue. Thus, the liver does not process the haemoglobin that comes from dying erythrocytes and the orange and yellow-coloured breakdown products build up in blood, tinting the skin and eyes yellow. Normal liver tissue processes carbohydrates and proteins and manufactures bile, which is used for fat absorption and the absorption of fat-soluble vitamins. The normal liver also manufactures clotting proteins. Finally, as blood flow through the liver is restricted by cirrhosis, abdominal and oesophageal venous pressure increases, which leads to the distortion of the oesophageal veins.

Multiple choice

1. b. inflammation of stomach mucosa
2. b. ulcerative colitis
3. b. coeliac disease/malabsorption syndrome
4. d. diverticulitis
5. d. prognosis is good, with an 85% cure rate
6. c. most often caused by diabetes
7. b. chronic alcoholism
8. a. cirrhosis
9. a. *Candida albicans*
10. c. cholecystitis

True or false

1. False
2. True
3. False
4. True
5. True
6. False
7. False
8. False
9. False
10. True

Fill-ins

1. amoebic dysentery
2. Crohn's disease
3. hernia
4. endoscope
5. C
6. cholelithiasis
7. bile duct
8. ascites
9. mouth
10. large intestine

Labelling exercise

1. Ileocaecal sphincter
2. Caecum
3. Haustrum
4. Ileum
5. Appendix
6. Right and Left hepatic ducts
7. Cystic Duct
8. Gallbladder
9. Duodenum
10. Common hepatic duct
11. Bile duct
12. Pancreatic duct
13. Sphincter of Oddi

Chapter 10
DISEASES OF THE RENAL AND URINARY SYSTEMS

Cases for critical thinking

1. Jane may occasionally notice blood in the urine because of the monthly menstrual cycle, but the pain is not normal. Because of a short urethra in females the urinary bladder is commonly contaminated by infection. The appropriate antibiotic agents, like the fluoroquinolones or older drugs like sulphonamides, may relieve the condition. If medication is ineffective, then a cystoscopic examination could be performed.

2. Britany has developed oedema over the past 2 weeks because of a sequela-type event. Following the streptococcus infection of the throat, it has occupied the glomerulus of the kidney, causing glomerulonephritis. This inflammation is caused by an antigen–antibody complex that congests the glomerulus and reduces the filtration process.

   Treatment includes antibiotics such as penicillin to reduce any underlying infection, ACE inhibitors and/or NSAIDs to reduce protein loss, and antihypertensive medication if needed.

3. This patient has a renal tumour, and haematuria suggests tissue breakdown. A nephrectomy can be performed to remove the kidney and the growth. Unfortunately, the tumour is usually well advanced before it is detected, and has therefore usually metastasised. Cancer therapy usually follows the surgery.

Multiple choice

1. d. diabetes mellitus
2. a. pyelonephritis
3. c. pyelitis
4. d. uraemia
5. b. usually exhibit dysuria, urgency and frequency
6. a. peritoneal dialysis
7. b. incontinence
8. a. protein
9. c. decreased plasma protein
10. b. aging

True or false

1. False
2. True
3. True
4. True
5. True
6. True
7. True
8. False
9. False
10. True

Fill-ins

1. Pyuria
2. Diabetic nephropathy
3. kidney stones
4. Lithotripsy
5. Polycystic kidney
6. oliguria
7. nocturia
8. bacteria
9. recessive
10. IVP

Labelling exercise

1. Kidney
2. Ureter
3. Urinary bladder
4. Urethra

Chapter 11
DISEASES AND DISORDERS OF THE REPRODUCTIVE SYSTEM

Cases for critical thinking

1. The condition is endometriosis; its cause is unknown. Treatment includes pain relievers, hormone therapy and surgery.
2. Trichomoniasis is a possible diagnosis. Tests and procedures would include pelvic examination, microscopic visualisation, culture and laboratory and pH tests. Antiparasitic medication is the available treatment.
3. Possible diagnoses include benign prostatic hyperplasia or prostate cancer. A digital rectal examination, PSA test and biopsy might be performed. Treatments include watchful waiting, surgery and hormone therapy.
4. Decreasing transmission includes monogamy, use of condoms and dental dams and regular pelvic examinations. Taking antiviral medication on a regular basis may decrease transmission of the virus.
5. Because prostate cancer often grows very slowly, some men (especially those who are older or who have other major health problems) may never need treatment for their cancer.
6. Cryptorchidism is the name of the disease, and complications can include infertility and testicular cancer. Hormone therapy or surgery are possible treatments.

Multiple choice

1. c. uterine fibroids
2. d. *Treponema pallidum*
3. c. syphilis is only transmitted by sexual contact
4. a. chlamydia
5. d. menorrhagia
6. c. rectocele
7. b. dysmenorrhoea
8. c. cryptorchidism
9. b. fimbriae
10. c. human chorionic gonadotrophin hormone
11. b. progesterone
12. d. ovotestis
13. b. Menarche

True or false

1. True
2. False
3. True
4. False
5. True
6. True
7. True
8. True
9. False
10. False

Fill-ins

1. seminiferous tubules
2. Orchitis
3. chlamydia
4. prostate gland
5. Prostatitis
6. Trichomoniasis
7. 1; 2
8. Cystocele
9. Amenorrhoea
10. Erectile dysfunction

Labelling exercise

1. Ovarian ligament
2. Myometrium
3. Endometrium
4. Fundus of uterus
5. Isthmus of Fallopian tube
6. Uterine (Fallopian) tube
7. Ampulla
8. Ovarian follicles
9. Ovarian vessels
10. Corpus luteum
11. Fornix
12. External os
13. Vagina
14. Cervix
15. Cervical canal
16. Uterosacral ligament
17. Internal os
18. Ovary
19. Fimbriae
20. Infundibulum
21. Uterine cavity
22. Broad ligament

Chapter 12
DISEASES OF THE ENDOCRINE SYSTEM

Cases for critical thinking

1. Diabetes type 1 is consistent with age of onset, high urine production and weight loss when the boy should be growing. It is possible that weight loss could be due to hyperthyroidism.
2. Cushing's syndrome occurs more commonly among women. High blood glucose and lipids, hypertension and poor wound healing (the patient's bruise) are consistent with Cushing's syndrome.
3. Addison's disease is consistent with this history and these signs and symptoms.

Multiple choice

1. c. anterior pituitary
2. b. parathormone
3. b. Addison's disease
4. b. Cushing's disease
5. c. diabetes insipidus
6. a. Graves' disease
7. d. adrenal
8. a. Addison's disease
9. a. absolute insulin deficiency
10. c. thyroxine

True or false

1. True
2. False
3. False
4. False
5. False
6. False
7. False
8. True
9. True
10. True

Fill-ins

1. gigantism
2. acromegaly
3. oxytocin, vasopressin (ADH)
4. diabetes
5. phaeochromocytoma
6. islet cells
7. parathyroid hormone
8. anterior pituitary
9. growth hormone
10. eunuchism

Labelling exercise

1. Thyroid gland
2. Follicle
3. Capillaries
4. Thyroid cartilage (Adam's apple)
5. Isthmus
6. Trachea
7. Follicular cells (site of hormone synthesis)
8. Colloidal material (storage of hormone)

Chapter 13
DISEASES OF THE NERVOUS SYSTEM AND THE SPECIAL SENSES

Cases for critical thinking

1. John has bacterial meningitis, which is a very serious disease that may be lethal. The signs and symptoms plus lumbar puncture fit the disease, and a course of action is to use a broad-spectrum antibiotic such as cephalosporins, given intravenously, analgesics for pain, antipyretics to reduce inflammation and diuretics for cerebral oedema.
2. Cataracts cause dimming of light and distortion of image formation on the retina. The lens should be replaced to prevent potential blindness because it is too thick and ineffectual. The prognosis is very favourable following lens replacement surgery.
3. Trevor had a viral infection from the common cold that has spread into the middle ear (otitis media) and typically leads to a pus-forming bacterial infection. The doctor examines the ear drum externally using an otoscope to observe the tension on the tympanic membrane and notice any drainage. A warm heating pad gives some comfort and a mild analgesia and antipyretic such as paracetamol is used to reduce pain and fever. Antibiotics kill the bacteria and stop bacterial growth, and this (combination) regimen approach is usually a successful treatment process.

Multiple choice

1. b. virus
2. d. all of these
3. d. heart rate and breathing
4. b. meningitis
5. a. it is caused by a virus
6. c. it results from a damaged myelin sheath
7. b. TPA
8. c. epilepsy
9. a. no dopamine
10. c. conjunctivitis

True or false

1. True
2. True
3. False
4. True
5. False
6. True
7. False
8. True
9. False
10. False

Fill-ins

1. Tetanus
2. electromyography
3. Multiple sclerosis
4. Essential tremor
5. L-dopa
6. Cluster
7. trigeminal neuralgia
8. Bell's palsy
9. ALS
10. Myelocele

Labelling exercise

1. Foresight, abstract thinking judgement
2. Motor area
3. Central sulcus
4. Sensory area
5. Speech
6. Hearing
7. Pain, temperature, touch, pressure, position, body image
8. Memory, visual and auditory association
9. Vision
10. Equilibrium, muscle tone, coordination

Chapter 14
MENTAL ILLNESS AND COGNITIVE DISORDERS

Cases for critical thinking

1. A full mental health evaluation would provide appropriate diagnoses and recommendations for Bill. These would include various personality tests, IQ tests, symptom inventory, a complete physical examination with neurological testing, and a complete evaluation by a psychiatrist. Bill's symptoms are suggestive of attention deficit hyperactivity disorder. As adolescents, untreated patients with ADHD may abuse drugs or exhibit impulsive behaviours. ADHD has a genetic basis, however, and without treatment the symptoms can continue to escalate.

2. Anne-Marie has signs of both depression and anxiety that may be caused by her current set of circumstances. If she has had significant weight loss, one would also have to consider anorexia nervosa as a possible diagnosis. Anne-Marie would benefit from a mental health evaluation. Further treatment may include medication for her depression and anxiety, and psychotherapy.

3. David is displaying symptoms of PTSD and depression. Symptoms of mental illness include withdrawal, regret, loss of interest in activities that he previously found enjoyable and history of abuse. Recommendations include approaching David with the subject of mental health counselling, stress management and/or a complete physical and mental health examination. A supportive spouse, counsellor and medication can often assist in recovery from PTSD.

Multiple choice
1. b. Franz Mesmer
2. c. DSM
3. d. dopamine
4. a. ADHD is limited to children
5. c. acetylcholine
6. a. persecutory
7. b. bulimia nervosa
8. b. bipolar I
9. c. stimulant medications
10. d. obsessions

True or false
1. False   6. True
2. False   7. False
3. True   8. True
4. True   9. False
5. True   10. False

Fill-ins
1. Psychiatry
2. neurotransmitters
3. dopamine
4. mental retardation
5. tic disorders
6. acetylcholine
7. compulsive use, cravings, tolerance and withdrawal
8. affect
9. Seasonal affective disorder
10. mania

Chapter 15
DISEASES OF THE MUSCULOSKELETAL SYSTEM

Cases for critical thinking
1. Osteoporosis is common in elderly women. Pain, height loss and kyphosis may all be caused by vertebral fractures and bone loss. Calcium supplements and mild

exercise such as walking with a cane or walker may increase muscle strength and thus prevent falls and fractures. Calcium-supplemented diet and weightbearing exercise throughout adolescence and adulthood can reduce risk of developing osteoporosis later in life.
2. History, physical examination and occupation suggests degenerative joint disease. X-ray can show joint damage.
3. This young woman reports pain in her bone, not in her joint. Bone infection would be accompanied by fever and systemic symptoms such as weakness. A tumour would also cause pain and weakness. An X-ray can rule out tumours and fractures and a blood test can rule out infections.

Multiple choice
1. c. vitamin D
2. d. the bones of adults
3. c. median nerve
4. d. Duchenne's muscular dystrophy
5. b. Degenerative joint disease
6. a. rheumatoid arthritis
7. d. gout
8. c. osteogenic sarcoma
9. c. myasthenia gravis
10. c. osteomyelitis

True or false
1. False   6. True
2. False   7. True
3. False   8. False
4. True   9. True
5. True   10. True

Fill-ins
1. Pott's disease
2. rickets
3. osteoporosis
4. gout
5. calcium, phosphate
6. osteoblasts
7. synovial
8. myasthenia gravis
9. gout
10. calcium

Labelling exercise
1. Closed fracture   4. Depressed fracture
2. Open fracture   5. Spiral fracture
3. Comminuted fracture   6. Greenstick fracture

Chapter 16
DISEASES OF THE INTEGUMENTARY SYSTEM

Cases for critical thinking
1. Impetigo is the diagnosis; *Staphylococcus aureus* or *Streptococcus pyogenes* are potential causes. Treatment is antibiotic medication.

2. Possible causes of the rash include tinea cruris, candidiasis, pediculosis and scabies. Visual examination and culture are the diagnostic tests performed.
3. Basal cell carcinoma or squamous cell carcinoma are possible diagnoses; treatment includes a visual examination and biopsy.
4. Hormones, overproduction of sebum, bacteria, lack of, or uneven exfoliation, of skin cells. Treatment may include topical antibiotics and antibacterials, retinoids, oral antibiotics, oral contraceptives and isotretinoin. Prevention of acne includes not overcleansing the skin, not using harsh scrubs, avoiding products with high concentrations of alcohol, and keeping the hands away from the face.
5. Cold sores caused by the herpes simplex type 1 virus. HSV-1 is spread by kissing, close contact with herpetic lesions or contact with skin that is shedding the virus. Can be treated with antiviral drugs.
6. The hard, thick patches are likely to be plantar warts, caused by the human papillomavirus.

Multiple choice
1. c. staphylococci
2. b. macule
3. b. cyst
4. a. epidermis
5. c. white
6. c. subcutaneous tissue
7. c. papules
8. c. hair follicles
9. a. parasitic
10. c. Sebum

True or false
1. False
2. False
3. False
4. False
5. False
6. True
7. False
8. False
9. True
10. False

Fill-ins
1. Melanin
2. Keratin
3. dermis
4. Herpes
5. Pediculosis
6. Psoriasis
7. Contusions
8. Haemangioma
9. Vitiligo
10. Tinea pedis

Labelling exercise
1. Folliculitis
2. Furuncle (boil)
3. Wart
4. Psoriasis
5. Vitiligo

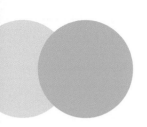

Appendix C
LABORATORY AND DIAGNOSTIC TESTS

Test	Normal value range (SI units)	Possible indications
Ammonia (NH$_3$) diffusion	Adult <40 μmol/l Healthy preterm <200 μmol/l	Abnormal levels of ammonia in the body are used to investigate severe changes in mood and consciousness and to help diagnose the cause of coma of unknown origin.
Ammonia nitrogen	11–32 μmol/l	The test for ammonia nitrogen is non-specific and does not indicate a cause. Higher than normal levels indicate the body is not effectively metabolising and eliminating ammonia.
Amylase	<100 IU/l	Amylase concentration depends on the collection method. An increased level may indicate disorders of the digestive or reproductive systems or cancer of the pancreas. Tubal pregnancies will also cause a rise in amylase levels. Decreased amylase levels may indicate damage to the pancreas and kidneys.
Anion gap $(Na^+ + K^+) - (HCO_3^- + Cl^-)$	6–16 mmol/l	A determination of electrolytes in the plasma fluid. Abnormal readings indicate a variety of factors. The test is non-specific. Some factors that cause an abnormal anion gap reading include ketoacidosis, starvation, kidney damage and ingestion of toxic substances such as antifreeze, excessive amounts of aspirin or methanol.

Bicarbonate:
  Arterial
  Venous
	
	21–28 mmol/l
	22–29 mmol/l
		See *Carbon dioxide content* below.

Bilirubin:
  Conjugated (direct)
  Total
	
	4 μmol/l
	Adult female <18 μmol/l
	Adult male <35 years <26 μmol/l
	Adult male >35 years <23 μmol/l
		Increased levels of bilirubin may indicate blockage to the liver or bile duct, hepatitis, trauma to the liver, adverse drug reaction or long-term alcohol abuse or inherited disorders, such as Gilbert's, Rotor's, Dubin–Johnson, Crigler–Najjar. Increased levels of bilirubin in newborns is a critical situation as excessive levels kill developing brain cells and may lead to mental retardation (kernicterus).

Calcitonin	Adult male <18.9 ng/l Adult female <5.5 ng/l	Increased levels of calcitonin in combination with a thyroid biopsy may be an indication of parafollicular hyperplasia, a premalignant stage in the development of familial medullary thyroid carcinoma.
Calcium, total Calcium, ionised	2.1–2.55 mmol/l 1–1.3 mmol/l	Increased levels of calcium in the body indicate defective calcium metabolism. Causes include hyperthyroidism, sarcoidosis, tuberculosis, excess Vitamin D intake, kidney transplant and high protein levels. Decreased levels may indicate primary hypoparathyroidism, pseudohypoparathyroidism, vitamin D deficiency or magnesium deficiency. If a tourniquet is used for too long while blood is collected, calcium levels may be high; in this case, free or ionised calcium remains normal.

(continued)

Test	Normal value range (SI units)	Possible indications
Carbon dioxide (plasma)	21–32 mmol/l	Higher levels indicate respiratory acidosis, particularly compensated, owing to poor gaseous exchange. Lower than normal CO_2 levels indicate a compensated respiratory alkylosis, metabolic acidosis in diabetes mellitus or renal failure, disrupting the acid–base balance, which can be an indication of several disorders.
Carcinoembryonic antigen (CEA)	<2.5 µg/l (non-smokers)	CEA is a protein that is found in embryonic tissues. Increased CEA levels can indicate some non-cancer-related conditions of inflammation of internal organs. Pregnant women who smoke tend to have embryos that have increased levels of CEA. In a normally healthy infant all detectable levels of CEA are gone by birth.
Chloride	95–110 mmol/l	Increased levels of chloride may indicate dehydration or increased blood sodium, acute renal failure or diabetes insipidus. Decreased levels of chloride occur with prolonged vomiting, chronic diarrhoea, emphysema or other chronic lung disease, and with loss of acid from the body.
Coagulation screen		Indicates clotting effectiveness in terms of quality and/or quantity of clotting factors.
Bleeding time	180–570 sec	
Prothrombin time	10–13 sec	
Partial thromboplastin time (activated)	2–37 sec	
Protein C	700–1400 U/ml	
Protein S	700–1400 U/ml	
Copper, total	11–25 µmol/l	Indication of liver disease
Corticotropin (ACTH: adrenocorticotropic hormone)	0800 hr <13.2 pmol/l	This test is used in conjunction with cortisol to determine if a patient has Cushing's syndrome or Addison's disease.
Cortisol	0900 hr 140–690 nmol/l 0000 hr <140 nmol/l	Abnormal levels of cortisol may indicate Cushing's syndrome (high) or Addison's disease (low).
Creatine kinase (CK)	Female 40–185 U/l Male 40–215 U/l	Creatine kinase is an enzyme found in the heart, brain, skeletal muscle and other tissues. Most increases are caused by diseases of skeletal or heart muscle. The body has specific types of CK which give an indication as to which muscles are affected.
Creatine kinase isoenzymes, MB fraction	Value varies depending upon the assay kit used. Specimens recording values (µg/l) higher than 99th centile in the presence of clinical ischaemia are suggestive of acute myocardial infarction	Depending on the ratio, the CK–MB fraction will indicate some form of muscle damage. The specific ratio can indicate whether the muscle damage is cardiac or skeletal. Remains a useful lab test for acute myocardial infarction.
Creatinine	Adult 60–120 µmol/l 0–4 days 30–90 µmol/l 4 days–1 year 20–35 µmol/l 1–12 years 30–65 µmol/l 12–18 years 40–90 µmol/l	Increased creatinine levels indicate a disorder with kidney function. Creatinine can also increase temporarily as a result of muscle injury. Low levels of creatinine are not common. They may been seen in persons with decreased muscle mass, such as comatose patients. Normal pregnancy will cause the creatinine levels to drop and are not a cause for concern.

(continued)

Test	Normal value range (SI units)	Possible indications
C-reactive protein (CRP)	Adults and children <10 mg/l Pregnancy <20 mg/l Neonate <4 mg/l	Acute phase protein synthesised in the liver in response to injury, infection, inflammation or malignancy.
Erythrocyte count (red blood cell, RBC)	Female $3.8–5.8 \times 10^{12}$/l Male $4.5–5.65 \times 10^{12}$/l	
Erythrocyte sedimentation rate (ESR)	<50 years 1–10 mm/h 50–70 years 1–30 mm/h >70 years 1–50 mm/h	A low ESR can indicate polycythaemia, extreme leukocytosis and some protein abnormalities. Elevated ESR is an indication of inflammation, anaemia, infection, pregnancy or advanced age.
Fibrinogen	1.8–4.6 g/l	Low fibrinogen levels indicate that the person may not be able to form a stable blood clot after injury. Chronically low levels may indicate an inherited condition such as afibrinogenaemia, or an acquired condition such as liver disease, malnutrition or some types of cancer. High fibrinogen may indicate acute infection, breast, kidney or stomach cancer, chronic DIC, inflammatory disorders, myocardial infarction, stroke or trauma. Fibrinogen concentrations may rise sharply in any condition that causes inflammation or tissue damage.
Follicle stimulating hormone (FSH)	Male 1–10 IU/l Female follicular 1–12 IU/l Female midcycle 2–24 IU/l Female luteal 1–10 IU/l Female menopausal >30 IU/l	Increased levels of FSH and LH (luteinising hormone) are consistent with primary ovarian failure, which is when ovaries themselves fail. In men this may be an indication of testicular developmental defects or injury. Decreased levels of FSH and LH are an indication of secondary ovarian failure, which results in problems with the pituitary or hypothalamic glands. In men this may be an indication of hypothalamic disorders.
Glucose, fasting	3.0–6.0 mmol/l: normal 6.1–6.9: impaired tolerance >7.0 mmol/l: diabetes mellitus	Indicates diabetes mellitus or prediabetes.
Glucose tolerance test (oral)	2 hours post drink: <7.8 mmol/l: normal 7.8–11 mmol/l: impaired tolerance >11.1 mmol/l: diabetes mellitus	Indicates diabetes mellitus or prediabetes.
Haematocrit (HCT) or packed cell volume (PCV)	Female 0.37–0.47 Male 0.4–0.52	Decreased haematocrit indicates anaemia, such as iron deficiency, but may have other causes such as vitamin or mineral deficiencies, recent bleeding, liver cirrhosis or malignancy. Increased haematocrit may be an indication of dehydration. Polycythaemia vera (greater than normal number of red blood cells in a person) can also cause a prolonged increase in the haematocrit levels. Higher than normal haematocrit levels are also seen in persons at altitude or with chronic pulmonary conditions or lung damage. The person's bone marrow will increase production of red blood cells to supply the body with oxygen in response to a deficient pulmonary system.
Haemoglobin A_{1C}	<7% target	Detects glycosylated haemoglobin and thus indicates control over an extended time period (8–12 weeks).

(*continued*)

Test	Normal value range (SI units)	Possible indications

Haemoglobin (Hb)
   Female
   Male
	
	 115–165 g/l
	 130–180 g/l
		Low Hb indicates anaemia, which can arise owing to multiple causes. Some types of anaemia are treated with iron, folic acid or vitamin B_{12} or B_6 supplements. It is normal for women of childbearing age to have temporary decreases during menstrual periods and pregnancy.

Haptoglobin	0.44–3.03 g/l	Decreased haptoglobin levels in combination with several other tests may be an indication of haemolytic anaemia. Haptoglobin is elevated in many inflammatory diseases, such as ulcerative colitis and acute rheumatic disease. Other causes include infection, tissue injury, malignancies and major depressive illnesses.
Leucocyte count (white blood cell count; WBC)	$4.0–11.0 \times 10^9/l$	WBC is elevated during pregnancy. Raised WBC levels may indicate infection, inflammation or cancer. Decreased levels may indicate autoimmune conditions, some severe infections, bone marrow failure or congenital marrow aplasia. Decreased levels may also occur with certain medications such as methotrexate.
Lipase	7–60 units/l @ 37°C	High lipase levels, with abdominal pain, may indicate acute pancreatitis; slightly raised levels can indicate kidney disease, salivary gland inflammation or peptic ulcer disease.

Lipids
   Total cholesterol
     Borderline high
     High
   High density lipoproteins (HDL)
   Low density lipoproteins (LDL)
	
	 <5.0 mmol/l
	 5.5 mmol/l
	 >5.5 mmol/l
	 >1.0 mmol/l males
	 >1.2 mmol/l females
	
	 <3.0 mmol/l desirable
		A person with high cholesterol has more than twice the risk of coronary heart disease as someone whose cholesterol is below 5.0 mmol/l.
		 Low HDL is considered a major risk factor for heart disease.

Lymphocytes	$1.0–4.0 \times 10^9/l$	Chronic high levels may indicate lymphocytic leukaemia.
Prostate specific antigen (PSA)	40–49 years <2.5 μg/l 50–59 years <3.5 μg/l 60–69 years <4.5 μg/l 70+ years <6.5 μg/l	PSA is a test indicating the level of specific protein the prostate cells are producing. The higher the PSA number, the more likely prostate cancer is present. Age, hormonal factors and medications can alter the test results so a high PSA alone is not a definitive indicator of cancer.
Testosterone	9–27 mmol/l	Reduced testosterone can be found in erectile dysfunction. Low–normal testosterone (less than 12 nmol/l) may still require replacement therapy as low and low–normal testosterone levels have been implicated in the metabolic syndrome, coronary heart disease and some male cancers.
Thyroid stimulating hormone (TSH)	0.3–5.0 mU/l	First-line thyroid function test. A high TSH result is often caused by acute or chronic thyroid dysfunction that causes the thyroid to be underactive. Although rare, a high TSH can also be an indication of secondary hyperthyroidism, which is a problem with the pituitary gland. A low TSH can indicate an overactive thyroid gland.

(*continued*)

Test	Normal value range (SI units)	Possible indications

Triglycerides
  Pregnancy
	<1.8 mmol/l
	First trimester 1.1–3.7 mmol/l
	  Second trimester 1.7–4.1 mmol/l
	  Third trimester 2.8–7.1 mmol/l
		Normal triglyceride levels vary by age and sex. A high triglyceride level combined with low HDL cholesterol or high LDL cholesterol seems to speed up atherosclerosis, the build-up of fatty deposits in artery walls. Atherosclerosis increases the risk for heart attack and stroke.

Urea, plasma (blood urea nitrogen, BUN)
  Pregnancy
	<60 years 2.5–6.5 mmol/l
	>60 years 2.9–7.5 mmol/l
	First trimester 1.9–6.2 mmol/l
	  Second trimester 1.8–6.5 mmol/l
	  Third trimester 1.6–5.0 mmol/l
		Increased BUN levels may be due to acute or chronic kidney disease, damage, or failure. Conditions that result in reduced blood flow to the kidneys, such as a recent heart attack, will also result in an increased BUN. Low BUN levels are rarely detected because they result from diseases or symptoms, such as dehydration or starvation, which do not warrant a BUN test.

Urinalysis pH	5.0–7.5	Urinary pH varies in contrast to blood pH. Extremes in urinary pH may indicate systemic acidosis or alkylosis.
Urinary specific gravity	1.001–1.030	Specific gravity of urine is a measure of the concentration of solutes in urine. Reduced specific gravity may indicate diabetes insipidus, certain renal diseases, excess fluid intake or diabetes mellitus. Raised specific gravity can indicate dehydration, adrenal insufficiency, nephrosis, congestive cardiac failure or liver disease.

INDEX